AF346501

XV Congrès International de Médecine

Lisbonne—19-26 Avril 1906

Section IX

CHIRURGIE

1.er FASCICULE

LISBONNE
Imprimerie Adolpho de Mendonça
1906

XV Congrès International de Médecine

LISBONNE, 19-26 AVRIL 1906

IX

XV Congrès International de Médecine

LISBONNE, 19-26 AVRIL 1906

Section IX

CHIRURGIE

LISBONNE
IMPRIMERIE ADOLPHO DE MENDONÇA
1906

Organisation de la section

Présidents d'honneur

MM.

BARDENHEUER, Geh. Medicinalrat, directeur de l'Académie de Médecine pratique de Cologne.

CARDENOL, directeur de l'Hôpital du «Sagrado Corazón» de Barcelone.

MARCOS BEZERRA CAVALCANTI, professeur de la Faculté de médecine de Rio de Janeiro.

LADISLAS DE FARKAS, médecin en chef, Budapest.

DAVIDE GIORDANO, chirurgien en chef de l'Hôpital de Venise.

A. W. MAYO ROBSON, D. Sc., F. R. C. S., Londres.

J. B. MURPHY, professeur de l'École de médecine de Chicago.

PAUL RECLUS, membre de l'Académie de médecine de Paris.

JEAN SABANEEFF, Odessa.

CH. WILLEMS, professeur agrégé à l'Université de Gand.

Comité d'organisation de la Section

Président	M. Oliveira Feijão.
Vice-Président	M. Manuel Moreira Junior.
Secrétaire responsable	M. Augusto de Vasconcellos.
Secrétaires adjoints	MM. Francisco Gentil et Paes de Vasconcellos.
Membres	MM. Clemente Pinto, Craveiro Lopes et Francisco Stromp.

Rapports officiels

1. — Infections péritonéales septiques. — Classification ; traitement.
    Rapporteurs : MM. Davide Giordano, Venise ; J. B. Murphy, Chicago.
2. — Les anastomoses gastro-intestinales et intestino-intestinales.
    Rapporteurs : MM. Hartmann, Paris ; Augusto de Vasconcellos, Lisbonne ; Hermann Schloffer, Innsbruck.
3. — Chirurgie artérielle et veineuse. Les modernes acquisitions.
    Rapporteurs : MM. Sousa Junior, Oporto ; D'Arcy Power, Londres ; Pierre Delbet, Paris.
4. — Chirurgie du grand sympathique.
    Rapporteurs : MM. T. Jonnesco, Bucarest ; Salazar de Souza, Lisbonne.
5. — Anastomoses des vaisseaux sanguins.
    Rapporteurs : MM. Alexis Carrel et C. C. Guthrie, Chicago.

XV CONGRÈS INTERNATIONAL DE MÉDECINE

LISBONNE — AVRIL 1906

SECTION DE CHIRURGIE

Rapports officiels

THÈME : CHIRURGIE ARTÉRIELLE ET VEINEUSE : LES MODERNES
ACQUISITIONS

(Recent advances in the surgery of the blood vessels)

Par M. D'ARCY POWER (London)

Surgeon to St. Bartholomew's Hospital

Many advances have been made of late years in connection
with the surgery of the bloodvessels and to these advances the
English-speaking races have contributed their fair share, though
fortunately surgery like science knows no nationality and every
improvement whether in theory or practice becomes at once the
property of all mankind.

Surgical knowledge is based upon pathology and pathology
itself is but a part of physiology. Improvements in physiology therefore, acting through pathology, lead to improvements in the
science and art of surgery. Physiologists have devoted much attention to the vascular mechanism and they have been so ably
assisted by histologists that we have now a tolerably clear idea
of the circulation of the blood and of the means by which it is
maintained and regulated.

Surgical shock & collapse

This knowledge, at first sight, would appear to be more useful
to the physician than to the surgeon but the surgeon has employed
it to advantage in elucidating the cause and the rational treatment
of collapse and shock, conditions which every surgeon has long
viewed with the utmost alarm because they so often put an abrupt
end to his best planned operations. You all know the sequence of

events as they occur in the surgery when a man is brought in with a railway smash, in the operating theatre during the administration of an anaesthetic and in the wards when a patient is dying with a gangrenous appendix. Such conditions are bad enough in hospital practice, they are worse when they occur in private, worst of all when they have to be faced at home. Need I draw you again the classical picture of a patient in a state of shock? A picture drawn so well by my old master Sir William Savory that I cannot improve upon it. «The patient lies in a state of utter prostration. There is a striking pallor of the whole surface, most marked in the face. Even the lips are quite pale and bloodless. There is a cold and clammy moisture upon the skin and often distinct drops of sweat upon the brow and forehead. The countenance has a dull aspect and appears shrunken and contracted. There is a remarkable languor in the whole expression and especially in the eye which has lost its natural lustre and is partially concealed by the drooping of the upper lid, whilst the pupil is dilated and reacts sluggishly. The nostrils, too, are usually dilated. The temperature is reduced so that the patient shivers from time to time and complains of cold. Muscular debility is extreme — apparent at a glance in the condition of the lips and hands — occasionally even in the relaxation of the sphincters. The pulse is generally frequent, sometimes irregular, always very feeble, perhaps quite imperceptible. In this latter case although the ear may detect the fluttering action of the heart the pulse does not reach the wrist. The respiratory movements are short and feeble or panting and gasping, «wanting the relief of sighs», sometimes imperceptible, although in the majority of cases some action of the diaphragm may be detected by careful observation. Vertigo with dimness of visions upervenes. As a rule there is not complete insensibility, but the patient is drowsy and bewildered, yet conscious and often rational when roused. Blissfully unconscious of his perilous condition he dreams away his end, or roused by the fruitless activity of his attendants he may ask «Is this death?» Sometimes the intellect is singularly clear and the senses are perfect, the hearing, occasionally, even peculiarly acute, whilst in the less extreme cases there are often nausea and vomiting with hiccough.»

Starting with such a picture in his mind Dr. Crile (¹) has carried out an important and elaborate research upon the blood pressure in Surgery and has thrown his results into the form of an essay which gained him the Cartwright Prize for 1903. The research, he says, was undertaken to study the cause of shock and collapse as it occurs in surgical practice and to obtain, if possible, some rational treatment for a condition which is of no rare occurrence in the practice of every operating surgeon.

The essential phenomenon in shock is a fall of blood pressure caused by exhaustion rather than by structural lesions and the fall is due to the blood accumulating in the veins and especially in the larger venous trunks. In shock, therefore, there is a condition of intravenous haemorrhage. When the fall of pressure occurs gradually the patient passes into a condition of shock: if it occurs suddenly, he is said to be in a state of collapse and a similar condition is produced by actual loss of blood as well as by other causes.

The tradition of different schools varies very greatly in the treatment of the shock and collapse following operations. One surgeon administers alcohol as a routine method after every severe operation, another gives it before as well as after the operation, whilst a third never gives it at all. One orders digitalis: another strychnia: others strychnia and its antagonist nitroglycerine at the same time: whilst others, again, give hypodermic injections of ether, even when the patient has been anaesthetised by ether. Atropin is injected hypodermically because the cutaneous circulation is thereby increased and in shock the patient has a cold skin. Others give caffein because it stimulates the heart. Ergotin is a favourite remedy in France: strychnia in Germany. We in England follow the German rather than the French plan and employ strychnia largely. But if the truth must be spoken and we examine the results obtained by those who stimulate their patients habitually and compare them with those obtained by surgeons who only resort to stimulation occasionally, it seems as though the better results were gained by the surgeons who reserve their remedies for really urgent cases.

The treatment of surgical shock and collapse therefore is clearly empirical at the present time and Prof. Crile has done a useful work in undertaking an investigation upon the blood pressure in surgery with a view to ascertain by experiment the conditions under which it varies, for until these conditions are known there can be no rational treatment.

The questions to be answered in connection with shock and collapse are the following:

To what is the fall of blood pressure due?

Is it caused by (a) exhaustion of the blood vessels i.e. the anatomical periphery: (b) exhaustion of the heart: (c) of the centres, vaso-motor, cardiac, or respiratory, and if it is due to failure of these centres is it the result of an exhaustion or failure of action on their part or is it caused by the blood plasma passing through the walls of the blood vessels? (d) if it is due to an exhaustion of one or more of these centres or organs would stimulation relieve the exhaustion or would further exhaustion follow the stimulation? in other words is it better to lash the tired horse or to rest it? If only some of the centres or organs are exhausted would it be advantageous to stimulate those which are not affected whilst the exhausted ones are allowed to rest? Would it be advantageous to restore the blood pressure in such cases by harmless mechanical means if it were found possible to do so? Are not the centres governing the circulation automatic in their action and are they not all stimulated automatically, moreover, are they not all stimulated to the point of exhaustion before the final circulatory breakdown known to us as collapse or shock? Is it better to depend upon drug stimulation of these exhausted centres or should reliance be placed upon their automatic stimulation?

Prof. Crile submitted these problems to the test of experiment and as far as possible subjected his experimental results to a clinical comparison in his surgical wards. He arrived by these means at the following noteworthy results which will be useful to every surgeon, for they deal with the various remedies we are accustomed to employ in the treatment of the more severe cases of shock and collapse.

ALCOHOL. — The administration of a moderate dose of alcohol to animals in varying conditions of shock was found to produce still further depression. In a few instances a considerable dose of alcohol in an animal suffering from profound shock was almost immediately followed by death. As a general rule the more profound the shock the more marked was the depressing effect of alcohol. This conclusion is of extreme interest, for it is the universal custom to give alcohol in every case of fainting, and syncope is the epitome of shock.

NITROGLYCERIN AND AMYL NITRITE. — In experiments in which the animals were in deep shock and the blood pressure was gradually falling there was no evidence to show that these drugs produced any decrease in the rapidity of the decline and it appeared on the whole that nitroglycerine and amyl nitrite increased the shock.

DIGITALIN. — Digitalis generally caused a rise in bloodpressure when it was administered to animals reduced to varying degrees of surgical shock, but when death occurred it was usually more sudden than in animals in a similar state which had not been treated with digitalis. It seemed on the average that cases of shock treated by digitalis did not survive quite so long as the controls, although the data do not allow a positive statement to be made. It may be stated with certainty that such animals did not live longer.

STRYCHNIA. — Strychnia causes a rise in bloodpressure proportional to the degree of shock when it is administered to animals in which varying degrees of shock had been artificially produced. When strychnia was injected into animals who were only in a condition of slight shock, the rise of blood pressure and its maintenance were correspondingly slight and a repetition of the dose did not usually cause any further rise. In cases where the shock was developed almost to the fatal extent a slight rise occurred after the injection of strychnia, but this lasted only for a few minutes, after which no amount of strychnia produced any farther rise. A therapeutic dose of strychnia caused an animal in any degree of shock to pass into a deeper shock when its effects had passed off.

SALINE INFUSION. — Saline infusions caused a rise in the blood pressure of every animal in a state of shock, the rise was gradual and was proportional to the degree of shock. The gain in bloodpressure was fairly well maintained in cases of moderate shock, whilst in animals suffering from profound shock the blood pressure was not maintained beyond a certain time, even if the infusion were continued. Blood counts and haemoglobin estimations showed that the blood was not much diluted by the saline infusion because the solution escaped from the blood vessels at a rate which was fairly equal to the rapidity of the infusion. The fluid which thus passed through the walls of the blood vessels accumulated in the walls and lumen of the stomach, intestines and abdominal cavity, in the respiratory tract, the cavity of the thorax and the subcutaneous tissues.

ADRENALIN. — Adrenalin raised the blood pressure in animals in every degree of shock and collapse and under all circumstances when it was given by intravenous injection. The latent period of the drug was twenty seconds and the duration of its effect two minutes. Clinically it was given continuously for eight hours to a patient who was dying of shock and in another case a human heart which had stopped beating for nine minutes was made to beat for thirty-two minutes by the combined effect of artificial respiration, rhythmic pressure upon the thorax over the heart and the intravenous infusion of adrenalin.

MORPHIA. — Morphia alone or morphia combined with ether reduces an animal's susceptibility to shock to a considerable extent. Morphia combined with ether forms an anaesthetic under which extensive operations can be carried out for longer times with less risk of shock than by means of ether or chloroform alone.

It follows from these observations that the essential phenomenon in shock and collapse is a fall of blood pressure due to an exhaustion of the vaso-motor centres rather than to any structural lesion. When this fall occurs gradually the patient passes into a condition of shock: if its onset is sudden, he is said to be in a state of collapse. The term collapse therefore is applied to the cases of more sudden fall of blood pressure due to haemorrhage, injuries of the vaso-motor centre or cardiac failure. In shock there is an exhaustion of the centre leading to a general fall of blood pressure because the blood accumulates in the veins and more especially in the larger venous trunks leading to a condition of intravenous haemorrhage; in collapse the fall is due to a suspended action of the vaso-motor centres.

The treatment varies with the condition. Stimulants may be serviceable in collapse, but they are useless in shock. To put this in a concrete form, if one animal is subjected to so great a degree of shock as to produce a marked decline in the blood pressure because the bulk of the blood is in the large veins and if another animal be bled until the blood pressure falls to the same extent, the symptoms will be identical though the cause is widely different. In the animal with the exhausted vaso-motor centre whose blood is in its veins (shock), neither stimulants nor saline solution will be of much assistance. But adrenalin might be of great service because it causes an enormous rise of blood pressure under every condition, even when the vaso-motor centres have been exhausted, when they have been cocainised and when they have been actually destroyed. The rise, too, occurs when both vagi and both nervi accelerantes have been divided and when the animal is under the influence of curare.

The most effective method of administering adrenalin is by the continuous intravenous infusion of adrenalin in salt solution, the strength varying from one part in fifty thousand to one part in a hundred thousand. Indeed so powerful is the action of the drug that Prof. Crile narrates the following extraordinary experiment: An ordinary laboratory dog was decapitated. The bleeding was stopped; adrenalin and saline solution were immediately and continuously administered and it was found possible by these means to control the blood pressure at will. The beheaded dog lived ten hours and a half and finally died of air emboli produced by artificial respiration.

The action of adrenalin in cases of shock can be supplemented by external pressure, which drives the blood towards the heart, if it be applied uniformly to the skin from the periphery to the centre. Prof. Crile has therefore invented a pneumatic suit which can be inflated until it exercises the required pressure.

Collapse may reasonably be treated by cardiac stimulants and by the injection of saline solution as well as by change of position, for the vaso-motor centres are not exhausted, though their action is temporarily suspended.

Prof. Crile sums up the results of his observations in the following words:

In many cases the control of the blood pressure is the control of life itself. Surgical shock is an exhaustion of the vaso-motor centre: neither the heart muscle, nor the cardiac centres, nor the respiratory centre are other than secondarily involved. Collapse is due to a suspension of the function of the cardiac or of the vaso-motor mechanism or to haemorrhage. In shock therapeutic doses of strychnia are inert: physiological doses are dangerous or fatal. When it does not cause death increased exhaustion follows the administration of strychnia. It is impossible to make any distinction between external stimulation of the vaso-motor centre — such as is produced by injuries and operation — and internal stimulation by such stimulants as strychnia. Each in sufficient amount produces shock and each with equal logic might be used to treat the shock produced by the other. Stimulants of the vaso-motor centres are not contraindicated in shock and collapse. But in shock cardiac stimulants have only a limited range of usefulness, whilst their action may prove to be injurious. Stimulants may be useful in collapse, because the centres are not exhausted.

Saline infusions are not very useful in shock, but they may

be very effective in the treatment of collapse. The blood only tolerates a limited dilution with saline solution and elimination soon begins to take place through the ordinary channels of absorption. The fluid which thus accumulates in the splanchnic area may be sufficient in quantity to lead to fixation of the diaphragm and moveable ribs causing death by respiratory failure. Saline infusion in shock raises but cannot sustain the blood pressure.

Adrenalin, as has been shown, acts both upon the heart and the blood vessels. It raises the blood pressure in every degree of shock, even when the medulla is cocainised and when it is absent as in an animal which has been decapitated. But adrenalin is so quickly oxidised by the body tissues and by the blood that its effects are very temporary. The drug must therefore be given continuously, and in excessive doses it stimulates the cardio-inhibitory mechanism, though the stimulation can be set aside experimentally by the injection of atropin.

A pneumatic rubber suit which can be inflated at will provides an artificial peripheral resistance, which is capable of controlling the blood pressure within a range of 25-60 mm. of mercury, and is a useful adjuvant to adrenalin in cases of advanced shock. By the continued use of artificial respiration, rhythmic pressure upon the thorax over the region of the heart and the infusion of adrenalin, animals which had apparently been dead for fifteen minutes were resuscitated. By the same means with the addition of the rubber suit a patient who had been conventionally dead for nine minutes after an injury to his brain was partially resuscitated for thirty-two minutes and during this time exhibited a strong heart beat and was able to move his head.

It is clear from these investigations that we are in a fair way to obtain a rational treatment for shock and collapse based, as all surgical advances should be based, upon a sound substratum of pathological knowledge gained by experiment.

The ligature of arteries in their continuity

Everyone who knows anything of the history of surgery knows that the modern method of stopping bleeding by the ligature of arteries is due to the labours of Ambroise Paré. The ligature of arteries was described by Celsus in A. D. 50 and by Galen in A. D. 130 and these surgeons recommended that the artery should be tied in two places and afterwards divided. Few people are aware of the amount of careful experimental work which has been performed to bring up the surgical technique of ligature to its present standard of excellence, though every surgeon knows the radical change of procedure which has taken place within the last twenty years. Then, a septic ligature passed round an artery was deliberately left with the ends hanging out of the wound that it might ulcerate through the vessel with a serious risk of secondary haemorrhage; now, a thin ligature of silk or of some animal tissue capable of being absorbed is cut short after it has been tied, and is buried in the wound in the full confidence that it will become disintegrated, and secondary haemorrhage is almost unknown.

In England many of the advances in our knowledge are due to the work of Messrs Ballance and Edmunds who published their conclusions in 1891 in a *Treatise on the Ligation of the Great Arteries in Continuity with observations on the nature, progress and treatment of Aneurysm* [2]. The scientific portion of the work deals with the physiological occlusion and the pathological obliteration of arteries as illustrated by the ductus arteriosus and by the changes taking place in syphilitic arteritis. Consideration is given to the conduct and fate of the corpuscles, of the clot, of the arterial coats and of the ligature after an artery has been tied. The choice of ligature and the kind of knot are then discussed together with the amount of force which should be exerted in tying the ligature.

The most important practical points are those connected with the choice of ligature, the character of the knot and the force employed. A perfect ligature must be sufficiently strong not to break: inelastic, round, smooth, pliable, and easily tied into a knot. It must not be too bulky: it should be capable of being absorbed, though not too readily. Lastly, a good ligature should be capable of being rendered absolutely sterile. These conditions are only fulfilled by a few materials and the choice of ligature must fall on ox peritoneum, goldbeaters skin, kangaroo tendon or boiled floss silk: failing these on boiled chinese twist silk, chromic catgut or silkworm gut. The reasons for arriving at this conclusion as regards the nature of the ligature may be given in the following terms: «The outer coat and sheath of an artery consist of white fibrous tissue and the most appropriate ligature, therefore, is prepared from this material, that is to say from tendon or peritoneal tissue of sufficient strength. These ligatures satisfy all theoretical requirements. They are strong, inelastic, round, smooth, pliable and are easily obtained of the proper size. They are slowly absorbed and are readily made aseptic. Peritoneum should be better than tendon because it resists absorption for a longer time. Floss silk is a smooth and trustworthy ligature. Ordinary silk and chromicised catgut are good, but their rough surfaces and the presence of mucous and muscular tissue in the catgut are defects, for it makes them more difficult to keep aseptic. Wire is too rigid and too difficult to handle to make it useful as a ligature; silkworm gut is not easy to manipulate round an artery unless it has been soaked for a long time in water and, moreover, several strands must be employed to make a ligature which will not cut the coats. This adds to the difficulty but when these obstacles are overcome silkworm gut makes a very beautiful ligature. Ox aorta must be rejected on account of its weakness, bulk and elasticity». For the practical purposes of everyday life in the operating theatre I prefer silk for the ligature of arteries and I direct that it shall be unwound from the wooden reels on which it is bought, rewound on glass reels in shorter lengths and then boiled for at least an hour. I have an abiding distrust of catgut even when it is most carefully prepared and I think that when tendon is used the first half hitch of the reef knot is apt to slip whilst the second turn is being made.

The knots ordinarily used for tying ligatures are the reef, the granny and the surgical knot. All are open to the objection I have just mentioned, that the first part of the knot may slip whilst the second part is being completed. There is thus «an uncertainty of occlusion» which applies not only to the tying of arteries but to the ligature of other structures, such as hernial sacs, and the pedicles of tumours. To overcome this difficulty Messrs. Ballance and Edmunds recommend the use of two ligatures passed round the vessel and tied as a «stay knot». The best method of tying the two ligatures is, they say, «to make on each separately and in the same way the first hitch of a reef knot (fig. 1) and to tighten each separately so that the loop lies in contact with the vessel but without constricting it: then, taking the two ends of one side together in one hand and the two ends on the other side in the other hand, to constrict the vessel sufficiently to occlude it and finally to complete the reef knot (fig. 2). The simplest method of completing the knot is to treat the two ends in each hand as a single thread and then to tie as if completing a single reef knot».

The principle on which this «stay-knot» depends is that the mutual support which the ligatures afford to one another by fric-

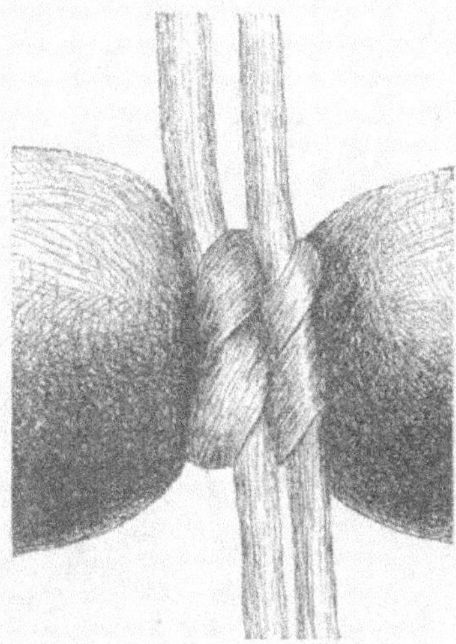

Fig. 1

tion and locking prevents the first hitches of the knot from

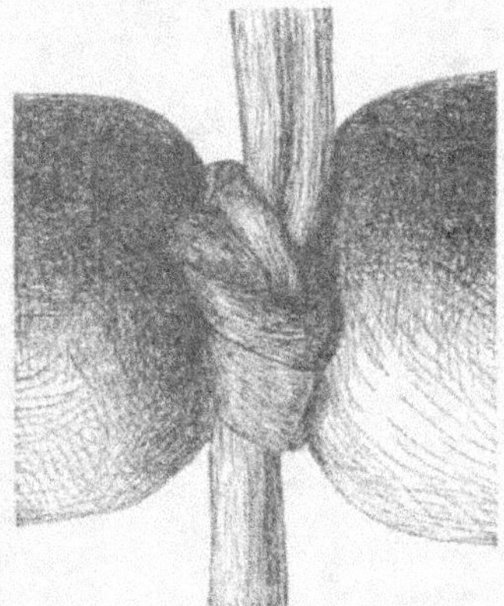

Fig. 2

slipping when the ends are relaxed as they must be to complete
the knot. The loops do not expand in the least and abundant

time is allowed to tie the second hitch without risk of the artery
being left imperfectly constricted.

Messrs Ballance and Edmunds make out a strong case both
on experimental and clinical grounds for the discontinuance of
the ordinary practice of rupturing the internal and middle coats
of arteries when they are tied in their continuity. They advocate
the occlusion of the lumen by bringing the intima into apposition
for some distance at the seat of ligature. The great disadvantage
attending rupture of the internal and middle coats as it is usually
practised in the ligature of an artery in its continuity is that the
vessel is seriously weakened. There is consequently a danger of
secondary haemorrhage and this accident has actually happened
after ligature of large vessels like the innominate even when there
has been no appreciable sepsis.

The surgical treatment of aneurysm

The operative treatment of aneurysm has been a matter of
interest to surgeons from the earliest times and it has always
been somewhat of an *opprobium chirurgi*. Antyllus at the beginning of the fourth century of our era was bold enough to incise
the sac, turn out the clot and ligature both ends of the artery.
But as we only know of him by repute it is impossible to
ascertain with what success he operated. Later surgeons, learning
by tradition how fatal was the operation either regarded all interference as useless or at most contented themselves with amputation when the aneurysm was conveniently situated as in the
arm or the leg. John Hunter's successful case of popliteal aneurysm cured by ligature of the main artery at a distance from the
sac created a new era in this part of surgery and his method is still
generally employed. The use of aseptic ligatures and the general adop-
tion of Listerian methods have rendered the operation peculiarly satisfactory and surgeons are now free from the old bugbears
of suppuration and secondary haemorrhage.

The exact choice of operation in cases of popliteal aneurysm
has been a matter of dispute of late years. Whether the artery
should be tied in two places a short distance apart and then divided, whether it should be tied in one place with rupture of the
inner and middle coats or whether it should be tied in one place
without rupture of the coats as is recommended by Messrs Ballance and Edmunds, and lastly whether it is better to tie close

to the aneurysm or at some distance away from it, have been the
chief points on which surgeons have agreed to differ. For some
years the method of tying the artery in two places and dividing
the artery between the ligatures was extensively followed. But
accidents some times took place because the surgeon did not make
sufficient allowance for the retractile power of the larger vessels or
did not tie the ligatures sufficiently tight. One or other of the ligatures
came off when the vessel was divided and the patient either bled
to death or was only saved with the utmost difficulty. Of late
years therefore surgeons have contented themselves with plac-
ing a single ligature round the artery to be tied in its continuity,
but instead of dividing the inner and middle coats as was formerly the constant practice, they have found it best to employ
the «stay-knot» (p. 11). This method is especially adapted for the
ligature of arteries of the first and second magnitude like the
innominate, carotid, subclavian and iliac arteries, for even when
there has been no suppuration these vessels are especially prone
to secondary haemorrhage when they have been ligatured. In
smaller arteries like the axillary, brachial, ulnar, radial and fe-
moral the older method of ligature with division of the inner coats
is still usually employed with good results.

Aneurysms treated by methods other than ligature

Much has been done of late years by physicians to treat aneurysm successfully without having recourse to the surgeon. Bel-
lingham's rest and diet method, advocated by Tufnell, combined
with the administration of potassium iodide in ten grain doses every eight hours sometimes makes a new man of a patient with an
aneurysm and enables him, at any rate for a time, to perform his
duties again. But the relief is too often only temporary and in
other cases it never occurs. Such desperate cases drift into the
surgical wards of hospitals and it is then our endeavour to do
by art what nature has failed to carry out.

Diagnosis by the Roentgen Rays.

Dr. Hügh Walsham *(The Clinical Journal,* vol. 18, 1901, p. 184,
and *The Edinburgh Medical Journal,* for 1901, vol. 1, p. 354) in
England and Dr. Guido Holzknecht *(Archiv und Atlas der normalen
und pathologischen Anatomie in typischen Röntgenbildern,* Hamburg, 1901) in Vienna have shown that the diagnosis of deeply
seated thoracic and cardiac aneurysms is sometimes greatly

assisted by the use of the screen and by radiographs. Dr. Walsham points out that to establish the diagnosis of an intrathoracic aneurysm the shadow must be in continuity with the heart or aorta and that the shadow of an intrathoracic new growth is quite different from that of an aneurysm. The variation in density between the heart shadow and the shadow of an aneurysmal sac is important from the point of view of prognosis. Fluid blood is almost completely transparent to the Röntgen rays whilst laminated clot is comparatively opaque. The greater the density of the aneurysmal sac in the radiograph, the more abundant therefore is the amount of laminated clot which it contains. Dr. Walsham also draws attention to the fact that the heart is often found to lie nearly transversely in the chest when there is an aortic aneurysm apparently, because it has been pressed into this position by the superincumbent weight of the aneurysmal sac.

An improved knowledge of pathology has shown the method by which nature attempts to cure an aneurysm and by following the clue thus given various forms of treatment have been adopted for aneurysms which are surgically inaccessible to the more simple plan of ligature. Foremost amongst these methods are the administration of gelatin or calcium chloride to increase the coagulability of the blood generally : acupuncture, electrolysis or wiring to promote coagulation locally. These methods have been tried chiefly in cases of intra-abdominal and intra-thoracic aneurysm and hitherto with so limited a degree of success as to show that some can be abandoned as useless, whilst others, with improved technique, may yet prove serviceable in cases which have been properly selected.

The injection of Gelatin.

The method of injecting gelatin was first recommended by Lancereaux in 1897 who based his recommendation upon experiments made by MM. Dastre and Floresco confirmed by Messrs Camus and Gley, that the injection of a solution of gelatin into the veins rendered the blood more coagulable. After reporting a single successful case in 1897 Dr. Lancereaux in 1898 brought forward the details of five other cases for three of which he claimed complete success whilst in the remaining two death took place, in one patient from rupture of the aneurysm and in the other from uraemia. He sums up the conclusions at which he has arrived in the following words :

«Gelatine introduced into the subcutaneous cellular tissue

penetrates into the blood which it renders more than normally
coagulable, and, since the blood encounters two conditions favou-
rable to coagulation in the sac of the aneurysm, viz: a slowing
of its current and a vascular wall which is often uneven, a more
or less abundant clot is formed which in time fills the sac. This
clot ultimately shrinks, the pouch in which is contained diminishes
in size and disappears. If the clot softens the blood penetrates
between it and the walls of the sac and the tumour is reproduced.
Under such conditions fortunately, coagulation again takes place
readily. Gelatine, therefore, constitutes an excellent therapeutic
agent, which, if it does not cure aneurysms, at any rate favours
the general process of cure».

Dr. Lancereaux has fixed experimentally the quantity of gelatine necessary to obtain a sufficient coagulability of human blood.
It is 250 cc. of a saline solution containing two grammes per 100
cc. of gelatine and he has found by experience that several months
are required to obtain satisfactory results and that during this
period at least twelve or fifteen injections are necessary. According to Dr. Huchard a one per cent solution of gelatin is safer
than a two per cent and it is advisable to leave a clear interval
of eight to ten days between each injection. As a general
rule it is not possible to introduce more than 100 cc. of the
gelatine solution into the subcutaneous tissue without causing
pain and even this amount should be injected slowly—over an interval of ten to twelve minutes — in order to avoid discomfort and
overdistension of the skin. A considerable swelling is formed at
the point of injection but it subsides entirely in from six to twelve
hours. The inner aspect of the thigh is found to be the most con-
venient place for the injection. The method of procedure consists
in filling a sterilised glass syringe with 100 cc. of the gelatine
solution made as follows: One ounce of gelatine, 131 grains of
sodium cloride and fifty ounces of sterile distilled water are
put into a flask plugged with cotton wool. The flask is allowed to
stand an hour or two for the gelatine to soften and it is then
heated in a waterbath until the gelatine is dissolved. The flask
is afterwards placed in a steamer for an hour and is subjected
to this treatment on three consecutive days.

Immediately before it is used the quantity to be employed 100
cc. is again resteamed. Every precaution is taken to secure complete asepsis not only of the solution but also of the skin of the
patient and the instruments employed. The necessity for com-

plete sterilisation of the gelatin is shown by the fact that two patients died of tetanus at Guy's Hospital whilst undergoing this method of treatment and it appears that commercial gelatine often contains tetanus germs. It is satisfactory to find that these germs are killed by boiling for three minutes and that boiling for this length of time does not affect the process of gelatinisation.

Iodide of potassium is given in ten grain doses three times a day concurrently with the gelatine injections and with it Dr. Guthrie Rankin (?) combines minim doses of a one per cent solution of nitroglycerine whenever the tension of the pulse becomes excessive or when there are symptoms of angina. The nitrogenous elements of the daily dietary are also reduced to the lowest extent and the amount of liquid allowed is kept within very narrow limits.

This method of treating aneurysms by the subcutaneous injection of gelatin is still upon its trial in cases of inaccessible aneurysm. It is by no means uniformly successful and it appears likely to fall into disuse.

Treatment by the introduction of foreign bodies into the sac.

When the aneurysm is small and is inaccessible to ligature without being surgically inaccessible and when there is only a small aperture so that the danger of embolism is diminished, attempts have made to cause coagulation locally in the sac by the introduction of foreign bodies.

Acupuncture.

Simple acupuncture without the use of electric currents was adopted at first upon the suggestion of Prof. Velpeau in France and of Mr. Benjamin Phillips in England. It has been employed by Mr. Christopher Heath and Mr. Chauncy Puzey. Three pairs of sewing needles are introduced into the sac where each pair are made to cross. They are left in position until the fifth day and are then withdrawn. Although some satisfactory results were obtained by this method it is not likely to be again adopted.

Wiring.

In 1864, Dr. Murchison and Mr. C. Moore (4) of the Middlesex Hospital passed a fine trocar and cannula into a large aneurysm of the ascending aorta which was protruding into the second and third intercostal spaces. Twenty six yards of fine iron wire were introduced into the sac of the aneurysm through the cannula, the end of the wire being pushed home with a blunt trocar. The operation lasted one hour and no anaesthetic was given. The patient seemed much relieved at first but died of sepsis on the fifth day. The post mortem examination showed that the sac was full of clot mostly post mortem, but Mr. Moore points out that there was firm adhesion between the fibrin enclosing the wire and the wall of the aneurysm, so firm indeed that the adhesion was inseparable without dissection and the mass of wire and fibrin together could only be removed by tearing it apart.

Loreta (¹) in 1885 was the first to apply this method to an abdominal aneurysm. He performed laparotomy and passed six feet of silvered copper wire into a large aneurysmal sac. The patient left the hospital ten weeks later with the aneurysm reduced to a hard non-pulsating mass of the size of a walnut. He died three weeks afterwards from rupture of the aorta below the aneurysm.

G. L. Hunner ( ) collected all the cases of this operation, both thoracic and abdominal, which had been published up to 1900. The list contains fourteen cases with three cures and eleven deaths. A necropsy was obtained in nine of the eleven patients who died and in all there was evidence that the presence of the wire had induced firm clotting within the sac. The cases which did best were those in which from five to ten feet of wire were introduced.

Several other aneurysms have been «wired» since this list was published, notably one by myself ( ) in which an attempt was made to improve the technique of the operation by the use of an ingenious instrument devised by my present house-surgeon Mr. G. H. Colt. The apparatus was designed to introduce a known quantity of silver wire into the sac of an aneurysm with complete asepsis, a maximum of speed and a minimum of disturbance. The instrument «snagged» the wire and caused it to coil within the sac. The simplicity of the operation defeated its own ends for the instrument worked so easily that in two minutes and a half I introduced eighty inches of silver wire into the aneurysm with a clotting surface of 3.7 square inches. The patient survived the operation fifty hours and at the post mortem examination a loop of silver wire seven inches long was found projecting into the arch of the aorta, the rest of the wire being coiled irregularly within the sac of the aneurysm and covered with blood clot some of which was certainly formed during the life of the patient. The aneurysm was thought to be formed on one of the branches of the coeliac axis but the autopsy showed that it was derived from the abdominal aorta, that it was of the size and shape of a large orange and that it projected forwards between the layers of the transverse mesocolon.

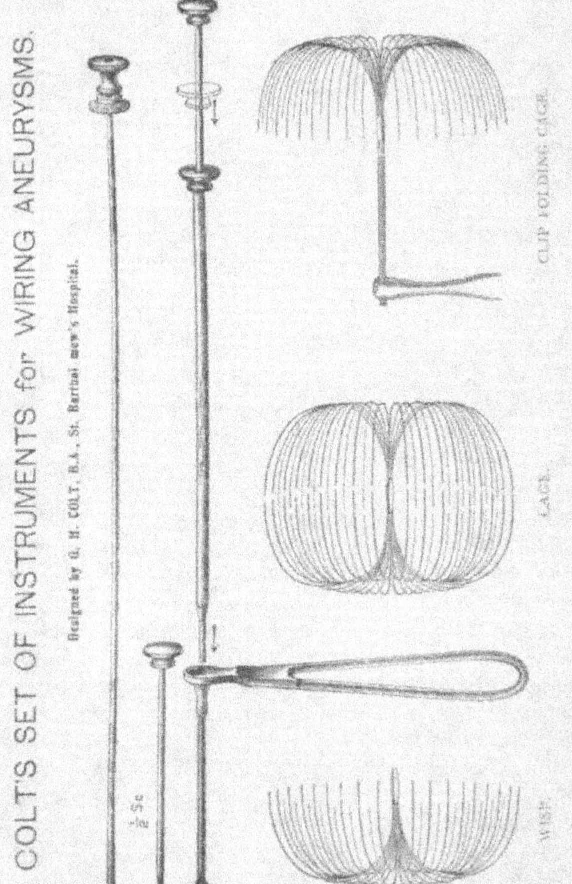

Mr. G. H. Colt afterwards invented a third instrument to prevent any risk of wire entering the aorta after it had escaped from the sac of the aneurysm; it is extremely ingenious as will be gathered from the description and illustration (fig. 3).

The apparatus consists of a trocar and canula, a ramrod, a cartridge and a wisp. The wisp consists of a number of fine steel wires soldered together at one end, each wire being curled over in a separate plane so that they readily expand as soon as they are at liberty to do so; though under ordinary conditions they are packed up into small bundles in which the wires lie parallel to each other. If it be preferred a cage can be used instead of a wisp. The cage consists of a bunch of fine steel wires caught together with solder at their midpoints so that when the wires expand the cage becomes spherical. Both the wisps and the cages are made in different sizes to suit different aneurysms. Each wisp or cage fits into a cartridge or hollow metal tube open at both ends, which can be adapted with ease and accuracy to the distal end of the canula. The cartridge just holds the wisp or cage in its compressed condition as a bundle of wires lying side by side. When the operation is performed, the sac of the aneurysm is exposed and if possible a purse string suture is run round the spot to be punctured. The trocar and canula are driven through the sac wall, the trocar is withdrawn and the cartridge containing a cage or a wisp is fitted to the canula. The contents of the cartridge are then gently pushed along the canula by means of the ramrod until the wisp or cage is safely delivered into the sac of the aneurysm. The canula and ramrod is immediately withdrawn and the pursuiting suture is simultaneously tightened and tied to close the puncture. When a wisp is used care should be taken to puncture the sac in a direction which as far as possible is estimated to be towards the plane of its opening, because the wisp expands and curls back directly it begins to emerge from the canula and there is consequently less danger of any of the wires projecting through the opening. When a cage is employed it will probably adapt itself better to the larger sac if the puncture be made in a direction parallel to the plane of the opening.

Mr. Colt claims for his instrument, and I think he claims justly, that it abolishes the three great dangers attending the wiring of an aneurysm, viz. sepsis, haemorrhage and the escape of some of the wire from the aneurysmal sac into the parent artery. The older method of tediously introducing a length of wire into an aneurysmal sac through the lumen of a small canula necessarily led to a serious risk of septic infection and there was a considerable loss of blood when the operation was prolonged. Mr. Colt's apparatus enables the operation to be performed in a few seconds and the whole apparatus can be thoroughly sterilised by boiling. By the older method there was no guarantee as to the position occupied by the wire within the sac of the aneurysm. In five cases where an aneurysm had been wired in the ordinary way and a post mortem examination was afterwards made the wire was found to have passed out of the aneurysm into the lumen of the artery. In my own case a loop of wire extended upwards from the abdominal aorta nearly to the arch, whilst in another case it had passed into the left ventricle and had remained there for nine months fortunately without causing any bad symptoms, for the patient seemed to be greatly benefited by the operation. Curiously enough it has been found impossible to predict when such an escape would occur, for the wire has sometimes passed through the narrow neck of an aneurysm, whilst in other cases where the communication with the artery has been large the wire has not escaped. The use of the umbrella shaped «wisp» or «cage» precludes the possibility of such an accident. The amount of wire introduced is regulated by the size of the aneurysm; thus wisp No. 1 presents a total surface of 1 ¾ square inches; wisp No. 2 of 2 ½ sq. in.; No. 3 of 3 ½ sq. in. and cage 4 of 3 ½ sq. in. It will be noticed that the wires of the wisp and cage are dull gilt and if they be examined under the microscope it will be seen that this makes them finely granular and enables the clot to adhere more firmly than if the wire were polished.

The apparatus has been used three times within the last few months and in every case the surgeon has expressed his complete satisfaction with the manner in which it worked.

The first case was operated upon by Major M. P. Holt R. A. M. C. at the Royal Infirmary, Dublin, on December 8th, 1903, and the notes are published in the *Journal of the Royal Army Medical Corps* for August 1904. The patient was a sergeant in the army who complained of increasing pain in the epigastrium, left costal margin and left lumbar region. The pain had existed for several months and was made worse rather than diminished by vomiting. He had a small tumour to the left of the middle line situated midway between the xiphisternum and the umbilicus. The swelling was about two and a half inches in diameter and had an indistinct, smooth, rounded, outline. There was well marked expansile pulsation and a loud harsh murmur over the tumour. The swelling gradually increased whilst the patient was under observation until it measured nearly five inches in diameter. The pain soon became intolerable, the patient rapidly lost flesh and colour and unceasingly implored that something should be done at any cost. The aneurysm was exposed on December 8th and was thought to be either an aneurysm of the aorta involving the coeliac axis or an aneurysm of the coeliac axis alone. It was determined to obtain access to it from above and the stomach was therefore drawn upwards and the small omentum torn through. The hepatic artery was then seen to be pulseless whilst the tumour was pulsating terrifically.

The canula and trocar of Mr. Colt's apparatus were pushed well into the sac, the trocar was withdrawn and was at once replaced by a cartridge loaded with No. 1 size wire wisp. The wisp was pushed slowly along the canula by means of the piston until it was safely delivered into the aneurysm not more than half a drachm of blood being lost in the operation. The canula was then withdrawn and although there was no escape of blood at the seat of puncture three Lembert sutures of catgut were inserted over the puncture. There was no shock: the evening temperature was normal with an unusually and undesirably strong pulse. On the following morning the patient became restless complaining of pain in the chest on inspiration. The respiratory symptoms became worse and the patient died of pneumonia about sixty hours after the operation. Major Holt has kindly given us the specimen which is placed in museum of St. Bartholomew's Hospital with the number 1551 e. The post-mortem examination showed that the operation area was clean, dry and apparently aseptic, for there was no blood or fluid in the peritoneum nor any signs of peritonitis. The aneurysmal tumour had shrunk to about a quarter its original size. It was removed entire with the aorta from the diaphragmatic opening above to the origin of the renal arteries below with the exception of a small area of about half an inch square on the posterior wall where it was firmly incorporated with the anterior surface of the body of the first lumbar vertebra, which was bare and slightly eroded over a corresponding area. The pancreas was firmly adherent to the front of the sac. The aneurysm, greatly contracted in size, contained a considerable amount of clot, much of which was firmly adherent to the wisp of wire which had expanded well within the sac. The aneurysm originated from the abdominal aorta immediately above the coeliac axis, it involved the coeliac axis itself, the origin of the superior mesenteric artery and the aorta immediately below the axis.

Major Holt is kind enough to conclude his paper with a high appreciation of Mr. Colt's apparatus. He says, «the operation itself demonstrated (i) the extreme simplicity of the working of the apparatus; (ii) the complete safeguarding of asepsis; (iii) the rapidity and accuracy with which a very large surface of wire, precisely determined beforehand, can be introduced through a pinhole opening; (iv) the complete absence of haemorrhage from the sac during and after the introduction, notwithstanding an inordinately high blood tension; (v) the complete avoidance of shock. The operation was one of no little interest and completely justified every point claimed for the apparatus».

Major Holt again writes to me on February 24th 1905: «I thought it might interest you to know that your wire apparatus has been used again twice, once three weeks ago by Mr. Lentaigne of the Mater Misericordiae Hospital here and again yesterday by Major Spencer at the Curragh Hospital». Three days later Surgeon Lentaigne wrote from Dublin: —«I am sure you will be glad to hear that I have recently employed the apparatus in a case of large aneurysm of the abdominal aorta. I operated on January 27th using No. 2 wisp and am glad to say that so far, with the exception of a rather troublesome stitch abscess apparently due to infection from the deep skin layer, the man has done very well indeed. Before the operation the patient suffered from very severe and almost constant pain especially in and below the left shoulder. All this has ceased for some time and the man now declares himself free from pain, the pulsation is much diminished though still present as, of course, must be expected».

It may be mentioned here that substances other than wire have been introduced into the sac of an aneurysm with a view to produce coagulation. Levis employed horsehair, Murray of Newcastle-on-Tyne catgut, and Schrötter of Vienna floss silk. It was supposed that with these substances a nidus for the deposit of fibrin would be offered with less risk of subsequent irritation and with a better prospect of the organised thrombus and sac wall becoming firmly contracted. It is not easy to estimate the exact utility of the agents so used as methods of cure, based on the earlier operations done as they were before the days of clean surgery, but it is certain that the results have not been so good as with wire.

Electrolysis.

Galvanopuncture was originally suggested by Pravaz the

younger who was always interested in the treatment of aneurysm, for he took as the subject of his graduation thesis at Paris in 1857 *Sur le traitement des anévrysmes par les injections de perchlorure de fer*, and for making these injections he introduced the little Pravaz syringe, though it has long been divorced from its original purpose.

Pravaz employed electrolysis for external aneurysms and in the form of galvanopuncture, but the method was soon taken up by Dr. Ciniselli (²) at Cremona, who used it in cases of thoracic and abdominal aneurysms, and he was followed by Drs. James and John Duncan in Scotland.

For galvanopuncture of aneurysms steel needles are employed five inches in length, insulated to an inch and a quarter of their point. Four cells of a Bunsen's battery are sufficiently effective and do not give rise to more than a bearable amount of pain. The battery should have a continuous current and the needles, if this method of operating be adopted, should be introduced from the same side, near the base of the external tumour, parallel to each other and one or two inches apart. The number of needles may be multiplied if the aneurysm is large and the action may be prolonged till pulsation ceases or till gas can be clearly detected on percussion. A *séance* of twenty minutes is generally enough for one application and this may be repeated according to the circumstances of the case.

The method of simple electrolysis has yielded good results, even though they were only temporary in several selected cases, but of late years it has given place to a combination of wiring and electrolysis which is now known as:

The Moore-Corradi method.

Prof. Corradi, the acomplished professor of the history of medicine at Pavia, suggested this combination of wiring and electrolysis to prof. Burresi (²) who employed it in a case of aneurysm of the ascending aorta in 1878. Barwell (¹º) suggested a treatment on similar lines independently of Corradi and the plan has since been followed up in America chiefly by Dr. D. D. Stewart (¹¹). The advantages claimed for the method are that instead of a soft unstable coagulum being slowly formed about the wire as is the case when wiring alone is employed, electrolysis almost immediately produces a tough clot of considerable size. Experience has shown that the strength of the current must be rather high — from 40-80 milliampères — and the *séance* long — from three quarters of an hour to an hour and a half. — It is better, too, not to have both poles in the aneurysm as was formerly the custom, but the anode or positive pole should always be the active electrode. This pole is connected with the wire which has been previously introduced into the sac and the negative rheophore should be a large clay plate or pad of absorbent wool placed upon the abdomen or under the back. The current is brought into circuit slowly, its strength being noted by an accurate milliampèrimeter. It is gradually increased for a few moments until the maximum strength, supposed to be necessary for the individual case, is reached and this maximum is then maintained until nearly the end of the séance when it is slowly reduced to zero. Mr. Colt has adapted his apparatus to this method of treating aneurysm by providing the ramrod with a binding screw by which the positive pole of a battery can be brought into electrical communication with the end of a wisp previously introduced into the sac of the aneurysm.

Dr. Guy Hunner ([6]) says that with the combined method (Moore-Corradi) there have been treated 23 cases, 17 thoracic and 6 abdominal. Four of these or 17 per cent. these thoracic or one abdominal have been cured: nine cases or 39 per cent showed amelioration of symptoms and prolongation of life. Death was probably hastened in the other 10 cases.

The venous system

It is difficult for us in 1905 to picture to ourselves the fear and abhorrence which surgeons felt towards any operation on the veins even so late as 1883. The third and last edition of Holmes' *System of surgery* published in that year says (vol. 3, p. 170): «Numerous operations are in use for the obliteration of varicose veins. They seek either merely to produce coagulation in the varix, to divide the venous channels above or below the varices or finally to remove the varicose part of the vein. These results can be obtained:—1st, by, the action of caustics applied over the course of the vessel: 2nd. by subcutaneous division of its walls: 3rdly by compressing it between a steel pin and a twisted suture, or by some similar contrivance or lastly by complete excision . . . Except in the cases which have been referred to, these operations are not to be recommended and the patient, if wise, will be content with the palliative measures of a more simple character». In England Mr. John Marshall, surgeon to University College Hospital, gave a clinical lecture in 1874 *On a case of varicose veins treated by a new operation*. He advocated in this lecture that a considerable length of the vein should be excised where it is most enlarged and the operation was performed in the following manner: — "The course of the vein having been marked with ink, a pin is passed under it at each end of the part to be removed. The limb is then emptied of blood by Esmarch's bandage, the skin is divided along the marked line and the vein, previously secured by figure of eight ligatures passed over the pins, is cut across at each end and dissected out, the wound is then dressed after Lister's method». This lecture, published in the *Lancet* of 23rd. January 1875, marks the first public recognition by hospital surgeons in England of the treatment of varicose veins by open incision, and it was not long before operations upon varicose veins became more numerous.

I find that at my own hospital — St. Bartholomew's — ten patients only were submitted to operation for the relief of varicose veins in 1875, and twelve in 1876. The results do not seem to have been satisfactory, for in 1877 only three cases are recorded and in 1878 five cases. The average number of cases admitted in the decennium 1875-1885 was 8.2, and in the years 1886-1893 it was 19. After this year the numbers increased rapidly and an average of 70 cases a year is now maintained.

The increasing confidence of surgeons in Listerian methods soon brought about modifications in the original operation. The underpinning of the veins was first omitted because it was not found necessary to make any attempt to limit the process of clotting and with aseptic wounds veins proved themselves as amenable to ligature as arteries.

The number and extent of the incisions necessary in an advanced case of varicose veins long militated against the success of the operation and a great step in advance was made by Trendelenburg in 1890 when he published his paper *Ueber die Unterbindung der Vena Saphena magna bei Unterschenkelvaricen*, from the surgical clinic at Bonn in the *Beiträge zur klinischen Chirurgie*, vol. 17. The operation recommended by Trendelenburg is so short, simple and effective, that I have been greatly interested in it and I have done various comparative operations in cases where the two legs have been pretty evenly affected. The results have been equally satisfactory on the two sides so far as I could get the patients to make definite statements. They preferred, as was natural, the operation in which there was but a single scar and with this conclusion no surgeon would quarrel, for multiple wounds mean multiple chances of sepsis. Trendelenburg's operation, however, like everything else has its limitations. In my hands it has not been of use in cases of extensive capillary varicose veins where the whole leg is mottled from the thigh to the foot as so often happens in young women, neither have I been satisfied in cases where there have been only one or two greatly enlarged veins, for in these cases the trunks have remained full of blood which has shown no tendency to clot or to disappear.

Varicocele

The operation on varicocele, like that of varicose veins, has also undergone a radical change of late years. The mental condition of the patients, as shown by their anxiety to have something done, has always caused operations for varicocele to be more numerous than those for varicose veins even in prelisterian days, but like varicose veins it was not a favourite operation with the last generation of surgeons, so that in 1881 only one case was operated upon in S. Bartholomew's Hospital, whilst last year there were no less than 85.

Similar changes have taken place in connection with the operation for varicocele as in that for the relief of varicose veins. With the advent of Listerian methods surgeons discarded the older palliative treatment by suspenders and the use of pewter rings passed over the scrotum and tightened above the testis to limit the blood supply and for a time they adopted an ingenious but somewhat dangerous treatment by underpinning the enlarged veins and by subcutaneous ligature. The subcutaneous operation was replaced about 1887 by ligature of the pampiniform plexus of veins through an open incision in the scrotum. An important modification of this method, which in England we attribute to Mr. Jacobson and Sir William Bennett, consists in shortening the spermatic cord by removing a considerable portion of the enlarged veins and afterwards uniting the cut extremities. The scrotal operation proved to be unsatisfactory in several ways. The incision was small and the surgeon was often unable completely to stop the venous bleeding from the smaller vessels. A haematom was frequently formed and this combined with the difficulty of rendering the rugose skin of the scrotum sufficiently

aseptic often led to suppuration, whilst the incomplete removal
of the varicocele allowed recurrence to take place with undue
frequency. Of late years, therefore, it has become the custom to
ligature and excise the spermatic veins rather than the pampiniform plexus through an incision above the pubis situated over the
external abdominal ring. The spermatic cord is shortened in the
same way as in the older operation by means of a double ligature, excision of the veins and subsequent union of their cut ends.
All interference with the vas deferens is rigorously avoided but
it is recognised that the whole of the enlarged veins must be
obliterated and not merely the main trunks, whilst the inclusion
of the spermatic artery in a ligature does not necessarily or even
usually lead to wasting of the testicle.

Haemorrhoids

The recent advances in surgery have left the operation for
piles less changed in appearance than almost any other surgical
procedure. Yet it has changed in everything that is essential except
the mere ligature. The parts are now washed, shaved, and rendered as aseptic as possible before operation, a carefully boiled ligature of floss silk is applied to each pile, and the pile itself distal
to the ligature is afterwards cut off. Ample reward is obtained in
return for the care bestowed on these details. The operation for
piles was formerly too often followed by suppuration, secondary
haemorrhage, cellulitis and pyaemia. It was therefore looked
upon as a serious operation, nowadays these sequelae are so
rare that a surgeon occasionally fails to warn his patient that such
risks are still unavoidable in every case and when they occur
and the patient dies he is surprised and calls it a surgical catastrophe.

Other methods than ligature have been used for the cure of
piles and foremost amongst these are the clamp and cautery,
excision of the haemorrhoidal mucous membrane, and the treatment by high tension currents.

The treatment of piles by excision of the rectal mucous mem-
brane has been strongly advocated by Mr. Walter Whitehead [19], of
Manchester, but the method has never been used very extensively
in this country owing no doubt to the severity of the procedure.
Mr. Whitehead describes the operation in the following words:
— «The sphincters are stretched to complete relaxation in order

to allow of the free descent of the haemorrhoids and any prolapse which may be present. By the use of scissors and dissecting forceps the mucous membrane is divided at its junction with the skin round the entire circumference of the bowel, every irregularity of the skin being carefully followed. The external and the commencement of the internal sphincters are then exposed by a rapid dissection and the mucous membrane and attached haemorrhoids, thus separated from the subcutaneous bed on which they rested, are pulled bodily down, any undivided points of resistance being snipped across and the haemorrhoids being brought below the margin of the skin. The mucous membrane above the haemorrhoids is now divided transversely in successive stages, and the free margin of the severed mucous membrane above is attached, as soon as it is divided, to the free margin of the skin below by a suitable number of sutures. The complete ring of pile-bearing mucous membrane is thus removed. Bleeding vessels throughout the operation are twisted on division.

Treatment of piles by high frequency currents.

There are always a certain number of patients whom it is undesirable to submit to a surgical operation. Those who suffer from piles are often singularly ill-suited to the various forms of surgical procedure in common use, either because their constitutions are broken from continued ill health or those still more unhappy persons whose minds are centred on themselves and whose condition is made worse rather than better by every attempt to alleviate their ailment. For all such persons Prof. Doumer, of Lille, advocated in 1897 the treatment of piles and of fissures of the anus by currents of high frequency. The treatment, he says, is painless, it involves no interference with ordinary occupations and it effects a cure in a large proportion of cases. Mr. T. J. Bokenham ([15]) has given the method a fair trial during the last two years and a half and he has applied Doumer's treatment to more than one hundred cases of rectal trouble. The results he has obtained leave much to be desired in the direction of complete cure but he believes that they are far superior to those obtained by any other means except operation.

Naevi

The treatment of the various forms of angeiomata, whether in connection with the blood vessels or the lymphatics, has undergone but little change within the last few years. When the operation is reasonably practicable, excision of naevi has almost completely replaced the older method of subcutaneous ligature. Electrolysis has come into more extensive use and attempts have been made to cure the superficial forms by using the Roentgen rays. But it has not been found possible to abolish «the port wine stain» naevus which may be the most conspicuous, as it is certainly the most persistent form of congenital vascular malformation. In the very slighest forms I have obtained good results by painting capillary naevi with a solution of corrosive sublimate, one part in seven parts of celloidin. This application is more satisfactory than the usual one of ethylate of soda.

My own experience with the large cystic lymphangiomata which occur in the necks of young children where they form a most unsightly swelling, has shown me that even the largest may be removed safely and with good prospects of success. The bleeding at the time of the operation is always less than would be expected in so large a dissection and even if the whole tumour be not removed the prognosis is not necessarily unfavourable, because the portion left behind often becomes completely atrophied, so that there only remains a nodule of fibrous tissue or a single enlarged lymphatic gland. The cystic hygromata or «barren cysts» are much less satisfactory to treat. Their attachments in the néck are so deep and they burrow so extensively that it may be impossible to dissect them out completely, yet if they are not wholly removed they will reappear sooner or later even when every attempt has been made to destroy the vitality of those portions of the cyst wall which have been unavoidably left behind.

CONCLUSIONS

It is clear from this summary of recent surgical work in connection with the vascular system that we have not reached a limit in any single branch. There is room for improvement in the treatment of shock: the method of ligaturing the larger arteries is by no means perfect: the cure of aneurysm is still at fault and even naevi cannot yet be treated satisfactorily. But neither has surgery itself attained to finality. Hosts of surgeons in every part of the world are enlarging its bounds and amongst them not a few are engaged in endeavouring to perfect the technique of the surgery of the bloodvessels.

March 15th, 1905.

BIBLIOGRAPHY

(¹) *Blood-Pressure in Surgery. An experimental and clinical Research*, by George W. Crile A. M. M. D. Professor of Clinical surgery Western Reserve Medical College, Cleveland, 8 vo. Philadelphia and London, 1903.

(²) *A Treatise on the Ligation of the Great Arteries in continuity, with observations on the nature and progress and treatment of aneurysm*, by C. A. Ballance and Walter Edmunds, 8vo. Lond. Macmillan & Co, 1891.

(³) *The treatment of Aneurysm by the subcutaneous injection of Gelatin*, by Guthrie Rankin M. D. *The Medico-Chirurgical Transactions*, vol. 86, 1903, p. 377.

(⁴) *On a new method of procuring the consolidation of fibrin in certain incurable aneurysms*, by Charles H. Moore and Charles Murchison M. D. *The medico-Chirurgical Transactions*, vol. 47, 1864, p. 129.

(⁵) Loreta, *Memoirs "Royal Academy.. Bologna*, vol. 5, series iv.

(⁶) *Aneurysm of the Aorta treated by the insertion of a permanent wire and galvanism (Moore-Corradi method) with a report of five cases*, by Guy L. Hunner M.D. *The Johns Hopkins Hospital Bulletin*, vol. No. 116, November 1900, p. 263.

(⁷) *A case of aneurysm of the abdominal aorta treated by the introduction of silver wire with a description of instruments invented and constructed by Mr. G. H. Colt to facilitate the introduction of wire into aneurysms*, by D'Arcy Power and G.H. Colt. *The Medico-Chirurgical Transactions*, vol. 86, 1903, p. 363, and *The Lancet*, 1903, vol. 2, p. 808.

(⁸) *L'Elettrolisi e le sue applicazioni terapeutiche*, opera postuma del Dottor Ciniselli Cav. Luigi, compilata dai dottori Ottoni cav. Gregorio e Omboni Vincenzo, Cremona, 1880.

(⁹) Burresi, *Lo Sperimentale*, April 1879, p. 445.

(¹⁰) Barwell, *The British Medical Journal*, vol. 2, 1886, p. 675.

(¹¹) *The treatment of sacculated aortic aneurysm by electrolysis through introduced wire*, by D.D. Stewart M.D. *American Journal of the Medical Sciences*, July-Dec. 1892, p. 422, and July-Dec. 1898, p. 170. See also *The Trans. of the Coll. of Physicians of Philadelphia*, 1897, p. 35.

(¹²) *Three hundred consecutive cases of haemorrhoids cured by excision*, by Walter Whitehead F.R.C.S.E. *The British Medical Journal*, 1887, vol. 2, p. 449.

(¹³) *The treatment of haemorrhoids and allied conditions by oscillatory currents of high tension*, by T. J. Bokenham. *The Lancet*, vol. 1, 1904.

—The blocks illustrating this report are kindly lent by Messrs Macmillan & Messrs Down.

THÈME 4 - CHIRURGIE DU GRAND SYMPATHIQUE

(La chirurgie du sympathique)

Par M. le Prof. SALAZAR DE SOUZA (Lisbonne)

Pour pouvoir juger de la valeur de la chirurgie du sympathique dans les différentes maladies où elle a été pratiquée, il faut d'abord connaître la physiologie de ce système nerveux. Pour ce qui concerne le sympathique cervical, ma tâche est accomplie.

puisque après le rapport de MM. Thomas Jonesco et Floresco (C. R. Acad. de Méd. 1 juillet 1902) basé sur l'étude des phénomènes produits par la sympathectomie exécutée sur 15 épileptiques, rien n'est venu changer nos connaissances. Quelques autres points relatifs au même sujet, je les ai développés dans un travail personnel publié à Lisbonne en 1904 (*A Cirurgia do Sympathico*). Je n'y reviendrai pas, pour ne point allonger mon rapport outre mesure.

Les connaissances de la physiologie du sympathique abdominal, surtout ce qui se rapporte au plexus solaire, se trouvent très bien étudiées et mises au point, dans la thèse de Laignel-Lavastine (*Recherches sur le plexus solaire*, Paris 1903). Quant à l'innervation vaso-motrice du tronc et des membres, il suffit de savoir, d'après Langley, qu'elle se décalque sur l'innervation sensitive; il y a la même disposition métamérique pour le tronc et la même disposition en bandes pour les membres. D'après Langley encore, l'innervation sympathique des organes génitaux externes, ainsi que de l'anus, provient du plexus sacré; et l'innervation de l'utérus et de ses annexes provient du plexus lombaire et aortique par les nerfs qui suivent les vases utéro-ovariens. La vessie est innervée par toutes les racines lombaires et sacrées, mais normalement, la seconde, la troisième et la quatrième sacrées, seules, entrent en fonction.

Pour ce qui concerne les réflexes de Goltz, Brown-Séquard, Cyon, etc., ils sont assez bien connus de tous les physiologistes, pour qu'il ne soit nécessaire de faire plus que de les nommer.

En supposant donc que tous ces faits relatifs à la physiologie du sympathique soient bien connus, il faut maintenant aborder un autre point. *Primum non nocere.* Donc est-ce que l'ablation du sympathique, n'apportera point de troubles d'un autre ordre, préjudiciables à l'individu?

Brown-Séquard, Vulpian, Legros, Mapurgo, Snellen, Arloing, Sinitzin, Roger, Morat-Doyon, Lodato, Ferani, Christiani, Wattbaum, Huet, Gaskell, Floresco, Schiff, Olge, Lapinski observèrent différents faits, qui peuvent être classés en trois groupes : 1 — Les faits relatifs aux infections, jadis très fréquentes, et qui apportèrent des altérations de caractère inflammatoire mais non simplement trophiques. 2 — Les faits relatifs aux dégénérescences secondaires à travers les centres nerveux, après l'extirpation du ganglion cervical; ces dégénérescences ne peuvent que montrer le trajet des fibres, et jusqu'où l'action du sympathique peut arriver. 3 — Les cas où se manifestent les troubles de nutrition, soit des téguments, soit de l'œil, soit des centres nerveux (à l'exclusion des dégénérescences secondaires), soit l'augmentation du poids, supérieur à celui des animaux témoins. Comment devons-nous interpréter tous ces faits? D'abord on doit prendre note du peu de gravité et bien souvent de leur caractère passager. Mais si à tous les faits nous joignons l'altération de composition des humeurs de l'œil (Lodato, Morat-Doyon), la plus grande résistance aux poisons et à la putréfaction (B.-Séquard), la cicatrisation plus rapide de la plaie expérimentale de l'oreille du lapin (Mapurgo, Snellen), les troubles de la sécrétion de l'urée (Floresco)... nous ne pouvons interpréter ces petites altérations que comme des stigmates, des troubles du métabolisme intime, sous la dépendance du sympathique. Mais tous ces troubles ont été produits expérimentalement; après les interventions sur l'homme, aucun opéré n'a présenté en général des altérations trophiques cliniquement appréciables. Ne pouvant pas essayer sur l'homme comme sur les animaux, nous recourrons à une méthode indirecte qui est d'observer si les altérations pathologiques du sympathique sont accompagnées d'autres troubles; cela veut dire que nous avons à faire un chapitre d'anatomie pathologique, bien pauvre en faits. Vulpian, dans un cas de plaie accidentelle, a observé une certaine asymétrie de la face, plus apparente que réelle et qui est due au rétrécissement de la fente des paupières.

Dans la pleurésie du sommet du poumon, le ganglion cervical inférieur peut être attaqué par la sclérose, ce qui se révèle par les symptômes oculaires, et dans un cas où l'on a fait l'autopsie et où il y avait de l'hémiatrophie de la face droite, on a observé que le ganglion cervical inférieur du même côté était attaqué par le procédé de pachypleurite (Jacquet). Roux a rassemblé encore quatre autres cas d'hémiatrophie: deux semblables à celui-ci; le troisième où la lésion, que l'on a supposée du sympathique, a été due à une blessure produite par une arme à feu; le quatrième, où elle a été due à la fracture du col de l'humérus et de la clavicule du fœtus pendant l'accouchement. Dans ces cas on n'a pas fait l'autopsie; cependant, les symptômes oculo-pupillaires faisaient admettre la lésion du sympathique. Chez un opéré de Chipault, un petit épileptique, qui plus tard a été vu par Déjerine, il y avait une certaine atrophie de la face; mais Chipault affirme qu'elle était préexistante.

On cite un cas de décollement de la rétine chez un opéré (pour glaucome).

Des lésions microscopiques (cellules granulées, pigmentées, etc., hyperplasie du tissu conjonctif) ont été rencontrées par Echeverria dans les ganglions réséqués à des épileptiques.

Chipault a rencontré un myxome du sympathique chez un épileptique. Bogdanick dit qu'on le rencontre fréquemment volumineux et ecchymotique dans l'épilepsie. Juvara rencontre le sympathique hypertrophié chez un basedowien, et Gérard Marchant, dans la même maladie, remarque dans un cas que le nerf du côté droit était plus gros et plus vascularisé que celui du côté gauche; il remarque dans un autre cas que le nerf et le ganglion sont extrêmement volumineux du côté gauche, et le sont moins du côté droit, quoiqu'ils soient d'un volume encore supérieur au normal; dans un autre cas encore, le ganglion cervical supérieur du côté droit est volumineux, ayant le double des dimensions de celui du côté gauche. Chez une opérée à moi, avec un goître exophthalmique, le sympathique du côté droit était beaucoup plus volumineux que celui du côté gauche.

Dans le glaucome, Lodato rencontre des foyers d'hémorrhagie et de sclérose dans le ganglion cervical supérieur.

Ball, dans deux cas, Allanvart, Schlie, Wagner, dans d'autres cas, ont rencontré différentes lésions de sclérose du ganglion venant de la capsule, ou alors périvasculaires, mais les cellules nerveuses restant normales. Dans la buphthalmie on a également vu des lésions du ganglion supérieur du sympathique que M. Athias a trouvées normales chez mon opéré. Hale White décrit normalement des cellules dégénérées dans le ganglion cervical supérieur et dans les ganglions semi-lunaires, que Vas lie à l'artério-sclérose. Comme on voit, les altérations rencontrées ne sont, ni très claires, ni caractéristiques, mais cependant elles indiquent quelque chose. Je n'ai pas parlé des cas où le ganglion cervical supérieur a été trouvé plus ou moins adhérent au pneumo-gastrique, parce que ceux-ci entrent dans la catégorie des anomalies anatomiques.

Les altérations de pigmentation et de volume doivent être remarquées avec plus de soin. Vas (cité par van Gehuchten) a observé qu'en excitant pendant 15 minutes le ganglion cervical du lapin, il y a eu une augmentation de $\frac{1}{3}$ du volume de la cellule, une diminution ou disparition du chromophile dans les proximités du noyau, s'accumulant dans la périphérie cellulaire;

tuméfaction et dislocation du noyau à la périphérie. Lauchart confirme seulement la partie qui regarde les troubles du chromophile. Marin confirme en tous points les résultats obtenus par Vas, attribuant les altérations du chromophile, non au changement dans la périphérie cellulaire, mais à la diminution de cet élément, principalement auprès du noyau. Lugaro trouve d'abord augmentation du corps cellulaire, avec une légère augmentation de la substance chromophilique, ensuite vient la fatigue et, comme résultat, la diminution progressive du volume cellulaire et de la substance chromophilique. Van Gehuchten fait remarquer que probablement ces altérations n'atteindront pas le même degré dans l'excitation physiologique, parce que celle-ci n'a pas une intensité égale à un courant appliqué directement.

Ces expériences sont d'accord avec ce que Obreja et Tatuse (Soc. Sc. Med. Bucarest, novembre 1898) ont observé, c.-à.-d. une diminution énorme du pigment dans un cas de tétanos spontané et dans le tétanos strychnique (chien) et ils ont au contraire trouvé des cellules très pigmentées chez les individus qui meurent après un repos très prolongé au lit.

Ce qui reste établi, c'est qu'il y a des altérations cellulaires, qui représentent une excessive activité cellulaire, et pour cela il serait d'un grand intérêt que tous les ganglions réséqués fussent examinés microscopiquement, pour que l'on puisse arriver à une conclusion.

Dans le tabes, J. Roux décrit les lésions trouvées, qui consistent dans une dégénération des fibres fines de myéline, qui passent dans la racine postérieure, semblant peut-être à une atrophie consécutive à l'atrophie de la propre racine.

Le fait est que cette altération permet, d'après Roux, d'expliquer quelques troubles de sensibilité viscérale, tels que: abolition de la sensibilité du testicule et de la glande mammaire (avec intégrité et quelquefois même avec hyperesthésie cutanée), les perturbations vésicales; les crises gastriques avec irradiation vers les côtés du thorax; l'absence du réflexe trachéal (Sicard); l'anesthésie épigastrique, qui peut arriver au point de la disparition du réflexe de Goltz.

Dans la mélanodermie, on a trouvé quelquefois lésé le plexus solaire (7 fois en 8 autopsies), laissant croire que non seulement peuvent en dépendre les lésions suprarénales, mais aussi les vasoparalysies abdominales. Dans les infections comme la vérole, la fièvre typhoïde, etc., on peut trouver dans les ganglions des altérations qui sont secondaires à l'infection.

Dans les péritonites aiguës, comme celles qui résultent de la perforation de l'estomac chez un individu apparemment bien portant, il apparaît des altérations des cellules des ganglions du plexus solaire (vacuolisation, achromatose, noyaux à la périphérie) qui peuvent contribuer à l'hypérémie des viscères abdominaux, le foie, le rein, capsules suprarénales, pancréas (Levastine). D'égales altérations congestives furent trouvées chez des paralytiques, présentant des lésions du plexus solaire. Gaupner, chez un malade avec un goitre exophthalmique, souffrant de diarrhée et de glycosurie depuis un an, trouve dans l'autopsie des lésions du sympathique cervical et des splanchniques.

Mais on a trouvé souvent des lésions du sympathique, sans qu'il y ait des symptômes qui pendant la vie les fassent soupçonner.

Tel fut le cas opéré par Glochner (Arch. Gyn. 1901 LXIII) d'un volumineux névrome du sympathique abdominal, et ceux de nodules tuberculeux et cancéreux trouvés parfois dans les ganglions du plexus, par Eulenberg et Guttman, sans que pendant la vie il y eût des perturbations intestinales.

Dans *la glycosurie*, dans les intoxications chroniques, comme la tuberculose, dans des états cachectiques, comme la sénilité, etc. on a quelquefois trouvé à l'autopsie des lésions des ganglions et des fibres, qui n'ont aucune influence sur la symptomatologie de la maladie en beaucoup de cas, excepté pour le saturnisme.

De tout ce que nous avons exposé, on voit que jusqu'à ce jour les données anatomo-pathologiques sur le système sympathique n'avancent pas beaucoup. Seulement, d'après les études microscopiques et d'après les expériences faites, on peut conclure qu'aux excitations aiguës (mécaniques, toxiques ou infectieuses) correspondent des dégénérescences des cellules nerveuses, et aux chroniques des lésions de sclérose interstitielle, avec neurophagie par les éléments mésodermiques (Laignel-Lavastine).

Épilepsie

Alexandre supposait d'abord que la stase sanguine dans le cerveau avec production d'œdème, etc., était la cause de l'épilepsie. De là son procédé de ligature des vertébrales qui, très bien reçu par quelques opérateurs, fut bientôt abandonné à cause des insuccès.

Les quelques cas dans lesquels il a obtenu un certain résul

tat semblent à Alexandre être ceux dans lesquels apparaissaient, consécutivement à l'intervention opératoire, les phénomènes oculo-pupillaires, montrant que le sympathique avait été lésé pendant l'intervention. Il a depuis essayé d'agir seulement sur le sympathique, et les résultats obtenus l'ont animé beaucoup plus que ceux de la ligature des artères.

Mais le sympathique excité est vaso-constricteur, la vaso-dilatation paralytique, consécutive à la section, a-t-elle une action favorable sur l'attaque?

Le moment est arrivé d'étudier l'influence des perturbations circulatoires sur la production de l'attaque épileptique.

On peut produire des convulsions chez les animaux par la ligature des carotides et des vertébrales (Cooper). Après une hémorrhagie abondante les convulsions peuvent apparaître.

L'excitation du sympathique produit des convulsions quand l'animal a d'abord été saigné (Nothnagel). Gutnikow a vu que posant un animal sur une table tournante, chez les animaux rendus épileptiques, la production de l'anémie augmentait les attaques, tandis que quand l'hypérémie se produisait, ceux-ci diminuaient.

Brown-Séquard trépanant des cobayes, ayant de l'épilepsie expérimentale, et leur produisant une attaque, vit le cerveau devenir exangue.

Chez l'homme, Doyen vit l'anémie se produire chez un trépané épileptique, qui eut une attaque pendant l'opération. On sait de longue date que l'anémie cérébrale est un irritant pour le cerveau. Le vaso-spasme est pour Krafft-Ebing un signe de l'insulte épileptique, se révélant par la pâleur de la face, ou à l'examen du fond de l'œil, et apportant dans les dernières phases de l'attaque une stase vasculaire. Knies, observant maintes fois le fond de l'œil chez un épileptique, a toujours pu vérifier que, d'abord, il y a un vaso-spasme, et après, quand l'accès passe, il y a une vaso-dilatation considérable. Magnan observant une femme après l'attaque, trouva toujours la dilatation des vaisseaux de la rétine.

Récemment, Ormea, dans le laboratoire de Cavazzani, étudiant les variations de pression du liquide céphalo-rachidien du chien, pendant l'attaque épileptique, reconnut, en épileptisant un chien, ou par l'électrisation du cortex, ou par l'absinthe, qu'il y a une augmentation de pression céphalo-rachidienne, atteignant le maximum pendant la phase tonique et pendant la première phase de la période clonique, qui vers la fin diminue avec de nombreuses et irrégulières oscillations. Les phénomènes post-épileptiques présentent une perturbation de la pression sub-arachnoïdée, qui persiste avec une intensité et une durée plus ou moins grande.

Cavazzani, étudiant la cause de cette augmentation de pression du liquide céphalo-rachidien des chiens rendus épileptiques, montre d'abord par l'action du curare, sur un animal trachéotomisé et soumis à la respiration artificielle, que ces variations sont indépendantes de celles qui peuvent résulter de la difficulté de circulation pendant la période tonique, due à l'arrêt de la respiration avec contraction brusque des muscles du thorax et de l'abdomen. Le même, étudiant la pression sanguine dans les vaisseaux du cerveau, voit que, tandis que dans l'aorte la pression augmente beaucoup pendant l'attaque épileptique, dans le polygone artériel de Willis elle diminue, ce qui peut seulement être obtenu par une forte vaso-dilatation active, parce que, si elle était passive et produite à peine par l'influx sanguin, il n'y aurait pas de diminution de pression, mais il y aurait équilibre. La correspondance des tracés de la pression du liquide céphalo-rachidien et de la pression sanguine de l'héxagone de Willis est telle qu'elle montre la connexité des deux phénomènes. Pour Cavazzani il y a donc une forte vaso-dilatation, avec diminution de la pression dans l'héxagone de Willis, et augmentation de la pression du liquide céphalo-rachidien.

Ainsi se trouve aussi expliqué pourquoi durant l'accès Ormea vit le liquide céphalo-rachidien devenir rosé, y trouvant avec facilité des globules rouges.

Bombarda se rapportant aux stigmates, qu'il classifie de nerveux, fait noter la facilité avec laquelle les vaso-moteurs réagissent sous des causes minimes.

Il dit: «La chaleur, l'alcool en doses minimes, les repas déterminent de notables rubéfactions de l'extrémité céphalique, qui démontrent la faiblesse des appareils nerveux respectifs. Cette simple faiblesse irritable des vaso-moteurs, apportant de faciles paralysies des vases de la face et probablement du cerveau, est le produit d'une excitabilité morbide des éléments nerveux» … Ceci montre l'importance qu'il donne aux perturbations vaso-motrices; mais il faut dire qu'il ne les considère pas comme cause productrice de l'attaque, car il est certain qu'il le dit encore plus clairement à la page 203 de son livre (*Epilepsia et pseudo-epilepsias*): «Les nerfs vaso-moteurs fonctionnent très fréquemment d'une manière déséquilibrée. Dans ceux-ci, comme chez d'autres dégénérés, est remarquable la facilité avec laquelle se produisent des paralysies vasculaires, étendues sous l'influence de causes minimes, l'alcool, etc. Je suis convaincu que beaucoup de perturbations cérébrales n'ont pas une autre origines; mais la page 257 complète sa pensée des relations possibles entre les altérations vasculaires et la production de l'attaque par les paroles suivantes: «On se rapporte généralement aux perturbations de la circulation cérébrale, mais celles-ci, qui me semblent un phénomène consécutif, nécessitent à leur tour une explication».

Le spasme vasculaire, qui apparaît au commencement de l'attaque, ou qui la précède même, et qui est suivi par la vaso-dilatation comme la décrit Krafft-Ebing, expliquerait pour quelques-uns tous les symptômes de l'attaque. Ainsi, pour Meyer, les phénomènes se passeraient de la manière suivante: La vaso-constriction produirait l'excitation convulsive, d'abord clonique, ensuite tonique, ce qui apporterait un épuisement des centres, qui ne pourraient plus réagir que par des convulsions cloniques, espacées; mais l'excitation violente des centres vaso-moteurs finirait par l'épuiser aussi, et une vaso-dilatation paralytique intense succéderait à la vaso-constriction.

Or, cette vaso-dilatation paralytique apporterait les symptômes d'une autre phase de l'attaque: à la lividité de la face succède la congestion, presque cyanose, qui dans le cerveau se fait remarquer par le coma, phénomène pseudo-paralytique, etc.

La bouche écumante serait la sialorrhée résultant de la congestion des glandes salivaires.

Mais, quoique les faits soient le mieux d'accord, il est seulement licite de dire que des phénomènes vaso-moteurs se succèdent à l'attaque et l'accompagnent, et plus encore, que l'épileptique, comme un dégénéré qu'il est, est sujet à divers désordres vaso-moteurs.

Il est facile de rencontrer des faits appuyant l'opinion contraire, cela veut dire que la congestion origine l'attaque. Excitant expérimentalement le cerveau par l'électricité, Fritsch, Hitzig, Corville, Duret, Ferrier, n'ont pas eu le vaso-spasme, mais la vaso-dilatation.

On cite des faits cliniques, dans lesquels l'élément congestion et stase produit la convulsion; ce fut suivant cet ordre d'idées qu'Alexandre proposa et fit la ligature des artères vertébrales.

Le propre B.-Séquard (Arch. Phys. 1891, page 216) écrit que l'anémie cérébrale, dans l'épilepsie, comme dans le sommeil, n'est

pas la cause de la perte de connaissance, mais que l'arrêt de
l'activité cérébrale doit dépendre d'un acte inhibitoire.

Ainsi, nous pouvons seulement conclure que l'épileptique
est sujet à de brusques troubles vaso-moteurs, et ceux-ci sont
constants pendant les attaques.

Ainsi, en tout et pour tout l'épileptique est un individu anatomiquement et physiologiquement mal constitué. Tous les stigmates l'indiquent.

Dans la cellule nerveuse, mettant de côté la gliose superficielle du cortex, ces altérations se produiront et se manifesteront
quant au fonctionnement.

Le prof. Bombarda dit, à la page 14 du livre cité: «Je veux
dire, quelle que soit la cause de la dégénérescence (et ici je me
rapporte à toutes les dégénérescences), l'impression qu'on reçoit
d'une soigneuse observation est qu'elles sont une véritable anoma-
lie, une production tératologique, qui a communiqué au cerveau
un fonctionnement spécial sans maladie actuelle... Or, chez l'épileptique, nous voyons que la cellule nerveuse, non seulement répond d'une manière anormale aux excitations, de quelque part
qu'elles viennent, mais le fait d'une manière incohérente et dis-
proportionnée. Un motif insignifiant, qui produirait peu d'impression sur un organisme normal, est, pour l'épileptique, un motif
suffisant pour le mettre en fureur».

Le professeur de l'Ecole de Lisbonne ajoute encore: «L'émo-
tivité des dégénérés est toujours sous tension; toutes les actions qui
sont indifférentes aux autres hommes, pour eux sont accompagnées par des impressions de plaisir ou de douleur, qui s'associent
même aux plus purs phénomènes intellectuels... On peut observer
chez le même individu la plus extrême variation d'état de l'esprit, des exaltations et des dépressions, se suivant sans cause ni
raison» *(loc. cit.).*

Ces variations brusques du fonctionnement de la cellule nerveuse sont aussi des stimulants brusques pour les vaso-moteurs;
le fonctionnement du cerveau étant désordonné, la réponse vaso-
motrice le devait être aussi, et elle doit l'être encore plus, vu que
ses centres reposent sur un encéphale mal constitué, car il m'est
difficile de supposer la sélection de la dégénérescence exclusive
pour les neurones de la région psycho-motrice.

Mais ces altérations brusques vaso-motrices, qui doivent être
disproportionnées au stimulant, ne peuvent pas avoir lieu sans
apporter de leur côté de graves troubles. Or, la sympathectomie

produisant un état permanent de dilatation vaso-paralytique, et empêchant ainsi ces altérations brusques vaso-motrices, ne pourra-t-elle pas être favorable à l'épileptique? La cellule nerveuse, ne pouvant être accompagnée, dans son fonctionnement désordonné, par le désordre vaso-moteur, est-ce qu'il ne résultera pas d'ici une phrénation dans son fonctionnement?

Voyons: B.-Séquard rendant épileptiques des cobayes, et leur réséquant les ganglions cervicaux supérieurs du sympathique, vit l'excitation de la zone épileptogénique produire l'attaque. Vulpian obtint le même résultat, ne remarquant aucune différence dans les attaques, avant et après avoir ôté le glanglion, soit que l'on prenne pour terme de comparaison le même animal avant et après l'opération, soit qu'on le compare aux animaux témoins rendus épileptiques mais non sympathectomisés.

Laborde (Soc. biol. 1 oct. 1898) vit, chez les cobayes, l'attaque se produire avec ses trois phases, tonique, clonique et comateuse, malgré la résection du sympathique. Il remarque cependant que, quand on fait d'abord la résection, et après quelques semaines on fait l'incision épileptogénique, l'attaque se produit de la même manière: suivant l'ordre inverse, il vit chez une des cobayes l'attaque à peine ébauchée. Cependant, dans la session du 31 décembre de la même année, recommençant à raisonner sur ce sujet, il présente trois cobayes, concluant des expériences auxquelles il a procédé que la résection du sympathique n'exerce aucune influence, ni préventive ni curative, sur l'épilepsie expérimentale. Kussmaul et Tenner, coupant le sympathique cervical, mais aidant la stase sanguine par la ligature des veines jugulaires n'ont pas réussi à produire l'épilepsie. D'autre part, sachant l'importance qu'on attache à l'intoxication, Vidal, de Périgueux, vit que la sympathectomie, augmente la résistance des cobayes aux poisons convulsivants; pour rendre convulsive une cobaye sympathectomisée, il est nécessaire une dose de macération de tabac beaucoup plus considérable que celle nécessaire pour les cobayes témoins.

Le contraire arrive, si l'opération qui a été faite est la ligature de la carotide, Vidal concluant que chez la cobaye la susceptibilité pour les poisons est en raison inverse de l'activité de la circulation cérébrale.

Si l'on peut raisonner pour l'homme par ce qui se passe chez l'animal, si l'on peut identifier l'épilepsie expérimentale avec l'épilepsie essentielle, nous voyons que les résultats obtenus par les expériences, sont ou douteux, ou défavorables à la sympathectomie. Est-ce que chez l'homme il arrive la même chose?

C'est à cela que l'analyse des observations nous permettra de répondre, mais il est intéressant de citer d'abord quelques opinions.

Déjerine-lui est absolument contraire, par ce qu'il a vu chez une malade opérée par Chipault. Chipault, venant à l'attaque, dans une autre session de la Société de Biologie, cite quatre épileptiques sur lesquels le bromure n'avait pas produit d'effet et qui virent disparaître les attaques avec l'opération. Déjerine ne se rend pas, et répond que les rémissions sont fréquentes dans le grand mal, et que les malades furent observés pendant peu de temps.

Vidal entend que la résection est indiquée pour les épilepsies causées par l'anémie cérébrale et par auto-intoxication. Pour voir si l'attaque est due au vaso-spasme, il propose que, quand l'accès est à son commencement, on fasse des inhalations de nitrite d'amyle, et que l'on opère seulement dans les cas où les inhalations se montrent favorables. Suivant cette pratique, il eut l'occasion de trouver indiquée une craniectomie (car il y eut augmentation du mal avec le nitrite) et de guérir la malade en ôtant une tumeur.

Souques, chez une épileptique de 48 ans, opérée depuis six mois, vit recommencer les attaques qui au commencement avaient disparu.

Jaboulay et Lannois virent des guérisons seulement chez les hystéro-épileptiques (16 cas qu'ils opérèrent) et ils ont conclu qu'il faut renoncer à espérer des améliorations sérieuses par l'ablation du sympathique.

Ricard, opérant une malade de Féré, ne vit les attaques se modifier en rien.

Donath réséque, chez trois malades, le ganglion cervical supérieur, sans résultat.

Toufher, en 1877, ôta le ganglion moyen sans résultat.

Alexander, sur 24 opérés, obtient six guérisons de 3, 2 et 1 an, et une de 4 mois, 10 améliorations, 5 insuccès et 2 aggravations.

Kümmel opère une femme en ôtant le ganglion cervical supérieur; 2 ans après, la malade se trouve bien, ayant eu à peine une attaque.

Jacksh, chez deux militaires, lie les vertébrales et coupe simultanément le sympathique, obtenant des guérisons qui se maintiennent respectivement pendant 2 et 3 ans.

Bogdanik obtient une guérison en ôtant le ganglion moyen.

Otero de Acevedo obtient avec la résection totale une amélioration relative.

Jonesco est celui qui se montre le plus enthousiaste; il fait la résection totale et, récemment, chaque fois que c'est possible, il ôte aussi le premier ganglion dorsal. En 1898, il avait opéré 35 épileptiques, desquels il avait pu suivre 15 pendant assez longtemps avec 4 guérisons, 4 améliorations et 2 résultats nuls. En 1900, il compte déjà, sur 49 cas, 12 guérisons (de 4, 3 et 2 ans) et 4 améliorations. En 1902, il relate 2 cas de longue observation (l'un d'eux de 6 ans), qu'il répute favorables, quoique les malades fassent usage de bromure.

On voit que les résultats varient d'un opérateur à l'autre. A côté de l'anathème lancé par Déjerine (qui n'opère pas), il y a le doute de quelques-uns, qui opèrent, et la ferme croyance d'autres.

Effectivement, dans l'épilepsie essentielle, qui est celle que nous visons, un pourcentage de 12 guérisons sur 49 cas, sans compter les améliorations, est un résultat encourageant.

Est-ce que nous avons de grandes ressources thérapeutiques ?

Je pense que la pensée générale est bien exprimée par Winter, par exemple, quand il dit que malgré tous les traitements, l'épilepsie est et continuera à être guérissable seulement par exception (Arch. f. Klin. Chir. 1902, 817).

Malheureusement il y a trois points qui rendent difficile l'étude du sujet. Le premier c'est que beaucoup de fois on n'indique pas dans les observations si la sympathectomie fut partielle ou totale, le second c'est que les observateurs se limitent à dire que le malade était un épileptique, sans justifier le diagnostic, quand il est certain que celui-ci n'est pas toujours facile (par exemple le cas d'épilepsie nasale de Lannois, et les troubles psychiques signalés par Garel, et relatés à la Soc. Méd. des Hôp. de Lyon, [Juin 1902]); le troisième c'est que le critérium suivi pour le diagnostic de la maladie et pour juger de la guérison, c'est le fait brutal de l'attaque.

Or, aujourd'hui on ne peut d'aucune manière admettre que l'on parle ainsi de l'épilepsie. Pour moi, un épileptique qui avec l'opération voit disparaître les attaques n'est pas un épileptique guéri, si les troubles psychiques persistent, mais un épileptique amélioré.

Est-ce que l'opération a quelque influence sur l'état psychique ?

Les observations nous disent peu sur ce rapport, comme nous verrons.

Je connais 231 cas d'opérations pratiquées sur des épileptiques, il semble que, après cela, il devait être facile d'établir un accord entre les opérateurs, mais il n'en est pas ainsi.

De ceux-ci on doit exclure 95, soit que l'on ne puisse pas bien juger, à cause du peu de temps qui s'est passé, soit qu'ils doivent être étudiés à part (6 cas).

Nous avons ainsi à juger 136 observations (je ne les publierai pas ici, me limitant à présenter les pourcentages rencontrés. Ces 136 observations peuvent être lues dans mon livre: *Cirurgia do sympathico* (Lisboa 1904).

Dans quelques-unes est indiqué le résultat sur les fonctions psychiques.

Résultats favorables quant aux fonctions psychiques:

A) Exclusivement — 3 cas.

B) Sur les fonctions psychiques et favorables aux attaques — 3 cas.

C) et encore sur les fonctions psychiques et plausiblement favorables aux attaques — 8 cas; total 14 cas.

Résultats favorables sur les attaques exclusivement; 21 avec les 3 cas du groupe B) — 24.

Résultats plausiblement favorables sur les attaques 18 — avec 8 du groupe C — 26.

Aggravations — 5 cas.

Morts — Bronchopneumonie le 3-ème jour 1 cas d'Alexander — Bronchopneumonie le 2-ème jour 1 cas de Braun — Pendant une attaque le 12-ème jour 1 cas de Donath — Pendant une attaque le 13-ème jour 1 cas de Jonnesco — Pendant une attaque quelque temps après l'opération 1 cas de Braun.

Par complication durant l'intervention (ligatures, perforations de la plèvre, etc., seulement dans les résections totales de Jonnesco): 4 cas.

Lésions qui produirent la mort indépendamment de l'opération (mort en état de mal) 1 cas de Lannois et Padiot.

Nous voyons ainsi que, en se bornant à la résection du ganglion supérieur et d'une partie du cordon du sympathique, dans des cas où les complications qui causèrent la mort des malades de Jonnesco ne sont pas citées, et si nous excluons encore les cas de Lannois et Padiot, dans lesquels les lésions rencontrées pendant l'autopsie expliquent l'état de mal, il reste seulement le cas d'Alexander et celui de Braun, de broncho-pneumonie ayant causé la mort; les cas de Donath et Jonnesco et celui de Braun devant être plutôt considérés comme aggravation du mal causé par l'opération de laquelle resulta la mort, plutôt que de la gravité de celle-ci comme acte chirurgical. Je veux dire que la mortalité due réellement à l'opération, si on ne fait pas la résection totale, est presque nulle.

Nous avons ainsi, faisant le pourcentage de 136 cas:

Améliorations exclusives sur l'état intellectuel (3 cas) 2,9 %.

Amélioration de l'état intellectuel et plus ou moins claire sur les attaques (11 cas) 8 %.

Résultats favorables sur les attaques exclusivement (21 cas) 15,4 %.

Résultats plausiblement favorables sur les attaques (18 cas) 13,2 %.

Ce qui donne: action plus ou moins favorable sur l'attaque en général (50 cas) 36,7 %.

Action sur l'état intellectuel (14 cas) 10,2 %.

Aggravation (5 cas) 3,6 %.

Ou, si nous ajoutons les cas de Donnath et Jonnesco et celui de Braun, et même ceux de Lannois et Padiot et de Mariani, 7,3 %.

J'ai toujours cherché dans mon appréciation plutôt à aggraver qu'à atténuer l'opinion faite par l'auteur de l'observation, classifiant quelquefois d'insuccès ce qui est désigné comme une légère amélioration, et d'amélioration ce qui est désigné comme guérison.

Malgré cela j'arrive à la conclusion que l'on peut obtenir des améliorations plus ou moins fermes dans 36 % des cas. Ce qui est plus important et mérite d'être pondéré dans les nouveaux cas que l'on peut opérer, c'est que 10 fois % les fonctions cérébrales s'améliorent beaucoup! Gravité de l'opération à peu près nulle!

Winter (Arch. of Clin. Chirurgery, page 861, 1902), prenant pour critérium de guérison définitive une période de 3 ans sans attaque, trouva 6,6 % de guérisons définitives, 17 % de guérisons temporaires, et 18,9 % d'améliorations, ou, additionnant le pourcentage de tous ces cas, dans lesquels il y a eu des améliorations plus ou moins claires, 42,5 %; cela veut dire un nombre proche de celui que j'ai trouvé.

Dans une maladie comme l'épilepsie est-ce qu'on doit mépriser un tel nombre? Je crois que non, et d'autant plus que ces nombres peuvent souffrir la comparaison avec les statistiques du remède réputé héroïque.

Ainsi la statistique de l'Asile sanatorium pour les épileptiques de Bielefeld donne par l'emploi du bromure:

Guérisons de 3 ans ou plus .... 1,72 %
Améliorations........................... 3,35 %
Ceci pour 8000 malades

Et celle de Bethel, avec le même traitement:

Guérisons de 1 ans ou plus .... 7,7 %
Améliorations..................... 22 %

Ces chiffres sont évidemment inférieurs à ceux de la statistique de la sympathectomie et c'est pourquoi Winter se déclare en faveur de la supériorité de celle-ci.

Pour moi, il reste cependant encore un point obscur, qui est le temps limité des observations existantes, qui fait que nous sommes obligés de nous maintenir dans la réserve que j'ai établie, réduisant à simples améliorations les cas désignés comme des guérisons. On sait qu'il y a des cas où les attaques, soit par l'emploi du bromure, soit spontanément, disparaissent pendant des années, pour apparaître après ce temps ou même ne pas reparaître, sans que pour cela l'individu cesse de commettre des actes de caractère épileptique: tel est le cas cité par Maudsley d'un homme de 62 ans, qui tua sa mère, quand depuis 42 ans il n'avait point d'attaques convulsives.

A Rilhafolles, le professeur Bombarda montre deux épileptiques, chez lesquels les attaques n'apparaissent pas depuis 9 à 12 ans.

Tout ceci fait considérer l'appréciation de l'élément «attaque» comme très faible.

Mais c'est celui-là que les observations présentent et c'est à lui que nous nous rapportons.

Du reste, l'on ne doit pas exagérer, et le fait de la suspension ou atténuation des attaques doit être considéré comme une amélioration, parce que l'attaque a une influence pernicieuse sur l'épileptique.

Continuant à apprécier les cas, je vois qu'il y a 13 interventions unilatérales, et par ces interventions les attaques furent 7 fois plus ou moins favorisées — une fois surtout l'état intellectuel fut influencé (cas de Chipault) — et il y a trois insuccès.

Évidemment, 13 cas c'est peu pour établir la statistique et pour établir des conclusions si telle opération est meilleure ou pire que l'autre; mais ce que ces cas favorables permettent de dire déjà, c'est qu'il n'est pas indispensable de recourir à la résection totale bilatérale pour obtenir des guérisons.

D'autre part, comparant les cas d'Alexander avec ceux de Jonnesco, il n'y a pas de supériorité.

J'ai choisi les statistiques de ces deux, parce qu'elles sont les plus longues, et parce qu'elles sont des partisans de deux interventions différentes: Alexander, résection bilatérale du ganglion supérieur, Jonnesco résection totale (3 ganglions) bilatérale, ou du moins résection très étendue.

Je me servirai de l'appréciation des observateurs mêmes pour classifier les résultats.

Alexander a 24 cas: de ceux-ci nous devons soustraire 4 pour différentes raisons, il en reste 20; il présente comme résultats plus ou moins favorables 14 observations ou soit 70 %.

Jonnesco en a 35: nous devons en soustraire au moins 5; il classifie comme résultats favorables 21 cas, ce qui donne 70 %. Dans cette appréciation je ne suis que favorable à Jonnesco; parce que l'on devait encore exclure 8 cas qui furent observés pendant peu de temps, ce qui donnerait 13 résultats favorables dans 22 cas; une différence minime.

Une plus grande difficulté, une complication possible d'hémorragie, la perforation de la plèvre dans un cas, et l'égalité des résultats font que je répudie la pratique de Jonnesco et que je préfère la section du sympathique (Jaboulay) ou la résection du ganglion supérieur. Cependant, en égard à ce que la résection du ganglion ne présente point une difficulté plus grande et qu'elle nous garantit de la régénération possible, ainsi que par le fait que les phénomènes physiologiques, consécutifs à la sympathectomie, sont plus accentués après la résection du ganglion qu'après la simple section du sympathique, qu'ils rétrocèdent plus lentement, et que, encore, le ganglion pourra acquérir une autonomie indépendante des connexions pré-ganglionnaires, qui lui viennent par le cordon du sympathique; en considérant tout cela, je préfère l'extirpation du ganglion cervical supérieur.

Si je voulais me servir des cas de Mariani, j'arriverais même à démontrer la supériorité absolue de l'opération d'Alexander sur celle de Jonnesco, dont se servent aussi Chipault, Mariani et Vidal. Comment interpréter les résultats obtenus?

Nous entrons dans le champ des hypothèses.

Il y a d'abord le groupe de ceux qui attribuent tout à la suggestion, se fondant principalement sur ce fait que c'est dans les cas qu'on peut soupçonner d'hystérie que les résultats sont meilleurs.

Or, il y a deux faits contraires à cette hypothèse; le premier c'est que l'on voit, dans quelques cas qui sont évidemment d'épilepsie, apparaître des résultats favorables; le second c'est que, en général, les améliorations viennent graduellement quand elles viennent, ce qui n'est pas ordinaire dans la suggestion. Un hystérique qu'on opéra et qui vit ses attaques apparaître comme avant l'opération, pendant quelque temps, développa dans son cerveau l'idée suggestive de l'incurabilité opératoire.

Vidal suppose que l'opération est favorable dans l'épilepsie comme intoxication, ou quand il y a de l'anémie cérébrale, parce que l'action convulsivante des toxiques est en raison inverse de l'irrigation cérébrale.

Le fait de Wheray, qui dans l'asile d'aliénés de Clarinda réduit à 1/3 le nombre des attaques et améliore l'état mental par l'usage permanent des vaso-dilatateurs (nitrites) chez les épileptiques, est favorable aux idées de Vidal; Jonnesco dit qu'elle agit de deux manières: 1.º la circulation sanguine se modifie; 2.º la transmission des excitations réflexes par le sympathique, venues des organs abdominaux et thoraciques, reste ainsi empêchée. Chipault créa la théorie de l'encéphaloclyse: activant la circulation cérébrale, les cellules se dégagent plus facilement des produits toxiques qui les surchargent.

Jojot croit que la sympathectomie peut agir à la longue modifiant l'état de la nutrition du cerveau, soit par l'action vaso-dilatatrice, soit par une action trophique.

Théorisons aussi; je pense que les résultats obtenus ne peuvent être dus à un seul facteur.

La vaso-dilatation passe, l'action trophique est très probable. C'est même ce qui concorde avec la guérison tardive et graduelle, exactement quand les phénomènes vasculaires tendent à disparaître. Cela suffirait pour mettre de côté l'idée exclusive de l'hyperémie cérébrale. Si cela était ainsi, comment expliquer les attaques qui tant de fois surviennent à l'opération? Je ne parle pas des cas où il y a augmentation du mal, parce que dans ces cas il n'y aurait pas d'anémie, il y aurait le contraire et l'opération serait contre-indiquée, mais de ceux où à une phase d'attaque suit une amélioration graduelle.

Pour moi la résection du sympathique sera favorable, parce qu'elle apporte un plus grand afflux de sang au cerveau; elle sera favorable tout de même parce qu'elle combattra une anémie irritante. Mais pour moi, ce que le symphatique coupé fait, c'est de finir avec les brusques troubles vaso-motrices, que nous avons vu être l'apanage des dégénérés, et qui ne se produisent pas sans grand risque pour le cerveau.

Cependant, d'ici je vois déjà l'objection: après avoir obtenu la vaso-dilatation paralytique, la physiologie montre que ce phénomène va disparaissant, et que par les plexus des parois des vaisseaux acquièrent nouvellement l'état de contraction en harmonie avec le reste de la circulation. C'est vrai: mais si ces plexus ont permis que les vaisseaux perdissent l'état de dilatation paralytique, ils sont impuissants pour permettre des variations, je ne dirai pas brusques mais d'ample calibre. Ce n'est pas une hypothèse, c'est à peine la conclusion que je tire des expériences et des observations.

Les expériences montrent que les phénomènes de la vaso-dilatation passent; mais elles montrent aussi, que, dans ces conditions, refroidissant ou réchauffant artificiellement l'oreille de l'animal, on peut faire apparaître des différences de température, qui apparemment n'existaient plus, entre les deux côtés. En refroidissant, la température baisse plus pour l'oreille du côté non opéré, parce qu'il se donne la vaso-constriction de défense, qui ne se donne pas au côté opéré: en réchauffant l'oreille du côté sain il se réchauffe plus, parce que la vaso-dilatation est plus grande.

Nous avons, la résection du sympathique agissant d'abord par la vaso-dilatation, activant la circulation cérébrale, et permettant l'encéphaloclyse, de Chipault.

Ensuite, et pour moi c'est beaucoup plus important, nous la voyons combattant par la stabilité, les brusques variations vaso-motrices, préjudiciables au propre cerveau. Le trophisme se ressentira favorablement de cet état; la cellule nerveuse obéit au principe général d'adaptation. Quand les conditions de milieu varient, elle doit également varier, si peu que ce soit, et cette variation peut seulement se traduire dans son fonctionnement.

On ne doit pas non plus mettre de côté l'action que la résection du sympathique peut avoir, par augmentation si petite qu'elle soit sur la température intracrânienne, et cela parce que aujourd'hui on sait que l'augmentation de la température locale sur le crâne favorise le fonctionnement cérébral.

Nous avons déjà ainsi divers facteurs à agir de manière à imprimer une nouvelle modification dans le fonctionnement cérébral; de cette manière s'explique aussi comment les opérations plus limitées, unilatérales, peuvent avoir des résultats peut-être supérieurs quelquefois aux bilatérales.

La raison en est que, en matière d'excitation et de fonctionnement cérébraux, la réaction n'est pas toujours proportionnelle à l'action.

De tout ce qui est écrit je crois pouvoir conclure: a) la sympathectomie peut donner des résultats favorables dans l'épilepsie; b) que l'on ne peut d'avance prévoir quels seront les cas favorables; c) que, vu la gravité du mal, dans les cas qui se montrent rebelles au bromure, on peut tenter l'intervention chirurgicale.

Goître exophthalmique

Les symptômes qui s'imposent le plus, dans la maladie de Basedow, sont ceux de la trinité de Graves: le goître, l'exophthalmie, et la tachycardie. Sachant depuis Cl. Bernard que, l'excitation du sympathique produit l'exophthalmie et l'accélération du pouls, on devrait s'attendre à ce que l'attention fût dirigée vers le sympathique; ainsi il entre en scène dans la production des symptômes de Basedow. Soit par l'excitation directe de son cordon ou des ganglions, le résultat sera le même. Mais quand on commence à observer minutieusement les symptômes, les difficultés apparaissent.

L'excitation du sympathique produit l'exorbitisme avec l'ouverture de la fente des paupières et la tachycardie; mais comme elle est aussi vaso-constrictrice des vaisseaux de la tête, comment expliquer la vaso-dilatation de ces vaisseaux?

Les carotides et toutes les artères qui dépendent du sympathique cervical sont dilatées, elles pulsent d'une manière exagérée; même par l'ophthalmoscopie on voit ce phénomène.

Ainsi l'interprétation est fausse; le sympathique agira par la vaso-dilatation, soit par la paralysie des vaso-constricteurs (paralysie du sympathique), soit par l'excitation des vaso-dilatateurs.

L'exorbitisme s'expliquait par la vaso-dilatation rétro-orbitaire, avec prolifération du tissu cellulaire dans la cavité orbitaire.

Dans ce cas la tachycardie serait d'origine pneumogastrique. Mais deux doutes s'élèvent; le premier c'est que l'exorbitisme n'est pas dû à la dilatation vasculaire. L'excitation du sympathique le produit, quoique accompagné de vaso-constriction; ensuite, chez les épileptiques auxquels on a fait l'opération d'Alexander, après l'incision, on observe l'exophthalmie, quoique l'on puisse parfois observer une vaso-dilatation paralytique. Cette lexophthalmie est due à la paralysie de la musculature lisse, Sappey, Müller (innervée par le sympathique), comme l'exophthalmie est due à la contracture de celle-ci.

Du côté de l'œil, il s'élève encore d'autres complications: l'excitation produit la mydriase; or dans le goître exophthalmique la pupille peut être en myose. La myose pourrait s'expliquer par la vaso-dilatation.

Dans la tachycardie d'origine pneumogastrique, il y a seulement une augmentation de pulsations (F. Frank); il n'y a pas une plus grande impulsion; or les caractéristiques de la tachycardie des basedowiens sont ceux de la tachycardie par l'excitation du sympathique.

Jaboulay se tire des difficultés en n'expliquant pas, ou plutôt n'analysant pas les symptômes, minutieusement, et dit que le goître exophthalmique, au moins par deux de ses symptômes l'exophthalmie et la tachycardie, représente une excitation intense du sympathique ou de ses centres. Ce fut à cause de cette considération qu'il opéra son premier cas, après les insuccès obtenus par d'autres interventions chirurgicales.

Abbadie prétend tout expliquer par une dissociation dans l'excitation du sympathique; ce seraient à peine les centres vaso-dilatateurs qui seraient excités. C'est pour affirmer cette théorie qu'il l'expose et la développe successivement au Congrès français de chirurgie en 1896, dans les articles de la *Presse médicale* (Mars et Juin 1897), à l'Acad. de Méd. 1897 (Juillet), à la Société de médecine de Paris (Novembre 1897), et qu'il publie le résumé de ces travaux dans les *Travaux de Neur. Chir. 1898*.

Trousseau avait déjà fait cette remarque fondamentale, oubliée depuis, «que les troubles vasculaires ne se font sentir que dans le territoire du sympathique cervical. Seules les carotides et les thyréoïdiennes sont animées de brusques mouvements d'expansion, tandis qu'au contraire les iliaques, les fémorales, l'aorte abdominale semblent se maintenir dans les conditions ordinaires. Il en serait tout autrement si l'excitation du sympathique était produite par l'introduction dans la circulation d'une substance élaborée en excès par la glande. Tout le réseau artériel devrait alors être influencé en son entier, et, dans toutes les régions, les gros troncs vasculaires devraient être animés de battements exagérés».

«Comment expliquer encore avec la théorie de l'hyperthyroïdisation, les cas de goître exophthalmique qui restent limités à un seul côté de la face? Une intoxication générale devrait toujours produire des effets bilatéraux. — La turgescence des vases thyroïdiens apportait en seconde place le goître, et la propre sécrétion thyroïdienne serait aussi défavorablement influencée, et exercerait à son tour une action toxique, qui apporterait les symptômes secondaires du basedowisme, que l'on peut attribuer à la sécrétion de la glande thyroïdienne».

Les vaso-dilatateurs de cette région ont leurs centres d'origine dans le bulbe, et dans la partie supérieure de la moelle cervicale, pouvant être intéressés les uns indépendamment des autres et donnant ainsi les explications des cas frustes.

Abbadie explique dans sa théorie la gravité des thyropexies par l'excitation que les manipulations sur la thyroïde apportent au sympathique, et qui, s'ajoutant à l'excitation déjà existante, constituerait une aggravation.

Les résultats favorables pourraient s'expliquer, non par l'ablation du corps thyroïdien lésé, mais par la section de fibres sympathiques.

Il trouve encore une confirmation dans le fait que l'exophthalmie est rarement influencée: «les interventions chirurgicales portant sur le corps thyroïde n'ont jamais modifié l'exophthalmie qui a toujours été aussi forte après qu'avant l'extirpation plus ou moins complète de la glande: preuves indéniables de l'indépendance absolue de ces deux symptômes». C'est pour cela que sa théorie pathogénique se résume dans la phrase suivante: «Dans le goître exophthalmique, tout semble se comporter comme s'il y avait une excitation permanente des fibres vaso-dilatatrices seules du grand sympathique cervical ou de leurs noyaux d'origine».

Jaboulay comprend difficilement cette dissociation, et pense que l'on doit seulement dire qu'il se passe des phénomènes d'une excitation intense du grand sympathique.

Or, si la théorie d'Abbadie explique tout, quoique ce soit pour faire trouver cette dissociation si extraordinaire; si elle explique les formes frustes, comme elle explique les cas brusques après de fortes émotions; si elle explique les formes réflexes, principalement celle du goître d'origine nasale; elle n'expliquera pas aussi clairement les goîtres basedowifiés.

Pourquoi est-ce seulement à un certain moment qu'un goître de longue date commence à exciter fortement les vaso-dilatateurs? Vraiment, les troubles du fonctionnement de la glande thyroïdienne ne peuvent pas être complètement mis de côté. Abbadie est intransigeant, parce qu'il juge que si ces troubles étaient les premiers, l'intoxication étant générale, attaquerait tous les centres. Cette argumentation me semble erronée, parce qu'on pourrait se rapporter à l'électivité.

Et, hors de cela, est-ce qu'il n'y a pas de troubles généralisés dans beaucoup de cas de basedowisme, de nature trophique et d'autres, montrant que ce ne sont pas seulement les centres au bulbe et à la partie supérieure de la moelle qui sont attaqués?

Ainsi, si la théorie d'Abbadie, ou plutôt la théorie de Rosenthal développée par Abbadie, explique presque tout, deux points restent plus obscurs; le premier c'est le singulier phénomène de la dissociation de l'excitation du sympathique, le second c'est l'existence de cas liés à la pathologie de la thyroïdienne. Le premier serait un fait que l'observation révèle; ainsi ce serait l'admettre comme certain. Pour le second, il n'en est pas ainsi.

La théorie de Gauthier, qui n'est point admise, est plus d'accord avec les faits que celle d'Abbadie.

Le point d'excitation pour cet auteur c'est le bulbe et, par la tachycardie qui en résulte, elle viendrait par le nerf de Cyon, la dilatation des vaisseaux du corps thyroïdien du cou et de la face donnant l'exophthalmie.

Cyon (Acad. des Sc. 28-VI-1897) relate que chez le lapin, le chien et le cheval, l'excitation du dépresseur peut, par une action réflexe, agir sur les accélérateurs cardiaques, sur l'appareil oculo-moteur, et par voie directe, sur la glande thyroïdienne. Cette diversité de fonctions du dépresseur, de même que la réciproque influence de la thyroïde et du cœur, permet à Cyon d'expliquer les principaux symptômes de la maladie de Basedow: goître exophthalmique, symptômes du côté du cœur, ainsi que la diarrhée persistante (paralysie des splanchniques).

La théorie de Cyon ainsi exposée me semble marquer le point initial du Basedow, ou la glande thyroïdienne ou le cœur, excluant le grand sympathique.

Est-ce là la pensée de Cyon?

Moi, j'interprète les symptômes d'après la même théorie, mais je n'exclus pas que la lésion puisse dans quelques cas pro-

venir d'abord du sympathique, comme je pense que Cyon exclut
cela.

L'exophthalmie résulte sans doute de l'excitation du sympathique et est indépendante de vaso-dilatation.

La tachycardie est aussi d'origine sympathique et non pneumogastrique. Un cœur battant 120 ou 130 et plus pulsations par
minute doit nécessairement appeler à son aide toutes les défenses,
qu'il peut avoir, et celles-ci sont l'excitation du centre du vague et
la vaso-dilatation (cela veut dire le réflexe par le nerf de Cyon).

L'excitation du vague caduque, si la cause excitante est forte
et permanente, parce qu'à égalité de circonstances le sympathique est plus excitable que le vague (Coutarde et Guyon, Soc. de
Biol. 2-vi-1902); il nous reste la vaso-dilatation. Mais ce n'est pas
une augmentation brusque de tension que le cœur a à défendre,
ce qu'il ferait facilement par les splanchniques. La tension n'est
pas augmentée; ce qui est nécessaire c'est de défendre le cerveau
des brusques variations résultant d'une tachycardie.

Le cerveau oscille avec la courbe du pouls, et ce ne sera certainement pas salutaire de lui faire subir ces variations brusques.
Comment le défendre?

E. Cyon nous enseigne que c'est par la vaso-dilatation de la
glande thyroïdienne. Mais par la troisième racine le nerf de Cyon
va au ganglion cervical supérieur. Est-il alors étonnant qu'il y ait
des phénomènes de l'excitation de ce ganglion: l'exophthalmie, le
signe de Graef et de Stellwag?

Voyons maintenant comment nous pouvons expliquer tous
ces cas.

I. — Dans le véritable goître exophthalmique (de Marie), celui
qui tant de fois vient après une brusque émotion, généralement
c'est la tachycardie qui apparaît d'abord. Marie pense même que
pour le Basedow classique, celui-ci est toujours le premier symptôme: «Je crois qu'il faut distinguer, au point de vue du traitement, la maladie de Basedow classique qui débute par la tachycardie et ne s'accompagne de goître qu'après un autre symptôme basedowien dans lequel le goître précède quelquefois
de 15 à 20 ans les palpitations». Ensuite par le nerf de Cyon
vient la dilatation vasculaire, principalement thyroïdienne, qui,
étant un phénomène de défense, apporte cependant des troubles
métaboliques de la thyroïdienne, et ceux-ci à leur tour produisent
les symptômes d'auto-intoxication thyroïdienne, qui accompagnent la maladie.

L'exophthalmie s'explique, comme nous voyons, sans l'attribuer à la vaso-dilatation.

Et la myose?

Celle-ci n'est jamais extrême, et sera réellement due à la vaso-dilatation de l'iris, mais on sait qu'elle ne dépend pas seulement d'un centre, et que, si nous supposons que le ganglion ciliaire et d'autres centres n'ont pas été atteints, elle aura la valeur d'une défense autonomique. Je ferai remarquer qu'elle n'est ni extrême ni même constante.

2. — Les goitres réflexes pourraient s'expliquer par une action à distance sur le bulbe, facilement transmise par la 5.ᵉ paire, depuis la muqueuse des fosses nasales.

Cette relation de la muqueuse nasale avec les centres bulbaires est si directe qu'il n'est pas étonnant qu'elle soit la plus fréquente dans tels réflexes; ce n'est pas seulement le goitre, c'est l'asthme réflexe et c'est aussi, ce qui pour moi a plus importance, la tachycardie réflexe. Celle-ci fut indiquée par Spencer Watson, tachycardie de 120, pénible et persistante, disparaissant avec l'extirpation de polypes muqueux des deux fosses nasales. Est-ce qu'elle n'indique pas le premier pas dans la production du Basedow réflexe? D'autant plus que, pour quelques-uns, comme Huchard, la tachycardie essentielle sans lésion organique sera aussi bien une forme fruste de Basedow qu'une névrose bulbaire.

3. — Maintenant supposons un goitre qui s'est basedowifié.

En règle, le premier symptôme c'est la tachycardie. Dans ces thyroïdiennes on a remarqué l'altération du parenchyme et il n'est pas étonnant que cette glande altérée soit un motif constant de l'excitation de ses nerfs; cette excitation suivrait la route des laryngés jusqu'au bulbe; si elle devient intense et permanente, la tachycardie et tout le reste viendront. La tachycardie est d'une importance primordiale pour les observateurs comme G. Sée, qui la considère comme pivot. Elle ne manque pas dans les Basedows frustes.

Et généralement elle est la première à apparaître.

Voyons ce que nous montrent d'autres faits, apparemment contradictoires.

Je coupe le sympathique ou j'enlève le ganglion cervical supérieur, j'obtiens principalement du résultat sur l'exophthalmie.

Une partie des filets cardiaques accélérateurs seront coupés si cela est assez pour réduire ou plutôt pour équilibrer l'action du vague avec ce qui reste encore du sympathique pour le cœur;

les symptômes de défense devront disparaître, parce que la tachycardie disparaît: ainsi la tachycardie et le goître rétrocèdent.

Mais qu'est-ce que Jonnesco montre exactement? C'est que les goîtres basedowifiés sont ceux où la tachycardie apparaît moins souvent, pouvant même persister après l'intervention.

Par la théorie déjà exposée s'explique que la thyroïde malade, étant le point de départ de l'excitation, vienne à agir sur le bulbe: de là, la tachycardie et les phénomènes consécutifs de défense. La section du sympathique aura une action seulement sur l'exophthalmie; peu ou même pas d'action sur le goître et la tachycardie. Mais faisons la thyropexie ou la strumectomie; c'est dans ce cas qu'elle donne un résultat; ce sont les cas que Tillaux et Marie et plusieurs autres classifient de goître chirurgiques; qu'est-ce qu'on remarque?

La tachycardie disparaît, parce que la cause excitante sur le bulbe a disparu: les phénomènes vasculaires de congestion de la face et du cou disparaissent, parce qu'ils n'ont rien à défendre. Et l'exophthalmie? Celle-ci disparaîtra ou persistera, parce que l'excitation permanente des filets sympathiques qui l'a produite peut avoir produit une lésion permanente, et ainsi elle forme maintenant, pour ainsi dire, une maladie à part.

Nous avons ainsi un groupe d'excitations et de réflexes formés par: des centres bulbaires, médullaires, et des ganglions sympathiques au cœur; de celui-ci à la glande thyroïdienne et à son tour de celui-ci au bulbe. Si je coupe le sympathique dans le cou ou si j'ôte ses ganglions, je puis interrompre la chaîne de deux manières et obtenir la guérison: ou parce que j'ôte la voie d'où vient l'excitation accélératrice pour le cœur, ou parce que je coupe l'accès au bulbe par cette voie. Et cela sera assez si tous les symptômes du côté de la thyroïdienne et du cœur sont la seconde étape de cette excitation.

Mais si la lésion est dans la thyroïde ou même dans le cœur, pour ceux qui admettent la névrose cardiaque?

Comme avec la section que j'ai faite je n'ai pas supprimé toutes les voies de conduction, nous avons une atténuation mais non une guérison des symptômes. C'est le cas des goîtres basedowifiés.

Est-ce que je mets de côté l'intoxication thyroïdienne? Non. Je me lie plutôt au dysthyroïdisme qu'à l'hyperthyroïdisme, mais celui-ci est la cause d'autres phénomènes, comme les mouvements fébriles, qui indiquent l'intoxication. La désassimilation exagérée des albuminoïdes est clairement dépendante de l'altération thyroï-

dienne. Ainsi Mathes, après avoir extirpé le goître à des basedowiens, vit la sécrétion d'azote, qui avant l'opération était de
14,2, tomber à 9,6 après l'opération pendant plusieurs jours.

En donnant une poudre préparée avec la propre glande qu'on
a extirpée, le pourcentage d'azote éliminé s'élève de nouveau jusqu'à
14,1. L'expérience était susceptible de répétition chez le même
malade et avec les mêmes résultats.

Finalement les crises de diarrhée que quelques-uns, comme
Samson, appellent crises pneumogastriques, ne pourraient-elles pas
s'expliquer par l'intermède des splanchniques?

La vaso-dilatation que le splanchnique apporte sera-t-elle suffisante pour donner des crises de diarrhée? Mais celles-ci peuvent
aussi être obtenues par l'action de la sécrétion thyroïdienne, elles
peuvent être dues à l'auto-intoxication.

Ce qui est hors de doute, c'est que la glande thyroïdienne,
le sympathique et le bulbe sont dans le mystère du syndrome
basedowien, et dans les cas où la médecine se déclare impuissante,
les chirurgiens, désireux de faire quelque chose d'utile, se sont
dirigés vers la thyroïde, mais avec des résultats peu encourageants. Ne pouvant attaquer le bulbe, ils enlèvent le sympathique,
et cette fois le sort les a favorisés.

L'opération est acceptée, sa conception s'adapte aux faits, les
résultats en sont supérieurs à ceux de la thyroïdectomie, surtout
dans les goîtres réputés médicaux, ce qui est important.

Dans les autres formes de goître exophthalmique, l'opération
faite par Tillaux a donné des résultats.

Les guérisons brillantes du Basedow présentées par Doyen
par la thyroïdectomie partielle, le sont ainsi, parce qu'il s'agit de
basedowisme secondaire.

Les résultats brillants présentés récemment par des chirurgiens
américains par les opérations partielles thyroïdiennes pour le
Basedow, doivent être bien analysés sous ce point de vue.

L'action favorable de l'intervention sur le sympathique sur
le tremblement et le caractère est en grande partie explicable de
la même manière que j'ai expliqué les altérations favorables dans
la fonction psychique des épileptiques.

Quelle est la gravité des interventions sur le sympathique
dans la maladie de Graves?

J'ai réuni 58 interventions, dont 3 sont personnelles, et dans
ce nombre on indique 10 cas fatals, mais de ceux-ci voyons quels
sont ceux que l'on peut attribuer à l'opération.

Dans un des cas de Jaboulay, le malade était complètement guéri de l'intervention, il était mieux, et le cas paraissait devoir être favorable, quand une grippe avec broncho-pneumonie le tua, plus d'une semaine après l'intervention.

Dans un autre cas de Jaboulay, une intervention intempestive, une cautérisation avec pâte de Canquoin sur la thyroïde, donna un résultat fatal, dans un cas où la guérison était presque certaine. Ce cas est bon comme enseignement, et il corrobore l'opinion que ce n'est pas seulement du sympathique que dépendent les accidents du basedowisme.

Un autre malade meurt quelques jours après l'opération (une semaine au moins) avec une congestion du poumon. On doit remarquer d'abord qu'on était au mois de Décembre, ce qui peut-être a eu quelque influence, mais nous devons aussi remarquer que les broncho-pneumonies et les congestions poumonaires sont des complications fréquentes des interventions thyroïdiennes. Reverdin en 93 cas de mort consécutive à l'intervention sur la thyroïdienne pour le goître, remarqua que la cause a été due, en 42 cas, à des troubles de l'appareil respiratoire (suffocation, asphyxie, pneumonie), et 6 fois à la syncope cardiaque. Dans un autre cas, une érysipèle récidivante emporta le malade le 18-ème jour après l'opération.

Les cas de Faure et un cas personnel sont des morts causées par une syncope cardiaque durant l'opération.

Dans le cas de Chauffard et Quénu, il y eut intoxication accidentelle avec de la digitaline, plusieurs mois après l'opération. Ce cas est douteux, quant au résultat qu'on pourrait obtenir.

Le cas de Peugniez est plutôt un cas d'insuccès thérapeutique; je ne crois pas qu'il soit facile d'attribuer la mort un mois et demi après à l'opération, et si nous admettons pour le Basedow la mortalité indiquée par Charcot de 21 %, je ne crois pas que ce cas sortirait hors de l'évolution qui lui serait normale.

Malgré cela je l'ai classifié d'aggravation post-opératoire, qui apporta la mort consécutive.

Pour le cas de Témoin, les mêmes considérations peuvent se faire: aggravation post-opératoire.

Dans le cas de Gérard-Marchant les accidents sont analogues à ceux qui apparaissent après les interventions sur le corps thyroïdien, et qui sont classés de thyroïdisme aigu.

Nous avons ainsi, en 58 interventions: une mort par congestion pulmonaire, quelques jours après l'opération; deux aggravations et morts en quelques semaines; une aggravation qu'on peut comparer aux accidents aigus dans les interventions sanglantes sur le corps thyroïdien et dans la thyropexie; deux morts par syncope cardiaque pendant l'opération.

Ce sont ainsi 3 morts et 3 aggravations.

Est-ce que l'on peut dire en vérité qu'il y a une mortalité spéciale due à l'opération? Est-ce que l'on peut comparer ce qui se passe ici avec ce qui se voit dans les thyroïdectomies pour la maladie de Basedow, où les morts brusques après l'opération s'élèvent, pour Allen Starr, à la proportion de 33 en 190 opérations? et nous devrions encore ajouter les nombreux cas d'insuccès (aggravations analogues à celles des 3 cas indiqués), qui dans les interventions sur la thyroïdienne sont beaucoup plus nombreux.

Il nous reste la congestion pulmonaire.

C'est vrai, mais nous avons déjà vu qu'elle n'est pas moins fréquente quand le corps visé par le canif est le corps thyroïdien.

Mais il nous reste la syncope, probablement causée par le chloroforme, n'est-ce pas?

Celle-là oui, mais pour montrer non pas la gravité spéciale de l'intervention, mais pour confirmer la gravité de l'anesthésie chloroformique sur des individus avec un cœur prompt à défaillir, et exténué par un travail exagéré de tachycardie. On doit préférer l'éther.

Même pour une autre intervention la gravité certainement ne serait pas moindre; l'opération n'est donc pas absolument grave, et si nous la comparons avec les interventions sur le corps thyroïdien, la bénignité ressort triomphante.

Pour évaluer les résultats, je les classerai en différents groupes: celui des guérisons complètes; celui des grandes améliorations où je ferai entrer les cas où la guérison serait certaine par la marche régressive des symptômes, mais qui à la date de la publication de l'observation ne pouvaient pas encore être groupés avec les guérisons absolues; celui des améliorations et des insuccès.

Je classerai comme des guérisons les cas où la tachycardie disparaît, ainsi que le tremblement, l'état général s'améliore et les fonctions psychiques deviennent normales, quoique l'exophthalmie et le goître ne soient pas disparus tout à fait; et cela parce que la permanence de ces symptômes dans le basedowisme donne comme résultat les hyperplasies, qui ne sont pas en rapport avec la maladie, et représentent seulement la manière de réagir d'un tissu devant l'excès de vascularisation, celles-ci une fois établies ne peuvent pas revenir tout à fait. Mon jugement, comme chirurgien, pour apprécier la guérison sans risquer de manquer à la vérité, ne peut être différent du jugement du médecin; or, à la page 1002 du vol. du *Traité de médecine* de Charcot, Bouchard et Brissaud (1re éd.) on lit:

«La maladie de Basedow peut guérir, c'est même la terminaison la plus ordinaire quand elle évolue sans que les accidents viscéraux éclatent. Les symptômes s'amendent mais ne disparaissent pas sans laisser des vestiges. Pour peu qu'elle ait duré, le goitre ne rétrocède pas totalement, et les yeux sont toujours un peu saillants et irréguliers. Il reste surtout un état de susceptibilité nerveuse tel que la guérison risque d'être compromise au moindre choc».

Et à la page 991 se rapportant à la tachycardie:

«Elle est capitale au point que, si elle a disparu pendant une longue période, on peut considérer le basedowisme comme guéri, alors même que d'autres signes persistent».

Comme on voit, je suis plus exigeant dans la classification de la guérison, parce que j'exclus seulement le léger exorbitisme et léger goitre qui ne peuvent pas rétrocéder tout à fait.

Suivant ce critérium, je classifierai dans le même groupe comme *des guérisons radicales et de grandes améliorations*, 23 cas; — *comme des résultats favorables*, 19 cas. De ceux-ci on doit exclure 8 cas, parce qu'ils ont peu de temps d'observation. Je dois également exclure le dernier cas de Jaboulay parce qu'il est d'une information incomplète. Le cas de Chipault, qui est évidemment le cas d'un goitre basedowifié, et 4 cas de Jonnesco de goitre fruste et secondaire formeront un groupe séparé.

Mais si ces observations ne doivent pas entrer dans le pourcentage des résultats favorables (qui doit être pris sur 43 cas), elles peuvent entrer dans le résultat établi pour la mortalité.

Aggravations: les cas de Peughiez et Témoin — 2 cas. *Insuccès*: les cas de Chauffard et Soulié (dans celui-ci la thyroïdectomie et la thyropexie ont eu le même insuccès) et un cas de Chipault — total 3 cas. *Morts vraiment imputables*, 3 cas.

Dans les cas du premier groupe nous avons à côté des guérisons absolues dont on ne peut pas douter de grandes améliorations que l'on pourrait appeler des guérisons; en tout cas, tout fait supposer qu'un grand nombre de ces améliorations deviendraient des guérisons. La guérison vient lentement et graduellement, et seulement le peu de temps écoulé entre l'opération et la publication du cas fait qu'on nomme amélioration ce qui deviendra une guérison.

C'est ce qui arriva dans un cas de G. Marchant, qu'il rapporta à l'Académie de médecine comme une amélioration, et qui, un an après, vint déclarer qu'il n'y avait pas de raison pour maintenir la même réserve:

«Cette malade a été revue en Juin 1898, les réserves que nous faisions en Juin 1897 dans notre communication à l'Acad. de Méd. n'ont plus lieu d'être maintenues aujourd'hui. Tous les symptômes ont disparu et cette malade peut être considérée comme radicalement guérie».

Gérard Marchant, dans la marche consécutive à l'opération, pense pouvoir établir trois périodes:

1. — Amélioration immédiate;

2. — Un arrêt de l'amélioration; un état douteux, pendant lequel on ne sait pas de quel côté marchera la maladie;

3. — Progression de l'amélioration jusqu'à la guérison définitive, ou, au contraire, aggravation.

Jonnesco au Congrès int. de Méd. 1900 dit avoir opéré jusqu'à cette date 15 goitres exophthalmiques, informant que tous les malades furent, ou guéris ou profondément améliorés. La guérison consiste dans la modification de l'état général et nerveux, dans la disparition de l'exophthalmie et du goitre, dans la disparition de la tachycardie.

En 1902, Jonnesco appelle nouvellement l'attention sur la résection du sympathique pour le goitre d'un malade à la Soc. de Méd. de Bucarest, session du 23 Janvier.

Dans cette communication il ne cite pas le nombre des nouveaux cas opérés, j'en ai tiré les passages suivants parce qu'ils m'intéressent:

«Dans ce cas encore j'ai observé une amélioration continue et progressive et c'est ainsi qu'agit toujours la résection du sympathique. Pour ce qui est des inconvénients de la résection du sympathique, je n'en ai observé aucun, ni avant, ni après l'opération».

Ensuite, en réponse aux objections de Bardesco:

«Presque aucun des malades opérés par moi n'a manqué d'un traitement médical prolongé avant de se soumettre à l'opération. Quelques-uns d'entre eux sont tombés en cachexie avancée, en

sorte que, uniquement par ce motif, l'opération paraissait contre-
indiquée. Eh bien, ceux-là aussi se sont guéris. J'ai répété plusieurs fois que la résection du sympathique agit d'une manière
réelle, lente, continue et progressive, les améliorations s'accen-
tuent et se transforment en guérisons».

C'est pour cela que je dis que les résultats par moi classifiés
comme grandes améliorations seront très probablement des guérisons futures.

Est-ce que les interventions sur le sympathique sont préférables à celles sur la glande thyroïdienne? De celles-ci la résection
totale est mise de côté, parce qu'elle apporte le myxœdème opératoire. Il nous reste l'énucléation intraglandulaire, la thyroïdectomie partielle, comme des interventions où il y a de la diérèse du
corps thyroïdien, et l'exothyropexie et la ligature des thyroïdiennes, comme des interventions qu'il faut aussi discuter.

Quant aux injections de liquides irritants ou caustiques,
quant à l'application de la pâte de Canquoin, etc., je ne ferai aucune considération à leur sujet; complètement abandonnées, il n'y
a pas de raison d'en parler.

L'énucléation intra-glandulaire peut seulement être appliquée
exceptionnellement au goître exophthalmique; plus d'un opérateur
jugeant un cas favorable à la strumectomie, se vit forcé à faire
une résection partielle (Lauré, Reverdin, Billroth, etc.) La récidive est fréquente, l'hémorrhagie peut être terrible, de manière
que l'on peut dire qu'elle n'est pas maintenant employée
pour le véritable goître ophthalmique; on emploie de préférence
la résection partielle. La gravité de cette opération pour le goître
exophthalmique est grande, et elle contraste avec sa bénignité relative pour le goître ordinaire et même pour le goître basedowifié.
Or, comme dans la plus grande partie des statistiques viennent
sous le nom de goître exophthalmique des cas de véritable goître
exophthalmique et de goître basedowifiés, il s'ensuit que les résultats
d'ensemble de ces statistiques sont plutôt favorisés qu'aggravés.

Allen Starr rencontre une proportion de 33 morts rapides sur
190 cas.

Mais Marie fait remarquer que l'on a opéré indistinctement
de véritables goîtres exophthalmiques et des goîtres basedowifiés.

«Or, il résulte de mes recherches que les décès se rapportent surtout aux sujets atteints de maladie de Basedow, tandis
que les guérisons concernent des sujets atteints de goître basedowifié».

On doit remarquer que les paroles de Marie que je transcris textuellement (Soc. Méd. des Hôp. 15 Janvier 1899), se rapportent à la même statistique d'Allen Starr, ce qui veut dire que dans celle-ci les morts subites dans les véritables Basedow opérés sont beaucoup plus de 33 en 190.

Dans d'autres statistiques les résultats sont plus favorables.

Buschram présente 6 cas de mort sur 80 (7,5 %) et 17 aggravations (20 %).

Frieberg donne 10 % de décès, et sa statistique se rapporte seulement aux goitres basedowifiés.

Doyen, qui se montre si enthousiaste de la résection partielle de la glande, doit ses succès à des goitres basedowifiés.

Jaboulay, dans le véritable Graves, vit le goitre se reproduire après des interventions partielles, tandis que pour les goitres vulgaires, et même pour les basedowifiés, la règle est de rétrocéder.

A la Société de Médecine de Hambourg (oct. 1897) on présente les désastres de cette intervention pour la maladie de Basedow; l'opération est considérée comme de résultat incertain et grave, donnant une mortalité au moins de 10 %, sans compter les aggravations.

Au XV-ème Congrès allemand de médecine interne, Eulenburg, rapporteur, conclut que la mortalité est loin d'être méprisable et les cas de mort subite ne sont pas rares, et, ce qui est plus, il fait remarquer que l'intervention est souvent inutile, parce que le goitre se reproduit fréquemment après l'opération. C'est le cas de Jaboulay.

Nous ne devons pas oublier que le propre Tillaux, qui le premier appliqua cette intervention pour le basedowisme, opéra un goitre basedowifié, et il fit immédiatement remarquer la différence, nommant le véritable Graves goitre médicinal, et le considérant hors de la portée du chirurgien.

Malgré cela, l'intervention se généralisa, et les cas de Allen Starr en montrent la gravité; c'est pour cela que la suivante remarque de Debove est naturelle:

«En présence de semblables accidents, je me demande si la thyroïdectomie peut être conseillée dans le goitre.

C'est surtout sur la tachycardie que cette intervention agit; l'exophthalmie est peu influencée.

Nous avons ainsi: une opération difficile, parce qu'elle est fréquemment compliquée par une hémorrhagie et des accidents asphyxiques (qui ont quelquefois obligé l'opérateur à faire la trachéotomie); elle est grave parce qu'elle apporte fréquemment la mort subite avec des symptômes d'intoxication aiguë; et même dans les cas où la mort ne survient pas il arrive des accidents fébriles et des congestions pulmonaires qui mettent le malade en danger.

C'est en vain que Tuffier prétend éviter le danger de l'auto-intoxication par l'emploi du thermo-cautère et la moindre malaxation possible du corps thyroïdien; la gravité est la même. C'est même pour éviter la diérèse du corps thyroïdien que Jaboulay exécuta l'exothyropexie, proposée par Poncet depuis 1873. La meilleure critique de celle-ci serait de dire que le propre exécuteur l'abandonne pour les interventions sur le sympathique, après avoir eu 3 morts avec des accidents aigus d'intoxication thyroïdienne en 15 cas, sans que les résultats consécutifs fussent tels qu'ils la rendissent supérieure à la thyroïdectomie, les récidives étant même fréquentes, principalement dans le véritable basedowisme.

Je ne peux pas manquer de faire une mention spéciale de la critique d'Ehrhart, dans le *Traité de Chirurgie* de Bergmann, Bruns, et Mikulicz.

Ainsi, la statistique de Ehrhart, en 230 opérations pour goître exophthalmique, compte 45 % de guérisons, 21 % d'améliorations remarquables, 11 % de petites améliorations, 10 % d'insuccès, 7,5 % où l'opération fut cause de mort. On ignore la terminaison des autres cas. Tous ces cas furent divisés en véritables et secondaires, mais l'unique indication donnée c'est que pour la forme primitive le nombre de guérisons est de 36 % et la mortalité plus grande que dans la statistique générale. Mais qu'est-ce que l'auteur considère comme guérison?

Il le dit textuellement:

Parmi les cas de guérison, on avait fait entrer ceux où les symptômes nerveux subjectifs avaient disparu presque complètement, où la tachycardie et le tremblement n'existaient plus, seulement une légère exophthalmie subsistait, car les symptômes subjectifs et l'exophthalmie, quand ils existent depuis longtemps, ne disparaissent que très lentement.

On voit aussi que les cas que je considère comme de grandes améliorations et que j'associe aux guérisons sont présentés sous le nom de guérisons dans cette statistique et dans le pourcentage de 36 % pour le Basedow primitif. Dans les sympathectomies ce pourcentage est de 56.

Des 5 cas de goîtres basedowifiés, qui apparaissent dans les observations que j'ai réunies; 4 s'améliorèrent, mais ne se guérirent pas; 1 resta dans le même état, ce qui ne montre pas un grand avantage de l'intervention. Mais quant au Graves primitif, est-ce que nous devons admettre comme certain le jugement d'Ehrhart, que les résultats des sympathectomies ne peuvent se comparer à ceux des strumectomies? Est-ce qu'on peut considérer la sympathectomie «sinon plus grave, au moins aussi grave» que la strumectomie? Je crois que non; et il faut encore remarquer que certaines circonstances qui sont générales dans les statistiques opératoires, dans ce cas aggravent plutôt la sympathectomie, loin de la favoriser.

Quant à la ligature des thyroïdiennes, elle n'est pas aussi en faveur; Kocher est le seul qui lui montre quelque sympathie; en tous les cas il a eu 10 % de morts immédiates. Lefort a réuni 31 cas avec 7 morts par hémorrhagie secondaire.

Il est vrai que Kocher donne pour cette intervention 90 % de guérisons et 3 % de morts subites, et encore 7 % de morts immédiates, dans les premières 24 heures et évidemment attribuables à l'opération; mais Bello de Moraes fait remarquer: «En beaucoup de guérisons figurent des cas que l'histoire de l'évolution morbide ne permet pas de distinguer de la véritable maladie de Basedow».

«Si dans beaucoup de cas le goître vulgaire ne fut pas pendant longtemps accompagné du reste du syndrome, et ceux-là pouvaient être nommés des cas de basedowisme secondaire ou faux, beaucoup d'autres cas réalisèrent le type morbide, que les partisans de la théorie gardaient pour la névrose».

Or, ces cas de faux basedowisme viennent surcharger favorablement la statistique, parce que les trois cas de mort subite qui sont propres au véritable Basedow ne leur appartiennent pas.

Ridigier en 1895 compte 22 opérations pour Basedow, en ligaturant les 4 artères thyroïdiennes sans accident; 20 fois les malades furent améliorés ou guéris. D'abord c'est la glande qui diminue, ensuite c'est le tremblement, la tachycardie et l'exophthalmie. Nous devons dire que le seul adepte pour la ligature des quatre artères c'est Ridigier, parce que tous, Kocher lui-même, craignent que le myxœdème survienne. De l'analyse de tous les faits, des résultats brillants de Kocher et Doyen opérant des goîtres, on tire la conclusion que, pour les goîtres basedowifiés, l'intervention directe sur le corps thyroïdien peut être faite sans grand danger et avec de grandes probabilités de réussite; mais dans le véritable Basedow, les doutes émis par Debove persistent. Or, justement dans ce cas, Jonnesco le dit et les observations le montrent, la résection du sympathique donne des résultats favorables.

Jonnesco obtint seulement des guérisons dans le véritable basedowisme, dans les faux goîtres exophthalmiques il obtint sur 4 cas 4 améliorations, mais point de guérisons.

Je pense que les interventions sur le sympathique dans le véritable goître exophthalmique sont indiquées, quand les traitements médical, pharmacologique, hydrothérapeutique, électrothérapeutique n'ont pas donné de résultat ou dans les cas qui vont s'aggravant brusquement.

Dans ces cas beaucoup de malades doivent la vie à la chirurgie et il n'est pas logique d'intervenir avant d'essayer d'obtenir la guérison d'une manière plus suave; il n'est pas aussi humain d'insister inutilement avec un traitement qui ne produit aucun bien, au lieu de recourir à la résection du sympathique, dont le résultat se montre si favorable. Quelle devra être l'intervention préférée?

Jaboulay est partisan de couper simplement le cordon sympathique ou de réséquer le ganglion supérieur. Il pense que c'est déjà beaucoup de paralyser le sympathique, et il se propose de modifier l'excitabilité du sympathique par l'étirement de ce nerf: «Ainsi la prochaine fois que j'aurai à opérer un malade atteint de goître exophthalmique, pratiquerai-je une opération simple qui ne fait que modifier l'excitabilité du nerf en respectant sa continuité: je pratiquerai l'allongement du sympathique». Il fit une fois seulement cette opération, et le résultat ne fut pas aussi complet qu'on le désirait.

Jonnesco, pour enlever tous les filets sympathiques qui donnent l'accélération au cœur, et suivant en cela les indications de Fr. Franck, fit chaque fois qu'il put la résection du dernier ganglion cervical, et dans quelques cas, celle du premier dorsal.

Voyons les résultats de l'un et de l'autre.

Jaboulay a 15 opérés; de ceux-ci on doit exclure pour les apprécier 4 cas de mort pour une cause différente de l'opération, et 1 cas parce que il se passa peu de temps après l'opération; malgré cela on remarquait tendance à une amélioration. Pour les 10 cas qui restent, il y a 5 guérisons, une grande amélioration (où on n'indique pas le résultat sur la tachycardie), 1 cas où la tachycardie se maintint à 100 (étant à remarquer qu'auparavant elle était 148), 3 cas qui sont trop récents et qui avec plus de temps d'observation seraient très probablement des guérisons; ce qui donne en 10 cas 5 guérisons certaines et 5 grandes améliorations, tous ayant été opérés, 7 par la sympathéctomie et 3 par résection du ganglion supérieur.

Jonnesco compte 15 opérations, toutes de guérisons et de grandes améliorations. En 2 cas il n'a pas fait la résection totale; dans un autre cas le procédé d'intervention ne vient pas indiqué.

Les cas de Jaboulay et Jonnesco sont tout à fait comparables. Nous avons déjà vu ce qu'étaient les cas de Jonnesco; quant à ceux de Jaboulay: «Toutes étaient atteintes de formes graves que nous n'avions opérées qu'après que les ressources de la médecine eurent été épuisées». Jonnesco juge que chez les malades de Basedow la résection totale est préférable à la résection partielle; parce que, quand on fait la résection partielle, on remarque, même chez les épileptiques, une accélération du pouls qui dure plus ou moins de temps. Après la résection totale, au contraire, le pouls se retarde et descend plus bas que la normale, en y revenant seulement après quelques jours (Soc. de chir. 1897).

En lisant les observations de Jonnesco, il semble vraiment que la guérison s'est établie plus régulièrement, mais la différence finale des résultats obtenus est si petite, si elle existe, qu'il est permis de demander s'il ne vaudrait pas la peine de nous limiter à une intervention plus modérée, telle que la section du ganglion supérieur ou du cordon, plutôt que de courir le risque de la résection totale. Pour un opérateur frappé dans ses interventions Jonnesco a tort; mais ne serait-il pas préférable de faire seulement la résection supéro-médiane, qui par les filets venus du ganglion du milieu agit plus directement sur la thyroïdienne, et permet d'atteindre également le nerf cardiaque du milieu?

Ne pourrait-on pas dans les cas où la tachycardie continue à faire souffrir le malade, aller chercher par une seconde intervention tardive le ganglion inférieur?

Je rappellerai encore que Jaboulay pense qu'il est possible d'extirper tardivement un goître qui ne rétrocède pas après la sympathectomie, sans courir le risque que cette intervention fait courir dans le Basedow.

Quel chemin doit-on suivre pour les goîtres basedowifiés?

L'intervention sur la thyroïde en tels cas est en règle de moindre gravité, mais cependant plus dangereuse que la résection du sympathique.

D'autre part, tandis que celle-là donne un bon résultat dans ces cas, celle-ci apporte seulement quelque amélioration. Le fait que la résection du sympathique diminue la gravité de la strumectomie est une conception théorique de Jaboulay, qui nécessite une confirmation pratique. Ainsi, si l'opérateur est habitué aux interventions sur la thyroïdienne, pour extirper rapidement un goître, sans grandes malaxations, je juge préférable de recourir à cette intervention, ou à la résection partielle.

Si nous voulons interpréter le mécanisme de la guérison, nous voyons que nous ne pouvons pas abolir tout le sympathique qui pourrait être intéressé dans la symptomatologie de la maladie, et malgré cela on obtient la guérison, mais lentement. Par l'abolition de la plus grande partie, nous arrivons à établir un équilibre que la 2ᵉ période de Gérard Marchant montre n'être pas complétement stable au commencement.

Quand je me rappelle que, dans les cas médicalement guéris, l'état spécial de nervosisme persiste, étant une menace de récidive (E. Boix), et voyant d'autre part que dans les cas les plus longtemps suivis l'amélioration de cet état nerveux s'accentue (dans mon 2ᵉ cas c'était évident), je demande si, pour établir l'équilibre définitif avec la guérison parfaite, l'amélioration graduelle de cet état ou également un meilleur fonctionnement des centres nerveux n'intervient pas, comme dans l'épilepsie, par le mécanisme que j'ai indiqué ?

LA NÉVRALGIE FACIALE

Dans les névralgies du trijumeau il y a toujours, à côté de l'élément douleur, des symptômes vaso-moteurs et sécrétoires qui montrent qu'il y a excitation des rameaux du sympathique et qui se font remarquer par la rougeur de la face, le larmoyement, l'augmentation du mucus nasal, la salivation et une sensation de chaleur exagérée de la face.

Ces paroxysmes, qui indiquent un trouble du sympathique, apparaissent à l'occasion du paroxysme douloureux.

Celui-ci est parfois précédé d'aura et accompagné d'une contracture brusque et involontaire des muscles de la face du côté malade; cela constitue le véritable «tic douloureux», considéré par quelques-uns comme analogue ou équivalent à une attaque épileptique.

Les névralgies du trijumeau peuvent dépendre d'une lésion

périphérique, une dent cariée, une affection du sac et du canal lacrymal, etc., mais si nous mettons de côté ces cas, où la guérison de la lésion apporte rapidement la guérison de la névralgie symptomatique, les doutes, quant à la nature intime de la névralgie faciale, restent les mêmes que pour les névralgies essentielles en général.

Pourtant les examens de beaucoup de ganglions de Gasser extirpés montrent que, si ce n'est pas constamment, c'est du moins très fréquemment que l'on rencontre des altérations pathologiques qui expliquent les phénomènes douloureux. Il y a des cas où l'extirpation du ganglion de Gasser n'apporte pas la guérison, et ceux-ci doivent être interprétés d'une autre manière.

Les interprétations peuvent être au nombre de deux: le ganglion ne fut pas complètement extirpé, ce qui arrive facilement, ou les lésions sont encore plus centrales dans le mesencéphale ou myélencéphale à côté des racines ascendantes du trijumeau.

Nous savons que le bulbe est une des origines des fibres préganglionnaires du sympathique, de même que les fibres sympathiques qui accompagnent les racines du trijumeau depuis le départ du pont y ont aussi leur origine.

Il n'est partant pas étonnant que dans les processus pathologiques dans lesquels ce nerf se voit embarrassé, on remarque aussi la participation des fibres sympathiques.

Les relations du trijumeau avec le sympathique, aussi bien que la constance des phénomènes de l'excitation de celui-ci pendant les paroxysmes douloureux, sans parler des troubles trophiques possibles, étaient de nature à mériter l'intervention sur le sympathique. Ce fut encore Jaboulay, le professeur distingué de clinique chirurgicale de l'École de Lyon, qui le premier fit la résection du ganglion cervical supérieur pour combattre la névralgie faciale.

Jaboulay fonde son jugement ainsi:

«L'extirpation du ganglion cervical supérieur fait, entre autres choses, atrophier et disparaître un centre sympathique situé à l'origine du trijumeau, de même qu'un autre centre situé entre les cinquième et huitième racines cervicales disparaît après la même opération, et encore un des noyaux du vagus de l'hypoglosse (Hoeben, Utrecht, 1896; Huet, Amsterdam, 1898), aussi bien que les fibres sympathiques annexées au trijumeau et à ses rameaux doivent disparaître. La suppression de ces nervi-nervorum est capable de modifier l'excitation du trijumeau».

Sa première intervention fut faite en Février 1899. Cavazzani, par des considérations presque analogues, et il semble sans avoir connaissance du cas de Jaboulay, intervient avec la même fin thérapeutique par la résection du ganglion cervical supérieur, en Novembre 1899. Il fonde son jugement sur les analogies du Basedow et de l'épilepsie avec la prosopalgie et les connexions du ganglion cervical supérieur avec le ganglion de Gasser et ainsi la prédominance trophique du premier sur le second.

Présentées ainsi les considérations qui portèrent d'abord Jaboulay et ensuite Guido Cavazzani à tenter la résection du ganglion cervical supérieur, il convient d'apprécier les cas opérés pour les comparer ensuite, en les analysant, avec les autres traitements chirurgicaux proposés pour cette maladie; et je dois dire traitement chirurgical, parce que je pense que le malade doit être soumis à l'intervention seulement quand les moyens médicaux ont été essayés. Nous avons 24 interventions et certainement ce n'est pas un matériel très abondant, et ce qui est pire, c'est qu'une partie de ces cas sont récents et sujets ainsi à une certaine réserve.

Je ne crois pas possible de présenter déjà une formule sûre et positive. La période actuelle ne peut, quant à la névralgie faciale, être considérée comme une période d'étude.

Il est indispensable de suivre, pendant des années, si cela est possible, les cas opérés, pour apprécier des récidives possibles.

Des 24 cas on peut immédiatement tirer les conclusions suivantes:

1.ª La récidive peut se produire;

2.ª L'intervention fut toujours favorable pendant un espace de temps plus ou moins long;

3.ª Qu'elle ne fut nuisible dans aucun cas;

4.ª Que les résections des nerfs douloureux faites à l'occasion même de la résection du sympathique ne montrent aucun avantage quant aux résultats (2 cas Delagenière);

5.ª Que l'amélioration définitive est souvent précédée d'une période de récidive post-opératoire;

6.ª Que la branche dentaire inférieure est celle sur laquelle l'intervention semble avoir le moins d'influence.

Voyons la première conclusion.

Le fait d'un malade de Cavazzani, considéré comme guéri pendant plus de deux ans, et qui présenta une récidive la troisième année, fait maintenir des réserves quant aux récidives tardives, mais, d'autre part, elle ne montre point l'incurabilité au moyen de cette intervention. Il est dommage que Cavazanni, dans l'aimable lettre qu'il m'adressa, ne m'indiquât point dans quelle branche la récidive se produisit; serait-ce dans la dentaire inférieur?

Nous avons ainsi une récidive partielle au bout de trois ans; une autre au bout de quelques mois, après une guérison apparente de cas Delbet). Ce cas peut laisser quelque doute, s'il ne s'agit point d'une récidive postopératoire passagère.

Disparition des douleurs pendant le temps d'observation de: un mois et deux mois (Jaboulay); quatre mois (G. Cavazzano); six mois, dix mois, plus d'un an (Jaboulay); un an et demi (Chipault). Améliorations très appréciables pendant le temps d'observation de: six mois, une année (Jaboulay); 18 mois (Poirier); plus de 2 ans (cas personnel). Il y a encore un cas de Jaboulay de grande amélioration suivi durant 16 jours, ce qui ne permet pas de pronostiquer quel serait le résultat final, le cas de Chipault qui est dans les mêmes conditions de doute, le cas de G. Cavazzani déjà cité comme une guérison de 3 ans, avec une récidive dans un des rameaux, au bout de ce temps. Le cas de Guido Cavazzani, dans lequel d'autres interventions auxiliaires contribuèrent à la guérison, celle-ci se maintenant pendant six mois d'observation. Le cas de Delbet sur lequel j'ai déjà fait des considérations, et finalement les cas de Delagenière, très intéressants pour démontrer l'inutilité de réséquer simultanément les nerfs douloureux et le sympathique. Il est même remarquable que de tous les cas ces deux sont les moins favorables.

Dans un des cas de Jaboulay, l'insuccès de l'arrachement des nerfs, fait d'abord, semble être réel, en tout cas il est dommage qu'il n'y ait pas un plus grand espace entre les deux interventions pour qu'il ne restât pas le moindre doute que le résultat favorable obtenu puisse être dû à l'arrachement.

Dans un autre cas de Jaboulay, quoique l'amélioration soit remarquable, c'est un cas de l'avenir duquel on ne peut pas encore juger.

Le plus remarquable est un autre cas de Jaboulay, dans lequel on voit d'abord l'insuccès complet de l'étirement, l'atténuation pendant 2 ou 3 mois à peine, par la résection du nerf maxillaire supérieur dans la fosse sphéno-palatine, ainsi que des incisions sous-cutanées faites au même point que les premières opérations, et des interventions faites, on voit que la plus avantageuse, celle qui apporte une guérison presque complète pendant un temps plus long, c'est la résection du ganglion cervical. Chez cet opéré, cette intervention peut souffrir, avec avantage, la comparaison avec les autres, les arrachements de Tiersch et l'extirpation du ganglion de Gasser.

Les névrotomies simples et les étirements produisent si fréquemment, et, ce qui est pire, avec tant de rapidité la récidive de la douleur que d'autres procédés ont été proposés et employés.

Toutes visent à inutiliser la plus grande partie possible du nerf, et l'une d'elles à l'ablation complète du propre ganglion de Gasser. Pour pouvoir apprécier la valeur comparée entre ces différents procédés et la résection du ganglion cervical supérieur, nous devons d'abord voir la valeur absolue de chacun d'eux. Ces procédés sont: l'étirement, la résection périphérique des nerfs, l'arrachement, la résection à la base du crâne et la résection du ganglion de Gasser.

L'arrachement proposé par Tiersch dans les névralgies faciales donne de bons résultats, mais il donne aussi des récidives. Il a en sa faveur de ne point être grave et d'être d'une exécution relativement facile. Avec soin on peut arracher le nerf presque complètement. Kareuski (de Berlin), en 9 cas, extirpa 4 fois complètement les rameaux du trijumeau et dans le *Traité* de von Bergmann, Bruns et Mikulicz nous trouvons une photographie d'un nerf maxillaire inférieur arraché par ce procédé qui montre bien jusqu'où peut arriver l'intervention.

On accuse cette méthode, qui permet avec tant de facilité et avec une incision si insignifiante d'extirper de grandes portions du trijumeau, d'avoir l'inconvénient de ne laisser d'autre ressource en cas de récidive que l'extirpation du ganglion de Gasser (Krause).

La peau reste anesthésiée dans la zone des nerfs arrachés, et dans un cas d'arrachement du supra-orbitaire Krause eut une kératite grave qui laissa la cornée opaque.

L'opération de Tiersch n'est point grave, elle n'apporte point de complications, elle donne plus de 65 % de guérisons et 30 % de récidives. Étant sans doute un bon procédé, on ne peut pas l'appeler idéal, parce que l'on remarque l'inconvénient d'être obligé en cas de récidive de recourir à la résection du ganglion de Gasser que Krause lui-même classifie de grave.

Nous reviendrons plus tard sur ce dernier argument. Quant au procédé propagé par van Gehuchten (l'arrachement brusque) il a besoin d'être expérimenté dans la pratique, car avec le procédé de Tiersch on arrive à ôter des portions du ganglion, ce qui laisse prévoir aussi la possibilité d'atrophies étendues.

Seuls les cas futurs sauront montrer sa valeur absolue et celle comparée au procédé de Tiersch.

Les névrectomies périphériques donnent des récidives non inférieures au procédé de Tiersch, et dans les cas où plus d'un rameau est affecté elles doivent être multiples. Les névrectomies plus ou moins étendues pratiquées plus proches du ganglion de Gasser, cherchant les nerfs à la base du crâne, sont des opérations délicates, et comme telles elles ne devraient être acceptées de préférence sur les autres que si la nécessité l'imposait.

Voyons cependant quelles sont les indications de ces névrectomies faites à la base du crâne en comparaison avec les névrectomies périphériques déjà citées. — Dans ces dernières les résultats ne sont point supérieurs à l'arrachement; elles doivent être étendues, et dans les cas de récidive douloureuse, si elles sont étendues et s'il n'y a point de régénération nerveuse, on peut être obligé, comme seule ressource, de procéder à l'arrachement du ganglion de Gasser.

D'où peut-on tirer quelque indication pour intervenir de manière à chercher les nerfs auprès du trou oval et du grand trou rond?

1.° Les cas où les résections périphériques étendues n'ont point donné de résultat;

2.° Les cas où la névralgie occupe des rameaux qu'il n'est pas possible d'attaquer par la périphérie, comme par exemple les nerfs palatins (Krause);

3.° Quand la douleur occupe la totalité de distribution de l'un de ces deux rameaux du trijumeau ou de tous les deux: maxillaire supérieur et inférieur.

Quels sont les résultats? Evidemment les résultats sont supérieurs à ceux des résections périphériques, cependant des récidives se produisent (Segond, Garré, Gerard Marchant, Deniu, Schwartz, Guinard, prof. Sabino Coelho). Aussi les rechutes ne sont-elles pas aussi rares que l'on pourrait supposer et, si après ces interventions il n'y a point de régénération nerveuse, la seule ressource qui reste, c'est de réséquer le ganglion de Gasser. Ainsi, je ne vois aucun avantage à les substituer à l'arrachement de Tiersch; quand celui-ci est praticable et bien exécuté, les résultats ne sont pas inférieurs. En outre, tandis que l'arrachement peut être fait dans un milieu quelconque et par un médecin sans grandes capa-

cités chirurgicales, ces interventions à la base du crâne exigent un
matériel et des aptitudes plus spéciales, ce qui fait qu'elles ne
peuvent se généraliser si facilement. Le pourcentage des guérisons
par la gasserectomie est élevé, mais on cite quelques récidives, et
dans quelques cas elle a même causé la mort de l'opéré, ou de
graves complications. Garré (XX° Cong. de la Soc. de Chir. Allem., 8 Avril, 1899) eut une récidive après l'extirpation du ganglion de Gasser. Ce cas qui avait déjà récidivé avec les névrectomies périphériques, avec la résection du nerf maxillaire supérieur à la base du crâne, est très intéressant, parce qu'après la
dernière récidive, en découvrant le trou oval, on y constata la régénération d'un filet délicat que l'on coupa, en obtenant ainsi la
guérison.

Friedrich (*Deutsche Zeitschr. f. Chir.*, LIII, 1899), dans un
cas qui avait résisté à quatre interventions périphériques, fit l'a-
blation du ganglion de Gasser, et eut une récidive au bout de 4
mois. Gérard Marchant et Herbert citent 4 cas de récidive, dont
quelques-uns partiels. Dans un cas communiqué par G. Marchant
(Soc. de Chir., 26 Août 1898), l'examen microscopique de ce qui
fut réséqué comme étant le ganglion de Gasser ne révéla point
de cellules nerveuses, partant l'opération ne fut pas exécutée.

Schwartz (Soc. de Chir., 12 Août 1898), dans une opération
compliquée, dans laquelle il y eut kératite neuro-paralytique de
l'œil gauche avec cécité consécutive, vit la récidive se produire au
bout de 15 jours, jugeant par cela que le ganglion ne fut pas extirpé complètement.

G. Cavazzani (*La Clinica chirurg.*, 1904), eut une récidive.
Perthes assembla 9 récidives sur 201 gasserectomies (Congr. Nat.
Allem., Oct. 1904). Krause (30° Congrès de la Soc. Allem. de Chir.,
10 Avril 1901) eut trois morts sur 25 cas opérés (1 par le chloroforme, un autre par collapsus cardiaque, le septième jour, et
un autre par hémorrhagie cérébrale). Tous les autres cas furent guéris, il y a huit ans de cela. L'intervention fut sans effet seulement sur un individu attaqué de douleurs neurasthéniques
simulant la névralgie faciale. Je ne peux pas juger jusqu'à quel
point ce cas doit être considéré comme un insuccès. Il remarqua
comme complications: une paralysie passagère des muscles de
l'œil (2 ou 3 mois); des troubles cérébraux généralment passagers, allant depuis une simple agitation jusqu'à l'aphasie et l'ictus
apoplectique.

Dans l'article de Bergmann, Bruns, Mikulicz, antérieure à

cette communication, sont assemblés 128 cas de différents opérateurs, avec 15, 6 % de mortalité.

Ainsi qu'on le voit, la récidive est possible; comment et dans quelles circonstances? Dans un cas de névralgie neurasthénique que l'on jugea être faciale (Krause); dans un cas où l'examen microscopique montra que le ganglion n'avait pas été extirpé (G. Marchant); dans un cas où l'on jugea que l'extirpation fut incomplète (Schwartz); dans le cas de Garré, où il y eut régénération d'un filet, l'extirpation fut incomplète.

Ceci fait supposer que si l'intervention était complète les récidives seraient plus ou moins nulles. Cela dépend de la difficulté inhérente à l'opération et de laquelle celle-ci est responsable.

Spiller, en coupant la grosse racine de la 5.ᵉ paire, dans des expériences maintes fois répétées sur les animaux, ne vit jamais la régénération nerveuse dans de tels cas (comme on ne la voit pas non plus quand on coupe quelque racine postérieure avant le ganglion spinal) et pour cette raison il proposa, depuis 1898, l'intervention. Ce ne fut qu'en 1901 qu'il opéra un malade par ce procédé et, un an après, il le présenta au Coll. Med. de Phil. (session du 1.ᵉʳ Octobre 1902) sans qu'il y eût eu récidive jusqu'à cette date (Frazer et Spiller publièrent encore 4 cas).

La résection du ganglion de Gasser (ou de la grosse racine) est une intervention que l'on peut considérer comme relativement sûre en ce qui concerne les résultats et c'est, sans doute, celle qui donne le moins de récidives; cependant, elle est plus dangereuse et l'on n'y doit avoir recours que comme dernière ressource. Je pense qu'avant d'y recourir nous en avons une autre moins dangereuse, je veux dire la résection du ganglion cervical supérieur.

Sa valeur est certainement inférieure à celle de la résection du ganglion de Gasser, mais il n'y a, peut-on dire, aucun danger.

Est-ce que les résultats en sont supérieurs aux étirements et aux névrectomies périphériques? Les cas observés jusqu'à présent sont trop peu nombreux pour répondre affirmativement à ce point.

Quant au procédé de Tiersch, je le trouve bon et il concorde avec ce que Marinesco et van Gehuchten nous enseignent.

L'argument qu'après cette intervention il n'y a pas d'autre ressource que la résection du ganglion de Gasser n'est pas convaincant, car je pense qu'on peut encore recourir au ganglion cervical supérieur. En résumé, il me semble qu'avec les observations actuelles un chirurgien est autorisé à attaquer le ganglion cervical supérieur du sympathique, opération relativement facile et bénigne, avant de chercher le ganglion de Gasser et que, pour ce qui concerne les résultats des autres interventions, on peut commencer directement par la résection du sympathique, ce qui n'empêche pas d'attaquer, en cas de récidive partielle, le rameau malade, comme dans un des cas de Cavazzani. Ou, en suivant l'ordre inverse, quand les interventions périphériques ne donnent point de résultat, au lieu de recourir aux interventions à la base, ou à la résection du ganglion de Gasser, on doit agir d'abord sur le ganglion du sympathique, parce que ce chemin est plus facile et moins grave et également sûr en comparaison avec les interventions à la base. Quand on a tout essayé, on doit recourir à l'opération intra-crânienne, la gasserectomie, dont on ne doit pas oublier la gravité.

GLAUCOME

On peut dire que le glaucome est la seule indication admise et suivie en ce qui se rapporte à la chirurgie du sympathique pour des lésions oculaires. Il est vrai que Jaboulay a publié une intervention dans un cas de myopie progressive, mais puisque les résultats de l'accommodation ne sont pas sûrs et surtout très faibles, je crois qu'il n'y a point d'ophthalmologiste qui recommande l'intervention dans des cas semblables.

Le prof. Abbadie fut le premier qui proposa l'intervention dans le glaucome (Mai 1897); mais ce fut le prof. Jonnesco qui la pratiqua dans cette maladie. Jaboulay, dans un article paru avant la communication d'Abbadie, se rapporte seulement à la myopie avec lésions oculaires et il ne fait pas une seule fois allusion au glaucome.

* * *

Si nous laissons l'humeur aqueuse s'écouler, comme dans une iridectomie, on voit la plaie de la cornée se cicatriser et l'humeur se régénérer. Pourtant, si l'humeur aqueuse se produit avec une si grande facilité, il faut admettre que le tonus oculaire sera maintenu pour que l'excédant de l'humeur s'écoule par les canaux, ou qu'il y ait une super-production d'humeur telle qu'elle entrave l'écoulement ou, finalement, que la composition de l'humeur soit altérée, en rendant l'écoulement par les schlemms plus difficile; dans tous ces cas, un excès d'humeur pourra s'accumuler et la tension oculaire monter, en rendant plus difficile la circulation sanguine dans l'œil et en produisant l'atrophie glaucomateuse de la rétine. Le glaucome peut se présenter aigu, subaigu ou chronique; à ces trois formes de glaucome il faut encore ajouter la forme hémorrhagique et la forme congénitale, le buphtalme. J'envisage seulement les glaucomes qu'on pourrait appeler essentiels et non ceux qui sont liés à une lésion oculaire, comme par exemple une inflammation des procès ciliaires, et dont l'évolution et le traitement sont subordonnés à la maladie qui en est la cause. La sympathectomie, au contraire, a été exécutée dans les glaucomes indépendants de toute maladie oculaire et constituant à eux seuls toute la maladie, c'est-à-dire le glaucome primitif. J'omettrai toutes les théories posées pour expliquer cette maladie et je mentionnerai seulement les relations du sympathique avec l'organe de la vision.

Le sympathique est chargé, en particulier, des fonctions de sécrétion et, pour ce qui concerne les humeurs de l'œil, je crois qu'on ne peut pas dire, avec Wecker, que son action est seulement hypothétique. Ainsi, par l'excitation du sympathique, le pourcentage de l'albumine augmente dans l'humeur vitrée (Morat, Doyon), et l'indice de refraction monte dans l'humeur aqueuse de 0,001 à 0,0015 par l'excitation et jusqu'à 0,025 par l'extirpation du ganglion cervical supérieur (Lodato). Je crois que ces troubles ne peuvent pas être attribués seulement aux perturbations vaso-motrices. Si par l'excitation du sympathique on obtient de l'hypertonie et par sa section l'hypotonie, on ne peut pas attribuer ces faits à l'influence exclusive des fibres musculaires lisses de Muller agissant comme muscles tenseurs du globe oculaire. Ainsi Lagrange, Pachon et d'autres, et moi-même, avons vu l'exophthalmie qui suit la sympathectomie persister, tandis que la tension oculaire, abord abaissée, monte à la normale. Donc, les deux phénomènes sont indépendants.

* * *

Voyons maintenant quelle est la théorie d'Abbadie. Je n'en ferai qu'un résumé puisqu'elle peut être lue dans les *Archives d'Ophthalmologie*, 1897, page 375. M. Abbadie croit que ni l'affaissement de l'angle irido-cornéen ou quelque autre altération permanente de cette région peut expliquer le glaucome, puisque celui-ci devrait alors être toujours permanent et ne pas présenter des oscillations fonctionnelles comme il peut arriver. Ainsi, Abbadie admet une influence nerveuse par les vaso-moteurs. Pour lui, il y a dans le glaucome une dilatation permanente des vaisseaux de l'œil: de cette vaso-dilatation résulte une hypertension et peut-être une hypersécrétion des humeurs de l'œil. Cette théorie est en désaccord avec ce que l'on sait des effets de la section du sympathique sur la dilatation vasculaire: ce que l'on voit à l'examen ophthalmoscopique, soit chez les épileptiques, soit chez les basedowiens, soit même chez les glaucomateux, après la sympathectomie, c'est la vaso-dilatation paralytique, et, au contraire, par l'excitation, la vaso-constriction. La tension dans le glaucome ne peut donc pas être due à la vaso-dilatation du fond de l'œil. Mais si la vaso-dilatation ne peut pas être admise, l'explication du prof. Jonnesco ne peut pas l'être davantage. Ce professeur admet que la constriction des vaisseaux de l'œil donne comme résultat une augmentation de la pression, ce qui favoriserait la secrétion. C'est une erreur qui résulte de vouloir appliquer la loi des pressions et de la vitesse à une circulation locale au lieu d'y appliquer le principe des vaisseaux communiquants. Ainsi, admettant une action pathogénique du sympathique dans la production du glaucome, on doit avec Laqueur, Dor, Wecker, le considérer comme le nerf régulateur de la sécrétion du procès ciliaire. L'irritation du sympathique produirait donc de l'exophthalmie, de l'hypertomie par hypersécrétion, de la dilatation pupillaire et une plus grande ouverture de la fente palpébrale. Est-ce qu'il existe dans le glaucome des signes de cette excitation? On peut répondre affirmativement; ainsi il y a toujours eu un certain degré d'exophthalmie, quoique moindre que dans le Basedow (ce que l'on peut expliquer par une participation moindre du sympathique cervical, plus grande du sympathique crânien, il y a de l'hypertension, il y a toujours de la mydriase et finalement (Gutter et Gibson) il y a l'existence du signe de v. Graef, quoique moins accentué que dans le Basedow (*Annals of Surgery*, n. 3, 1902). Cela est d'accord avec les considérations que j'ai faites à propos de l'exophthalmie et me permet d'établir le parallèle suivant: dans le Basedow les symptômes oculaires sont surtout sous le domaine du sympathique cervical; dans le glaucome sous le domaine du crânien. Ainsi, quelle que soit la nature intime de la maladie, quelle que soit sa pathogénie, seulement l'interprétation physiologique des symptômes autorise les interventions sur le sympathique.

Voyons maintenant si les résultats sont d'accord avec les hypothèses établies.

* * *

Lorsque j'ai publié mon travail sur la chirurgie du sympathique, en 1904, j'avais rassemblé 108 observations; pour la confection de ce rapport, je suis arrivé à en collectionner jusqu'à 143, sans que pour cela les conclusions aient changé, au contraire, les nouveaux cas ont confirmé ce que les autres avaient déjà établi. D'abord je dois faire remarquer que dans ces 143 cas un seul cas de mort par infection et broncho-pneumonie est rapporté, mais, si nous considérons que ces 143 cas se rapportent de bien près à des opérations des deux côtés, on voit que le pourcentage de la mortalité par la sympathectomie est bien minime. De ces 143 cas je dois écarter une observation de H. Price sur un malade que fut suivi seulement pendant 18 jours. Il reste donc 142 malades: de ceux-ci 80 furent favorablement influencés par l'opération, sur 47 le résultat a été nul, 4 se sont aggravés et 1 est mort d'infection et broncho-pneumonie. Parmi les résultats nuls j'ai considéré les observations dont le résultat est tout à fait passager ou minime. Si maintenant je considère, au lieu du nombre de malades, le nombre des yeux malades, j'ai 147 formes différentes de glaucome opérées par la sympathectomie, avec 94 résultats favorables et 48 nuls, 5 aggravations et 1 décès. Il ne reste que ces résultats qui méritent notre attention. Si nous comparons ces résultats à ceux fournis par l'iridectomie, et si nous nous rapportons à une statistique dont le nombre des cas est à peu près le même, comme la statistique de Haab (144 cas), on voit que dans 144 cas le résultat a été nul 51 fois. C'est-à-dire la différence n'est pas sensible: 35 % de résultats nuls pour l'iridectomie et 36 % pour la sympathectomie. Mais la valeur de l'iridectomie n'est pas la même pour toutes les formes de glaucome, et pour pouvoir juger dans quel cas l'intervention est indiquée, il faut analyser les résultats suivant la forme du glaucome.

Si nous nous rapportons à la statistique de Wygodski, de 1777 yeux iridectomisés depuis deux ans au moins, nous trouvons:

Glaucome aigu inflammatoire — bon résultat, 76 % — dans le même état, 5 % — mauvais résultat, 19 %.

Glaucome inflammatoire chronique — bon, 10 %; — nul, 40 % — mauvais, 50 %.

Glaucome chronique simple — bon, 0,96 % — nul, 10,5 % — mauvais, 88,5 %.

Voyons maintenant ce que donne la sympathectomie:

Glaucome aigu et sub-aigu, 18 malades, représentant 25 cas de glaucome: 12 malades correspondant à 17 cas de glaucome favorablement influencés, et 6 correspondant à 8 cas de glaucome sans résultat, ce qui donne 66 °/₀ de cas favorables par malades et 68 °/₀ par yeux glaucomateux.

Glaucome chronique simple, 60 malades, correspondant à 74 cas. Ont donné par la sympathectomie des résultats favorables en 37 malades, correspondant à 48 cas, et nuls 23 malades ou 26 cas, ce qui donne les pourcentages suivants : par malades, 61,6 °/₀ et 38,4 °/₀; par cas, 65 °/₀ et 35 °/₀.

Glaucome chronique irritatif, 49 malades ou 58 cas; on trouve des résultats favorables sur 33 malades ou 41 cas et nuls sur 16 malades ou 17 cas, c'est-à-dire, pour les malades semblables à ceux du glaucome simple on trouve de bons résultats, 34 °/₀, favorables 26 °/₀, nuls 40 °/₀ pour les malades, et 40 — 25 — 35 °/₀ pour les cas. Si nous nous rapportons à la statistique de Haab pour l'iridectomie, nous trouvons bons, 30,5 °/₀, favorables, 25 °/₀, nuls, 44,5 °/₀.

C'est-à-dire, résultat presque égal pour les deux opérations.

Glaucome congénital, 9 malades, 10 cas. On trouve deux insuccès, un cas d'aggravation malgré l'opération, et 5 cas influencés, quoique presque toujours très peu. Mais, considérant la gravité du mal, ces petits résultats doivent être pris en considération. Je dois faire noter l'innocuité de l'opération.

Dans le cas de glaucome congénital que j'ai opéré par la résection du ganglion cervical supérieur du sympathique, quoique le malade ne fût âgé que de onze mois (le plus jeune opéré jusqu'à présent), j'ai eu l'occasion de le revoir une année après, ne montrant pas de troubles trophiques qui puissent condamner l'opération. En tout cas, je dois avouer que le résultat sur le glaucome a été bien petit, quoique non tout à fait nul.

Glaucome hémorrhagique, 5 cas, 5 malades, dont quatre résultats satisfaisants, un d'eux étant même très notable, et un résultat à peu près nul. Mais si nous considérons que l'iridectomie est contre-indiquée chez de tels malades, et doit céder sa place à la sclérotomie, nous trouvons une véritable source dans la sympathectomie.

* * *

A propos des interventions sur le sympathique pour combattre le glaucome, je dois encore citer les interventions sur le ganglion ciliaire, qui doit être considéré comme appartenant au sympathique crânien. Rohmer a exécuté l'extirpation du ganglion ciliaire dans des cas de glaucome douloureux, où la vision était tout à fait perdue, au lieu de pratiquer l'énucléation ou la névrotomie opto-ciliaire.

L'opération fut pratiquée sept fois par Rohmer, et une fois par Aubaret et Lagrange; dans ce dernier cas on fut obligé de recourir à l'énucléation six semaines après.

Des sept cas de Rohmer, six ont été favorables et un donna un insuccès. Cette opération est donc une ressource à considérer avant de se décider pour l'énucléation.

* * *

Considérant dans l'ensemble tous les cas de sympathectomie cervicale, voyons maintenant quelle est la gravité de cette opération.

Epilepsie: 4 cas de mort par résection totale avec des complications opératoires. Deux cas de mort par broncho-pneumonie.

Basedow : Deux cas par broncho-pneumonie; deux cas, syncope cardiaque; un cas, hyperthyroïdisme aigu.

Glaucome : Un cas par broncho-pneumonie.

Nous avons donc cinq cas par broncho-pneumonie, deux par syncope cardiaque et quatre par complications opératoires. L'hyperthyroïdisme, je ne le considérai pas comme gravité générale opératoire.

On trouve donc 11 décès opératoires sur 456 opérés, soit 2,5 %; mais en considérant que dans 67 cas, où la résection totale fut pratiquée, se trouvent cinq cas de mort, soit 7,4 %, on voit que le pourcentage de mortalité pour la résection du ganglion cervical supérieur est bien petit.

Elle se réduit vraiment à cinq cas sur 389 opérés, soit 1,23 %; et il faut encore prendre en considération que le nombre de cas se rapporte au nombre d'opérés, quoique, dans le plus grand nombre des cas, l'opération fût bilatérale.

LE PLEXUS SOLAIRE

Je ne connais que deux observations, dans lesquelles on ait pratiqué tout exprès des interventions chirurgicales afin de modifier le fonctionnement du plexus solaire.

Leur valeur, en tant que pièces de conviction, est insignifiante.

La première observation ne nous a montré que des améliorations appréciables; dans la deuxième, ces améliorations ont été si remarquables qu'on peut presque les considérer comme une demie guérison. La valeur de ces deux observations est définie par Jaboulay lui-même :

Je n'attache pas d'importance à l'amélioration qui a suivi, étant donné le terrain manifestement nerveux sur lequel on agissait. Cette opération, qui a été faite le 28 Janvier 1899, est seulement intéressante, parce qu'elle démontre la possibilité de son application aux maladies vraiment graves, dont nous avons parlé plus haut.

Dans la deuxième observation de Jaboulay il faut remarquer l'influence de la constipation habituelle. Il y a réellement, surtout chez les neuro-arthritiques, des constipations accompagnées de douleurs abdominales violentes, si rebelles que les malades seraient peut-être influencés favorablement par la modification du fonctionnement du plexus solaire, au cas où d'autres moyens n'auraient pas de prise sur eux.

En attendant, il ne nous reste qu'à attendre de nouveaux cas de cette phase opératoire, pour qu'on puisse se faire une opinion sûre. Donc, je ne ferai aucune considération sur de telles interventions, et je me limite ainsi à citer des faits.

LE SYMPATHIQUE LOMBAIRE ET SACRÉ

La conception des interventions chirurgicales dans le sympathique lombaire et dans le sympathique abdominal appartient toute à Jaboulay. Giuseppe Ruggi imagina aussi une intervention dans les sympathiques abdominaux en des cas spéciaux de névralgie des annexes ; sa façon d'opérer lui est propre ; mais la priorité des interventions en dehors de la région cervicale est due au distingué chirurgien de Lyon. Il y a peu de documents ; quant à présent, nous devons nous limiter à réunir des faits pour voir si nous pouvons tirer de leur interprétation des déductions pratiques et des indications utiles.

En conséquence, je vais transcrire tout l'article de Jaboulay, dans lequel il appuie la chirurgie du sympathique sacré sur les névralgies pelviennes.

Il faut entendre sous le nom de névralgie pelvienne une série de désordres subjectifs atteignant surtout les organes génitaux internes, où ils déterminent l'hyperesthésie vulvaire et le vaginisme sans qu'une lésion constante puisse être rencontrée. Le toucher vaginal, lorsqu'il est possible, provoque au contact du col et des culs-de-sac une sensation douloureuse extrême.

En même temps que les douleurs, des troubles fonctionnels existent ; dysmérrhée, ménorrhagie ou aménorrhée. Ces désordres sont d'habitude propres aux nullipares. Ils s'accompagnent d'irradiations sur l'état général, qui est celui des névropathes ou des neurasthéniques.

Ces troubles sensitifs et fonctionnels de l'appareil génital féminin doivent être rattachés à une altération du sympathique sacré et ne pas être confondus avec des lésions de l'utérus, des ovaires, des trompes, du vagin et de la vulve, ni être subordonnés ou rapportés à elles. D'ailleurs, les auteurs sont bien rares qui aujourd'hui croient à la névralgie pelvienne. Et ceux-là ont pour seule thérapeutique la castration totale ou tubo-ovarienne ou bien l'hystérectomie vaginale, c'est-à-dire, une opération grave.

Il en va ici comme pour le goître exophthalmique, où les chirurgiens, entraînés par le nom même de la maladie, s'adressaient à l'objet qu'ils croyaient malade. Or, un utérus qui n'a pas le flux menstruel, celui dont le flux menstruel est trop abondant ou très douloureux, souvent n'est pas un utérus malade, mais un utérus qui fonctionne mal. Les agents qui président à son fonctionnement en sont cause, et c'est à eux qu'il faut s'en prendre. Mais, on ne confondra pas: le système nerveux qui préside aux phénomènes menstruels et commande la sphère génitale est le système de la vie végétative et non pas le système myélinique; ça a été une erreur de Simpson de proposer, par exemple contre le vaginisme, la section d'un nerf à fibres blanches, le nerf honteux interne.

Sur le sympathique sacré soit à la fois sensitif et moteur, qu'il préside à l'hyperesthésie et à la contracture des organes pelviens, le fait n'est pas douteux; on connaît en outre des observations dans lesquelles à lui seul il a présidé aux fonctions de la parturition et de l'accouchement. On a vu des femmes à colonne vertébrale fracturée, continuer leur grossesse et accoucher; on a coupé la moelle à des femelles d'animaux qui ont pu être fécondées et mettre bas.

Aussi nous conseillons, en présence d'une névralgie pelvienne véritable, rebelle et intolérable, d'agir sur le sympathique sacré. Ce n'est pas que des succès n'aient pu être obtenus à l'aide de l'hystérectomie vaginale et de la castration; il suffit de lire les observations où ces opérations ont été pratiquées pour être convaincu du contraire; celles-ci ont amélioré la situation et cela ne peut pas plus être nié que les succès qui ont été signalés pour le goître exophthalmique après les thyroïdectomies. Mais précisément dans l'un comme dans l'autre état morbide il est nécessaire de rapprocher deux considérations; d'abord qu'il s'agit d'opérations graves, ensuite que l'amélioration consécutive peut être expliquée non pas par la suppression d'un organe que l'on croit être malade, mais bien par les sections qu'elles provoquent dans le plexus sympathique périphérique de leur territoire. Dès lors, s'il est possible de faire autrement et plus simplement, en obtenant le même résultat, il est obligatoire de le faire.

Voilà les conceptions de Jaboulay; mais, et c'est lui-même qui le dit, les gynécologistes modernes ne sont pas très disposés à accepter des lésions pelviennes idiopathiques, c'est-à-dire, sans lésions des organes. Jaboulay, donc, envisage les névralgies pelviennes comme dépendantes du plexus sacré.

Giuseppe Ruggi parle d'un autre ordre de faits. C'est une chose connue, et même fréquente, que les castrations pour guérir de l'ovarialgie ne donnent pas de résultat lorsque cette dernière ne dépend pas d'une lésion locale de l'ovaire. Aujourd'hui on n'opère plus ces ovarialgies essentielles et l'on attribue l'insuccès de cette opération à l'hystérie; quelquefois, s'il y a des lésions dans les ovaires, on peut expliquer l'insuccès par un autre mécanisme. Labadie Lagrave dit: «Les nerfs de l'ovaire pourraient présenter des lésions de névrite ascendante, qui expliqueraient la persistance des douleurs après la castration.» Frish admet des «exsudats péduculaires» qui reculent pour longtemps l'effet de l'opération. Ruggi attribue la douleur à l'irritation des filets nerveux du sympathique qui, accompagnant les vases utéro-ovariens, arrivent à l'ovaire après avoir suivi la trompe. Ces filets viennent du plexus rénal et lombaire-aortique. Donc, il a eu l'idée d'attaquer cette partie du sympathique, comme traitement des névralgies qui résistent à la castration et même comme une méthode générale pour modifier l'éréthisme des altérations veineuses des organes génitaux internes de la femme. Comme on le voit, Jaboulay cite des cas de névralgies utérines, qui s'étendent aux membres inférieurs, et de vaginisme, etc., dans la sphère du plexus sacré; tandis que les cas de Giuseppe Ruggi se rapportent principalement aux névralgies des annexes, même si ces névralgies se rattachent à quelques lésions pathologiques, comme l'oophorosalpingite. Dans ce cas, l'intervention chirurgicale serait complétée par l'ablation des filets sympathiques utéro-ovariens, employée comme mesure prophylactique pour empêcher une récidive névralgique. Au cas où la névralgie serait indépendante des lésions qui auraient besoin de l'inutilisation de ces organes, la simple résection des nerfs donnerait le résultat cherché, tout en épargnant les ovaires et les trompes.

Mais ce n'est pas seulement en France et en Italie que cette idée de la névralgie du sympathique est mise au jour. En Allemagne, Max Buch (*Nord. Med. Archiv*, XXXIV, 3 4, 1902) attribue à une névralgie du sympathique la cause de douleurs dans les annexes, d'une dysménorrhée douloureuse, de gastralgie, etc.

Il présente les signes caractéristiques suivants des névralgies du grand sympathique: une sensation spéciale, presque indéfinible, rappelant la colique intestinale; la contraction utérine ou même l'angine de la poitrine; et des irradiations qui généralement occupent une vaste étendue, pouvant atteindre des régions et des organes très éloignés, et pouvant être réveillées très facilement par la compression du sympathique au siège de la douleur.

Par la réunion des travaux du professeur de Lyon et du professeur de Modène une nouvelle ère d'espoir s'ouvre pour ces malheureuses que Richardot nous décrit rivées au lit, ne pouvant plus travailler, ni faire aucun mouvement, et envers lesquelles la médecine est impuissante, la plupart des fois, aussi bien que la chirurgie. On est arrivé à recourir à la castration totale, opération très grave, mais les douleurs sont revenues, et avec elles le découragement des opérateurs.

Un remarquable chirurgien de Venise, G. Cavazzani, ayant opéré deux malades par le système du professeur Ruggi, généralise l'application de cette nouvelle intervention, ablation du plexus utéro-ovarien sans castration, aux cas d'hystérisme ou de nervosisme dépendant de la sphère génitale, qui sont accompagnés de névralgies intolérables irradiant des annexes.

On sait qu'on a fait sans aucun résultat des mutilations des organes génitaux internes, afin de combattre ce nervosisme.

Ce n'était pas seulement pour la grande hystérie que l'inutilité de cette intervention chirurgicale était démontrée; les ressources de la médecine valaient peu ou rien, et ce qui est pire c'est que cet état de nervosisme, arrivant à être intolérable pour les malades et pour leurs proches, les force à réclamer nos soins.

Or, c'est à ces malades que Cavazzani veut appliquer, en toute confiance, l'indication opératoire. Après les deux interventions par la méthode du professeur Ruggi, sur deux malades qui souffraient des annexes, il dit textuellement dans une nouvelle publication :

... dai risultati ottenuti era lecito arguire, come una simile operazione si sarebbe potuto utilizzare contro una serie di malattie indefinite, nelle quali la sindrome sintomatica supera le alterazioni somatiche, o resta sproporzionata affatto alle medesime. Fra queste trova luogo quella svariatissima serie di passioni isteriformi, così complesse, così poco determinate, considerate dagli uni vere e reali malattie costituzionali, ribelli a tutti i mezzi dell'arte, ritenute dagli altri ingegnose simulazioni o quanto meno fantastiche esagerazioni, atte solo a far ammattire i sanitari ingenui e di buona fede.

Ensuite, accentuant que la castration des ovaires ne sert à rien, sauf dans un cas d'hystérisme à base matérielle ovarique :

Il che poi equivaleva quasi ad escluderla, perché molte ovariche non hanno punto disturbi nervosi e molte nervosiche non sono punto affette da alterazioni degli ovari.

L'état des malades empire, sans perdre l'aspect hystérique, malgré les mutilations des ovaires.

...non perdevano nulla l'aspetto isterico, anzi peggio.

et les résultats sont passagers dans la forme hystérique et hystéro-épileptique.

Pour garantir la véracité de son raisonnement il avait encore les effets sur l'état nerveux général, effets obtenus dans les premières interventions, comme il l'a fait remarquer dans son premier article:

...Fin d'ora io devo segnalare una curiosa osservazione, fatta dai miei assistenti, dalla R. Suora, dalle infermiere o da tutte le malate della sala, che entrambe le operate, irrequiete, fastidiose o modeste prima dell'operazione, divennero quiete, tranquille e mansuete subito dopo, e questo tanto più sorprese quanto meno si attendeva.

Evidemment, une nouvelle voie pleine d'espoir s'ouvre devant nous; mais, ne peut-on pas craindre que ce ne soit qu'un rayon éphémère?

Est-ce qu'on est sûr de la non venue de récidives après un ou deux ans?

Seul l'avenir nous le dira; nous ne pouvons pas faire des prophéties; on ne doit faire remarquer que le peu de gravité de l'intervention et les résultats immédiats favorables pour qu'on ne trouve pas inutile de suivre cette voie, accompagnant les malades le plus possible; car le point noir de l'opération c'est la récidive, et les cas sont encore trop récents et trop peu nombreux pour qu'on puisse s'en faire une opinion solide et définitive.

* * *

Parlons encore de la paralysie du plexus sacré dans la névralgie sciatique. Il est clair que, le principe étant établi, les interventions sur le sympathique dans les névralgies en général doivent constituer un chapitre nouveau de la chirurgie des nerfs.

La distribution du sympathique, suivant Langley, se superpose à celle des nerfs sensitifs, comme nous l'avons vu. Il est tout naturel de chercher si, dans la névralgie d'un certain nerf blanc, les filets sympathiques qui l'accompagnent restent indifférents.

La réponse n'est pas difficile. Depuis que l'observation a été dirigée vers le tableau morbide des névralgies, ces altérations ont été remarquées. La douleur, les contractions fibrillaires des muscles, les perturbations vaso-motrices ou sécrétoires sont considérées comme des symptômes pathognomiques. Les perturbations vaso-motrices consistent tantôt en spasmes vasculaires, qui peuvent faire baisser de quelques degrés la température locale, tantôt en une vaso-dilatation avec hyperthermie.

Cependant, ce phénomène ne peut être bien observé que dans le tic douloureux : c'est là, également, que les altérations sécrétoires sont plus évidentes, liées, non à la vaso-dilatation, mais, selon Vulpian, à l'irritation réflexe des nerfs dont l'excitation provoque la sécrétion glandulaire. La sécrétion de la sueur est souvent excessive dans toutes les formes de névralgie (Leroboullet).

La névralgie peut être accompagnée de phénomènes paresthésiques et de quelques analgésies cutanées, et aussi de diverses altérations trophiques.

Par conséquent, on ne peut pas douter que dans les névralgies se passent des phénomènes qui prouvent que ce ne sont pas seulement les fibres sensitives myéliniques qui entrent en scène, mais aussi les sympathiques.

Ce qu'on ne peut encore dire c'est la relation qu'il y a entre les unes et les autres dans le procès névralgique. On peut aussi bien dire que les perturbations vaso-motrices résultent d'un réflexe que la névralgie est le produit de brusques perturbations vaso-motrices.

Mais, puisque nous savons que dans le tic douloureux l'attaque peut être produite souvent par un léger souffle sur le visage, devons-nous nous étonner que des altérations du calibre des vases puissent donner le même résultat au moyen d'un procès exclusivement mécanique sur le nerf sensitif malade?

Par tout ce que j'ai exposé, je pense que, jusqu'à présent, nous pouvons seulement affirmer qu'il y a une participation du sympathique et des nerfs sensitifs dans le procès morbide, sans qu'on puisse établir aucune liaison entre eux par rapport à la production de la maladie.

* * *

Jaboulay fait dépendre de la pathologie des organes pelviens certaines affections articulaires du membre inférieur, et prétend guérir ces affections au moyen de la paralysie du sympathique sacré.

Jaboulay est un professeur et un chirurgien distingué; la conception de l'intervention n'appartient qu'à lui seul, aussi bien que son application pratique; c'est pourquoi je crois d'une grande utilité de transcrire ses considérations:

Une série d'affections articulaires, jusqu'ici encore mal déterminées, doivent être rattachées à des perturbations fonctionnelles du sympathique sacré.

Les trois grandes articulations peuvent être prises: l'articulation de la hanche, celle du genou, ou bien celle du cou de pied. On y observe tantôt de la simple raideur due sans doute à la contracture des muscles péri-articulaires occasionnée elle-même par la douleur, tantôt une véritable hydarthrose, etc.

Outre ces perturbations décrites par Jaboulay, je pense que tout un groupe d'affections caractérisées par des altérations vaso-motrices et trophiques du membre inférieur doit rester dépendant des interventions chirurgicales dans le sympathique sacré. C'est à cause de ces considérations que j'ai fait à mon premier malade, atteint du mal de Raynaud, le décollement du rectum (et que je sache, ce cas est le seul où l'on ait fait ce décollement). Effectivement, il y a un groupe ou ensemble symptomatique appelé *acroparesthésie* (Schultz), névrose vaso-motrice (Nothnagel), érythromélagie, maladie de Raynaud, asphyxie des extrémités, œdème angionerveux, etc., où il y a, en même temps que des perturbations vaso-motrices continuelles, des perturbations sensitives, sécrétoires, trophiques.

A. Carrier *(Centralb. f. Nervenk.*, 1900) considère comme le type classique de ces maladies la maladie de Raynaud, et présente la synopse suivante de ces groupes symptomatiques:

1.º. Symptômes vasculaires:
Syncope locale — Asphyxie locale — Hyperhémie locale.

2.º. Symptômes sensitifs:
Paresthésie — Douleurs — Thermoparesthésie — Thermalgies — Anesthésies — Hyperthésies.

3.º. Symptômes sécrétoires:
Anhydrose — Hyperhydrose.

4.º. Symptômes trophiques:
Gangrène locale — Atrophie et hypertrophie de certaines parties — Sclérodermie (pour ma part, j'ajouterai encore: — et le mal perforant).

L'auteur déduit de son exposition plusieurs conclusions, dans le but de montrer que ces symptômes peuvent apparaître en diverses maladies nerveuses, et aussi pour différencier ces symptômes des lésions artérielles; mais il affirme que l'entité autonomique de l'acroparesthésie ou névrose vasomotrice ou érythromégalie, etc., doit être admise.

On comprend à présent que la diérèse du sympathique, dominant les perturbations vaso-motrices et montrant le mauvais fonctionnement de cette organe, donne un bon résultat, surtout quand la perturbation ne consiste pas dans une hyperhémie active, sans stase veineuse.

On comprend encore que l'idée d'agir sur le sympathique pour guérir le mal perforant était toute naturelle; et Jaboulay l'a mise en pratique, mais, comme la lésion du mal perforant était très limitée, au lieu de faire son intervention dans le plexus sacré, il alla jusqu'aux branches du sympathique qui accompagnent l'artère fémorale, en la mettant à nu au triangle de Scarpe, et en arrachant «les nerfs vasculaires qui passent sur elle à ce niveau».

C'est le moment de parler d'une autre intervention proposée et exécutée la première fois par Chipault pour guérir le mal perforant — l'allongement des nerfs blancs — et, ensuite, généralisée par lui-même aux ulcères chroniques de la jambe et à d'autres affections trophiques.

Chipault appuye son traitement sur des faits cliniques et expérimentaux. Par la lecture de plusieurs observations relatives à l'allongement des nerfs (1875-1890) pour guérir des névralgies, des douleurs fulgurantes, tabétiques, des contractures, la lèpre, etc., il vit que la guérison ou l'amélioration des perturbations trophiques qui accompagnaient les symptômes à cause desquels on avait fait l'allongement était très fréquente; et l'idée lui vint d'appliquer ce système aux lésions simplement trophiques et d'abord au mal perforant.

Il vérifia expérimentalement sur des cobayes que les plaies accidentelles ou spontanées des membres postérieurs étaient guéries plus rapidement quand on faisait l'allongement du sciatique. Les observations cliniques publiées depuis cette affirmation confirment les espérances qu'on a conçues. En 79 cas de mal perforant on a fait 72 fois l'allongement, obtenant 61 guérisons, dont 14 primitives et 55 secondaires.

Or, puisqu'il est établi que l'allongement agit à la façon d'une section partielle, serait-il logique de faire, au cas d'un mal perforant, cet allongement des nerfs épinaux, dans un but de guérison? Dans la névralgie on comprend qu'on doive le faire, mais dans le mal perforant en aucune façon.

Alors le résultat ne s'obtiendra-t-il par l'allongement de ces nerfs?

Nous savons, d'après Langley, que les filets sensitifs sont accompagnés jusqu'à leur dernière ramification par des fibres du sympathique.

Nous savons que, sans myéline tout autour, minces et plutôt isolés que réunis dans un cordon résistant, ces filets sont beaucoup moins résistants que les nerfs du système cérébro-spinal; par conséquent, quelle raison y a-t-il pour ne pas admettre que ce sont les fibres sympathiques qui accompagnent le nerf blanc celles qui perdent la continuité?

S'il en était ainsi, les résultats d'une intervention seraient les mêmes que si l'on agissait sur le sympathique. Or, à joindre aux observations du mal perforant, il y a celle de Jaboulay qui n'a agi que sur les filets vasculaires. S'il y a des névralgies sciatiques guéries par le hersage et par l'allongement du sciatique, il y en a d'autres guéries par le décollement du rectum. A joindre à l'observation de De Buck (perturbations angioneurotrophiques du membre inférieur gauche) et à celle de Dubois (maladie de Raynaud) étirant les nerfs blancs, où l'amélioration a été très lente, il y a ma première intervention dans laquelle j'ai aboli le sympathique, obtenant ensuite une amélioration rapide. C'est pourquoi je pense avec Buck et Chipault que la chirurgie de l'allongement dans les lésions trophiques est une manière indirecte de faire la chirurgie du sympathique. On comprend donc qu'une intervention chirurgicale dans le sympathique et l'allongement puissent donner des résultats égaux, tandis que ce dernier et la résection du nerf sensitif donnent des résultats tout opposés sur le trophisme.

Mais, s'il en est ainsi, ce qui étonne c'est qu'on ne se fût pas décidé à agir plutôt sur le sympathique pour obtenir la guérison de plaies rebelles à la cicatrisation; car il y a déjà longtemps que les physiologistes ont fait remarquer que l'ablation du sympathique cervical des lapins fait guérir les plaies produites tout exprès sur les oreilles de ces animaux. Par conséquent, quand les lésions pour la guérison desquelles Chipault emploie l'allongement s'étendent sur plus d'un territoire nerveux, je crois que nous devrions faire le décollement du rectum au lieu de faire, par exemple, l'allongement du sciatique.

Faut-il dire que, pour les névralgies et les perturbations trophiques et vaso-motrices des membres supérieurs, Jaboulay a l'intention d'agir sur le sympathique qui accompagne ces gros vases, soit en mettant à nu la subclavière, soit en inutilisant, à la hauteur du cou, les branches communiquantes depuis la cinquième paire cervicale jusqu'à la première paire dorsale?

S'il n'a pas encore fait cela, c'est parce qu'il n'en a pas encore eu l'occasion.

Tito Cavazzani, plus heureux que lui, a eu déjà l'occasion d'intervenir sur le sympathique cervical dans un cas «d'acinésie algera», avec un résultat partiel.

Un autre cas est pris comme un cas de douleur névralgiforme et il est aussi suivi pendant peu de temps. Donc, il ne reste qu'un cas où le malade a été observé pendant dix mois et demi, la guérison se maintenant toujours; ce qui faisait dire au malade, très content: «Je ne suis plus le même homme!»

Mon observation mérite une mention spéciale, parce qu'on a obtenu immédiatement, pour ainsi dire, la guérison sur tout le trajet du sciatique, sauf sur le sciatique poplité externe, ce qui me força à une nouvelle intervention sur ce nerf. J'ai colligé 15 opérations de décollement du rectum, dont 13 ont été exécutées par Jaboulay et les autres par moi-même. De cet ensemble d'opérations, sept ont eu pour but de combattre la névralgie sciatique. On a obtenu dans ces sept cas des résultats favorables, et parmi eux l'on peut compter cinq guérisons complètes. Trois de ces dernières montrent que le décollement est favorable, mais elles ne permettent pas d'établir une opinion positive sur la stabilité de la guérison, parce qu'on n'a pas pu les suivre pendant le temps nécessaire. Si la névralgie avait été limitée exclusivement aux autres branches du sciatique, j'aurais obtenu un cas de guérison remarquable à cause de la rébellion aux autres traitements essayés avant.

Mais, puisque le procès névralgique occupe toutes les branches, quelle raison y a-t-il pour expliquer cette sélection si spéciale dans le mécanisme de la guérison?

Il n'y avait pas de motif pour que le décollement du rectum, c'est-à-dire, la paralysie chirurgicale du plexus sacré, eût agi sur certaines branches du sciatique, sans agir sur les autres. Il n'y a que deux hypothèses pour expliquer un cas si étrange: 1. Le sciatique poplité externe ne reçoit pas de filets du sympathique; mais les études de Langley ne nous laissent pas admettre cette hypothèse; 2. les fibres sympathiques qui proviennent du sciatique poplité externe ne partent pas du plexus sacré.

Nous savons par Langley que la distribution des nerfs sensitifs des membres et celle des branches vaso-motrices du sympathique sont entièrement superposées, ou, pour mieux dire, elles suivent le même trajet initial aux racines médullaires. Voyons donc de quelles racines partent les fibres nerveuses du sciatique poplité externe. Si l'on a recours au schéma de Thornburn, on voit que le trajet innervé par le sciatique et par son rameau sciatique poplité interne appartient à la deuxième et troisième racines sacrées, et que le côté postéro-externe de la jambe, tout le pied jusqu'à la moitié externe du premier doigt, c'est-à-dire le territoire de l'innervation cutanée par les rameaux cutanés du muscle cutané et cutané péronier partent de la cinquième racine lombaire. Par conséquent, je conclus que la branche communicante du sympathique qui doit emporter les fibres qui passent dans le sciatique poplité externe ne doit pas être atteinte, puisque le décollement s'est limité au sacrum.

Mon observation est donc très intéressante, parce qu'elle présente la contre-épreuve de la valeur de l'intervention sur le sympathique. Analysons d'autres observations. En voici deux : la première, de vaginisme, accompagné de douleurs pelviques et de souffrances du côté de l'utérus ; la seconde, de vaginisme et douleurs pelviques, principalement à la fosse iliaque droite. Dans la première il y a eu récidive, dans la deuxième guérison. Une observation sur une névralgie pelvique doit être exclue comme incomplète.

On peut dire que la cause de la récidive chez la première malade doit être le tempérament névropathique, mais on peut aussi parler d'un autre facteur : l'utérus. Soit que la souffrance ait été déjà sous la dépendance d'une perturbation du sympathique, soit qu'il s'agissait réellement d'une métrite, le fait est que, si l'on admet que le vaginisme est sous la dépendance de la lésion utérine qui existait, on s'explique très bien la guérison passagère suivie de récidive. En effet, Langley montre que les organes génitaux externes sont sous la dépendance du plexus sacré, mais que les organes génitaux internes dépendent des nerfs lombaires par le plexus utéro-ovarique ; c'est pourquoi le décollement du rectum a été une opération incomplète.

Dans le deuxième cas il semble que les symptômes de vaginisme existaient avant l'apparition des douleurs hypogastriques et c'est pour cela qu'elles cédèrent entièrement à l'abolition du plexus sacré.

Il y a à présent une observation récente qui est remarquable parce qu'elle se rapporte aux douleurs tabétiques, contre lesquelles les ressources de la médecine sont très faibles. Tous les symptômes de tabes ont continué ; les lésions anatomo-pathologiques qui apporteront avec elles l'atrophie de la racine postérieure doivent continuer, tandis que les douleurs fulgurantes ne sont pas revenues. Cela porterait à mettre ce symptôme, au cas où des faits de cet ordre se répéteraient, sous la dépendance du sympathique, ainsi que J. Roux l'admet pour d'autres observations.

Il y a, finalement, trois observations qui, bien qu'elles ne puissent pas être superposées, ont cependant un facteur commun: ce sont les perturbations vaso-motrices.

En effet, une des observations de Jaboulay est mise sous la rubrique «Troubles vaso-moteurs et articulaires dans le membre inférieur gauche»; une autre, aussi de Jaboulay: «Troubles névralgiformes et vaso-moteurs du membre inférieur gauche, d'origine probablement utéro-ovarienne».

Dans cette observation qui, par un manque involontaire d'asepsie, donna la mort à la malade, on voit que les douleurs ne sont pas revenues.

Mon observation, qui entre dans le tableau de Carrier, était principalement constituée par les troubles vaso-moteurs; on comprend alors que l'opération eût donné un bon résultat, faisant disparaître l'asphyxie et la contracture, jusqu'à la mort accidentelle par diarrhée verte, quelques semaines après.

C'est dommage que, m'étant absenté pour quelques jours, cette coïncidence m'ait empêché de faire l'autopsie.

Ce que j'ai dit sur la névralgie sciatique ne me suffit pas.

Quel doit être le mécanisme de la guérison?

Quand j'ai parlé de la névralgie faciale j'ai montré quel devait être le mécanisme de la guérison, sans avoir recours à l'idée d'une origine sympathique de la névralgie. Le même fait se produira-t-il avec la sciatique?

On ne peut pas admettre pour des procès morbides analogues (névralgie faciale et sciatique) des mécanismes différents. Quand j'expliquais la guérison de la névralgie faciale sans admettre que la maladie provenait du sympathique, mais bien du trijumeau (comme une gassérite), il me coûtait d'être forcé à admettre une théorie sympathique pour la névralgie sciatique ou à généraliser (puisque Jaboulay admet cette méthode comme une méthode générale pour le traitement des névralgies) la nature sympathique de toutes les névralgies, sauf celle du trijumeau. Mais on n'a pas besoin de cela.

J'ai déjà dit plus d'une fois qu'il y a des fibres appartenantes au système du sympathique qui naissent des cellules contenues dans la base de la corne antérieure et dans la corne latérale et qui vont passer par les racines postérieures; mais il y en a encore d'autres qui nous intéressent davantage: ce sont les fibres afférentes qui pénètrent dans la moelle par leur racine postérieure, et dont le centre trophique existe dans les ganglions et dans les plexus sympathiques et qui, par leurs arborisations terminales, sont en relation avec les cellules de la colonne de Clarke. Toutes ces fibres dégénèrent si l'on coupe leur racine postérieure, aussi bien que par l'ablation de la branche communicante. Bechterev (loc. cit. pag. 23) dit, en parlant de ces fibres qui partent du sympathique et qui pénètrent par sa racine postérieure:

> . . . nous avons déjà vu que la section expérimentale de cette dernière ne peut pas les mettre en évidence, mais il faut remarquer par contre que la résection d'un ganglion sympathique entraîne une dégénération partielle de plusieurs dorsales.

Il est vrai que les troubles doivent se faire sentir sur les cellules de la corne latérale et sur la base de la corne antérieure, de même que sur la colonne de Clarke.

On sait aujourd'hui que la dégénérescence d'un neurone peut apporter avec elle la dégénérescence d'un autre en relation avec lui (altération tertiaire, de Bechterev); on sait aussi que dans la colonne de Clarke elle-même on rencontre la terminaison de plusieurs collatéraux courts venant des cordons postérieurs (du moins ceux de la zone radiculaire moyenne, de Flechsig) de même qu'il y a d'autres collatéraux qui vont finir à la corne antérieure et à sa base; ainsi nous voyons que, par l'abolition du sympathique, nous allons produire des troubles exactement dans la zone de ramification des collatéraux courts des fibres myéliniennes qui pénètrent par leur racine postérieure et dont le centre trophique est dans le ganglion spinal. Ces troubles suffiraient à eux seuls à expliquer la modification dans le neurone sensitif et par les troubles dynamogéniques admis par Marinesco. Mais il y a plus: Nous avons vu qu'il y avait des cellules du type sympathique dans le ganglion spinal (Dogiel); outre celles-là, Dogiel décrit encore des cellules unipolaires, dont le plus grand prolongement se ramifie énormément dans le ganglion lui-même et qui doivent être en connexion avec les fibres sympathiques (vidé van Gehuchten, pag. 385, Bechterev, pag. 23).

Donc, il doit y avoir dans le ganglion des troubles consécutifs à la destruction du sympathique, en relation avec ce dernier.

Par conséquent, je pense que l'explication, ou mieux le mécanisme dont on peut se servir pour agir sur le nerf sensitif par l'intermédiaire du sympathique, est toujours le même, soit qu'on ait affaire au sciatique, soit au trijumeau. Pour ce dernier on doit agir sur le bulbe et sur le ganglion de Gasser (Jaboulay-Cavazzani). Pour le sciatique on doit agir sur la moelle et sur les ganglions spinaux.

Les pratiques chirurgicales (rallongement, névrotomies) appliquées dans la névralgie faciale ont été également appliquées à la sciatique et à d'autres névralgies. La résection du ganglion de Gasser et de sa racine se trouve encore représentée ici par la résection des racines postérieures faite dans des cas de névralgie des moignons d'amputation (Chipault) et dans les névralgies dues à un cancer utérin inopérable (Faure). Ce sont des interventions graves qui ne doivent être faites qu'en des cas rebelles à tout autre traitement.

Or, il y a encore deux formes d'intervention qui ont été appliquées dans la sciatique, une qui est toute récente et qui entre dans la catégorie des interventions médicales: la première, c'est le hersage; la seconde, les injections d'air stérilisé.

Le hersage, proposé et appliqué par Delagenière (du Mans) dans les sciatiques variqueuses, donne des résultats même quand cet élément vient à manquer. Les études expérimentales de Marty montrent que cette opération «provoque, anatomiquement, la section de quelques tubes nerveux, la disparition d'autres, et la sclérose diffuse de la gaine du nerf, avec la séparation des tubes; elle supprime momentanément les fonctions sensitives, tout en conservant les fonctions motrices, etc.»

Ces expériences, pour être complètes, devaient être accompagnées d'une étude sur les cellules nerveuses des ganglions spinaux et sur les troubles dans les racines postérieures jusqu'à la moelle; mais, somme toute, on voit qu'il y a disparition et trouble des fibres sensitives, ce qui implique un trouble secondaire du neurone.

Les injections d'air stérilisé, sur les points douloureux, ont été appliquées non seulement dans la sciatique, mais encore en d'autres névralgies.

Cadier, de Lyon, fut le premier à les proposer et à les appliquer. L'idée qui le porta à faire ces injections fut exactement celle d'obtenir un allongement des filets nerveux douloureux, sans recourir à une intervention sanglante.

Sur 25 malades (sciatique) il obtint la guérison de 13, au bout d'une à cinq sessions, et l'amélioration de six. Il est indubitable que l'injection de l'air au niveau des points douloureux des ramifications nerveuses doit faire allonger ces dernières, et qu'il doit

se produire des troubles dans le neurone, comme dans l'allongement à ciel ouvert. Le mécanisme de la guérison est, par
conséquent, toujours analogue.

* * *

Comme nous l'avons dit, Ruggi, attribuant les douleurs qui
continuent après la castration ovarienne à l'excitation des filets
sympathiques qui accompagnent l'artère utéro-ovarienne, attaqua
cette partie du sympathique; nous avons vu aussi qu'il croit pouvoir produire de cette façon-là une modification de l'éréthisme
nerveux des organes génitaux internes. Si la pathogénie signalée
par Jaboulay dans certaines névralgies pelviques avec des troubles de menstruation est vraie, l'indication d'agir suivant le conseil du professeur de Modène est plus conforme à ce que nous
savons de l'intervention sympathique que le décollement simple
du rectum.

Nous avons dit aussi comment G. Cavazzani a été amené à appliquer la même intervention aux états névropathiques dépendants
de la sphère génitale. Il ne nous reste qu'à apprécier les observations de ces deux chirurgiens italiens et celles de Toschine,
leur compatriote, observations que je n'ai pas fait suivre immédiatement à celles du décollement du rectum, pour plus de commodité dans l'étude.

Nous avons donc à apprécier 16 observations, dans lesquelles
on a fait l'extirpation du plexus utéro-ovarien. Dans quelques-uns
de ces cas cette opération a été accompagnée d'autres, ce qui lui
ôta une partie importante de la valeur dont elle avait besoin
scientifiquement pour nous convaincre de son efficacité. Quant à
moi, je suis absolument sûr que toute personne habituée à la rébellion de ce genre de malades aux interventions même les plus
radicales, ne pourra pas ne pas remarquer que l'extirpation du
plexus utéro-ovarien a été, sinon le facteur principal de la guérison, du moins un puissant auxiliaire. Il serait d'un grand intérêt
scientifique de réunir des cas de ceux où l'on faisait anciennement l'opération de Basey, et qu'on n'opère plus aujourd'hui, et
d'opérer les maladies en n'extirpant que le plexus sympathique et
en épargnant les ovaires, pour voir ensuite quel résultat il y aurait sur les douleurs. Mais ces interventions sont encore à l'étude
et je ne dois analyser que les éléments qu'on me fournit et la manière dont on me les fournit.

Sur les 8 opérations de Ruggi il y en a sept où il faut remarquer que les malades avaient déjà souffert d'autres interventions sur les organes génitaux internes, ce qui met de côté le facteur de la suggestion dans les résultats obtenus par la sympathectomie abdominale. Pour deux observations le résultat obtenu doit être attribué à la sympathectomie et non à l'oophoro-salpingectomie droite; car les irradiations douloureuses étaient, du côté opéré d'abord, sans résultat, montrant qu'on y devait chercher le procès névralgique.

Une autre observation de Ruggi mérite les mêmes considérations quant au côté gauche; mais quant au côté droit, il y a eu plusieurs interventions qui ôtent quelque valeur à l'observation.

Deux autres observations montrent encore plus l'importance de l'opération de Ruggi. Elles appartiennent à la catégorie de ces cas rebelles qui se moquent des interventions les plus radicales.

Il y a une observation qui, étant démonstrative à cause de la brutalité des symptômes douloureux qui disparurent, nous laisse cependant quelques doutes (parce que la malade tombait en syncope très facilement) quant à la possibilité d'hystérie et de la facilité de suggestion du sujet.

Dans l'avant-dernière observation de Ruggi la sympathectomie a été faite pour guérir une névralgie pelvique droite, la malade ayant été opérée auparavant, pour d'autres raisons, du côté gauche. Il faut remarquer que, bien que l'on respectât l'ovaire droit, la malade fût guérie de la névralgie du côté gauche.

Dans la huitième et dernière observation, la valeur de la sympathectomie apparaît en pleine lumière, laissant dans l'ombre l'ovariotomie simple, impuissante à combattre la névralgie qui s'améliora remarquablement avec l'opération de Ruggi.

Des cinq observations de Cavazzani nous devons retenir ceci:

Dans la première, l'idée de suggestion doit être mise de côté, et Cavazzani l'éloigne soigneusement en parlant de l'état de la malade, le soir de l'opération:

Alla sera l'ammalata si lodava assai del suo stato, ed assicurava che i suoi dolori erano affatto cessati, esclusa ogni suggestione, perché nulla, proprio nulla era stato promesso all'ammalata, nemmeno dalle infermiere, trattandosi d'operazione del tutto nuova, e perché, a motivo della sordità, l'ammalata non si prestava a delle facili confabulazioni

Mais cette observation de Cavazzani ne doit pas être exclue; il y avait des lésions suffisantes pour qu'on pût expliquer la

guérison par l'intervention chirurgicale, même sans sympathectomie; en outre, il y avait du liquide dans le péritoine, liquide qu'on
a retiré, en faisant après la toilette de la membrane.

Il n'y a contre cela que l'impression personnelle de l'opérateur, mais en science ce n'est pas assez.

Tuttavia credo di poter asserire cosa nota a quanti hanno pratica di chirurgia addominale, che non incontro ogni giorno un'ammalata laparotomizzata, che
nella sera medesima dell'operazione dichiari di sentirsi completamente sollevata
dei suoi dolori; ciò che si deve quindi attribuire non già all'estirpazione dell'ovario,
in sè stessa, ma sibbene alla resezione del plesso.

Dans la seconde observation de Cavazzani nous retrouvons
les mêmes conditions que celles des deux premières de Ruggi; et
l'on doit attribuer le résultat à l'intervention sur le sympathique
et non à l'extirpation de l'autre ovaire:

Va notato che le sofferenze di questa paziente erano costantemente a destra
e que l'ovario rimasto era a sinistra, ma ovario e tuba erano in completa fase di
involuzione e non esisteva traccia di processo morboso in corso o progresso.

La troisième observation est plus démonstrative par l'inefficacité des opérations antérieures.

Dans la quatrième la démonstration de la valeur de la sympathectomie, est plus claire; là guérison de cette malade a été
obtenue en respectant les annexes et l'utérus qui étaient sains, et
on remarque une modification frappante dans l'état psychique du
malade.

Dans la dernière opération, l'extirpation des deux ovaires, en
atrophie, ôte quelque valeur au cas comme pièce à conviction.
Nous pouvons supposer seulement que la sympathectomie a eu
des avantages, par la fréquence de l'inutilité de l'ovariotomie
bilatérale, sur des malades avec des manifestations névralgiques
aussi intenses que celles de la malade dont je parle.

Voyons les trois observations de Ruggi.

Dans la première, le résultat a été meilleur du côté où l'on
n'a fait que l'opération de Ruggi que du côté où l'on a retiré
l'ovaire. Dans la seconde, les douleurs continuèrent, après la
castration utéro-ovarienne, vaginale, et il y eut des attaques hystériques; mais on a obtenu la guérison radicale, observée pendant
deux années, en appliquant le système de Ruggi.

Dans la troisième on n'a fait que l'opération de Ruggi, laissant
les annexes, et la malade a été guérie des douleurs et des attaques.

En résumé: Nous avons 14 opérations (j'en exclus la première et la dernière de Cavazzani) dans lesquelles l'intervention sur le sympathique a été favorable. De celles-ci les plus démonstratives sont une de Ruggi, une de Cavazzani et une autre de Foschini, dans lesquelles on a conservé les organes génitaux internes.

Mais, si l'observation de Ruggi et la troisième de Foschini perdent une partie de leur valeur, parce qu'on peut faire intervenir en elles la suggestion — car la malade de Ruggi tombait en syncope avec facilité, ce qui pourrait être en rapport avec l'hystérie, et celle de Foschini a eu des attaques hystériques —, la 21ª de Cavazzani est, au contraire, très démonstrative, et l'idée de suggestion doit être entièrement mise de côté, la malade ayant déjà souffert des traitements antérieurs, et même avec un intervalle de trois mois. On peut dire la même chose de la 2ᵉᵐᵉ opération de Foschini. Dans les autres, l'insuccès d'interventions considérées comme radicales montre également que, dans cet ordre de faits (même s'il y a des lésions supposées des annexes), la sympathectomie du plexus utéro-ovarien est un puissant élément de guérison.

Quant à la douleur, m'appuyant seulement sur un si petit nombre de cas, je crois pouvoir conclure que: 1.ª — Au cas où l'on intervient sur des lésions utéro-ovariennes ou annexiales douloureuses, avec des irradiations, l'extirpation du plexus utéro-ovarien est un complément de l'opération qui donnera à celle-ci plus de garanties de guérison; 2.ª — Attendu le peu de gravité de l'intervention chez les malades avec des névralgies annexiales et qui irradient jusqu'à l'abdomen et aux cuisses, etc., cas où l'intervention sur les annexes est contre-indiquée, parce qu'ils sont sains, la sympathectomie doit être tentée en désespoir de cause, avec quelques probabilités de succès.

Si, sans aucun doute, les 16 opérations que j'ai citées nous mènent à poursuivre dans cette voie, pleine d'espoir, nous manquons de la sanction du temps et d'un plus grand nombre d'observations pour avoir une opinion solide sur la stabilité de la guérison. Les cas de Foschini, suivis pendant une ou deux années, et ceux de Ruggi, suivis plus longtemps, nous permettent de la prophétiser; et je terminerai en transcrivant quelques lignes de Ruggi, où il parle de ses observations:

I fatti tutti annotati sono oltremodo eloquenti, essendo destinati a far conoscere che l'operazione di simpatectomia da me consigliata in questi speciali eventi, riesce sempre efficace perchè quando non guari perfetamente le ammalate ne migliorò in modo sensibilissimo le loro condizioni.

In tute le predette inferme finalmente la mia operazione riuscì del tutto innocua, essendo tutte le malate guarite senza complicazioni e fatti successivi fastidiosi.

THÈME 3 — CHIRURGIE ARTÉRIELLE ET VEINEUSE. LES MODERNES ACQUISITIONS
Par M. le Dr. PIERRE DELBET (Paris)

INTRODUCTION

La réunion par première intention des plaies vasculaires, qui assure non seulement l'hémostase mais encore la perméabilité du vaisseau sectionné, telle est dans cet ordre d'idées la grande acquisition moderne.

J'étudierai d'abord, en m'appuyant sur les expériences, les conditions qui permettent de réaliser la suture efficace des artères et des veines, puis, dans une seconde partie, j'envisagerai les indications des sutures vasculaires, indications encore vagues et incertaines, mais qui deviendront, peut-être nombreuses et variées.

Chacun sait que l'idée de suturer les artères date du milieu du XVIIIe siècle. Lembert [1] l'a exprimée et sur son conseil, le 15 juin 1758, Hallowell ferma par une suture entortillée une artère humérale piquée au cours d'une saignée. L'hémorrhagie fut arrêtée, l'épingle tomba le 14e jour et le malade guérit.

En 1772, Assmann [2] fit quatre expériences de suture entortillée sur des artères fémorales de chien. Les deux animaux survivants furent sacrifiés au bout d'un mois et demi. Les artères étaient complètement oblitérées.

Après ces tentatives audacieuses et lointaines, la suture vasculaire tomba dans l'oubli comme bien d'autres problèmes de chirurgie dont la solution n'était possible que par l'asepsie.

À partir de 1823, on reprend peu à peu l'étude des sutures vasculaires. Les veines où la pression est moindre et dont les parois souples sont plus maniables sont l'objet des premiers efforts. On essaie les ligatures latérales et même les sutures. Mais, à l'époque où les hémorrhagies secondaires décimaient les opérés, ces tentatives ne pouvaient donner de grands résultats.

---

[1] Lembert, Med. Obs. and Inquiries. T. 2, p. 360. Londres, 1762.
[2] Assmann, Inaug. Dissertatio (Groningue) 1773.

Avec l'antisepsie, la question change de face. Les sutures veineuses acquièrent d'abord droit de cité. Puis, les sutures artérielles tentent les expérimentateurs et bientôt les chirurgiens. Je ne veux pas refaire cet historique qui se trouve partout. Je me borne à indiquer les grandes étapes du progrès. Après les tentatives de Gluck [1], de Postempsky [2], Jassinowsky [3] établit définitivement en 1889 la possibilité des sutures latérales. En 1892, Durante [4] pratique la première chez l'homme.

La même année, Niebergall [5] essaie expérimentalement les sutures circulaires. En 1887, Murphy [6] les réalise par un procédé spécial : l'invagination.

Abbé [7] (1894), Nitze [8] (1897), Gluck [9] (1898), Payr [10] (1900), imaginent de rapprocher les deux bouts des artères sectionnées avec le secours de tubes prothétiques.

En 1902, les travaux de San Martin [11], de Carrel [12], de Jaboulay [13] ouvrent la question des anastomoses artério-veineuses.

En 1903 paraissent de beaux travaux parmi lesquels il faut citer celui de Jensen [14] sur la suture circulaire, et les remarquables recherches de Hoepfner qui établissent la possibilité des greffes vasculaires.

Dès qu'on a conquis le moyen, c'est-à-dire la suture efficace, on a tenté et réalisé en quelques années les anastomoses et les greffes vasculaires. Ce sont là les divers chapitres que j'aurai à étudier. J'exposerai d'abord, je le répète, les conquêtes progressives que nous devons à la chirurgie expérimentale, puis les applications qu'on en a faites à la clinique.

---

[1] *Gluck*, Archiv f. klin. Chirurgie, 1882, T. XXVIII.
[2] *Postempsky*, Congrès de Rome, 1886.
[3] *Jassinowsky*, Inaug. Dissert, Dorpat, 1889.
[4] *Durante*, T. de Pathologie et Thérapeutique chirurgicale, T. VII, p. 293.
[5] *Niebergall*, Deutsche Zeit. f. Chirurgie, T. XXIII.
[6] *Murphy*, Med. Rec. N. York, 16 janvier 1897, et Congrès de Moscou, 1897, T. V, p. 514.
[7] *Abbé*, N. York M. J. Janvier 1894.
[8] *Nitze*, Congrès de Moscou 1897.
[9] *Gluck*, Archiv für klin. Chirurg. 1900, T. 28, et Berliner Klinik, 1898.
[10] *Payr*, Archiv für klin. Chirurg. 1900.
[11] *San Martin*, Madrid 1902. Communication à l'Acad. Royale de Médecine.
[12] *Carrel*, Lyon Medical 1902.
[13] *Jaboulay*, In-Lecercle. Thèse de Lyon 1902.
[14] *Jensen*, Archiv f. klin. Chirurg. 1903, T. 69, p. 939.

PREMIÈRE PARTIE
Résultats des recherches expérimentales
SUTURES ARTÉRIELLES ET VEINEUSES

Pour suturer une artère blessée, il faut naturellement suspendre le cours du sang dans son canal pendant toute la durée de l'opération. Étudions donc d'abord les moyens d'hémostase temporaire, condition indispensable de la suture.

A — 1° Hémostase temporaire.

L'usage de la bande d'Esmarch a établi depuis longtemps la possibilité de suspendre la circulation dans tout un membre sans compromettre sa vitalité et sans amener de coagulations intra-vasculaires.

Cependant, la bande d'Esmarch n'est peut-être pas toujours sans inconvénient et d'autre part elle est inapplicable dans la plupart des régions où les sutures vasculaires sont intéressantes. C'est seulement pour les grosses artères qu'il peut être avantageux de substituer la suture à la ligature, fémorale commune, iliaque, axillaire, sous-clavière, carotide. Or, au pli de l'aine, dans l'aisselle, au cou, on ne peut appliquer la bande, et il ne saurait en être question pour les artères viscérales.

Pour rendre pratiques les sutures artérielles, il fallait donc assurer l'hémostase temporaire en agissant directement sur les deux bouts du vaisseau blessé.

Or, les expériences ont heureusement prouvé que le degré de compression qui suffit pour arrêter complètement le cours du sang dans une artère n'y détermine aucune lésion lorsqu'il est bien appliqué.

Les artères peuvent même supporter une pression très forte sans que leur vitalité soit gravement compromise. Bothézat(¹) place sur des fémorales de chiens des pinces à forcipressure ordinaires et les laisse en place pendant des temps variables. Quand il enlève la pince au bout d'une demi-heure, voici ce qui se passe. La circulation se rétablit brusquement, la paroi amincie se laisse distendre et il se fait une légère dilatation anévrysmale. Mais

---

(¹) *Bothézat*, Archives de Méd. expérimentale et d'Anatomie pathologique, T. 6, p. 473, 1894.

cette dilatation ne persiste jamais. Un nodus se forme autour du segment forcipressé et les parois altérées se réparent complètement sans oblitération de la lumière du vaisseau. Bolhézat nous dit même qu'une fémorale étreinte pendant trois heures dans les mors d'une pince retrouve sa perméabilité.

Il va sans dire que pour faire une suture, on ne doit jamais serrer une artère avec cette brutalité. Je rappelle ces expériences parce qu'elles sont intéressantes à un autre point de vue. Il est bien clair que la striction violente d'une pince à forcipressure entraîne des lésions graves de la paroi artérielle et particulièrement de la tunique interne. Si l'artère recouvre cependant sa perméabilité, c'est donc que ces lésions se réparent sans entraîner de coagulation oblitérante. C'est un point d'une extrême importance sur lequel j'aurai à revenir.

Ces expériences montrent encore qu'entre la striction suffisante pour arrêter le cours du sang et celle qui entraîne des lésions irréparables, il existe une large marge.

On doit évidemment employer toujours la pression minima. Comment peut-on la réaliser?

Il est un procédé simple qu'on emploie couramment dans les laboratoires de physiologie. Il consiste à passer sous le vaisseau un fil en anse dont un aide tend les deux chefs rapprochés. On soulève ainsi le vaisseau, on le coude, on l'aplatit de telle sorte que les deux parois s'adossent. C'est l'artifice qu'a recommandé Ch. Nélaton pour les anévrysmes de la sous-clavière. Il est inoffensif, mais il faut reconnaître que pour faire une suture, il n'est pas commode. On est obligé de passer un fil sous chaque bout du vaisseau sectionné, et il faut un aide spécial pour tenir les quatre chefs de ces deux fils, un aide dont l'attention ne se relâche pas un instant. En outre si on place ces fils près de la plaie à réparer, ils gênent considérablement les manipulations et dans les sutures circulaires, ils rendent difficile le rapprochement des deux bouts. Il faudrait donc aller dénuder le vaisseau loin du point malade, ce qui serait au moins une perte de temps. En somme, quand il s'agit de sutures artérielles, ce n'est qu'un pis aller.

On peut en dire autant de la compression digitale effectuée dans la plaie. Les doigts de l'aide qui comprime gênent l'opérateur même lorsqu'il s'agit d'une suture latérale. Ils rendent très difficiles les sutures circulaires pour lesquelles il faut pouvoir manœuvrer librement le vaisseau.

La ligature temporaire donne à ce point de vue une grande aisance, mais appliquée directement sur le vaisseau elle est dangereuse. Même lorsqu'elle est faite avec un fil large, la ligature directe, en fronçant le vaisseau à l'excès, produit des déchirures longitudinales de la tunique interne. Si on veut employer la ligature, il faut non seulement se servir de fil large, mais encore interposer entre le vaisseau et le fil soit une mince compresse de gaze souple, soit une feuille ou un tube de caoutchouc.

Pour assurer l'hémostase temporaire, la plupart des expérimentateurs se sont servis de pinces. Gluck, Jassinowsky, Payr, Crile, Hoepfner [1] en ont fait construire de modèles spéciaux. Ces instruments peuvent être commodes, mais ils ne sont pas indispensables. On réalise une hémostase temporaire parfaite, sans danger pour le vaisseau, avec n'importe quelle pince à mors souples bien garnis de caoutchouc.

2.º Dénudation du vaisseau.

C'est là une question extrêmement importante sur laquelle les recherches modernes ont profondément modifié les idées communément admises autrefois.

C'était récemment encore un principe fondamental de la médecine opératoire qu'il ne fallait dénuder une artère à lier que sur une étendue de quelques millimètres, tout juste pour permettre le passage du fil. On croyait qu'une dénudation plus étendue, en détruisant les vaso-vasorum, compromettait la vitalité du vaisseau, ce qui était d'ailleurs parfaitement vrai quand il s'agissait de plaies septiques. Danna [2] déclarait que si une dénudation d'un demi-centimètre n'avait pas d'inconvénient, une dénudation de 1 centimètre amenait la coagulation du sang et qu'une dénudation de trois centimètres entraînait une dégénérescence de la tunique moyenne et une thrombose étendue. L'enveloppement des artères avec une mince feuille d'or même sur une faible étendue, avait toujours entraîné une nécrose totale. En 1899, Dœrfler [3] redoutait encore les dénudations étendues.

Les expériences récentes ont montré que dans une plaie aseptique on peut dénuder une artère sur une étendue de plusieurs centimètres sans compromettre sa vitalité. Comme il est bien pro-

---

[1] *Hœpfner*, Archiv f. klin. Chirurg., 1903, T. 70, p. 417.
[2] *Danna*, J. of Am. Med. Assoc., 1905, T. 45, p. 393.
[3] *Dœrfler*, Beiträge zur klin. Chirurg., 1899.

bable qu'après une dénudation de plusieurs centimètres l'artère ne peut plus être nourrie par les vaso-vasorum venant de la portion restée en connexion avec sa gaîne, la conservation de sa vitalité dans de telles conditions prouve que de rapides anastomoses peuvent s'établir entre les fins vaisseaux de la gaîne et ceux des parois artérielles, c'est-à-dire qu'une artère est susceptible de se greffer.

Hoepfner en a donné la preuve expérimentale complète en réséquant sur un chien un segment de carotide et en le replaçant en sens inverse. Je reviendrai sur cette expérience importante qui a ouvert la question si intéressante des greffes vasculaires.

En somme, il est acquis aujourd'hui que dans les plaies aseptiques les artères supportent sans dommage une dénudation étendue. Ce n'est point à dire naturellement qu'il faille les dénuder inutilement, inconsidérément. Toute dénudation inutile est blâmable parce que, sans compromettre fatalement le succès, elle en diminue cependant les chances.

Les expériences récentes ont montré en outre que les vaso-vasorum d'une artère sont capables d'assurer la nutrition du vaisseau sur une étendue de 5 à 8 millimètres. Payr a en effet imaginé un mode de suture dont l'un des temps fondamentaux consiste à entourer un des bouts du vaisseau sectionné d'un tube de magnésium, et par ce procédé Hoepfner a obtenu de magnifiques résultats expérimentaux avec des tubes d'une longueur de 5 à 8 millimètres.

3.° Thrombose.

C'est sur ce point que les recherches récentes ont modifié le plus profondément les idées anciennes. On a cru longtemps que la présence d'un corps étranger dans un vaisseau devait fatalement amener une thrombose oblitérante.

Il faut remarquer tout de suite, et c'est là un point capital pour les sutures vasculaires, que physiologiquement le sang n'est en rapport qu'avec le seul endothélium des artères, des veines et des capillaires. Pour lui, tout ce qui n'est pas cet endothélium (sauf peut-être l'endothélium de certaines séreuses) est corps étranger. Ainsi, pour le sang, les fibres conjonctives élastiques ou musculaires de la tunique moyenne des artères sont aussi bien corps étrangers qu'un fil de catgut ou de soie. Nous retrouverons cette notion lorsqu'il s'agira de choisir une technique de suture.

Lorsqu'on étudie en bloc les résultats des expériences de

suture vasculaire, ils paraissent singulièrement capricieux et même paradoxaux. Avec toutes les techniques on a obtenu des succès; avec toutes on a eu des échecs, de telle sorte que les résultats paraissent dépendre surtout des conditions autres que celles dont on s'est particulièrement préoccupé.

La nature des fils, la manière de les placer et d'obtenir l'affrontement, le rétrécissement du vaisseau, tout cela a certes une importance, mais seulement une importance de second plan.

Les deux conditions de succès qui dominent toutes les autres, sont l'asepsie et l'intégrité de l'endothélium, et ces deux conditions sont dans une certaine mesure connexes.

Clermont ([1]) est le premier qui ait attribué la thrombose opératoire à l'infection. C'est Jensen ([2]) qui a démontré le rôle de cette dernière.

Étudiant les expériences de Murphy, qui a noté l'état des plaies, il constate que sept sutures avec un décours cliniquement aseptique ont donné 4 succès, tandis que, sur 9 cas où la plaie était infectée, il s'est produit 8 thromboses.

Dans une de ses propres expériences, il a observé un thrombus pariétal qui s'était développé du côté correspondant à un petit abcès.

Il a ensemencé des thrombus et toujours il s'est développé des colonies de micro-organismes: streptocoques, staphylocoques, quelquefois des bâtonnets dont le rôle est incertain.

Il a fait des coupes des artères thrombosées et sur ces coupes il a toujours trouvé des microcoques nombreux, sauf dans un cas où il n'a pu voir que deux diplocoques. Dans un autre cas où l'animal avait été conservé 66 jours, il y avait encore dans le caillot de nombreux cocci. Et on ne peut penser qu'il s'agisse de caillots primitivement aseptiques, secondairement envahis par les microbes, car ceux-ci existent au niveau de la suture, et c'est autour des fils qu'ils sont le plus nombreux. Dans un cas même, il y avait des microbes dans le fil bien qu'il n'y eût pas de caillot. La suture était entourée d'une gaine fibreuse qui l'avait isolée de la lumière du vaisseau.

Enfin, l'innocuité du corps étranger aseptique est démontrée péremptoirement par les expériences suivantes:

---

[1] *Clermont*, Presse Médicale, 1901, p. 329, n. 42.
[2] *Jensen*, Archiv f. klin. Chirurg., 1903, t. 69, p. 989.

La première est celle que Raymond Petit a communiquée à la Société de Biologie le 25 janvier 1896 :

«Le 5 avril, on dénude la veine saphène gauche d'un chien, on introduit dans sa lumière deux centimètres de catgut que l'on fixe à l'extérieur de la veine par un nœud. Le 10 mai, on trouve la veine perméable. Il n'y a plus de catgut. Cette expérience a été répétée deux fois».

Jensen (¹) a fait sur une artère une expérience plus démonstrative encore. Un catgut stérilisé fut placé diamétralement dans la carotide primitive, traversant les deux parois et noué à l'extérieur. 18 jours après il n'y avait pas trace de caillot. Le catgut était libre dans le vaisseau. Il paraissait plus épais à ses extrémités qu'au milieu, et avait la même apparence que la tunique interne comme s'il était recouvert d'endothélium.

Il devait être en effet engaîné de cellules endothéliales.

Voici comment on peut concevoir la succession des phénomènes. On admet que la coagulation est due à une diastase qui vient des globules blancs et qui transforme le fibrinogène du plasma en fibrine insoluble. Cette diastase, thrombine ou fibrioferment, préexiste-t-elle dans les leucocytes ou bien n'est-elle produite, secrétée en quelque sorte que sous l'influence de l'irritation produite par le contact de corps étrangers? Il nous importe peu. Le fait important au point de vue qui nous occupe, c'est que la thrombine n'est mise en liberté que par les leucocytes qui entrent en contact avec un corps étranger.

Qu'il existe une petite lésion de la tunique interne, ou qu'un corps étranger fasse saillie dans la lumière du vaisseau, les conditions réalisées sont identiques au point de vue de la coagulation. Dans l'un et l'autre cas, il existe dans le vaisseau, en contact avec le sang, une surface dépourvue d'endothélium où les globules blancs s'arrêtent; que la plaie soit septique ou non, ces leucocytes en contact avec un corps étranger déversent de la thrombine dans le sang.

Si la surface dépourvue d'endothélium est petite, la quantité de thrombine mise en liberté est minime et la masse du sang sans cesse renouvelée qui passe au point lésé est trop considérable pour qu'il se produise une coagulation massive. Il ne se forme qu'une coagulation microscopique.

(¹) Jensen, Arch. f. klin. Chirurg., 1903, T. 69, p. 684.

La rapidité de la circulation intervient donc pour limiter la coagulation. Et ceci nous indique qu'une bonne méthode de suture ne devra pas retarder le cours du sang dans le vaisseau. Ce point sur lequel ont insisté Eberth et Schimmelbusch [1] est d'autant plus important que le nombre des globules blancs qui s'arrêtent est proportionnel au ralentissement du courant.

Dans le premier phénomène la septicité n'intervient pas, ou, du moins, ne joue pas le rôle prépondérant. En effet, les ruptures sous-cutanées des artères, lorsque la lésion est étendue, entraînent en milieu aseptique des coagulations oblitérantes.

Revenons à la petite lésion ou au petit corps étranger sur lequel il s'est formé un coagulum. Certains expérimentateurs en examinant à la loupe la face interne des vaisseaux suturés et oblitérés ont vu ces petites coagulations.

Si les lésions restent en cet état, tout se passe comme dans un vaisseau dont la paroi est malade : le coagulum, d'abord microscopique, grossit ; il devient d'abord rétrécissant, puis oblitérant.

Pour que la coagulation s'arrête, il faut que le petit coagulum qui s'est formé sur la plaie ou sur le corps étranger soit recouvert par des cellules endothéliales. Tikhow [2] a mis ce fait en évidence en étudiant les sutures veineuses.

C'est ici qu'intervient la septicité.

L'endothélium vasculaire a une extraordinaire puissance de pullulation. Mais une infection, même légère, suffit à l'empêcher de proliférer. Quand la plaie est infectée, les cellules endothéliales ne se multiplient pas et la thrombose se produit.

Mais si l'infection joue dans la production des thromboses consécutives aux sutures vasculaires un rôle prédominant, elle n'en est pas la seule cause. Il est d'autres conditions qui sont singulièrement adjuvantes et qui même sont capables, lorsqu'elles sont poussées à l'extrême, de produire à elles seules l'obstruction du vaisseau.

C'est la prolifération rapide de l'endothélium qui arrête la coagulation. Une bonne suture doit donc respecter son intégrité. Or, à côté de l'infection, il est deux autres causes qui peuvent la compromettre : des causes mécaniques et des causes chimiques.

---

[1] Eberth et Schimmelbusch – Fortschritte der Medizin, 1885, et T.⁰ de Médecine (Charcot et Bouchard t. V. p. 3 4.

[2] Tikhow – Chirurg. Letop. St. Petersbourg 1894 – Cent. f. Chirurg. 1895 p. 110

Les causes mécaniques, frottements, pincements, décollements, sont capables d'altérer gravement l'endothélium. Que ces altérations mécaniques puissent produire la thrombose, nous en avons la preuve dans les contusions des artères. Chacun sait qu'on observe souvent à leur suite une obstruction suivie de gangrène.

Les causes chimiques sont les lavages avec les solutions antiseptiques. J'ai étudié autrefois avec la collaboration de MM. Bresset et de Grandmaison (¹) les lésions qu'elles produisent sur l'endothélium péritonéal. Il ne me paraît pas douteux qu'elles engendrent des lésions du même ordre sur l'endothélium vasculaire; et ces lésions, en troublant sa vitalité, l'empêchent de proliférer. Ainsi, les antiseptiques sont une cause sérieuse d'échec des sutures vasculaires. Je ne serais pas étonné que bien des insuccès soient dus à leur emploi. Comme le conseille Densen, il ne faut se servir en fait de liquide au cours de l'opération que de la solution salée physiologique, et on peut poser comme règle que la suture artérielle doit être une opération rigoureusement et exclusivement aseptique.

4° Des injections anticoagulantes intra-vasculaires.

Pour empêcher la thrombose, on pourrait peut-être recourir aux injections intra-veineuses anticoagulantes. Ces substances sont assez nombreuses; mais il en est qu'on ne peut songer à employer, soit à cause de leur toxicité, soit à cause de la fugacité de leur action, ainsi: les oxalates, les fluorures, les citrates d'alcalis. Les fluorures sont très toxiques. Les oxalates et les citrates ont une action très momentanée; leur effet ne dure que quelques minutes chez le chien. En outre, ils amènent un abaissement de la pression sanguine, qui serait peut-être avantageux pour la suture, mais qui ne le serait pas pour le malade.

La peptone, et particuliérement les protéoses qui constituent la peptone de Witte, injectées dans le sang à la dose de 0 gr. 3 par kilog. en solution dans l'eau salée à 7 ‰ (10 grammes de peptone pour 100 cc. de solution) rend le sang incoagulable pendant deux heures. Elle agit sur le chien, mais non sur le lapin. Agirait-elle sur l'homme? Arthus (²), dont on connaît la compétence sur ces questions me dit qu'il n'en sait rien! En tout cas, elle produit chez le chien une sorte de coma avec abaissement énorme de la pression sanguine. Il est à craindre qu'elle ait le même effet sur l'homme.

(¹) Annales de Gynécologie et d'Obstétrique 1889.
(²) M. Arthus — Communication orale

L'extrait de tête de sangsue n'aurait pas ces inconvénients. Il provoque l'incoagulabilité pour une période de deux heures environ et cette période peut être prolongée par une deuxième injection. Peut-être cette substance rendrait-elle des services. Il ne faut pas toutefois s'imaginer qu'elle permettra à elle seule de réussir toutes les sutures artérielles. On ne peut en effet prolonger indéfiniment l'incoagulabilité. Quand elle cessera, si la ligne de suture est infectée, l'endothélium ne sera pas régénéré et la coagulation se produira. Mais, en cas d'infection très légère, elle permettrait peut-être la séquestration des fils, leur énucléation hors de la lumière du vaisseau.

B. — TECHNIQUE DES SUTURES VASCULAIRES.

Les notions brièvement exposées ci-dessus permettent d'apprécier la valeur des divers procédés techniques qui ont été imaginés.

Avant de les étudier, il convient de choisir le matériel commun à tous les procédés.

1° Matériel des sutures.

a) Les aiguilles. — Djemil-Pacha (¹) et Viart (²) ont pu mener à bien sur l'homme des sutures latérales avec de fines aiguilles de Reverdin. Cependant, ces aiguilles, en général excellentes, présentent pour cet usage un grave inconvénient. Elles ont les bords tranchants et font par suite des plaies relativement considérables. Je m'en suis servi pour des expériences de suture circulaire sur des chiens, et j'ai toujours vu les points perforants faits avec ces aiguilles donner une hémorrhagie notable et souvent difficile à arrêter. Si donc on voulait se servir de ces aiguilles, il faudrait commencer par en faire faire qui ne soient pas tranchantes.

Même avec cette modification, elles ne seraient point encore très bonnes pour les sutures artérielles, car en raison de la pièce mobile on ne peut les faire très fines.

Tous les expérimentateurs sont d'accord sur ce point : les meilleures aiguilles pour suturer les vaisseaux sont les fines aiguilles rondes. Suivant le genre de suture que l'on pratique, il peut y avoir avantage à les prendre droites, légèrement courbes ou très courbes.

(¹) Djemil Pacha, Congrès de Moscou 1897.
(²) Viart, Soc. de chirurgie 1903.

b) Fils. — Sauf le crin de Florence, on a employé toutes les variétés de fils utilisés en chirurgie : tendons, catgut, fil de lin et soie. C'est la soie qui a été le plus souvent employée tant sur l'homme que sur les animaux. Sur 21 sutures chirurgicales, Landais [1] en compte 13 faites à la soie, 6 au catgut et 1 au fil de lin.

Le catgut a séduit certains expérimentateurs par deux qualités. Il est résorbé et il gonfle au contact de liquides aqueux. Cette augmentation de volume le rend capable d'obturer les trous par lesquels il a passé. Ce n'est point là un avantage bien considérable, car lorsqu'on emploie des aiguilles appropriées, l'hémorrhagie qui se fait par les points perforants, lorqu'on enlève les pinces qui assurent l'hémostase temporaire, est toujours aisément arrêtée par une compression légère.

Certains craignent que sa résorbabilité, bien loin d'être un avantage, soit un inconvénient. Ils redoutent que la résorption s'achève avant que la réunion soit solide. Je ne crois pas que cette crainte soit justifiée. Dans une plaie aseptique, le catgut ne se résorbe pas si vite. Jensen, dont j'ai rapporté la mémorable expérience, l'a retrouvé au bout de 18 jours. C'est plus qu'il n'en faut pour assurer la solidité de la cicatrice.

Un reproche plus sérieux, c'est qu'on trouve malaisément des catguts très fins et qu'à égalité de diamètres, ils sont moins solides que la soie.

En voici un autre qui me paraît avoir son importance. Le catgut est souvent stérilisé par des procédés chimiques et celui-là même qui l'est par la chaleur est conservé dans l'alcool ou dans la benzine. Bref le catgut est plus ou moins imprégné de substances qui peuvent être toxiques pour l'endothélium. Aussi je crois qu'il est bon lorsqu'on s'en sert de le laver dans la solution salée physiologique. Durante [2] et Heidenhain [3] ont déjà recommandé cette précaution pour assurer le renflement hygrométrique du fil.

La soie a rallié les suffrages de la majorité des expérimentateurs et des chirurgiens qui ont eu l'occasion de suturer des artères. Les expériences de Tikhow [4] ont montré qu'elle n'a aucune tendance à passer dans la lumière du vaisseau. Bien au contraire,

---

[1] *Landais* — Thèse de Paris 1903-1904.
[2] *Durante* — T. de Pathologie et Thérap. chirurg. T. VII p. 195.
[3] *Heidenhain* — Cent. f. Chirurg. 1895 n° 30.
[4] *Tikhow* — Chirurg. Leçto St. Petersbourg 1894 — Cent. f. Chirurg. 1909, p. 110.

elle est en quelque sorte énucléée, rejetée excentriquement par un mécanisme qu'il est facile de saisir après ce que j'ai dit de l'enrobement des corps étrangers par un mince coagulum qui est rapidement recouvert d'un vernis endothélial.

On sait que, hors des vaisseaux, le sang se coagule plus lentement dans un vase à parois lisses que sur des surfaces irrégulières ou anfractueuses. La coagulation est encore plus lente lorsque les parois sont telles que le sang ne les mouille pas. C'est ainsi qu'on la retarde énormément en enduisant le vase de paraffine. Y aurait-il un avantage à paraffiner ou à vaseliner les fils destinés aux sutures artérielles? En tout cas, comme cet artifice ne pourrait avoir aucun inconvénient il mérite d'être essayé.

2.° Sutures latérales.

Les sutures latérales se font toujours par affrontement direct des bords de la plaie.

Le point qu'on a le plus discuté à leur sujet, c'est la manière de passer les fils. Doivent-ils traverser de part en part toute l'épaisseur de la paroi vasculaire, ou n'en prendre qu'une partie? Doivent-ils être perforants ou non perforants?

Jassinowsky [1] fait remarquer que les points non perforants évitent les hémorrhagies qui se font par les trous des points perforants. C'est un petit avantage car lorsqu'on emploie des aiguilles convenables, la petite hémorrhagie qui se fait par les trous est toujours facilement arrêtée. Tous les auteurs qui ont fait des sutures perforantes sont unanimes sur ce point.

Garré [2] reproche aux points non perforants d'être moins solides et craint qu'ils n'exposent aux hémorrhagies secondaires.

La grosse affaire, c'est de savoir si les points perforants exposent plus à la thrombose que les non perforants. Jacobsthal [3], Doerfler [4] avaient déjà soutenu que la saillie des fils dans la lumière du vaisseau n'entraîne pas la thrombose. Les expériences de R. Petit [5] et de Jensen [6] ont démontré l'innocuité des fils aseptiques. Il semble donc qu'il n'y ait pas d'inconvénient à faire des sutures perforantes.

---

(1) *Jassinowsky* — Inaug. Dissert. Dorpat 1889 et Archiv f. klin. Chirurgie 1891 T. 42 p. 816.
(2) *Garré* — Cent. f. Chirurgie 1899 n.° 18 — Münch. med. Woch. 1901 n.° 16.
(3) *Jacobsthal* — Beiträge zur klin. Chirurg. 1900.
(4) *Doerfler* — Beiträge zur klin. Chirurg. 1899.
(5) *Raymond Petit* — Soc. de Biologie. Janvier 1899 p. 7.
(6) *Jensen* — Archiv f. klin. Chirurgie 1903. T. 69 p. 938.

                PIERRE DELBET

Mais Jensen, qui a le mieux démontré le rôle de l'infection, pense justement que les sutures non perforantes exposent moins à la thrombose parce que les fils sont en rapport moins direct avec le sang. S'il y a une différence à ce point de vue, elle est plus théorique que pratique. Si les fils sont infectés de microbes virulents, le résultat ne sera pas meilleur qu'ils passent ou non dans l'intérieur du vaisseau. Il faudrait que leur virulence fut singulièrement atténuée pour que cette condition pût avoir une importance, d'autant que, même avec des points non perforants, il n'est pas certain que le fil n'est pas apparent dans la lumière du vaisseau. L'affrontement de la tunique interne n'est pas toujours si étroit que le sang ne puisse arriver jusqu'au contact des fils.

Je n'ai pas besoin d'ailleurs de discuter plus longtemps cette opinion émise par Jensen. Lui-même la considère sans doute comme plus théorique que pratique, puisque pour les sutures circulaires il donne la préférence aux points en U, qui sont nécessairement perforants.

Le fait pratiquement important, c'est qu'on peut faire sans danger des points perforants pourvu qu'ils soient aseptiques. S'il en eût été autrement, la suture vasculaire ne serait jamais devenue chirurgicale, car on ne peut pas être sûr que l'un des fils d'une suture n'intéresse pas la tunique interne.

Si les circonstances obligeaient à faire une suture avec de mauvaises aiguilles, trop grosses, trop coupantes, certes il faudrait s'appliquer à faire des sutures non perforantes, parce que l'hémorrhagie qui se produirait par les trous pourrait être difficile à arrêter. Mais, lorsqu'on dispose d'un bon matériel, aiguilles fines et rondes, fils appropriés, le tout bien aseptique, on peut faire sans danger des sutures perforantes.

Jusqu'à quelle étendue les plaies incomplètes sont-elles justiciables de la suture? Cela dépend de leur direction. Il n'y a pour ainsi dire point de limite à la longueur des plaies parallèles au grand axe du vaisseau. Pratiquement, elles ne sont jamais bien étendues et il est toujours possible de les suturer.

Il n'en est pas de même des plaies circulaires, c'est-à-dire perpendiculaires à l'axe. Jassinowsky (¹) déclare que dès qu'elles dépassent la demi-circonférence du vaisseau, il faut renoncer à la suture latérale qui amène un rétrécissement trop marqué. Quand

-----

(¹) Jassinowsky, Inaug. Dissertat. Dorpat, 1889, et Archiv. f. klin. Chir. 1891, T. 42, p. 425.

la plaie est plus étendue, à plus forte raison quand il ne reste plus qu'un point unissant les deux bouts du vaisseau, il vaut mieux compléter la section et faire une suture circulaire.

Les plaies obliques sont plus embarrassantes. Il est difficile d'indiquer une limite à l'étendue justiciable de la suture: tout dépend du degré d'obliquité. C'est donc affaire de coup d'œil dans chaque cas particulier. Ce qui les rend plus embarassantes, c'est que quand elles sont trop étendues pour être suturées, on ne peut les transformer directement en plaies circulaires complètes. Pour arriver à ce résultat, il faut réséquer un segment du vaisseau. Nous aurons à chercher à propos des anévrysmes quelle étendue on peut donner à cette résection sans compromettre la suture circulaire.

Les plaies à lambeaux se composent en somme de deux sections obliques. Les mêmes considérations leur sont applicables.

En dehors de la question des points perforants, il y a peu de chose à dire de la technique proprement dite.

Quand la plaie est étendue, surtout quand elle est à lambeaux, il faut unir d'abord, par un point séparé, le milieu de ses deux lèvres. Si on suturait en cheminant progressivement d'un angle à l'autre, on pourrait tirer plus une lèvre que l'autre, ce qui produirait au niveau du dernier angle un froncement fâcheux.

Pour assurer complétement l'affrontement, faut-il faire une suture à points séparés ou une suture en surjet?

Les uns prétendent que les points séparés assurent mieux l'hémostase; d'autres attribuent cet avantage à la suture en surjet.

Il est certain que des points séparés bien placés et suffisamment rapprochés donnent un bon affrontement et une hémostase sûre. D'ailleurs, si le sang suinte entre deux points, il est aisé de placer un point complémentaire.

La suture en surjet est peut-être plus difficile à bien faire. Si on la serre trop, elle fronce et rétrécit. Si on ne la serre pas assez, elle laisse suinter le sang. Il faut serrer juste, ce qui peut être assez délicat. Mais elle est un peu plus rapide.

Pour les petites plaies que deux ou trois points séparés suffisent à aveugler, la question du surjet ne se pose même pas.

Pour les lésions plus étendues, je ne vois aucune raison péremptoire de donner délibérément la palme à l'un plutôt qu'à l'autre mode de suture. C'est affaire d'habitude et de préférence personnelle.

3.º *Réunions circulaires.*

Robert Abbé [1] (1894) est le premier qui ait tenté de réunir les deux bouts d'une artère complètement sectionnée. Il introduisait un mince tube de verre dans chacun des deux bouts et après avoir amené pardessus le tube les deux extrémités en contact, il les fixait par deux ligatures dont les deux chefs étaient réunis l'un à l'autre pour empêcher le glissement. Abbé n'a fait qu'une autopsie, et il a trouvé l'artère thrombosée. Mais il avait ainsi réuni des aortes de chats, et convaincu qu'aucune circulation collatérale ne pouvait suppléer l'aorte, il considérait la survie de l'un des chats comme la preuve indiscutable de la perméabilité du vaisseau. Jensen [2] remarque justement qu'une autopsie aurait été plus probante, et on peut admettre avec Gluck [3], qui a lui-même essayé cette méthode, que c'est tout au plus si elle peut assurer la circulation dans une artère pendant quelques heures. Ce n'est donc point pour son intérêt pratique que j'ai rapporté cette tentative; c'est parce qu'elle est la première en date et qu'elle a ouvert toute une ère de recherches audacieuses.

Bien des appareils ont été imaginés pour réunir les deux bouts d'une artère coupée. Quelques-uns sont fort compliqués. Nitze a employé sur des carotides de chiens un cylindre creux en ivoire qui a pour but d'adosser l'une à l'autre les tuniques internes des deux bouts. Jensen, qui a voulu expérimenter cet appareil déclare que son mode d'emploi est resté pour lui énigmatique.

Payr [4], outre les tubes que je décrirai plus loin, en a imaginé d'autres qui fonctionnent un peu à la manière des boutons anastomotiques intestinaux.

Il me paraît tout à fait inutile de donner la description de ces appareils qui ont été à peine expérimentés.

D'ailleurs, quand on étudie les travaux de ces dernières années, on voit que l'on en vient de plus en plus aux procédés simples et il semble que l'avenir ne soit pas aux appareils compliqués.

Pour éviter les redites fastidieuses que nécessiterait la description chronologique des divers procédés employés, je les réu

---

[1] *Abbé*, N. York Med. Journal Janvier 1894.
[2] *Jensen*, Archiv f. klin. Chirurg, 1903, T. 69, p. 938.
[3] *Gluck*, Archiv f. Kinderheilkunde, 1897, T. 31 — Berliner Klinik, 1898.
[4] *Payr*, Archiv f. klin. Chirurg, 1903, T. 68, p. 97 et 1901.

nirai en trois groupes: a) Les sutures invaginantes, b) Les réunions sur des appareils prothétiques, c) Les sutures bout à bout.

a) Sutures invaginantes. — La méthode qui consiste à invaginer par des sutures le bout central dans le bout périphérique a été imaginée par Murphy [1], dont elle porte le nom. Quel que soit le sort que l'avenir lui réserve, on n'oubliera pas que c'est Murphy qui avec sa méthode d'invagination a fait la première suture circulaire chez l'homme. Voici en quoi elle consiste essentiellement.

Des fils en anse prennent sans le perforer le bout central de l'artère. Les deux chefs de l'anse sont conduits dans l'intérieur du bout périphérique dont ils traversent la paroi de part en part et de dedans en dehors à une certaine distance (1 centimètre, 1 centimètre ½) de la surface de section. Trois ou quatre anses sont placées de la même façon à égale distance, de telle sorte que le bout central est engaîné dans un réseau de six ou huit fils qui vont le conduire dans le bout périphérique où ils pénètrent eux-mêmes.

Lorsqu'on tire simultanément sur les anses le bout central est en effet entraîné dans le bout périphérique où il s'invagine.

Malheureusement, les calibres des deux bouts étant égaux, l'invagination ne se fait pas toujours sans difficulté.

Dans ses premières expériences, Murphy passait les anses sur le bout central perpendiculairement au grand axe du vaisseau, comme des points en U. Ces anses étant placées à une certaine distance de la section, l'invagination était laborieuse, et pour la faciliter, il était obligé de faire sur le bout périphérique un débridement longitudinal, parallèle à l'axe du vaisseau.

Ultérieurement, il a placé les anses sur le bout central, non plus perpendiculairement, mais au contraire parallèlement à son grand axe. Il fait cheminer le fil dans l'épaisseur même de la paroi (sans perforer la tunique interne) de telle sorte que, pénétrant à une certaine distance de la surface de section, il ressorte tout près d'elle. L'invagination devient ainsi plus facile. Bouglé [2] était de son côté arrivé à la même technique sans connaître les travaux de Murphy.

---

[1] *Murphy*, Med. Rec. N. York, 16 janvier 1897, et Congrès de Moscou, 1897, T. V, p. 38.
[2] *Bouglé*, Soc. Anat. 1920, p. 764. Archives de Méd. expérimentale, 1921 (Mars) et Chirurgie des artères, veines, etc., 1 vol. Paris 1921, p. 63.

Lorsque les fils sont serrés, le bout central est invaginé dans le bout périphérique, et les surfaces accolées sont larges. Murphy complète la coaptation en fixant par quelques points séparés le bord du bout périphérique invaginant au bout central invaginé. Ces points ne prennent qu'une partie de l'épaisseur du bout central et perforent de part en part le bout périphérique, mais en un point où il ne peut plus être en rapport avec le sang.

Dans quelques cas, Murphy a en outre récliné l'adventice sur le bout central invaginant, puis, l'invagination faite, il l'a rabattue sur la ligne de suture et fixée par quelques points.

Quand l'opération de Murphy est terminée, aucun fil n'est apparent dans la lumière du vaisseau. C'était là, je crois, le but principal que se proposait l'auteur, car à l'époque où il faisait ses recherches, en 1897, on redoutait encore la présence de corps étrangers comme agent de coagulation.

Mais, s'il n'y a pas de fil dans le canal artériel, en revanche, la surface de section du bout central (invaginé) baigne dans le sang. Comme elle est dépourvue d'endothélium, elle joue le rôle de corps étranger à l'égal d'un fil, et, tant qu'elle n'est pas revêtue d'un vernis endothélial, elle peut être un point d'appel pour la coagulation. La méthode de Murphy n'atteint donc pas le but qu'elle se propose.

Elle a cependant des avantages. Elle assure parfaitement l'hémostase immédiate. Elle doit donner des réunions d'une extrême solidité puisqu'au point réuni, la paroi est double.

Mais elle rétrécit fatalement le vaisseau. Le rétrécissement n'est peut-être pas définitif, puisque dans une des expériences de Jensen (¹), au bout de 54 jours, la lumière de l'artère a paru normale, ou, si elle était modifiée, c'était plutôt dans le sens de l'élargissement. Il n'en est pas moins vrai que le rétrécissement du début favorise la coagulation.

Enfin, cette méthode d'invagination est d'une exécution difficile. C'est une considération dont il faut tenir compte, non pas en raison de la difficulté même, mais parce que les manœuvres prolongées peuvent entraîner des altérations de la précieuse tunique interne.

Elle n'a pas donné, entre les mains des expérimentateurs, de succès bien éclatants. Sur onze expériences faites avec son pre-

---

(¹) *Jensen*, Archiv f. klin. Chirurg., 1902, T. 66, p. 938.

mier procédé, Murphy a eu huit thromboses et trois artères perméables mais rétrécies.

Doerfler [1] a fait quatre expériences sur des chiens. Trois fois l'artère s'est thrombosée; le quatrième animal est mort le troisième jour d'une hémorrhagie qui s'est faite non par l'artère mais par une veine blessée au cours de l'opération. L'artère était encore perméable.

Bouglé avec la première technique de Murphy a toujours échoué. Jensen qui l'a essayée ne la recommande pas.

En somme, les avantages de cette méthode ne paraissent pas compenser ses inconvénients.

b) Réunion sur des appareils prothétiques. — J'ai déjà parlé succinctement des tentatives faites par Abbé de suturer les artères sur des tubes de verre. On s'est servi aussi comme soutien de tubes caramel qui n'ont d'autre but que de faciliter la suture car ils fondent en quelques minutes dès que le courant sanguin est rétabli.

Toutes les prothèses endovasculaires sont complètement abandonnées aujourd'hui.

Payr [2] se sert de prothèse extra-vasculaire et sa méthode se distingue de toutes les autres en ce qu'elle ne comporte aucune suture.

L'appareil se compose d'un simple tube de magnésium pourvu de rainures. Hoepfner [3], qui a fait de très belles expériences par cette méthode, a légèrement modifié les tubes de Payr. Il les a raccourcis de manière à proportionner leur longueur à leur diamètre. Voici les dimensions qu'il a adoptées. Il donne aux tubes de trois millimètres de diamètre une longueur de 5 mm. et place la rainure à trois millimètres d'une extrémité. Il augmente la longueur avec le diamètre, mais dans une faible proportion, si bien que les tubes de 12 millimètres de diamètre ne mesurent que 8 millimètres de long. En outre, l'épaisseur du tube a été réduite autant que possible.

Voici la manière de se servir du tube de magnésium. Il reste complètement en dehors du vaisseau. Cette prothèse est donc, je le répète, extra-vasculaire. C'est le bout central de l'artère que le tube doit entourer.

---

[1] Doerfler, Beiträg. zur klin. Chirurg., 1899.
[2] Payr, Arch. f. klin. Chir., 1900, T. 62, et 1901
[3] Hoepfner, Arch. f. klin. Chir., 1903, T. 70, p. 415.

Le vaisseau étant bien libéré et les pinces destinées à l'hémostase temporaire mises en place, on passe dans le bout central près de la surface de section trois fils régulièrement espacés qui traversent la paroi de part en part.

On conduit les trois fils dans le tube métallique et on entraîne l'artère à leur suite, de façon que la surface de section dépasse le cylindre de magnésium. Celui-ci se trouve donc placé autour de l'artère comme une bague autour d'un doigt.

Pour maintenir le tube en place et l'empêcher de glisser, Hœpfner a fait construire une pince spéciale qui est sans doute très commode, mais on peut se servir d'une pince ordinaire.

On confie l'un des fils à un aide, l'opérateur saisit les deux autres. En exerçant des tractions simultanément sur les trois fils, on retourne le bout artériel qui dépasse le tube, de telle façon que sa face externe vienne reposer sur le métal, et que la face interne regarde au dehors. La bague métallique est donc coiffée de l'artère retournée, et pour maintenir cette dernière, on la lie par un fil circulaire qui doit entrer dans la rainure. Les chefs de ce fil sont coupés au ras du nœud.

On arme ensuite le bout périphérique de trois fils comme on avait fait pour le bout central. En se servant de ces trois fils pour élargir le vaisseau, et l'attirer, on le fait passer par-dessus le bout central retourné. En d'autres termes, on invagine le bout central dans le bout périphérique, mais comme le premier a été retourné, ce sont les tuniques internes qui sont au contact. Le bout périphérique est entraîné jusqu'au-delà de la portion retournée du bout central, et on le fixe là par une ligature circulaire qui se trouve plus près du cœur que la première.

Les anses de fils passés dans la paroi servent uniquement à manier les deux bouts du vaisseau et sont enlevés.

Ainsi, par cette méthode, on obtient un large affrontement des tuniques internes, et cela sans suture, avec deux simples ligatures circulaires. Elle est incontestablement fort ingénieuse.

Son auteur dit en avoir obtenu de bons résultats, mais il n'a pas donné le détail de ses expériences. Il l'a employée une fois sur l'homme pour une plaie opératoire de la fémorale. Le malade est mort le troisième jour de pneumonie : l'artère n'était pas thrombosée.

C'est Hœpfner (1) qui a le plus et le mieux expérimenté cette

---

(1) *Hœpfner*. Archiv f. klin. Chirurg. 1908. t. 70 p. 434.

méthode et il a obtenu avec elle des succès remarquables. Il l'a employée non seulement pour des sutures circulaires, mais aussi pour des greffes très intéressantes sur lesquelles j'aurai à revenir. Je ne donnerai ici que le résultat de ses sutures circulaires.

Elles sont au nombre de six. Deux fois l'artère s'est thrombosée. Dans les deux cas, la réunion avait été faite avec des tubes de 2 millimètres de diamètre. Hoepfner pense que la cause de ces deux échecs est dans l'étroitesse du vaisseau. Il ajoute que, dans ces deux cas, il avait essayé d'employer des tubes plus gros, ce qui avait amené des lésions de la tunique interne. On peut, il me semble, négliger ces deux échecs, car je ne crois pas que, chez l'homme, on ait jamais intérêt à faire la suture d'un vaisseau aussi petit.

Dans les quatre autres cas où la réunion a été faite avec des tubes de 3 et de 5 millimètres, l'artère est restée perméable. Il existait naturellement un léger rétrécissement dû au tube métallique, mais il n'y avait pas de caillots visibles sauf dans l'angle formé par les deux tuniques internes adossées où on pouvait en découvrir de très petits en cherchant à la loupe. Ces petits caillots n'allaient pas jusqu'à la lumière du vaisseau.

Il convient de dire que dans un cas, exclu par Hoepfner de sa statistique, il s'est produit une hémorrhagie mortelle. La réunion avait été faite sur la carotide d'un chien. Le cinquième jour, par erreur, on a lâché l'animal qui a manifesté sa joie par de violentes gambades. Le lendemain matin, on le trouva inondé de sang. Le bout périphérique avait glissé et s'était en partie détaché du bout central rétracté.

Il est intéressant de savoir ce que deviennent les tubes de magnésium. Le magnésium est résorbé, mais, sur la rapidité de la résorption, on ne peut rien tirer des expériences de Hoepfner. Ainsi, il a constaté que la durée de la résorption chez le même animal n'est pas la même au cou et à la patte. Il semble qu'elle soit plus rapide dans les régions très mobiles. Il a vu le tube fragmenté au bout de deux semaines, tandis que dans d'autres cas il ne l'était pas après plusieurs mois.

Les transformations chimiques qui amènent la résorption du magnésium produisent quelquefois de petits kystes gazeux. Hoepfner ne les a observés que dans les cas où l'artère s'était thrombosée. Il pense que les pulsations du vaisseau facilitent leur résorption.

J'ai dit que Hoepfner avait obtenu de magnifiques succès avec la méthode de Payr tant pour les simples réunions circulaires que pour les greffes.

Présente-t-elle donc de réels avantages sur les sutures?

Avec elle, aucun fil n'est saillant dans la lumière du vaisseau. Seule, la tunique interne de l'artère est en contact avec le sang. C'est là une condition incontestablement excellente.

Mais on peut se demander si dans la portion retournée du vaisseau, la vitalité n'est pas profondément troublée par la couture à angle très aigu. On peut se demander même si au niveau de l'angle saillant il ne se produit pas des éraillures profondes de la tunique interne. On peut se demander en somme si la perfection des résultats est due à la méthode ou à l'expérimentateur.

Toutes les expériences de Hoepfner ont été aseptiques. En lisant son mémoire et le détail de ses observations, on est frappé des soins minutieux qu'il y a apportés.

Jensen ([1]) n'a point été satisfait de la méthode de Payr. Il a essayé des cylindres en os, et a obtenu le retournement du bout central et l'adossement des tuniques internes en passant des points en U d'une manière ingénieuse, mais qu'il est fort difficile de faire comprendre sans figure. Il n'a pas obtenu de bons résultats de cette modification. Les sutures lui en ont donné de meilleurs, mais qui sont cependant inférieurs à ceux que Hoepfner a obtenus avec la méthode de Payr.

D'autre part, d'après Amberg ([2]), Stubenrauch, docent à Munich, a fait des expériences sur des fémorales de gros chiens avec les tubes de Payr, et, dans tous les cas, l'artère s'est thrombosée.

En somme, il est singulièrement difficile de porter un jugement sur la méthode de Payr. D'accord avec la grande majorité des chirurgiens, je suis peu enclin à remplacer les sutures par des appareils prothétiques, mais il est impossible de ne pas être très frappé des bons résultats de Hoepfner.

c) Sutures directes. — Quelle que soit la manière dont on veuille placer les points de suture, il est bon d'employer un petit artifice qui a été recommandé par Jensen ([3]) et par Carrel ([4]). Il consiste à placer d'abord deux, trois ou quatre points équidistants

([1]) Jensen, Archiv f. klin. Chirurg. 1903, T. 69, p. 934.
([2]) Amberg, Deutsche Zeit. f. Chirurgie. 1903, T. 68.
([3]) Jensen, Archiv f. klin. Chir., 1903, T. 69, p. 938.
([4]) Carrel, Lyon Médical, 1902, T. 98, p. 859.

qui fixent les deux bouts dans les rapports qu'ils doivent conserver et qui permettent de tendre le segment compris entre chacun d'eux de telle sorte que la suture en devient beaucoup plus facile. Jensen place aussi deux points cardinaux. Carrel en préfère trois, Floresco [1] quatre. Cet artifice, précieux pour les sutures artérielles, l'est encore davantage pour les sutures veineuses. Sans lui, la paroi des veines, trop flasque, est très difficile à manier.

On peut faire la suture circulaire d'une artère par de simples points séparés qui affrontent les deux surfaces de section.

Pour appuyer cette suture un peu fragile, surtout quand on ne fait pas de points perforants, Gluck [2] a imaginé le procédé suivant.

Il commence par réséquer un petit segment annulaire de l'artère et il le fait passer comme une bague par-dessus l'un des bouts. Il réunit les deux extrémités par un petit nombre de points séparés qui ne prennent que les deux tuniques externes. Puis, ramenant l'anneau réséqué sur la ligne de suture, il le fixe par quelques points tout à fait superficiels.

Cet anneau enserre la suture en exerçant une certaine striction. Il la maintient et assure l'hémostase immédiate.

D'après Gluck, on pourrait se servir de même d'anneaux d'os décalcifié, de caoutchouc ou de segments d'artères et de veines provenant d'un autre animal.

Tous ces artifices ont été abandonnés. Depuis Jensen, je ne connais aucun expérimentateur qui les ait essayés. On marche de plus en plus vers la simplicité.

Pour affronter les surfaces de section, on peut naturellement remplacer les points séparés par un surjet.

Quelques expérimentateurs donnent la préférence au point en U. Cette technique a été employée pour la première fois par Brieau et Jaboulay [3] (1896). Salomoni [4] s'en est servi sans connaître les travaux des deux auteurs précédents. Jensen [5], Amberg [6] la considèrent comme la meilleure.

On passe à une petite distance des surfaces de section des

[1] *Floresco*, Journal de Physiologie et de Pathologie générale, 1905, p. 37 et 47.
[2] *Gluck*, Archiv f. Kinderheilkunde, 1897, T. 44.
[3] *Brieau et Jaboulay*, Soc. de Sc. Méd. de Lyon, 1898 9 et 15 février.
[4] *Salomoni*, La Chirurg., Milano 1900, T. VIII, p. 241, et Gaz. degli osp. 1900, T. 21, p. 872.
[5] *Jensen*, Archiv. f. klin. Chirurg., 1903, T. 69, p. 939.
[6] *Amberg*, Deutsche Zeit. f. Chirurg., 1903, T. 68.

points en U, qui, lorsqu'ils sont serrés, affrontent les tuniques internes en éversant les bords des deux bouts. La suture terminée, il se forme donc un bourrelet circulaire comme celui qui sert à joindre les tuyaux de fonte.

Tel est le principe; il y a quelques variantes dans l'application.

Il est toujours commode de placer d'abord deux ou trois points cardinaux qui facilitent beaucoup la suture dans les espaces compris entre eux.

On peut suturer ces espaces intermédiaires soit par des points en U séparés, soit par une suture continue en passant alternativement le fil du bout central vers le bout périphérique, et du bout périphérique vers le bout central.

La suture terminée, on peut encore réunir par un surjet la partie saillante des deux bouts éversés. C'est ce qu'a fait Clermont[1] pour les sutures veineuses. Il exécute une suture continue en U, puis affronte par un surjet les bords des deux bouts éversés et donne à cet ensemble le nom de suture rabattue.

Briau et Jaboulay ont fait d'abord par leur procédé sur des carotides de chiens des expériences qui ont toutes échoué. Dans tous les cas, l'artère s'est thrombosée. Puis, ils ont opéré sur une carotide d'âne avec un succès complet. Trois semaines après, l'artère était perméable.

Salomoni a suturé l'aorte d'un chien avec un résultat parfait constaté également au bout de trois semaines.

Sur neuf expériences, Jensen n'a obtenu que trois artères perméables.

Pour les sutures veineuses, les prothèses ne semblent pas avoir donné de bons résultats. Bien qu'il ait réussi deux fois à conserver la perméabilité avec des anneaux d'os, Jensen ne les recommande pas.

La suture en U est plus difficile à pratiquer que sur les artères, mais elle est excellente. C'est là surtout que deux ou trois points cardinaux, qui permettent de tendre les segments compris entre eux, rendent des services.

Le simple surjet, toujours avec deux ou trois points cardinaux séparés, est plus simple et rapide. Jensen le préfère, bien qu'il expose à un léger rétrécissement.

---

[1] Clermont, Presse Médicale, 1901, p. 229, n° 40.

Quel que soit le mode de suture que l'on emploie, il est un certain nombre de précautions qu'il faut prendre, car le succès en dépend en grande partie.

J'ai déjà dit que l'opération doit être rigoureusement aseptique. Les solutions antiseptiques sont toxiques pour l'endothélium dont le rôle est si important. Aucune ne doit le toucher. Pour enlever les caillots, il faut se servir uniquement de la solution salée physiologique stérilisée. Et il vaut mieux la faire couler doucement que de frotter avec des tampons, car les frottements sont capables de détacher des cellules endothéliales.

Il est une cause physique d'altération dont on ne se gare pas toujours assez, c'est le desséchement. Hoepfner [1] a fait très justement remarquer qu'il amène une certaine rétraction des bouts artériels où la circulation est suspendue et qui sont mis à nu. Il est probable qu'il flétrit l'endothélium. Lorsqu'on se sert d'appareils prothétiques qui nécessitent des manœuvres d'une certaine durée sur l'un des bouts seulement, il faut bien prendre soin, pendant tout le temps qu'elles durent, d'envelopper l'autre bout d'une compresse imbibée de solution salée. Si l'on fait la suture directe, il est bon d'humecter de temps en temps la plaie avec la même solution.

Il faut éviter à l'artère tout traumatisme inutile. J'ai dit qu'on peut la dénuder sans danger sur une certaine étendue, mais il faut le faire avec précaution, éviter de la prendre dans des pinces, surtout dans des pinces à griffes.

Enfin, la suture de l'artère terminée, il est bon d'y ajouter une suture d'appui. Jassinowsky [2], Lindner [3], Silberberg [4] conseillent de suturer l'adventice; c'est un excellent moyen d'arrêter la petite hémorrhagie qui se fait par les points ou entre eux. Murphy [5] et Doerfler [6] recommandent de suturer la gaine. Gluck [7] suture les fascia et les muscles. Bref, il faut faire en sorte que les vaisseaux réunis soient bien entourés de tissus vivants et non pas isolés dans un espace mort.

---

[1] *Hoepfner* — Archiv f. klin. Chirurgie 1903, T. 70, p. 417.
[2] *Jassinowsky* — Inaug. Dissertat. Dorpat 1889 et Archiv. f. klin. Chirurg. 1891, T. 42 p. 816.
[3] *Lindner* — Berliner klin. Woch. 1895 p. 1023 — Berliner Klin. Avril 1898.
[4] *Silberberg* — Inaug. Dissertat. Breslau 1890.
[5] *Murphy* — Med. F. New-York (6 juin. 1896 — Congrès de Moscou 1897, T. V. p. 368.
[6] *Doerfler* — Beit. z. klin. Chirurg. 1899.
[7] *Gluck* — Archiv f. Kinderheilkunde 1897 T. 22.

C. — Anastomoses vasculaires.

Je ne sache pas que les anastomoses artério-artérielles aient jamais été tentées. Bien rares sont les régions où elles seraient possibles. Y a-t-il des cas où il y aurait avantage à anastomoser la thyroïdienne inférieure, la vertébrale, la carotide primitive l'une avec l'autre, ou bien des artères abdominales? Ces cas sont singulièrement rares. Il y a là cependant une possibilité qu'il faut avoir présente à la mémoire pour le cas où l'on se trouverait en présence de lésions où elle pourrait rendre service.

Les anastomoses veino-veineuses sont souvent pratiquées par les physiologistes. Tout le monde connaît l'anastomose de la veine cave avec la veine porte ou fistule d'Eck. Cet expérimentateur, après avoir enlevé le foie de chiens, a également anastomosé la veine porte avec la veine rénale droite. Mais, je ne crois pas que des anastomoses veino-veineuses aient été tentées chez l'homme, et on ne voit guère dans quelles circonstances elles seraient indiquées.

En revanche, les anastomoses artério-veineuses ont été l'objet dans ces dernières années de nombreuses et intéressantes recherches.

On a fait des tentatives très diverses sur la nomenclature desquelles on ne s'entend pas. Aussi, est-il indispensable de fixer la valeur des termes pour être compris.

J'appellerai anastomose artério-veineuse l'opération qui consiste à aboucher une artère dans une veine.

Quand on substitue un segment de veine à une artère, on ne fait plus une simple anastomose, mais une véritable greffe. J'étudierai cette question dans le chapitre consacré aux greffes. Il ne sera donc question ici que des anastomoses.

Anastomoses artério-veineuses. — Deux types de ces anastomoses ont été étudiés, les anastomoses latéro-latérales et les anastomoses termino-terminales ou bout à bout.

Gluck [1] a réalisé dès 1898 l'anastomose termino-terminale de la carotide avec la jugulaire sur un chien.

Les premières tentatives d'anastomoses latéro-latérales pa-

---

[1] Gluck, *Berliner Klinik*, 1898.

raissent avoir été faites par François-Frank en 1881 et 1883 [1]. Elles avaient pour but d'étudier la physiologie pathologique des anévrysmes artério-veineux.

Il semble que dès qu'un orifice est ouvert entre une artère et une veine, le sang artériel, en raison de sa haute tension, doive s'y précipiter et le maintenir béant. On va voir qu'il n'en est rien.

Dans les premières tentatives, Frank mettait à nu les vaisseaux fémoraux sans ouvrir leur gaine et par conséquent sans séparer l'artère de la veine. Puis, par une collatérale veineuse, il introduisait une fine lame pour sectionner à la fois les deux parois adossées de l'artère et de la veine. Il n'a jamais réussi par ce procédé à établir une communication entre les deux vaisseaux.

Dans une seconde série d'expériences, il a fait l'opération en deux temps. Le premier temps consistait simplement à promener une sonde cannelée entre l'artère et la veine pour produire entre elles des adhérences. Le second temps était exécuté comme dans les expériences précédentes. Cette méthode en deux temps a donné à François-Frank quelques succès.

Raymond Petit [2], qui a fait avec succès des anastomoses véino-veineuses, n'a jamais réussi à anastomoser une artère avec une veine.

C'est San Martin y Satrustegui [3] qui a abordé l'étude de cette question avec un but clinique. Son important travail contient 40 expériences d'anastomoses bout à bout. Les pièces ont été examinées de 48 heures à 20 jours après l'opération. Toujours, la communication était obstruée par un caillot. Dans un seul cas, le vaisseau resta perméable pendant plus de deux jours. Ces expériences ont été faites en 1898.

Deux ans après, il essaya des anastomoses latéro-latérales de la carotide et de la jugulaire. Il suivit la même technique que pour une entéro-anastomose, mais en faisant un seul plan de suture. Trois expériences ont été faites sur des chèvres. Aucune ne semble avoir atteint le but. Sur l'une des chèvres, qui fut sacrifiée au bout de trois mois et demi, il semble qu'un orifice ait persisté, mais il était obstrué par une sorte de formation valvulaire. En

---

[1] *François Frank*, Soc. de Biologie, 1896.
[2] *Raymond Petit*, Soc. de Biologie, 1898, p. 70.
[3] *San Martin y Satrustegui*, Madrid, 1902 (Communication à l'Académie Royale de Médecine).

tous cas, des injections poussées vigoureusement ne purent faire passer d'eau d'un vaisseau dans l'autre.

Lecerclé (¹) mentionne dans sa thèse (1902) les tentatives de Bérard et Carrel qui lui ont été communiquées oralement. Il rapporte également que Carrel et Morel ont anastomosé bout à bout la carotide et la jugulaire sur deux chiens. L'une des expériences amena un phlegmon, l'autre a été couronnée de succès.

La même année (1902), Carrel publia dans le «Lyon Médical» un article très court où il parle d'une tentative de greffe d'un rein par anastomose de l'artère et de la veine rénale avec la carotide et la jugulaire. Malheureusement, il ne donne aucun détail et ne mentionne pas le résultat.

En la même année 1902, Vignolo (²) réussit l'anastomose artério-veineuse chez le chien.

Frantz (³) reprend la question en 1905; il publie le résultat de ses recherches dans un très beau mémoire sur les anévrysmes artério-veineux.

Dans une première série d'expériences, il opère en deux temps.

Le premier temps consiste à suturer sans les ouvrir l'artère et la veine fémorale sur une étendue de deux centimètres. Huit jours après, il ponctionne la veine avec un fin couteau et sectionne les deux vaisseaux au point adhérent. L'orifice de la ponction est fermé par un point de suture. Jamais la communication ne s'est établie. Vignolo avait également échoué par ce procédé.

Dans une deuxième série d'expériences, il procède comme San Martin. Les surjets lui paraissent préférables aux points séparés. Vignolo s'était appliqué à mettre les nœuds en dehors de la lumière vasculaire. Frantz n'attache aucune importance à cette précaution. Comme Jassinowsky, Silberberg, Doerfler, il a constaté que les fils de soie saillant dans le vaisseau n'amènent pas la thrombose. Ce procédé lui a donné des succès.

Goyanès (⁴), dans un travail très documenté paru en 1905, rapporte quatre expériences d'anastomose bout à bout de l'artère dans la veine fémorale. Dans un cas la suture n'a pas tenu, l'artère s'est détachée de la veine. Dans les trois autres cas, l'anastomose s'est complètement obstruée et transformée en un bloc cicatriciel.

(¹) *Lecerclé*, Thèse de Lyon, 1902.
(²) *Vignolo*, Pisa, 1902 (monographie).
(³) *Frantz*, Archiv f. klin. Chirurg, 1905.
(⁴) *Goyanès*, Revista de Med. y Cirugía Practicas, 1905.

En Août et Novembre 1905, puis en Décembre de la même année, Carrel [1] publie de courtes notes, où il procède par affirmations sans donner le moindre détail. Dans l'un de ses articles, il écrit :

«Pendant le seul mois d'Août 1905, C. Guthrie et moi avons pratiqué treize anastomoses artério-veineuses sans avoir un seul échec [2].»

Il ne donne d'ailleurs aucune technique nouvelle.

De cet ensemble d'expériences, il résulte qu'il est moins facile qu'on aurait été tenté de le croire, mais cependant possible d'anastomoser les artères avec les veines.

Il reste à savoir si le chirurgien peut tirer de cette possibilité quelque avantage pratique. C'est ce que nous chercherons dans la partie de ce rapport consacrée aux applications cliniques.

II. — GREFFES VASCULAIRES

Théoriquement, on peut concevoir quatre variétés de greffes vasculaires.

1.º — Le remplacement d'un segment d'artère par un segment d'une autre artère, que l'on peut appeler greffe artério-artérielle.

2.º — Le remplacement d'un segment d'artère par un segment de veine ou greffe artério-veineuse.

3.º — Le remplacement d'un segment de veine par une autre veine ou greffe veino-veineuse.

4.º — Le remplacement d'un segment de veine par un segment d'artère. Il est bien évident que cette dernière variété est purement théorique, et ne peut avoir aucun intérêt pratique.

1ª Greffe artério-artérielle.

C'est Hoepfner [3] qui a inauguré cette question des greffes vasculaires. Il y a été conduit par ses études sur la dénudation. C'est pour démontrer l'innocuité de la dénudation qu'il a fait sa première greffe artérielle, et le résultat en a été si parfait qu'elle a tranché du premier coup la question.

Il a mis à nu la carotide sur presque toute son étendue et

---

[1] *Carrel*. Soc. de Biologie, 9 déc. 1905. Presse Médicale, 30 déc. 1905. American Medic. 12 août et 30 nov. 1905.

[2] *Carrel*. Presse Médicale, 1905, p. 843.

[3] *Hoepfner*. Archiv f. klin. Chirurg. 1903 T. 70. p. 447.

il en a réséqué un segment de quatre centimètres et demi. Ce segment a été complètement détaché, et gardé dans une compresse imbibée de solution salée, pendant qu'on armait le bout central de la carotide laissé en place du tube de magnésium. Ce greffon fut lui-même muni d'un tube prothétique, puis replacé entre les deux moignons de la carotide, mais retourné, son bout primitivement central, étant placé près de la bifurcation. D'ailleurs ce retournement n'ajouta rien à l'intérêt de l'expérience.

Quatre semaines plus tard, le vaisseau fut mis à nu. Il était engainé de tissu cicatriciel, mais battait dans toute sa longueur comme un vaisseau normal. Ayant senti deux noyaux durs qu'il prit pour les tubes de magnésium, Hoepfner plaça une ligature au-dessus et une ligature au-dessous, croyant réséquer toute la greffe. En réalité, il avait enlevé la moitié seulement de la greffe et deux centimètres et demi environ de carotide saine. Cette erreur a rendu la démonstration bien plus éclatante, car la ligature s'est trouvée placée sur la greffe. Il a d'abord constaté que la portion qu'il venait d'enlever ne présentait pas de modification appréciable de calibre. La tunique interne était partout lisse et brillante.

Huit semaines plus tard, Hoepfner mit de nouveau la région à nu. Il ne faut pas oublier que la ligature avait été placée involontairement à peu près au milieu du greffon. C'est ainsi qu'on put constater d'une part que le greffon était capable de faire les frais de l'hémostase définitive et d'autre part que le point d'implantation était capable de résister à ces conditions nouvelles de circulation. Il n'y avait en effet au niveau de la ligature qu'un caillot très court et il n'existait aucun dépôt au point d'implantation.

Dans une autre expérience, Hoepfner (1) a réséqué sur le même chien deux segments de même longueur, l'un sur la carotide, l'autre sur la fémorale, et il les a intervertis; c'est-à-dire qu'il a greffé la fémorale au cou et la carotide à la cuisse. Des deux côtés le résultat fut parfait: pas de caillot, ni dilatation, ni rétrécissement des segments transplantés. Mais, chose singulière dont j'ai déjà parlé, les tubes prothétiques étaient résorbés à la jambe, ils ne l'étaient pas au cou.

Ces deux expériences établissent la possibilité de transplan-

---

(1) *Hoepfner*, Archiv f. klin Chirurg. 1903. T. 70, p. 417.

ter des segments d'artère d'un point à un autre sur un même animal.

Hoepfner (¹) a montré ensuite que la greffe réussit entre deux animaux de même espèce. Il a pris deux chiens de même taille, et il a remplacé un segment de carotide de l'un par un segment de fémorale de l'autre et réciproquement. La plaie fémorale ayant suppuré, l'artère se thrombosa. Au cou, au contraire, le résultat fut parfait. Au bout de 45 jours, l'artère ne présentait aucune modification de calibre : il n'y avait aucun caillot ; l'endothélium était partout lisse et brillant.

Hoepfner conclut justement de ses expériences que la greffe d'artère est possible entre deux animaux de même espèce. La dimension du transplant n'est pas limitée. La grosse affaire est d'avoir des tissus sains pour le recouvrir et l'envelopper complètement de façon qu'il se greffe aussi bien par sa surface que par ses extrémités. Il a gardé le transplant jusqu'à trois heures hors du corps en l'enveloppant de compresses imbibées d'eau salée. En cas d'inégalité de calibre, il vaut mieux que le transplant soit plus petit que le vaisseau qu'il doit remplacer.

Ces expériences sont incontestablement du plus haut intérêt, mais il est bien clair qu'on n'en peut guère tirer d'applications chirurgicales, car les circonstances où l'on peut disposer d'un segment d'artère sain sont bien rares. Cependant, le hasard pourrait les réaliser, si par exemple, dans un service de chirurgie, on avait en même temps à faire une amputation et à traiter un anévrysme ou un écrasement d'artère.

Il n'est pas douteux que la greffe artérielle aurait plus de chance de devenir pratique si l'on pouvait faire des greffes hétéroplastiques d'une espèce animale à une autre espèce.

On sait malheureusement que pour aucun tissu, les greffes hétéroplastiques n'ont donné de résultats durables. Aussi, est-ce sans grande confiance que Hoepfner a tenté des greffes hétéroplastiques d'artères.

Il a pris l'aorte abdominale d'un lapin et de deux chats, et a transplanté ces vaisseaux sur trois chiens à la place de la fémorale réséquée. Dès le second jour, les pulsations n'étaient plus perceptibles au travers de la peau. Dans tous les cas, le vaisseau s'est thrombosé. L'un des chiens est mort d'hémorrhagie au dou-

---

(¹) *Hoepfner*, Archiv f. klin. Chirurg., 1903, T. 70, p. 439.

zième jour. Chez un autre, au quatorzième jour, l'aorte du chat
n'était plus représentée que par un mince cordon fibreux se continuant avec la fémorale thrombosée. Chez le troisième chien,
qui fut gardé cent cinq jours, l'aorte du chat transplantée entre
les bouts de la fémorale avait complètement disparu dans le tissu
cicatriel.

Le résultat de ces dernières expériences est conforme à ce
que l'on pouvait prévoir. Le chimisme des tissus diffère trop d'une
espèce à l'autre pour que ceux de l'une puissent vivre sur l'autre.

2.º *Greffe artério-veineuse.*

La difficulté serait tournée, et la greffe vasculaire deviendrait
capable de rendre des services, s'il était possible de remplacer
un segment d'artère par un segment de veine.

Gluck (1) a essayé de substituer la jugulaire à la carotide.
Il ne s'est pas produit d'hémorrhagie, mais le vaisseau s'est thrombosé.

Hoepfner (2) a poursuivi dans cette voie la série de ses belles expériences. Mais aucune de ses tentatives n'a été couronnée
de succès. Se servant toujours de la méthode de Payr, il a d'a-
bord greffé simplement un segment de veine à la place d'un segment d'artère. Dès qu'on rétablissait le cours du sang, le segment
veineux se laissait fortement distendre. Son diamètre devenait
double de celui de l'artère.

Attribuant la thrombose à cette dilatation qui modifiait le
cours du sang à la manière d'un anévrysme, Hoepfner doubla la
paroi veineuse, c'est-à-dire que par-dessus le segment à transplanter, il glissa et fixa une seconde veine d'égale longueur. La dilatation fut beaucoup moindre, mais le vaisseau ne s'en thrombosa
pas moins.

Il transplanta des veines plus étroites que l'artère sans plus
de succès.

Enfin, il sutura étroitement les tissus circonvoisins autour
du transplant de manière qu'ils puissent lui fournir un bon point
d'appui. C'est cet artifice qui lui a donné le meilleur résultat.
Tandis que dans les précédentes expériences, les battements n'é-
taient plus perceptibles le troisième jour, chez le chien opéré de

---

(1) *Gluck*, Berliner Klinik, 1898.
(2) *Hoepfner*, Archiv f. klin. Chirurg., 1903, T. 70, p. 443.

cette façon on les sentait encore le sixième. Mais il se produisit un hématome et l'animal finit par mourir d'hémorrhagie.

Hoepfner attribue la difficulté de remplacer un segment d'artère par un segment de veine à l'insuffisance de résistance de la paroi veineuse. La pression exagérée amènerait la dégénérescence et celle-ci la thrombose.

Goyanès [1] a étudié cette question sous le nom d'angioplastie. Il a exécuté vingt et une transplantations incomplètes qui sont en somme des greffes à pédicule permanent. Elles consistent à anastomoser deux fois l'artère avec la veine correspondante. Après avoir réséqué un segment artériel, il sectionne à ses deux extrémités un segment d'égale longueur de la veine voisine et suture les deux bouts artériels aux deux bouts veineux sans dénuder la partie intermédiaire du transplant auquel il laisse ses connexions naturelles. C'est là ce qu'il appelle l'artérioplastie veineuse.

Six expériences ont été faites sur les vaisseaux iliaques et fémoraux. Un animal est mort pendant l'opération. Un second a succombé à des phénomènes infectieux, et l'état de la plaie ne permit pas d'étudier les vaisseaux. Dans les quatre autres cas, le vaisseau a été obstrué par des caillots et lorsque les animaux ont été conservés assez longtemps, on n'a plus trouvé à la place de la veine transplantée qu'un tissu de sclérose imperméable.

Les quinze autres expériences ont été faites sur l'aorte et la veine cave. Trois d'entre elles n'ont pu être menées à bien et se sont terminées par des ligatures. Huit animaux ont succombé le jour même ou le lendemain de l'opération.

Restent quatre expériences. Dans l'une d'elles la pièce fut enlevée le treizième jour sur l'animal vivant. La greffe était perméable. Il y avait seulement un léger revêtement fibrineux sur la suture. Les trois autres animaux sont morts: un le cinquième jour d'infection péritonéale, la greffe était perméable, — un le dixième jour d'hémorrhagie par désunion partielle de l'anastomose supérieure, — un le quatorzième jour: l'autopsie montra la perméabilité des anastomoses. Aucun renseignement n'est donné sur la cause de la mort.

Carrel [2] a repris ces expériences en collaboration avec Guthrie. Il a employé la suture avec trois points cardinaux, procédé dont j'ai déjà parlé. Il a obtenu des résultats merveilleux et les a publiés

[1] Goyanès, Revista de Med. y Cirugia Practica, 1905.
[2] Carrel.—Presse Médicale, 1906, p. 843.

plusieurs fois dans l'*American Medicine*, à la Société de Biologie, dans la Presse médicale, mais toujours sous forme de note d'une extrême brièveté, et sans donner le détail de ses expériences.

Il a fait des transplantations complètes, et des transplantations incomplètes.

Voici la note la plus complète qu'il ait donnée sur la greffe complète, sans pédicule :

«Un jeune chien de taille moyenne est éthérisé. Une incision découvre la veine jugulaire gauche, qui est disséquée sur une étendue de six centimètres et réséquée. Le segment veineux extirpé est alors soigneusement lavé et placé dans une solution isotonique de chlorure de sodium à la température du laboratoire. Après quelques minutes, l'artère carotide primitive est découverte et un petit segment de sa partie moyenne réséqué. Le segment veineux est alors interposé entre les bouts sectionnés de l'artère, et la circulation immédiatement rétablie. La paroi veineuse résiste très facilement à la pression artérielle. Les pulsations de la partie périphérique de l'artère sont plus faibles que celles de la partie centrale, sans doute parce que le segment veineux joue le rôle d'un sac élastique où s'épuise l'onde systolique. La plaie est fermée, et un pansement occlusif appliqué. Le cinquième jour après l'opération, l'état des pulsations n'a pas changé. Mais le treizième jour, on trouve que les pulsations du bout périphérique sont aussi fortes que celles du bout central. On pense alors que des modifications importantes sont survenues dans la constitution de la paroi du segment veineux. Le quatorzième jour, après éthérisation, l'examen direct et le tracé confirment l'examen clinique. Le vaisseau est alors extirpé. Les anastomoses sont excellentes, l'endothélium sain et la paroi veineuse reste béante à la loupe comme une artère. Elle s'est adaptée à ses nouvelles fonctions en s'épaississant beaucoup. L'épaisseur de la paroi veineuse est actuellement de 2mm88 à 4mm55, suivant les régions (l'épaisseur de la paroi de l'artère carotide étant 1mm25). L'examen histologique montre que l'hypertrophie porte surtout sur les éléments conjonctifs de la paroi.»

On voit combien ce résultat diffère de ceux obtenus par Hoepfner [1]. Un pareil épaississement de la paroi veineuse en quatorze jours, c'est merveilleux.

De toutes ces recherches, dont quelques-unes ont peut-être besoin de confirmation, il résulte que les greffes artérielles autoplastiques et homoplastiques sont possibles. Les greffes artérielles hétéroplastiques n'ont pas donné de succès jusqu'ici, et il est probable qu'elles n'en donneront jamais.

Les greffes autoplastiques de veines sur des artères n'ont donné de succès qu'entre les mains de Carrel. Quant aux greffes

<hr>

[1] *Hoepfner*, Archiv f. klin. Chirurgie, 1903. T. 70, p. 439

homo ou hétéroplastiques de veines, je ne sache pas qu'elles aient été tentées.

Il est un petit point sur lequel je voudrais attirer l'attention avant de terminer la première partie de ce rapport. Lorsqu'on fait des greffes vasculaires, et même de simples sutures, il est difficile d'éviter qu'il ne reste de l'air dans les segments vasculaires compris entre les deux pinces. Cette colonne d'air ne pourrait-elle aller former des embolies gazeuses quand le courant sanguin se rétablit? A la vérité, cet accident n'a jamais été signalé. Il est probable que l'air étant en petite quantité se dissout dans le sang. Toutefois, il peut être bon, surtout lorsqu'on fait des greffes, de le chasser en remplissant la partie du vaisseau comprise entre les deux pinces de solution salée physiologique.

DEUXIÈME PARTIE

Applications chirurgicales

La chirurgie artérielle sort à peine du domaine expérimental; par bien des points même, elle n'en est pas encore sortie. Il est donc singulièrement malaisé de fixer les indications des diverses opérations que les expériences ont montré possibles, et on peut craindre qu'il ne faille un temps fort long pour sortir de cette incertitude.

C'est qu'en effet il est difficile de se rendre compte des résultats des opérations pratiquées sur les vaisseaux chez l'homme. Après une suture artérielle, l'absence de gangrène, le rétablissement de la circulation, ne prouvent nullement que la suture a donné ce qu'elle devait donner, c'est-à-dire un vaisseau perméable. L'existence de battements artériels en un point périphérique par rapport à la suture ne suffit pas à prouver la perméabilité du vaisseau. La circulation collatérale suffit quelquefois à les produire. Ainsi, la persistance du pouls radial après une suture de l'axillaire ne prouve rien sur l'état du vaisseau suturé. L'absence de gangrène est moins probante encore, car il n'est pas d'artère dont la ligature amène fatalement la nécrose du membre correspondant.

La persistance des battements au point suturé a certainement plus d'importance, mais il y a bien des régions où ils ne sont pas perceptibles. Et alors même qu'on les sent, on ne peut être absolument sûr de la perméabilité du vaisseau. Hoepfner a constaté au cours de ses nombreuses expériences que des collatérales rapidement développées sur le trajet du vaisseau suturé se manifestent parfois par des battements perceptibles. On n'est à l'abri de cette cause d'erreur que si les pulsations n'ont cessé à aucun moment.

On voit combien d'incertitude comportent forcément les appréciations sur les résultats des opérations vasculaires.

A priori, on est tenté de se demander si les données acquises par les expériences sur les animaux sont applicables à l'homme. Je suis tenté de croire pour ma part que les résultats seront meilleurs, que la proportion de succès sera plus considérable, parce que l'asepsie y joue un rôle capital, et qu'il est plus facile de la réaliser sur l'homme que sur les animaux.

Je passerai en revue les diverses lésions au traitement desquelles on peut appliquer les modernes acquisitions de la chirurgie vasculaire. Ce sont: les plaies des artères et des veines, — les contusions des artères, — les gangrènes, — les embolies, — les anévrysmes artériels et les anévrysmes artério-veineux. Puis je consacrerai un court chapitre aux greffes de membres et d'organes.

Je dois faire remarquer que depuis deux ans les observations de suture artérielle sont devenues plus rares qu'elles ne l'étaient auparavant. Cette rareté est-elle réelle et due à une sorte de mouvement de recul? Est-elle apparente et due à ce que les chirurgiens au lieu de publier leurs cas en ont conservé la primeur au Congrès? Si cette dernière interprétation est exacte, le travail des rapporteurs est singulièrement ingrat.

I — PLAIES DES ARTÈRES

La question est de savoir si l'on doit remplacer le traitement classique, la ligature, par la suture.

Elle ne se pose que pour les artères de gros volume. La ligature des vaisseaux moyens n'entraîne jamais de troubles circulatoires; il est inutile de chercher mieux que cette opération simple et sûre qu'est la ligature. Félicitons-nous qu'il en soit ainsi, car tous les expérimentateurs sont d'accord sur ce point que par la suture la perméabilité est d'autant plus difficile à conserver que le vaisseau est plus petit. Au-dessous de trois millimètres, il est difficile de réussir; au-dessous de deux millimètres, l'échec est à peu près certain.

Une bonne suture assure l'hémostase immédiate aussi bien qu'une ligature, ce qui veut dire tout simplement qu'une suture bien faite est étanche. Les expériences et les faits cliniques ne laissent aucun doute sur ce point.

Si la suture permet d'obtenir l'hémostase primitive, met-elle à l'abri des hémorrhagies secondaires? Sur les animaux, les expérimentateurs ont observé des hémorrhagies secondaires assez nombreuses, ce qui n'est pas surprenant étant donné la difficulté de réaliser une bonne asepsie dans les recherches expérimentales.

Dans les quelques sutures faites chez l'homme, il s'est bien produit une hémorrhagie secondaire, mais elle est survenue à la suite d'un érysipèle. Ce sont des conditions où l'on en peut observer quel que soit le mode d'hémostase employé. On peut admettre, je crois, qu'une suture aseptique met aussi bien à l'abri de l'hémorrhagie primitive et des hémorrhagies secondaires que la ligature.

Pour qu'elle ait les mêmes avantages que la ligature, il faut encore que la cicatrice soit solide, et qu'elle n'expose pas à la formation d'anévrysme.

Burchi après des sutures latérales a observé de petites dépressions en cul de sac de la cicatrice ; je crois qu'il est le seul. On n'a jamais observé d'anévrysme ni chez les animaux ni chez l'homme; mais, chez les premiers, le temps d'observation est trop court, chez le second, les faits ne sont pas assez nombreux pour que l'on puisse porter un jugement définitif.

Les examens histologiques de la cicatrice artérielle peuvent-ils nous renseigner sur sa solidité? Les résultats n'en sont pas très concordants. Jacobsthal [1] insiste sur la régénération des fibres élastiques. Salvia [2] au contraire trouve que tous les tissus des artères ont une tendance marquée à la restitution complète, sauf les fibres élastiques. Ce dernier conclut d'ailleurs que, par la suture, la structure du vaisseau est peu changée. Bouglé [3] admet que la restauration de la couche musculaire est possible.

Hoepfner [4] déclare que la forte prolifération de tissu conjonctif qui se fait autour de la suture, assure contre l'anévrysme.

Gluck [5] a insisté sur ce fait que la résistance normale des

[1] *Jacobsthal* — Beiträge zur klin. Chirurgie, 1906
[2] *Salvia* — Wiener klin. Wochen. 1902 p. 841
[3] *Bougle* — Archives de Méd. expérimentale. Mars 1901
[4] *Hoepfner* — Archiv f. klin. Chirurg. 1903 T. 70 p. 417
[5] *Gluck* — Archiv f. Kinderheilk. 1897

parois artérielles est bien plus considérable qu'il n'est nécessaire. Tandis que la pression du sang dans une carotide de chien est seulement de quinze à dix-neuf millimètres de mercure, l'artère ne se rompt que sous une pression de sept à onze atmosphères. Chez l'homme sain, la carotide se rompt sous une pression de sept ou huit atmosphères. Athéromateuse, elle ne cède encore qu'à une pression de trois à cinq atmosphères. On en conclut que la cicatrice n'a nul besoin d'être aussi solide que la paroi normale. Cette conclusion est tout à fait illégitime. La résistance à une pression brusque est d'ordre purement mécanique. Au contraire, la résistance prolongée de la paroi artérielle à la pression sanguine et à ses modifications est d'ordre vital. Ce n'est pas par des considérations de ce genre que nous arriverons à savoir si la cicatrice due à la suture met en garde contre l'anévrysme.

Nous n'avons pas de certitude sur ce point, et il se passera de longues années avant que nous puissions en avoir. Ce que l'on peut dire dès maintenant, c'est que ce danger, s'il existe, est minime, qu'en tous cas il n'est pas tel qu'il doive faire renoncer à la suture, si cette dernière présente à d'autres points de vue des avantages sérieux.

Le grand avantage de la suture, son but même c'est tout en assurant l'hémostase de conserver au vaisseau sa perméabilité.

Ce but on ne l'atteint pas toujours. Pouvons-nous savoir, même approximativement, dans quelle proportion la suture assure le libre cours du sang? Je ne le crois pas. Dans la première partie de ce rapport consacré aux recherches expérimentales, j'ai cité un certain nombre de chiffres. Il ne servirait à rien de les grouper, car les méthodes employées sont trop nombreuses. On ne peut non plus se renseigner exactement sur la valeur relative des diverses méthodes, et parce que, pour chacune d'elles, les faits ne sont pas assez nombreux, et surtout parce que la différence des résultats parait tenir bien plus à l'expérimentateur, aux conditions de l'expérience qu'à la méthode employée.

Le fait principal qui se dégage de toutes les recherches expérimentales, c'est que la principale condition du succès est l'asepsie.

Un grand nombre d'expérimentateurs ont émis cette opinion que la suture, alors même qu'elle entraînerait la thrombose, rendrait encore des services. L'oblitération progressive qui se produit alors laisserait à la circulation collatérale le temps de s'établir. Elle exposerait moins à la gangrène que l'arrêt brusque causé par la ligature-

Il est fort probable qu'une thrombose qui, d'abord rétrécissante, devient lentement et progressivement oblitérante peut laisser aux collatérales le temps de se dilater, mais une autre question intervient, celle des embolies. N'est-il pas à craindre que des fragments du caillot se détachent et aillent emboliser des vaisseaux plus petits?

Ce danger n'est point purement hypothétique. Chez le malade de Ferguson (1), il ne semble pas douteux qu'il se soit produit une embolie dans le mollet au bout de 41 heures. La gangrène en résulta. Étant donné le petit nombre de sutures qui ont été pratiquées chez l'homme, ce fait prend une grande importance. Bien qu'il n'y ait pas eu de gangrène dans le cas de Wiart il semble bien qu'il se soit produit aussi une embolie.

Il ne faut pas oublier que le but de la suture, c'est de diminuer les chances de gangrène. Or, avec les ligatures, ces chances sont extrêmement faibles. Ce serait faire un marché de dupe que de ne pas les diminuer et surtout de les augmenter par une opération délicate et longue.

La lenteur de l'obstruction après suture, comparée à la brusquerie après ligature, n'a peut-être pas autant d'avantage qu'on l'a dit. Je me demande si ce faible avantage peut être mis en balance avec le danger des embolies. Il est possible que cela dépende beaucoup de l'artère blessée et c'est ce que je chercherai à déterminer plus loin. Mais d'une manière générale, il ne me semble pas de nature à faire préférer la suture quand les conditions sont telles que la perméabilité du vaisseau soit gravement compromise. En d'autres termes, quand on ne peut espérer d'une suture d'autre résultat que d'amener une oblitération progressive du vaisseau, je me demande si on est en droit de la préférer à la ligature et parce que l'avantage de la lenteur de l'obstruction n'est pas considérable, et parce que le danger des embolies est réel.

Nous avons vu que la septicité est la principale cause de la thrombose. Or, dans les plaies accidentelles, on ne peut jamais être sûr de l'asepsie. Aussi, est-on conduit à se demander dans quelle mesure on est autorisé à suturer une plaie accidentelle. Cela dépend évidemment de la proportion dans laquelle la ligature expose à la gangrène et cette proportion varie singulièrement avec chaque artère, ainsi que je le disais tout à l'heure. S'il fallait

---

(1) Ferguson — Annals of Surgery, 1903 May.

adopter une conclusion générale, je me rangerais volontiers à celle que Lejars a ainsi formulé: «Si l'on n'est pas en mesure de réaliser une asepsie complète, mieux vaut encore faire la ligature».

Je donnerai ici le résultat de quelques sutures artérielles que j'ai pu relever, en les rangeant par artères.

1.º *Plaies des artères de l'avant-bras.*

Je ne crois pas qu'il y ait jamais avantage à suturer les artères de l'avant-bras, car il est sans exemple que leur ligature ait amené la gangrène.

Si j'ai ouvert ce chapitre, c'est uniquement pour rapporter l'observation de Delanglade ([1]) qui a suturé la radiale et la cubitale simultanément coupées à un travers de doigt au-dessous de leur origine. Cette double suture n'a certainement pas atteint son but. On n'a jamais pu sentir les battements de la radiale dans la gouttière du pouls. Il s'est produit une plaque de sphacèle superficielle à la partie antéro-supérieure de l'avant-bras. Cette gangrène cutanée ne peut guère s'expliquer par une insuffisance de la circulation et il y a lieu de se demander si elle n'a pas été produite par de petites embolies.

2.º *Plaies de l'humérale.*

C'est sur l'humérale qu'a été faite la première suture artérielle par Hallowell ([2]) en 1758. L'artère avait été piquée au cours d'une saignée. Hallowell fit une suture entortillée avec une seule épingle. Celle-ci se détacha le 14.º jour. Le pouls radial était perceptible.

Depuis l'ère antiseptique, je trouve sept sutures de l'humérale, trois pour les anévrysmes que nous retrouverons plus loin et quatre pour des plaies accidentelles. Dans tous les cas, il s'agit de suture latérale. En voici un court résumé:

Garrè ([3]). Plaie par coup de fourche au-dessus du coude. La moitié de la circonférence antérieure de l'humérale est atteinte. Suture transversale avec quatre points perforants à la soie. Le pouls a persisté mais plus faible que du côté sain.

([1]) *Delanglade.* Soc. de Chirurgie. Séance du 24 Avril, 1905.
([2]) *Hallowell,* cité par Lambert. Med. obs. and inquiries, t. 2, p. 360. London, 1762.
([3]) *Garrè.* Cent. f. Chirurgie, 1889, n.º 48.

Torrance [1]. Plaie contuse du bras. Hémorrhagie secondaire. Suture latérale. Guérison.

Torrance [2]. Plaies par grains de plomb de l'artère humérale et de la veine basilique. Suture de la veine. Suture de l'artère par un seul point. Mort le jour même d'une autre blessure.

Matas [3]. Plaie de l'humérale par coup de couteau. Suture au catgut. Guérison.

On ne peut tirer aucun enseignement de ces quelques faits. Nous ne savons pas si l'artère est restée perméable. L'absence de gangrène ne prouve rien, car la ligature de l'humérale n'amène guère de troubles circulatoires. La suture dans ces conditions n'est qu'un exercice de virtuosité. Quand la plaie est infectée, il vaut mieux s'en abstenir.

3.° *Plaies de l'axillaire.*

J'ai relevé neuf cas de suture de l'artère axillaire dont huit latérales et une circulaire. C'est Murphy qui a exécuté cette dernière:

Murphy [4]. Plaie par balle de la partie supérieure de l'artère axillaire. La plaie est incomplète, mais, comme elle ne se prête pas à la suture, Murphy réséque un quart de pouce du vaisseau. Suture par invagination. On perçoit de faibles pulsations dans la radiale le lendemain et le surlendemain de l'opération. Un mois et demi après, le pouls radial n'était plus perceptible.

Ce résultat n'est pas surprenant, car la plaie était infectée au moment où la suture a été faite.

Des huit sutures latérales, six ont été faites pour des blessures chirurgicales, l'artère ayant été lésée au cours du curage de l'aisselle pour des adénopathies consécutives à des cancers du sein. Voici un court résumé de ces observations:

Heidenhain [5]. Blessure de l'axillaire par un coup de ciseaux pendant une opération pour cancer du sein. Plaie longitudinale d'un bon centimètre. Suture perforante au catgut en un seul plan. Guérison. Les battements ont persisté, et on a pu constater au bout de six mois qu'il n'y avait aucune dilatation anévrysmale.

[1] *Torrance*, Annals of Surgery, Juillet 1904.
[2] *Torrance*, American Medicine, 1902, p. 1038.
[3] *Matas*, cité par *Hoepfner*, Arch. f. klin. Chir., 1903, t. 70, p. 430.
[4] *Murphy*, Med. Rec., 16 Janvier 1897.
[5] *Heidenhain*, Centr. f. Chirurg. 1895, n.° 49.

140 PIERRE DELBET

Durante (1) a fait une suture dans les mêmes conditions. Au cours d'une opération pour récidive axillaire de cancer du sein, l'artère fut blessée sur une longueur d'un centimètre. La plaie était oblique. Elle fut suturée par des points non perforants au catgut. Le résultat fut très satisfaisant.

Djemil-Pacha (2) a suturé deux artères axillaires également blessées au cours du curage de l'aisselle. Dans un cas la plaie avait 15 millimètres de long et fut fermée par cinq points perforants de soie passés avec une aiguille de Reverdin. Le résultat fut très satisfaisant. La persistance de battements dans la radiale et l'axillaire fut constatée après l'opération; il n'y avait aucun trouble deux ans et demi après.

Dans un second cas, la plaie, un peu moins grande, mesurait un centimètre. Elle fut fermée par quatre points passés de la même manière que dans la précédente observation. Le résultat fut très satisfaisant. Cependant, deux mois après, les battements dans l'axillaire et dans la radiale étaient plus faibles que du côté opposé.

Ricard (3) a fait dans les mêmes conditions la ligature de la veine et la suture de l'artère au catgut. Le malade a été présenté à la Société de chirurgie le 24 Mai, quatre semaines après l'opération. Le pouls radial était conservé. La malade ayant succombé quelques mois après à la généralisation cancéreuse, l'autopsie démontra la perméabilité de l'artère.

Dans le cas de *Halstead* (4) la blessure était plus étendue. Elle intéressait les deux tiers de la circonférence du vaisseau. La première suture faite à points non perforants fut appuyée d'une seconde suture portant sur le tissu conjonctif périvasculaire. La guérison se fit sans aucun trouble et deux mois après les pulsations étaient identiques dans les deux radiales.

Deux autres sutures latérales ont été faites dans des conditions différentes mais également aseptiques.

Ricard (5), en faisant une large arthrectomie pour une luxation ancienne de l'épaule, blessa l'artère axillaire sur une longueur de trois millimètres environ. La plaie était longitudinale. Il la sutura en suivant une technique un peu particulière. Il ne put

---

(1) *Durante*, Tr. de Pathol. et Thérap. chirurg., t. VII, p. 298.
(2) *Djemil-Pacha*, Congrès de Moscou 1847.
(3) *Ricard*, Soc. de Chirurgie, 24 mai 1899, et 1901, p. 349.
(4) *Halstead*, Med. Rec., 29 juin 1901.
(5) *Ricard*, Soc. Chirurgie, 1900, p. 1012.

pas placer de pince ou de fil à distance pour faire l'hémostase provisoire. Il semble qu'on ait mis la pince sur la plaie elle-même. «Le surjet, dit Veau [1], qui a rapporté l'observation, est amorcé à l'une des extrémités de la plaie, puis M. Ricard piqua les bords de la plaie au-dessus de la pince, en ayant soin d'entrer l'aiguille le plus près possible de la tranche afin d'éviter le rétrécissement. Il repasse au-dessus de la pince, qui n'est enlevée que lorsque l'aide est maître de serrer le surjet. Ce fil est arrêté par un point complémentaire.» L'intention de Ricard était de faire des points non perforants, mais quelques-uns ont traversé toutes les tuniques. Douze jours après, l'axillaire et la radiale battaient normalement.

Koerte [2] fut moins heureux. Au cours de la réduction d'une luxation de l'épaule, une collatérale de l'axillaire fut arrachée au niveau de son origine. Koerte ferma la plaie vasculaire par un premier plan comprenant quatre points, puis il fit par-dessus un second plan de deux points. Vingt et un jours après, une hémorrhagie secondaire obligea à faire la ligature. L'avant-bras se gangréna partiellement.

Cet accident jette un voile sombre sur l'ensemble de ces faits d'ailleurs peu nombreux. Au point de vue de la gangrène, le cas était mauvais, puisqu'il s'agissait de l'arrachement d'une collatérale. Le vaisseau arraché était perdu pour le rétablissement de la circulation.

L'artère axillaire est une de celles pour lesquelles on a encore discuté, il n'y a pas très longtemps, l'opportunité de la ligature à distance. Derocque [3] distingue à ce point de vue deux portions dans le vaisseau, la première qui s'étend de la clavicule à la naissance de la sous-scapulaire; la seconde qui va de la sous-scapulaire à la terminaison de l'axillaire. La ligature de la seconde portion condamnerait à la gangrène.

Soupart [4] déclare même que les suites de la ligature dans cette zone dangereuse ne peuvent s'expliquer que par une division prématurée de l'axillaire, et recommande la ligature de la sous-clavière.

Je n'ai pas besoin de dire qu'il faut bien se garder de suivre ce conseil, et que jamais, pour une plaie artérielle, on ne doit

[1] *Veau*, Gaz. des Hôpitaux 1901, p. 297.
[2] *Koerte*, Archiv f. klin. Chirurg. 1902.
[3] *Derocque*, Gaz. des Hôpitaux 1897, p. 1121.
[4] *Soupart*, Belgique Médicale 1898, p. 453.

faire de ligature à distance. Lier les deux bouts, au point blessé, telle est la doctrine universellement admise en fait de plaies des artères.

D'ailleurs, ces considérations théoriques n'ont pas de fondement sérieux. La ligature aseptique n'entraîne pas l'oblitération des collatérales. Voilà le point capital. Or, les anastomoses entre les scapulaires, les circonflexes et l'humérale profonde sont assez nombreuses pour assurer le rétablissement de la circulation.

Et les faits sont là qui prouvent que la gangrène est extrêmement rare après la ligature de l'axillaire. Bergmann [1] nous dit que, dans les temps antiseptiques, les ligatures de l'axillaire et de la portion terminale de la sous-clavière pour plaies par piqûre n'ont donné que de bons résultats. Koch [2] a réuni quarante-cinq ligatures dont aucune n'a troublé la circulation.

Aussi, ne peut-on s'empêcher d'éprouver quelque hésitation à remplacer la ligature, opération brutale, antiphysiologique, mais qui donne de bons résultats, par la suture, plus élégante, plus rationnelle, mais qui n'a pas encore fait ses preuves.

Certainement, dans les plaies latérales aseptiques on ne résistera pas à la séduction de la suture qui est alors facile et sûre. Mais pour les sections complètes qui nécessiteraient une suture circulaire, il faut attendre l'enseignement des faits.

4.° Plaies des carotides.

La carotide primitive et la carotide interne sont parmi les rares artères dont la ligature est inquiétante. La suture rendrait un signalé service si elle mettait à l'abri des accidents cérébraux.

Je n'ai pu relever que six cas récents de suture de ces vaisseaux. Dans les six cas, il s'agissait de suture latérale. Tous se sont terminés par la guérison. Trois portent sur la carotide primitive.

Dans le fait de *Seggel* [3], la plaie, due à un coup de rasoir, était transversale et mesurait trois à quatre millimètres. Elle fut fermée par deux plans de trois points à la soie. Aucun des points ne fut perforant. L'artère est restée perméable.

Au cours d'une intervention sur le cou, la carotide fut piquée par une pince à dissection. Depage [4] ferma la toute petite plaie

---

[1] *Bergmann*, cité par *Hoegfner*, Archiv f. klin. Chirurg., 1903, t. 70, p. 418.
[2] *Koch*, Langenbecks Archiv, 1869. In *Oberst*, Beiträge zur klin. Chirurg., 1904, t. 41, p. 439.
[3] *Seggel*, Münch. Med. Woch. 7 et 14 Août 1900.
[4] *Depage*, Annales de la Soc. belge de chirurgie 1902.

par deux points non perforants à la soie. Le pouls carotidien reparut immédiatement et persista.

Launay [1] en extirpant une tumeur du corps thyroïde fit à la carotide primitive une plaie longitudinale de quinze millimètres de long. Il la sutura par un surjet perforant au fil de lin. Il fallut ajouter deux points complémentaires. Le rétablissement du pouls fut immédiat. Quatre mois plus tard, les battements étaient perceptibles dans tout le domaine de la carotide externe, mais ils paraissaient moins forts que du côté sain.

Les trois autres sutures ont porté sur la carotide interne.

En disséquant des ganglions cancéreux du cou, Garrè [2] blessa la carotide interne. Il ferma la petite plaie par un surjet à la soie fine. Le malade guérit mais il succomba trois mois après aux progrès de son néoplasme. L'autopsie ne fut pas faite.

Dans le cas de Gluck [3], il s'agissait d'une thrombophlébite de la jugulaire. Au cours de l'extirpation de la veine, la carotide fut intéressée puis suturée. Le malade a guéri.

Le résultat fut également satisfaisant dans le cas de Ziegler [4] où il s'agissait d'une piqûre.

Il n'y a rien à conclure d'un aussi petit nombre de faits. Cependant, ils sont encourageants.

C'est une grande satisfaction pour le chirurgien qui se trouve en présence d'une plaie minuscule de la carotide de pouvoir éviter la ligature brutale.

Je n'ai pas trouvé d'observation de plaie suturée de la sous-clavière.

5.º *Plaies de la poplitée.*

Je n'ai relevé que cinq cas de suture de l'artère poplitée, et dans l'un d'eux il s'agissait d'un anévrysme artério-veineux de sorte qu'il n'en sera pas question ici [5].

Durante [6] en extirpant un chondrosarcome fait à l'artère poplitée une blessure d'un centimètre et demi. Il la ferme par une suture continue au catgut à points non perforants. Le pouls persiste. La récidive de la tumeur ayant obligé à amputer la cuisse

[1] Launay, Soc. chirurg. 1901, p. 672.
[2] Garrè, Cent. f. Chirurg. 1899.
[3] Gluck, Archiv f. klin. Chirurg. 1900.
[4] Ziegler, Münchner med. Woch. 1897, p. 733.
[5] Koerte, 33.º Congr. de la Soc. allemand. de chirurg. 1904.
[6] Durante, Fortschritte d. Chirurgie 1896, p. 283.

dix-sept mois après, on vit la perfection du résultat. On ne put constater aucune modification sur la poplitée ni à l'œil nu, ni au microscope.

C'est aussi au cours d'une opération que la poplitée avait été blessée dans le cas d'Orloff [1]. La plaie mesurait de cinq à sept millimètres. Orloff la ferma par trois points perforants de suture de pelletier. Il ajouta sur l'adventice et la gaine deux points séparés. Le résultat fut satisfaisant. Plus tard, l'amputation étant devenue nécessaire, on constate que la poplitée était perméable, mais rétrécie.

Dans le cas de Rotter [2], la poplitée avait été blessée au cours d'une résection de l'extrémité supérieure du tibia sarcomateux. Par la suite, le malade, comme les deux précédents, dut être amputé, et l'on constata que l'artère était thrombosée.

Dans le dernier cas, le seul où à ma connaissance on ait fait la suture circulaire, les conditions étaient moins favorables. Il s'agissait non plus d'une plaie chirurgicale aseptique, mais d'un coup de feu qui avait complètement sectionné l'artère.

Ferguson [3] réséqua les bouts déchiquetés de l'artère et fit la suture par invagination. Les articulaires supérieures externe et interne avaient été détruites par la balle. Tout semblait aller à merveille quand, brusquement, quarante et une heures après l'opération, une embolie s'arrêta dans le mollet. Les orteils se gangrénèrent, et l'on fit l'amputation médiotarsienne. Quatre mois et demi après, en excisant une bride dans le creux poplité, Ferguson constata que l'artère était perméable au niveau de la suture.

Il ne faut pas oublier que ce cas était nettement défavorable. La destruction de plusieurs articulaires rendait problématique le résultat de la ligature. D'autre part, la septicité probable de la plaie rendait la suture aléatoire. Le malade s'en est tiré avec sa jambe et la moitié de son pied; c'est un succès. Mais c'est en même temps un avertissement du danger des sutures, puisqu'il s'est produit une embolie. Ce qui est fort singulier, c'est que l'embolie se soit produite, et que l'artère soit restée perméable au niveau de la suture. Faut-il admettre que, le caillot qui a été emboliser les vaisseaux plus petits une fois détaché, il ne s'en est pas produit d'autre?

[1] *Orloff*, Cent. f. Chirurg. 1897, p. 605.
[2] *Rotter*, Deutsche med. Woch. 1901.
[3] *Ferguson*, Annals of Surgery, May 1903.

Doit-on supposer que l'artère s'est thrombosée et que le caillot obturateur s'est secondairement canalisé? Il est impossible de le savoir.

Ces quatre cas sont en somme satisfaisants. Et s'il est vrai, comme le dit Jensen [1], que les blessures de la poplitée entraînent la gangrène dans 54,5 % des cas, il n'est pas douteux qu'il faille les traiter par la suture.

6.° Plaies des artères fémorales.

Chez un alcoolique invétéré, Heinlein [2] ne put mener à bien une suture latérale de l'artère fémorale. Tous les fils coupaient le vaisseau altéré et il fallut en faire la ligature.

C'est malheureusement lorsqu'elle serait le plus nécessaire que la suture des artères devient impossible. Comme l'a fait remarquer Israel [3], chez les athéromateux, dont les vaisseaux sans élasticité se prêtent mal à l'établissement de la circulation collatérale, la friabilité des parois s'oppose à la suture, et chez les gens jeunes et sains, où la suture serait facile, on peut lier les artères sans danger.

Parmi celles dont la suppression est sans conséquence, il faut ranger la fémorale superficielle. Les succès qu'ont donné les quelques sutures faites sur elle n'en sont pas moins intéressants.

Dans le cas de Camaggio [4], la blessure était due à un coup de couteau et mesurait de trois à quatre millimètres. La veine était également intéressée. La suture de l'artère fut faite à la soie par points séparés non perforants. Le malade a été revu quinze mois après : l'artère était perméable.

Tuffier [5] a suturé une plaie de moins d'un centimètre qui était due aussi à un coup de couteau. Il a fait trois points séparés et par dessus un second plan de suture. Le résultat a été excellent.

C'est encore un coup de couteau qu'avait reçu le malade d'Henderson [6] qui a également bien guéri.

Enfin, Heinlein [7] a cité à la Société médicale de Nuremberg un cas de suture couronné de succès. La plaie avait été aveuglée

[1] *Jensen*, Archiv f. klin. Chirurg., 1903, t. 69, p. 938.
[2] *Heinlein*, Nürnberg. med. Gesellschaft 1900, in Hoepfner p. 429.
[3] *Israel*, Berliner klin. Woch. 1893 n. 32.
[4] *Camaggio*, Rif. Med. 1898 p. 304.
[5] *Tuffier*, Soc. Chirurg. 1904 p. 977.
[6] *Henderson*, American Med., Philadelphia 1903, t. 2, p. 53.
[7] *Heinlein*, Münch. med. Woch. 1900, n. 20.

par trois points de soie. Je ne sais s'il s'agissait de la fémorale superficielle ou de la commune.

Et je le regrette, car la fémorale commune est de toutes les artères des membres celle dont la ligature trouble le plus gravement la circulation. L'ancienne statistique de Schmidt [1] leur imputait 57,1 % de gangrène. Raabbe [2], qui distingue les blessures de paix et les blessures de guerre, arrive pour les premières à 19 pour 100, et pour les secondes à 21 % de gangrène.

Les ligatures simultanées de l'artère et de la veine sont encore plus graves. Ziegler [3] trouve 48,3 % de gangrène. Steiner [4] arrive à 55 %. Bergmann [5] avait donné antérieurement la proportion de 60 %.

Moulinier [6], dans sa thèse sur la ligature simultanée de l'artère et de la veine fémorale à la base du triangle de Scarpa, trouve sur dix cas traumatiques trois gangrènes ayant nécessité l'amputation. Les cas pathologiques qui sont au nombre de 23 ont donné de plus mauvais résultats encore. Onze malades seulement ont guéri, douze sont morts. Parmi ceux qui ont guéri, un a été amputé pour gangrène, un autre a eu du sphacèle de la plante du pied. Parmi ceux qui sont morts, cinq ont eu de la gangrène.

Mahé [7], avec juste raison, étudie à part les plaies opératoires. Sur huit ligatures de vaisseaux inguinaux, il trouve deux gangrènes. Sur neuf cas, où on a lié les vaisseaux inguinaux et les vaisseaux fémoraux profonds, six se sont terminés par la gangrène.

L'extrême gravité du pronostic donne un puissant intérêt au succès de la suture.

Gluck a cité un peu brièvement à la Société de médecine de Berlin, le 15 Juillet 1895, un cas de Zoege Manteuffel [8] où le bénéfice de la suture ne paraît pas discutable. Bien que l'opération ait été entreprise pour un anévrysme artério-veineux, il est tout à fait indiqué de la citer ici. Zoege Manteuffel fit au cours de cette opération la suture latérale de la veine fémorale, la double ligature

[1] *Schmidt*, Militärärztl. Zeitschrift 1876 p. 677.
[2] *Raabbe*, Deutch. Zeitschrift f. Chirurg. t. 5, p. 116.
[3] *Ziegler*, Münchener med. Woch. 1897 p. 731.
[4] *Steiner*, Cité par Hoepfner, Archiv f. klin. Chir., 1903, t. 70, p. 416.
[5] *Bergmann*, Cité par Hoepfner, Archiv f. klin. Chir., 190 t. 70 p. 416.
[6] *Moulinier*, Thèse de Toulouse 1893-94.
[7] *Mahé*, Thèse de Paris 1893-94.
[8] *Von Zoege Manteuffel*, Berliner klin. Woch. 1895 n° 36.

de l'artère fémorale profonde et la suture latérale de l'artère fémorale commune. Il est bien probable, presque certain, que si on avait lié les trois vaisseaux intéressés, le malade aurait eu de la gangrène. Or, il a guéri sans accident. Cette guérison peut être comptée franchement à l'actif des sutures artérielles.

Dans le cas de Sabanajeff [1], le résultat de la suture peut être vérifié.

Une femme de 28 ans atteinte d'endocardite ulcéreuse consécutive à une fièvre typhoïde, présenta des accidents d'embolie de l'artère fémorale. La gangrène envahit le pied et menaça la jambe. On incisa longitudinalement l'artère fémorale dans le triangle de Scarpa pour la déboucher, mais on la trouva perméable à ce point. Après l'avoir suturée, on pratiqua l'amputation de Gritti, et la malade succomba 19 jours après. La suture avait été faite à points non perforants. A l'autopsie, l'artère fut trouvée perméable; il y avait cependant au niveau de la suture un petit caillot long, mince et peu adhérent.

Murphy [2] a fait en 1897 la double suture de l'artère et de la veine. C'est le premier cas de suture circulaire d'une artère chez l'homme. Le malade avait reçu un coup de feu au-dessous du ligament de Poupart. L'opération fut faite 20 jours après l'accident. La veine fut suturée latéralement, ce qui réduisit son calibre d'un tiers. La plaie de l'artère mesurait douze millimètres. Murphy réséqua 16 millimètres et fit sa suture par invagination. La guérison suivit sans incident. Le pouls fut senti dans le pédicule quatre jours après l'opération.

C'est encore une double plaie de l'artère et de la veine que Lindner [3] a suturée chez un homme de 66 ans. En opérant une fistule stercorale dans la région du canal crural, il dénuda la veine fémorale commune. Comme les sutures ne tenaient pas sur les tissus altérés, il réséqua deux centimètres du vaisseau et le lia. C'est au cours de cette resection qu'une petite artère fut arrachée au ras de son origine dans la fémorale. Lindner ferma le trou par de petits points perforants à la soie et fit un second plan de suture sur l'adventice. Le malade a bien guéri.

L'observation de Kummel [4] montre qu'on peut réséquer un

[1] *Sabanajeff*, Cent. f. Chirurgie 1896 p. 928.
[2] *Murphy*, Med. Rec. 1897, p. 1093.
[3] *Lindner*, Berlin. Klinik. Avril 1895.
[4] *Kummel*, Münch. med. Woch. 1899 et Beit. zur klin. Chir. 1900.

segment considérable de la fémorale commune sans compromettre les sutures. Une femme de 52 ans présentait une adénopathie cancéreuse du pli de l'aine. L'artère était perméable, mais entourée par le néoplasme et très adhérente. Kummel la réséqua sur une étendue de 4 à 5 centimètres. La section inférieure était à un centimètre au-dessus de l'origine de la fémorale profonde. En fléchissant le membre, il arriva à rapprocher les deux bouts sans tension. Il invagina un demi-centimètre du bout supérieur dans l'inférieur. Après l'ablation des pinces, il se produisit une petite hémorrhagie qui fut arrêtée par une suture de l'adventice. La suture fut encore recouverte par un muscle. Par-dessus, la plaie fut laissée ouverte et tamponnée. La veine qui était envahie par le néoplasme se thrombosa. Les pulsations furent constatées dans la poplitée. La malade succomba quatre mois après à la récidive du cancer. L'autopsie ne put rien apprendre sur le résultat de la suture, car l'artère avait été complètement détruite par le néoplasme [1].

Ortiz de la Torre [2] a eu à soigner, chez un homme de 30 ans, une blessure de l'artère fémorale faite par un clou. La plaie avait 1 cm. de long. En raison du voisinage de l'artère fémorale profonde, il rejeta la ligature et fit la suture. Un premier plan à points perforants fut fait au catgut. Il ajouta deux autres plans à la soie. La guérison se fit sans trouble.

Matas [3] a traité avec succès par la suture un anévrysme artério-veineux de la fémorale dans le triangle de Scarpa. Je n'ai pu trouver aucun détail sur ce cas.

C'est certainement pour les vaisseaux du pli de l'aine que l'avantage de la suture se marque avec le plus de netteté. La ligature simultanée de l'artère et de la veine fémorale commune amène la gangrène dans une proportion qui oscille dans les diverses statistiques entre $\frac{1}{4}$ et $\frac{1}{2}$ des cas. Quelques statistiques donnent même une proportion plus élevée.

Or, nous trouvons cinq cas traités par la suture où les deux vaisseaux étaient intéressés. Zoege Manteuffel a fait la suture

<hr>

[1] *Landais* rapporte dans sa thèse (Paris 1902-1903) un cas de Krause avec l'indication bibliographique : Deutsche medicinische Wochenschrift 1902. Je n'ai rien pu trouver sur ce cas, ni dans ce journal, ni ailleurs. Voici ce qu'en dit Landais : Résection d'un morceau de l'artère fémorale au cours de l'ablation d'une tumeur cancéreuse. Invagination et suture à la Murphy. Le pouls semble se rétablir, mais la gangrène survient. Amputation.

[2] *Ortiz de la Torre*, in Cent. f. Chirurg. 1902, p. 637.

[3] *Matas*, cité par Hœpfner, Archiv f. klin. Chir. 1903, t. 70 p. 450.

latérale de l'artère et de la veine, plus la ligature de la fémorale profonde. Murphy a fait la suture latérale de la veine et la suture circulaire de l'artère. Lindner suture l'artère et résèque la veine. Kummell fait une suture circulaire de l'artère après résection d'un segment de quatre à cinq centimètres. La veine envahie par un cancer se thrombose. Matas fait la suture latérale des deux vaisseaux.

Ces cinq cas se terminent par la guérison sans gangrène. Si l'on songe au pronostic habituel de la ligature simultanée des deux vaisseaux, on ne pourra nier que la suture ait rendu dans ce cas de signalés services.

7 — Plaies des artères iliaques.

Je ne connais que deux cas de suture des artères iliaques. L'une a porté sur l'iliaque primitive, l'autre sur l'iliaque externe.

Au cours d'une opération pour pérityphlite suppurée, l'iliaque primitive fut prise dans une pince et déchirée obliquement sur les deux tiers de sa périphérie. Israel ([1]) fit la suture avec cinq points de soie en partie perforants. Il n'y eut aucun trouble circulatoire. Le malade fut suivi deux mois. Ce résultat est d'autant plus remarquable que la suture a été faite dans un foyer septique. On ne peut affirmer, il est vrai, que la circulation ait persisté dans le vaisseau.

Dans le cas de Wiart ([2]), l'iliaque externe avait été déchirée pendant une cure radicale de hernie inguinale. La blessure avait quatre à cinq millimètres. Wiart fit trois points perforants à la soie fine avec une aiguille de Reverdin et ajouta deux plans de suture sur l'adventice. La circulation persista au niveau de la suture, mais il semble qu'il se soit fait plus tard une oblitération au niveau de la division de la fémorale, sans doute par une embolie. Il n'en résulta d'ailleurs aucun trouble dans la circulation du membre.

Conclusions. — De l'examen de ces faits, pouvons-nous tirer des conclusions fermes et définitives? Bien certainement non. Ce serait tout à fait prématuré. On ne peut tirer de ces quelques cas que des indications vagues et provisoires.

Il semble que le résultat des sutures soit meilleur chez les hommes que chez les animaux, et ceci était à prévoir pour la rai-

---

[1] Israel, Berliner klin. Woch. 1896 n° 34.
[2] Wiart, Soc. de chirurgie 1903.

son que j'ai déjà dite, c'est que l'asepsie est plus facile à réaliser dans les conditions cliniques que dans les conditions expérimentales. Cependant, il ne faut pas être trop optimiste. Il est possible qu'il n'y ait là qu'un trompe l'œil. Les résultats expérimentaux sont des résultats d'autopsie. Ils sont certains. On a vu l'artère suturée, on sait si elle était oblitérée ou non. Les résultats cliniques comportent une grande part d'incertitude. Dans les cas heureux, on ne sait qu'une chose avec certitude, c'est que la circulation s'est rétablie et qu'il n'y a pas eu de gangrène. Mais s'est-elle rétablie par l'artère suturée ou par les voies collatérales? Nous avons vu qu'il est souvent bien difficile de l'affirmer, et par conséquent difficile aussi d'affirmer le bénéfice de la suture.

Il y a cependant quelques cas où les amputations nécessitées ultérieurement par la récidive de néoplasme ont permis de vérifier chez l'homme le résultat des sutures latérales. Durante [1] ayant amputé un malade dix-sept mois après une suture latérale de la poplitée put constater que l'artère ne présentait aucune modification. Dans des conditions analogues, Orloff [2] a trouvé le vaisseau perméable, mais rétréci. Par contre, dans le cas de Rotter [3], il était thrombosé, bien qu'il ne se fût produit aucun trouble circulatoire.

Nous n'avons pas de renseignements aussi précis sur les sutures circulaires. Je n'en ai relevé que trois cas sur les grosses artères. Le malade de Kummel [4] est mort au bout de quatre mois, mais le cancer avait envahi la région où la suture avait été faite, et l'artère était méconnaissable.

Jusqu'ici rien ne peut faire douter de la solidité de la cicatrice obtenue par la suture. Quelques malades ont été suivis pendant plusieurs mois. Djemil Pacha [5] a revu les siens deux ans et demi après la suture. Dans aucun cas, il n'y avait de dilatation.

En somme, ces résultats dans leur ensemble sont satisfaisants. Il est certain que la suture est un bon moyen d'hémostase provisoire et définitive. Il est certain qu'elle permet, dans un nombre de cas qu'il est actuellement impossible de préciser mais qui paraît considérable, de conserver la perméabilité du vaisseau.

Il est vrai que dans la majorité des cas, il s'agit de suture

---

[1] *Durante*, Fortschritte der Chirurgie 1896 p. 8..
[2] *Orloff*, Cent. f. Chirurgie 1897 p. 68.
[3] *Rotter*, Deutsche. Med. Woch. 189..
[4] *Kummel*, München med. Woch. 189.
[5] *Djemil Pacha*, Congrès de Moscou 1897

latérale, et l'on a tendance à traiter ces sutures avec un certain dédain. Mais il ne faut pas oublier qu'à défaut de la suture, une plaie même étroite d'une grosse artère oblige à la ligature tout comme une section complète. Le service rendu par la suture est donc le même.

Il n'y a qu'une ombre au tableau, l'embolie. Il ne semble pas douteux que dans le cas de Ferguson (1) la gangrène ait été due à une embolie. Il en est peut-être de même dans le cas de Koerte (2); et dans celui de Wiart (3), où d'ailleurs il n'y a pas eu de gangrène, on ne peut guère expliquer autrement l'oblitération tardive de la fémorale.

Il me semble qu'il faut tenir compte du danger des embolies pour poser les indications de la suture.

Au niveau de la ligne de réunion, quelque artifice que l'on emploie, il s'arrête toujours quelques globules blancs, avant que l'endothélium, en proliférant, ait recouvert de son vernis tout ce qui joue le rôle de corps étranger, fils ou tuniques artérielles.

C'est un appel à la coagulation, et si le sang est très coagulable, il peut se former un caillot volumineux et mou susceptible de se détacher pour aller former embolie. Or, il est une condition qui rend le sang très coagulable, c'est l'hémorrhagie. Tous les physiologistes connaissent ce fait, et je l'ai moi-même observé bien souvent chez les chiens. Si on saigne un animal et qu'on recueille le sang dans différents vases, on constate aisément que le dernier recueilli se prend beaucoup plus vite que le premier. Aussi, je crois qu'il faut se défier de la suture chez les blessés qui ont perdu une grande masse de sang. Non seulement la longue durée de l'opération pourrait leur être fatale, mais encore ils seraient par la suture plus exposés que d'autres à l'embolie, et les injections de sérum, bien loin de diminuer la coagulabilité du sang, l'augmentent encore.

L'autre condition qui expose aux coagulations étendues, c'est la septicité. Dans les plaies infectées il faut donc se défier des sutures.

Y a-t-il là des raisons de proscrire absolument la suture? Faut-il la proscrire résolument chez tous les malades exsangues,

---

(1) *Ferguson*, Annals of Surgery, May 1903.
(2) *Koerte*, Langenbeck's Archiv 1902.
(3) *Wiart*, Soc. Chirurgie 1903.

chez tous les malades septiques ? C'est affaire de degré, et c'est affaire d'artère.

A ce point de vue, il faudrait distinguer les artères en artères liables et artères dangereuses. S'il s'agit de petites artères, il vaut mieux lier. S'il s'agit de la brachiale, de la fémorale superficielle, qui parmi les grosses est le type de l'artère liable, si le malade a beaucoup saigné, si la plaie est septique, il vaut mieux lier.

Mais s'il s'agit d'une artère dangereuse, la carotide, la fémorale commune, la poplitée, le tronc tibio-péronier, l'embarras devient extrême. Il faudra des faits nombreux et précis pour nous permettre de porter un jugement. Pourrait-on suturer le tronc tibio-péronier ? Y aurait-il plus d'avantage à suturer qu'à lier la carotide primitive ? Nous ne le savons pas. Pour la fémorale commune, nous sommes mieux documentés. Sa ligature est si dangereuse que je la suturerais dans tous les cas.

Dans les plaies aseptiques, et ce sont surtout les plaies faites au cours d'opérations, je crois qu'il faut préférer, si l'on est bien outillé, la suture à la ligature.

II — RUPTURE SOUS-CUTANÉE DES ARTÈRES

Les ruptures sous-cutanées des artères sont extrêmement graves. Elles entraînent la gangrène dans la proportion de 88 %, trente fois sur trente quatre cas réunis par Lejars [1]. Le chirurgien ne peut rester simple spectateur de ce drame qui se termine par l'amputation et quelquefois par la mort.

Pourquoi la gangrène, qui est si rare après la simple ligature des artères, est-elle si fréquente après la rupture sous-cutanée ? Il y a à cela trois ordres de causes.

Les contusions graves des artères sont toujours le résultat de traumatismes considérables. Aussi la grosse artère dont on constate la lésion n'est pas la seule endommagée. Les artères musculaires, les branches collatérales sont également altérées, et c'est là ce qui rend difficile le rétablissement de la circulation par les voies de détour. Contre cette attrition des branches artérielles moyennes ou petites, nous sommes complètement désarmés; nous ne pouvons rien pour leur rendre leur perméabilité.

---

[1] *Lejars*, Soc. Chirurgie 1902, p. 60.

Une seconde cause de gangrène, qui me paraît réellement importante, c'est l'hématome. Les grosses tumeurs sanguines fortement tendues apportent un obstacle considérable à l'établissement de la circulation collatérale, car elles compriment les vaisseaux par où cette circulation pourrait se faire. Quand la rupture artérielle est complète, et que l'hématome est pulsatile, quand il existe, comme on disait autrefois, un anévrysme faux, cette cause de gangrène devient tout à fait prépondérante. Aussi, je considère que l'hématome commande une intervention immédiate. Il faut inciser sur le foyer, et évacuer les caillots aussi complètement que possible. Mais l'hématome n'est pas constant, il peut être insignifiant et même manquer tout à fait quand la rupture ne porte que sur la tunique interne.

Le troisième facteur de sphacèle, c'est l'embolie. J'ai insisté, il y a longtemps, sur le rôle des embolies dans les anévrysmes. Il est plus considérable encore à la suite des ruptures artérielles et surtout des ruptures incomplètes. Le caillot qui se développe au niveau de la zone traumatisée n'est pas d'emblée oblitérant. Il peut se fragmenter sous la pression du sang. Des parcelles se détachent qui vont emboliser des artères plus petites. Et ce qui fait la gravité particulière de ces embolies, c'est qu'elles s'arrêtent souvent sur des éperons de bifurcation, au niveau des carrefours vasculaires si nécessaires au rétablissement de la circulation.

Contre ces embolies, nous avons un remède simple et efficace, c'est la ligature au-dessous du point traumatisé.

La double ligature qui isole complètement le segment d'artère écrasé, c'est le moins que l'on puisse faire. Et cette intervention doit être aussi précoce que possible. C'est une opération d'urgence, car les embolies sont parfois très précoces.

«Chez notre blessé, dit Lejars, nous sommes convaincus que dès le début, un gros fragment du caillot a été se loger dans la poplitée (il s'agissait d'une rupture de la fémorale). Une demi-heure après l'accident, il ressentait une brusque et violente douleur au mollet, et dès le lendemain le mollet était tendu, dur, comme prêt à se rompre; le pied était insensible et inerte, et le blessé avait fort bien remarqué que cette insensibilité avait débuté aussitôt après la douleur brusque du mollet».

Peut-on faire plus? Lejars l'a essayé le 1.er Mars 1902. Il est tombé sur des lésions étendues et du siège le plus fâcheux. «L'artère est dure, noire, épaissie sur une longueur de 5 centimètres; et le segment contus commence à un centimètre environ au-dessous de l'arcade et finit à deux centimètres au-dessous de l'origine de la fémorale profonde. Cette dernière présente le même aspect sur une longueur d'environ deux centimètres. Une ligature d'attente, sous-tendue par un demi-drain, est placée sur le bout supérieur de la fémorale; j'incise alors l'artère au bistouri, longitudinalement sur une longueur de un centimètre et demi; je traverse une tunique adventice, au moins triplée d'épaisseur, noire, et totalement imprégnée de sang, puis une tunique moyenne, friable, comme effritée et écaillée sur la face interne, aussi infiltrée de sang, et je pénètre dans la lumière de l'artère, occupée par des caillots noirs, mous, irréguliers; j'en extrais quelques-uns avec une pince, et à ce moment, un jet de sang rouge, peu saccadé, surgit du bout inférieur. Une seconde ligature temporaire sur un demi-drain est placée le plus bas possible sur le bout inférieur, et j'achève d'extraire les caillots en comprimant légèrement le vaisseau de bas en haut. Je puis aller passer un stylet librement dans le bout inférieur de la fémorale et aussi dans la fémorale profonde. La perméabilité était donc rétablie de ce côté, mais en haut il n'en est pas de même, et la ligature d'attente enlevée prudemment, le sang n'apparaît pas. Je replace la ligature d'attente, et je prolonge l'incision artérielle jusqu'à lui donner une longueur totale d'environ trois centimètres, en dépassant la limite supérieure du segment contus; par la pression de haut en bas, je fais sortir deux caillots moulés, gros ensemble comme l'index. Cette fois, l'artère était libre aussi au niveau de son bout supérieur. » Lejars a terminé par la suture de l'artère. Malheureusement, le membre s'est gangréné, et il a fallu faire une amputation haute de la jambe.

Est-il possible de rendre à l'artère sa perméabilité en la débarrassant de ses caillots? C'est bien peu probable. Les caillots enlevés, les conditions qui les avaient produits, c'est-à-dire les lésions de l'artère persistent; ils vont se reformer dans les mêmes conditions, et peut-être envoyer de nouvelles embolies.

Seule, la résection du segment altéré permettrait de rétablir la perméabilité du vaisseau, et s'il est une lésion où les récentes conquêtes de la chirurgie vasculaire doivent rendre des services, c'est bien la rupture sous-cutanée des artères. Là, il n'y a pas comme pour les plaies incertitude dans l'indication, et il n'y en aura pas non plus dans l'appréciation des résultats. La gangrène est si fréquente dans ces conditions que tout résultat heureux pourra être mis sans grande chance d'erreur à l'actif de l'intervention.

Ce qui fait de la rupture sous-cutanée le plus chirurgical de tous les traumatismes artériels, c'est que le foyer n'est pas infecté. On peut faire une opération aseptique. Mais il faut reconnaître qu'elle présentera dans la majorité des cas d'extrêmes difficultés.

La présence de collatérales importantes se détachant du segment écrasé est fort embarassante. Ce n'est pas qu'on augmente le danger en les liant, puisqu'elles sont oblitérées. Mais, après la résection, on se trouve en présence de deux bouts artériels de calibre différent et la suture peut devenir très difficile, voire même impossible.

Une autre difficulté vient de l'étendue des lésions. La première condition pour rétablir la perméabilité du vaisseau, c'est de réséquer toute la partie altérée. Cette résection faite, la suture sera-t-elle possible? Nous ne savons pas ce qu'on peut réséquer d'une artère sans compromettre le rapprochement des deux bouts. Salvia (¹) a réséqué plusieurs fois un centimètre de fémorale de chien. Sur un bélier il réséqua 25 millimètres de carotide commune et trois centimètres de la même carotide sur un âne. Murphy a réséqué 25 millimètres de carotide sur un veau et 20 millimètres sur un chien. Kummell a réséqué de 4 à 5 centimètres de la fémorale commune et suturé les deux bouts.

La situation des artères du côté de la flexion permet de satisfaire leur élasticité et de gagner une notable longueur en pliant le membre. Il semble donc qu'on puisse en réséquer une étendue relativement considérable.

Si l'étendue de la résection doit être telle que la suture bout à bout soit impossible, ou ne puisse se faire qu'au prix de tractions qui compromettraient son résultat, faut-il tenter la greffe vasculaire?

La greffe artério-artérielle qui donne les meilleurs résultats n'est pas possible, car, où prendre le transplant? Il y a certainement des artères qu'on peut lier avec la presque certitude de l'impunité, ainsi l'artère brachiale, ainsi la fémorale superficielle. Mais, serait-on autorisé sur l'homme à sacrifier une artère saine pour réparer une artère malade? Peut-être, si le résultat de la greffe était certain, mais il ne l'est pas.

Reste comme dernière ressource la transplantation veineuse. Quand la veine, voisine de l'artère lésée, est saine, on peut faire

---

(¹) Salvia, Wiener klin. Woch. 1902, p. 84.

la transplantation incomplète, c'est-à-dire remplacer le segment artériel traumatisé par le segment veineux correspondant sans le dénuder. Encore, faut-il pour cela que la veine puisse être supprimée, en tant que veine, sans inconvénient.

S'il s'agit d'une veine importante, comme la veine fémorale commune, ou bien encore, si la veine est lésée en même temps que l'artère comme il arrive parfois, cette ressource manque. Faudrait-il alors aller chercher dans une autre région un segment de veine saine pour le suturer aux deux bouts de l'autre: faudrait-il en d'autres termes faire une transplantation veineuse complète? Dans l'état actuel de la question, je ne le crois pas, car les résultats obtenus jusqu'ici par cette méthode sont bien peu encourageants.

Quant à faire passer le courant artériel par les canaux veineux, je dirai plus tard pourquoi il n'y faut pas songer.

En somme, un seul point me paraît acquis. C'est qu'en cas de rupture artérielle, on doit faire une intervention aussi précoce que possible. Il ne faut pas attendre que la gangrène se manifeste. Dès qu'elle commence, il est trop tard. Quoiqu'on fasse, on ne peut plus revivifier les parties sphacélées, et si la gangrène est due à des embolies, on ne réussira même pas à arrêter sa marche.

Dès que l'arrêt ou seulement l'insuffisance de la circulation est constaté au-dessous du point traumatisé — et cette insuffisance se manifeste par la faiblesse des battements dans les artères périphériques, par le refroidissement du membre, par la lenteur avec laquelle un point comprimé reprend sa coloration rosée — il faut mettre à nu l'artère traumatisée.

Chemin faisant, s'il y a un hématome, on enlève les caillots aussi complètement que possible, et par là, on rend déjà service au malade.

Dans certains cas, lorsque la tunique interne seule est rompue, l'altération de l'artère n'est pas toujours nettement apparente par sa face externe. Mais, en la palpant avec le doigt, on sent un noyau dur plus ou moins étendu. C'est là que la tunique interne s'est recroquevillée. Le moins qu'on puisse faire, c'est de lier au-dessous et au-dessus du point lésé. Mais on peut faire mieux. Dans les conditions de lésion bien limitée, il me semble nettement indiqué, si l'on est convenablement outillé, de faire la résection de la partie malade, suivie de la suture circulaire.

Lorsque la lésion est assez étendue pour rendre la suture impossible après résection, la question de la greffe veineuse se pose; mais il serait prématuré de la conseiller.

III — Gangrènes

Il est fort peu scientifique d'étudier les gangrènes en bloc, même au point de vue du traitement. Les étudier séparément, c'est s'exposer à bien des répétitions. Et puis, dans le langage chirurgical courant, on ne fait pas toujours bien exactement les distinctions que commanderait la pathogénie. Ainsi, on appelle gangrènes diabétiques toutes celles qui surviennent chez les glycosuriques; or, il est certain, comme plusieurs orateurs l'ont fait remarquer en 1901 à la Société de chirurgie, que bon nombre de celles-là sont dues à des artérites.

Il ne sera naturellement pas question dans ce chapitre des gangrènes d'origine septique, je ne m'occuperai que des gangrènes par oblitération artérielle.

Elles ont fait l'objet de tentatives chirurgicales de deux sortes. L'une se propose de déboucher l'artère obstruée par un caillot, l'autre de remplacer les artères par les veines, c'est-à-dire de faire passer le courant sanguin artériel par les vaisseaux veineux.

Il y a deux manières de désobstruer l'artère. L'une consiste à inciser le vaisseau et à enlever les caillots; j'en ai déjà parlé à propos des ruptures artérielles, j'y reviendrai en parlant des embolies. L'autre, dont il sera seulement question ici, est le cathétérisme des artères.

1.° *Cathétérisme des artères.* — C'est SéVéréanu, qui en a eu l'idée. Il a communiqué au Congrès de Rome en 1894 sa première opération qui remontait à une dizaine d'années. Il s'agissait d'un homme de 50 ans, atteint de gangrène du pied, consécutive à une embolie cardiaque. L'artère ne battait que très haut, et il semblait indiqué de faire l'amputation de la cuisse. SéVéréanu fit l'amputation de la jambe au lieu d'élection; il introduisit une fine sonde urétrale en gomme dans l'artère, et exécuta des mouvements de va et vient jusqu'à ce que le sang commençât à couler. Lorqu'il retira la sonde, l'onde sanguine fit sortir des caillots cylindriques, et le cours du sang se rétablit. Les lambeaux ne se sont pas gangrénés, et la réunion par première intention fut obtenue.

SéVéréanu ajoute qu'il a employé plusieurs fois cette manœuvre et qu'il s'en est toujours bien trouvé.

Il faut remarquer que ce premier cas était exceptionnellement favorable, puisqu'il s'agissait d'une gangrène par embolie.

Guinard (¹) s'est servi d'un artifice un peu différent dans des gangrènes par artérite. L'amputation faite, il a introduit dans la fémorale une longue pince qui lui permit d'extraire des caillots fibrineux. Il a employé deux fois cette manœuvre «qui rend saignant un moignon qui ne saigne pas» et s'en félicite.

Martin (d'Angers) (²) a communiqué à la Société de chirurgie une observation qui est intéressante par les détails. Le malade, âgé de 57 ans, avait une artérite oblitérante de la fémorale gauche, d'origine grippale. La gangrène avait envahi presque toute la jambe. Bien que l'artère ne battît pas à la base du triangle de Scarpa, Martin fait d'abord l'amputation au tiers inférieur de la cuisse. «La section reste presque exsangue, les muscles ont une couleur très pâle. Aucun jet artériel ne sort de la tranche. La fémorale est oblitérée par un caillot déjà ancien, gris violacé, adhérent aux parois de l'artère. Je remonte le niveau de l'amputation, et scie le fémur sous le trochanter. L'artère est oblitérée, mais la veine est libre, et le suintement sanguin un peu plus abondant... Je cherche à désobstruer l'artère avec une sonde en gomme n.º 18; je cathétérise l'artère; le caillot cède, et laisse pénétrer la sonde. Par des mouvements de va et vient, je désagrège le caillot, et la sonde sortant de l'artère entraîne ses débris. Après un véritable ramonage, je creuse ainsi un canal dans le caillot, et le sang commence à couler en bavant; bientôt, un jet plus fort chasse les derniers débris du caillot encore adhérent aux parois artérielles; la fémorale donne enfin à plein jet. En même temps, les artérioles musculaires et la fémorale profonde se mettent à saigner. Celles-ci n'étaient pas oblitérées, et il a suffi de déboucher la fémorale pour rétablir la circulation.» La plaie s'est réunie par première intention. Martin affirme que pendant le séjour du malade à l'hôpital, les battements de la fémorale ont été constatés à diverses reprises. Ultérieurement, l'artère s'est de nouveau oblitérée, mais le moignon est resté solide et indolent.

Ce qui me paraît particulièrement intéressant dans cette observation, c'est que le débouchage de la fémorale a ramené la circulation dans la fémorale profonde et dans les branches musculaires.

En effet, il semble que dans les oblitérations par artérite, les branches qui se détachent du tronc principal doivent être obstruées

<hr>

(¹) Guinard, Soc. Chirurgie, 1901.
(²) Martin (d'Angers), travail déposé à la Soc. de Chirurgie en 1901 et resté inédit.

au moins à leur origine, et on se demande à quoi peut bien servir le débouchage de ce tronc. Le fait de Martin prouve qu'il n'en est pas toujours ainsi, et que le cathétérisme peut quelquefois rétablir réellement la circulation. Les cas ne sont pas toujours aussi favorables. J'ai essayé deux fois le cathétérisme des artères. Dans un cas, je n'ai pas obtenu la moindre goutte de sang. Évidemment, la sonde n'avait pas dépassé la limite supérieure du caillot. Dans l'autre, il est venu un peu de sang qui s'écoulait en bavant. Il est certain que l'artère a recomplété son oblitération dès que la sonde a été enlevée, et que le cathétérisme n'a rendu aucun service au malade.

Mais, lorsqu'on réussit à désobstruer le vaisseau, et qu'il verse du sang à plein jet, n'est-il pas à craindre que la perméabilité ne soit bien temporaire? Martin nous dit que tant que son malade est resté à l'hôpital, la fémorale a continué à battre. C'est un résultat fort heureux, mais qui doit être bien rare : car, si le cathétérisme supprime le caillot, il ne supprime pas la cause qui l'a produit, au moins quand il s'agit d'artérite. L'artère reste malade, et l'obstruction doit rapidement se reproduire. C'est seulement dans le cas d'embolie que le cathétérisme peut donner des résultats durables.

Il est d'ailleurs fort difficile de juger de l'efficacité pratique du cathétérisme des artères. La réunion par première intention ne prouve rien en sa faveur, car des lambeaux, en apparence exsangues, peuvent avoir une vitalité suffisante. Schwartz ([1]) a rapporté le cas d'un diabétique qu'il a amputé de jambe au lieu d'élection. «Pas une artère ne donna. La réunion per primam fut parfaite.»

J'ai le souvenir d'une amputation pratiquée dans des conditions analogues. Pas un vaisseau ne fut lié. Le résultat fut excellent.

Le cathétérisme peut-il être dangereux? Certains chirurgiens ont paru craindre qu'il ne détermine des lésions de l'endothélium. Si l'on peut affirmer qu'il n'en produira jamais, on est cependant en droit de penser qu'elles ne seront jamais considérables, car un instrument mou et souple comme une sonde en gomme ne peut être bien traumatisant. Or, nous savons que dans une artère saine, des lésions limitées et septiques de l'endothélium ne sont pas

---

[1] Schwartz. Soc. Chirurgie 1901.

dangereuses. Dans le cas de gangrène par embolie, il ne semble
donc pas qu'il puisse être dangereux. Dans une artère malade, ces
lésions paraissent être plus fâcheuses; mais, en cas de gangrène
par artérite, les lésions produites par la sonde ne seront rien à
côté des altérations préexistantes.

En somme, le cathétérisme des artères fait avec une sonde
en gomme ne me paraît pas dangereux. Comme il est peut-être
capable de rendre des services dans quelques cas, je crois qu'on
est autorisé à l'employer sans lui accorder trop de confiance.

2.° *Anastomoses artério-veineuses.* — C'est San Martin (¹), dont
j'ai précédemment rapporté les expériences, qui a fait sur l'homme la première opération ayant pour but de faire passer le
sang artériel par les veines. Cette opération c'est l'anastomose
artério-veineuse.

Voici un court résumé de sa première observation qu'il a
publiée en 1902.

Il s'agissait d'un homme de 52 ans. La gangrène avait envahi
les deux premiers orteils, et empiétait sur le métatarse. San Martin pratiqua l'anastomose latérale de l'artère et de la veine fémorale un peu au-dessus du canal de Hunter. La pince enlevée, la
veine ne changea pas de couleur. Six jours après, on fit une amputation de jambe au lieu d'élection à lambeau postérieur. Le
sang qui sortait de la veine était noir. Le cathétérisme de l'artère
ne réussit pas à amener un véritable jet de sang. On dut ultérieurement amputer la cuisse au tiers moyen, et le malade succomba treize jours après la première opération. L'observation ne
renferme pas de renseignements précis sur l'état de l'anastomose.

San Martin répéta la même opération sur un homme de 73
ans. Pour traiter une entorse, un bandage serré avait été appliqué par un charlatan. Quand on enleva la bande le 3° jour, trois
orteils avaient pris une couleur livide. Quelques mois après, on
fit la désarticulation des deux dernières phalanges de ces orteils.
Le malade entra à l'hôpital avec les moignons gangrénés. San
Martin fit l'anastomose artério-veineuse au même point que dans
le cas précédent. L'artère était calcifiée. «Craignant, dit l'auteur,
qu'elle ne résistât pas à la suture, je me contentai de la ponction-
ner et de coudre l'adventice à la moitié antérieure de l'incision
veineuse. Les deux vaisseaux étaient très adhérents. On prati-

---

(1) *San Martin*, Academia Real de Medicina de Madrid 1902.

qua une amputation de Syme. Les lambeaux ne se sont pas gangrénés.

Avec ce que nous ont appris les expériences de François-Frank [1] et celles de Frantz [2], on peut être certain que, dans ce cas, la communication entre l'artère et la veine ne s'est pas établie.

Jaboulay [3] a exécuté la même anastomose, la même année, le 14 juin 1902.

Son malade, âgé de 47 ans, présentait depuis un an des phénomènes de claudication intermittente. Puis survient une gangrène sèche à évolution lente. On pratique l'amputation de Chopard le 14 Mars 1902. Le lambeau se gangrène, et on ampute la cuisse droite à la partie moyenne le 1ᵉʳ Mai. Quelques jours après, des symptômes de gangrène apparaissent sur le membre opposé. Le 14 Juin 1902, Jaboulay tenta l'anastomose artério-veineuse dans le triangle de Scarpa. «On pratique la suture à la soie fine de l'adventice des deux vaisseaux, sur leurs bords adjacents; le long de cette ligne de suture, ces vaisseaux sont alors longitudinalement ouverts par une incision de 3 à 4 centimètres sur leurs faces latérales adjacentes...... Dans la lumière artérielle est engagée une plaque d'athérome, remontant trop haut pour pouvoir être extirpée par l'incision vasculaire. Une deuxième ligne de suture à points séparés à la soie réunit l'endartère à l'endoveine, dans leur partie postérieure, et un 3ᵉ rang, ces mêmes tuniques en avant. Des fils superficiels réunissent en dernier lieu les adventices en avant de l'anastomose.»

Je laisse de côté une partie très obscure de cette observation, où il est dit qu'un fil «noué en amont sur l'artère est légèrement desserré, mais laissé cependant en place, de façon à diminuer l'afflux sanguin pendant quelques heures.»

Le résultat de cette intervention fut nul. «Les pulsations n'apparurent pas dans les veines. On crut en percevoir le soir et le lendemain matin dans la veine poplitée, mais elles ne persistèrent pas; la saphène se distendit nettement, mais par gêne de la circulation en retour, ne se remplissant que de bas en haut à l'épreuve du doigt. Jamais on ne perçut de thrill à la palpation.»

Le sphacèle progressa et atteignit le genou sans sillon net d'élimination. Un mois après, le 12 Juillet, on fit l'amputation de

[1] François-Frank, Soc. de biologie 1896.
[2] Frantz, Archiv f. klin. Chirurg. 1905.
[3] Jaboulay, in Gallois et Pinatelle, Rev. de Chirurg. 1903.

la cuisse gauche. Les gros vaisseaux étaient obstrués. Ils ne donnèrent pas une goutte de sang.

Cinq jours après cette seconde amputation, le malade mourut brusquement, probablement d'une embolie cérébrale.

Aucune de ces trois opérations n'a donné de résultat. Peut-on attendre mieux de cette méthode dans l'avenir?

Pour justifier sa tentative, San Martin cite le malade de Perthes qui vécut près d'un an avec une communication entre l'artère pulmonaire gauche et l'aorte. Il est certain que le mélange du sang artériel avec le sang veineux n'entraîne pas de trouble grave. Les anévrysmes artério-veineux ne sont pas sans inconvénient, mais ces inconvénients ne sauraient être mis en balance avec ceux de la gangrène. Si l'on pouvait sauver un membre au prix d'un anévrysme artério-veineux, il n'y aurait pas à hésiter. Mais la question est de savoir si l'on peut sauver le membre à ce prix, s'il est possible de rétablir la circulation en faisant passer le sang artériel par les canaux veineux.

En faveur de cette possibilité, Lecercle [1] rappelle les circulations dérivatives signalées par Muller en 1846, par Claude Bernard en 1855, par Sucquet en 1862, par Arnold et Hoyer en 1877. Niées par Sappey et Vulpian, elles ont été de nouveau décrites par Bourceret en 1885. Plus récemment, en 1895, Debierre et Girard auraient vu des anastomoses diverses entre les artères et les veines. Que ces circulations dérivatives, que ces anastomoses existent ou non, cela ne me paraît avoir aucune importance pour la question qui nous occupe. Le sang arrivant sous la pression artérielle dans une grosse veine peut-il cheminer dans cette veine du centre vers la périphérie, et aller traverser les capillaires pour revenir par d'autres vaisseaux veineux? Voilà la question.

Il y a une vingtaine d'années, à l'École pratique, nous faisions parfois la facétie suivante. Après une amputation circulaire, nous placions une canule dans la veine principale non pas du moignon mais du membre amputé, puis, chargeant une seringue de liquide coloré, nous invitions un néophyte à pousser l'injection vigoureusement. Si le jeune élève y allait de bon cœur, il recevait une douche, et n'oubliait plus jamais le rôle des valvules; en effet, le liquide injecté arrêté par les valvules refluait par toutes les veines et veinules de la surface de section. En disséquant, on

---

[1] Lecercle, Th. de Lyon, 1902.

pouvait constater que le liquide coloré ne pénétrait jamais à plus de 3 ou 4 centimètres dans le membre.

Tout le monde sait d'ailleurs qu'il est impossible d'injecter les veines par voie rétrograde. Il faut cependant le rappeler, car qu'est-ce qu'on se propose par l'anastomose artério-veineuse appliquée au traitement de la gangrène si ce n'est une injection rétrograde.

Gallois et Pinatelle (¹) ont repris avec une précision expérimentale ce que je présentais tout à l'heure comme une facétie d'école.

Ils poussent par la jugulaire interne une injection d'eau colorée sous une pression de 2ᵐ,20 à 2ᵐ,30. Le liquide revient immédiatement par toutes les veines profondes et superficielles (jugulaire interne du côté opposé, jugulaire externe, plexus vertébral, veines musculaires, veines superficielles). Quand on aveugle toutes les voies d'échappement, l'écoulement s'arrête «sans que les capillaires soient franchies, sans que du moins leur traversée se révèle par un suintement des carotides.»

Du membre supérieur au membre inférieur, l'injection poussée par la veine principale a le même sort. Ils essaient alors une injection vigoureuse de paraffine liquide. Le résultat est le même. «La pièce disséquée nous montre, disent-ils, qu'aucune valvule n'avait été forcée, quoique la veine fortement distendue eût presque triplé de volume ainsi que les affluents du segment veineux injecté.»

Gallois et Pinatelle semblent croire que les choses se passent autrement sur le vivant. En faveur de la pénétration rétrograde du sang, ils invoquent les battements que l'on perçoit parfois très loin dans les veines en cas d'anévrysme artério-veineux. Il y a là une confusion. Les battements indiquent des modifications de pression, et pas du tout le cheminement du liquide. Les pulsations peuvent être très nettes en un point d'une veine où il n'arrive pas une goutte de sang artériel.

Le fait a d'ailleurs été constaté par Frantz (²) au cours de ses expériences sur les anévrysmes artério-veineux. Sur deux chiens, il a mis à nu une veine en un point où elle battait. Elle était de couleur bleu foncé. Il l'a incisée, et il en est sorti du sang manifestement veineux.

(¹) *Gallois et Pinatelle*, Revue de Chirurgie, 1903.
(²) *Frantz*, Archiv. f. klin. Chirurgie 1905.

Frantz a étudié très minutieusement le mouvement de tourbillon qui se produit au point où les courants artériels et veineux se rencontrent. Ce point se déplace peu à peu vers la périphérie et, en général, il atteint au bout d'une heure un niveau où il reste ensuite un certain temps.

D'après Frantz, la distance à laquelle pénètre le courant artériel dans le bout périphérique de la veine dépend de la différence de pression entre l'artère et la veine. «Dans les deux tiers des cas, dit-il, je constate, même pendant les opérations de longue durée, que la limite inférieure à laquelle on peut voir le courant artériel dans la veine est située à deux ou trois centimètres au-dessous de la partie inférieure de l'orifice de communication Toutefois, on peut constater dans le cas IX que déjà pendant l'opération le sang artériel pénètre jusqu'à la gouttière des adducteurs. Pour trancher cette question, je fis chez le chien XVI une fistule artério-veineuse, et découvris la grosse veine saphène. Elle renfermait du sang artériel jusqu'au milieu de la jambe. La limite entre le sang artériel et le sang veineux n'était pas nette, mais floue. Au contraire, la veine poplitée n'était remplie de sang artériel qu'à deux centimètres au-dessous du point où se détache la veine précédente. Là, la limite était très nette. Mais la réplétion si lointaine de la veine par le sang artériel n'est pas toujours le cas, ainsi que le prouve l'examen des chiens XXII et XXX. Chez ceux-là aussi, après l'établissement de la fistule, la veine saphène fit une forte saillie; je l'ouvris, il s'en écoula du sang foncé....»

Frantz a constaté un fait très curieux. Parfois, surtout dans le bout central de la veine, la violence du courant sanguin fait un effet de trompe; et les veines qui s'abouchent à angle droit dans le tronc principal, loin de se remplir de sang artériel, sont vidées par aspiration.

Il me semble que tous ces faits prouvent surabondamment que les conditions circulatoires créées par une anastomose artério-veineuse latérale ne peuvent en aucun cas modifier l'évolution de la gangrène d'un membre.

L'anastomose bout à bout n'a pas été pratiquée chez l'homme. Aurait-elle plus de chances de succès? Certainement non.

On a beaucoup discuté sur la résistance des valvules. Braun a vu que celles de la saphène résistent à une pression de 18 centimètres de mercure. J'ai moi-même constaté que, sur les cadavres de sujets jeunes, non variqueux, elles ne se laissent pas forcer par une colonne d'eau de deux mètres cinquante. On peut se demander si sur le vivant, la veine ne se laisserait pas distendre peu à peu, même au niveau des valvules. En tous cas, cette distension ne pourrait être que le résultat d'un travail lent pendant lequel le membre aurait le temps de se sphacéler.

Mais laissons de côté cette question des valvules. Admettons que toutes les valvules soient forcées, admettons qu'il n'en existe pas, et que le sang, sous la pression artérielle, arrive à plein canal dans la veine principale d'un membre ; je dis que même dans ces conditions, d'ailleurs irréalisables, jamais le sang n'ira traverser les capillaires de manière à nourrir efficacement le membre. Dans un organe à circulation terminale, ce serait peut-être possible ; nous ne le savons pas. Mais, dans un membre, c'est absolument impossible, et voici pourquoi. Les anastomoses entre les veines moyennes sont si nombreuses que le système veineux constitue un véritable réseau. Le sang trouvera toujours des voies centripètes multiples, où la pression sera faible et jamais il n'atteindra dans les veines la pression nécessaire à la traversée des capillaires. Pour qu'il puisse l'atteindre, il faudrait que la pression dans le cœur droit arrive au même taux que dans le cœur gauche, et si cette condition était réalisée, le cœur droit ne pourrait plus se contracter.

Je crois donc qu'il faut abandonner tout espoir de faire circuler le sang dans les veines du centre vers la périphérie, et par conséquent, d'arrêter la gangrène par une anastomose artério-veineuse.

IV — EMBOLIES

Les embolies fourniraient sans doute les plus beaux succès de la chirurgie artérielle, si on pouvait diagnostiquer d'une manière précoce leur existence et leur siège, et si elles ne survenaient trop souvent chez des asystoliques. Car, quoi de plus simple que d'inciser une artère d'ailleurs saine pour enlever un caillot arrêté par son volume ou par la rencontre d'un éperon de bifurcation.

Je ne parle pas des embolies qui se produisent au cours des endocardites franchement infectieuses. Les caillots sont alors septiques, ce qui suffirait à ruiner l'efficacité de l'incision artérielle, si déjà la gravité de l'état général ne contre-indiquait toute intervention. Quelle que soit leur cause, on ne peut non plus rien attendre de la chirurgie dans les petites embolies viscérales, du rein, de la rate, du foie, du cerveau.

Mais les embolies dues aux cardiovalvulites rhumatismales banales, et qui s'arrêtent dans les artères des membres, dans les mésentériques, voire même dans l'aorte, bénéficieront des récents progrès de la chirurgie vasculaire.

Il importe de faire un diagnostic extrêmement précoce. Si l'on attend que la gangrène ait fait son apparition, le succès restera toujours incomplet, car en admettant qu'on arrête la gangrène, on ne la fera pas rétrocéder. En outre, au point de vue du rétablissement de la circulation, l'opération aura d'autant moins de chance de succès qu'elle sera faite à une époque plus éloignée de l'arrêt de l'embolie, et cela pour deux raisons. Dans certains cas, il se produit des coagulations étendues qui peuvent rendre impossible le débouchage du vaisseau ; et toujours la présence de l'embolie amène des altérations secondaires de l'artère telles que, le caillot enlevé, un autre devra forcément se former.

Tout dépend donc de la précocité de l'intervention.

Pour qu'elle soit prompte et facile, il faut encore diagnostiquer le siège de l'embolie.

Voyons d'abord si, par leur siège habituel, ces embolies sont accessibles. J'étudierai rapidement les embolies des membres, celles des artères mésentériques et celles de l'aorte.

1.° *Embolies des artères des membres*. Les membres inférieurs sont bien plus souvent atteints que les membres supérieurs.

Pour les membres inférieurs, Barié [1] donne les chiffres suivants. Quinze fois, l'embolie occupait les artères tibiales ; douze fois, les artères fémorales ; neuf fois, les artères iliaques ; sept fois, la poplitée, et une fois la pédieuse.

Laissons de côté la pédieuse qui n'a pas d'importance. Les embolies qui s'arrêtent dans les artères tibiales, et particulièrement au niveau du carrefour tibio-péronier, où toutes les obstructions sont graves, sont difficilement accessibles. Mais, dans la poplitée, dans la fémorale, dans l'iliaque, il serait fort simple d'aller chercher un caillot.

Aux membres supérieurs, cinq fois l'obstruction siégeait sur l'artère humérale, quatre fois sur les artères de l'avant-bras, trois fois sur la sous-clavière, deux fois sur l'axillaire.

Les embolies de l'artère de l'avant-bras n'amènent pas de gangrène grave à moins qu'elles ne soient multiples. Et dans ce

---

(¹) *Barié*. Presse Médicale 1906, p. 73, n° 11.

dernier cas, elles échappent à l'intervention. Celles des autres artères ne donneraient lieu à aucune difficulté opératoire.

Il arrive quelquefois que l'embolie n'accuse pas nettement sa présence. Le malade ressent, pendant quelques jours, ou même pendant des semaines, des fourmillements, des douleurs erratiques. Dans les cas de ce genre, qui sont rares, il est difficile de localiser l'obstacle et par conséquent d'intervenir.

Le plus souvent, le début se marque brutalement par une douleur atroce au point où l'embolie s'arrête. Le membre est paralysé, immobile et insensible. Il pâlit, se refroidit, et l'on constate que les artères ont cessé de battre. C'est alors qu'il faudrait intervenir sans tarder. La localisation suffisamment précisée par la douleur permet de le faire. Si on ne trouve pas l'embolie, comme cela est arrivé à Sabanajeff (1), on n'aura pas nui au malade. Si au contraire on enlève le caillot, on pourra sauver le membre.

Je sais bien que la gangrène n'est pas fatale, que la circulation peut se rétablir par les collatérales. Mais cette éventualité est exceptionnelle. En attendant qu'elle se produise, on compromet le résultat de l'intervention, car, encore une fois, on ne fera pas rétrocéder la gangrène, on ne revivifiera pas les tissus sphacélés.

Sans connaître d'observation qui vienne à l'appui de ma manière de voir, je conseille formellement d'intervenir aussitôt que le diagnostic est posé, et le cas échéant, je n'hésiterais pas à le faire.

2.º *Embolies de l'aorte.* C'est aussi par un début brusque que s'annoncent habituellement les embolies de l'aorte abdominale : paraplégie soudaine ou au moins très rapide accompagnée de violentes douleurs avec absence des pulsations artérielles dans les deux membres. Il s'y ajoute parfois des troubles viscéraux qui dépendent sans doute du point où le caillot s'arrête. Souvent le cœur s'affole et devient asystolique. Si l'on a signalé quelques cas de guérison, presque toujours la mort achève le tableau. Elle est en générale rapide. Quand la vie se prolonge assez, les membres inférieurs se gangrènent.

Dans une affection qui comporte un semblable pronostic, il ne semble pas douteux qu'on soit autorisé à intervenir, si grave que soit l'état du malade. Ouvrir largement l'abdomen, explorer

---

(1) *Sabanajeff*, Cent. f. Chirurg, 1895, p. 990.

l'aorte au point où les battements cessent, l'inciser après avoir accusé l'hémostase, enlever le caillot, et suturer. Tel est le seul traitement qui me paraisse rationnel.

3.º *Embolies des mésentériques.* Plus embarassantes sont les embolies des artères mésentériques.

Leur gravité est extrême, peut-être plus considérable encore qu'on ne le dit, car on peut se demander si, dans les quelques cas qui ont guéri, le diagnostic était bien exact.

C'est la mésentérique supérieure qui est le plus souvent frappée. En 1902, Wilhelm Neutra [1] comptait 77 embolies de la supérieure pour 9 de l'inférieure.

Litten a montré que l'artère mésentérique supérieure, bien que pourvue à ses deux extremités de nombreuses anastomoses, se comporte cependant comme une artère terminale. Les voies collatérales sont plus anatomiques que physiologiques. Avec la pression normale du sang, elles sont insuffisantes ou inutilisables, de telle sorte que l'obstruction du tronc principal amène la gangrène de l'intestin.

L'obstruction est causée parfois par des caillots qui mesurent seulement quelques millimètres de long. Ce sont les cas les plus favorables pour l'intervention. Mais on a rencontré aussi des embolies multiples, et dans quelques cas, l'artère était oblitérée sur toute sa longueur depuis l'aorte jusqu'à ses divisions intestinales. Ce sont là des résultats d'autopsie. Il est bien probable qu'il s'agissait de coagulations secondaires et qu'au début la lésion était limitée.

L'affection a un début brutal. Brusquement, éclatent de violentes douleurs à forme de coliques. Leur localisation n'est pas toujours précise. Kussmaul [2] pense que les douleurs qui siègent dans la région ombilicale indiquent l'obstruction de la mésentérique supérieure, tandis que les douleurs à prédominance sacrée indiqueraient l'obstruction de la mésentérique inférieure.

Bientôt s'installe de la diarrhée. Les selles, composées d'abord de matières fécales, deviennent liquides, aqueuses, puis sanglantes. Et ces hémorrhagies s'accompagnent souvent d'abaissement de température. Litten [3] pense que d'après les altérations du

---

[1] *Neutra.* Grenzgebiete der Medizin und Chirurgie, 1901, pag. 705, 777, 788, 830, 855.
[2] *Kussmaul,* Würzburger med. Zeitschrift, 1864, Band V.
[3] *Litten,* Virchow Archiv, 1875, T. 63.

sang, on peut localiser l'obstacle. Le sang très altéré indiquerait l'obstruction de la mésentérique supérieure. Le sang frais celui de la mésentérique inférieure. Trübel (1) a fait remarquer que des altérations peuvent tenir simplement au temps pendant lequel le sang a séjourné dans l'intestin avant d'être évacué. Le ténesme cependant indiquerait que l'artère inférieure est intéressée.

Malheureusement, les diarrhées hémorrhagiques ne sont pas constantes. Wilhelm Neutra ne les a notées que dans 30 % des cas. Il fait bien remarquer que cette rareté relative peut être due à l'insuffisance des observations; il n'en est pas moins vrai qu'on ne peut compter sur ce symptôme. Toutefois, quand il existe, on peut admettre avec Gallavardin (2) qu'il a une grande importance pour le diagnostic.

Dans certains cas, la constipation s'installe dès le début. C'est ce qui avait conduit Deckart (3) à distinguer la forme diarrhéique de la forme paralytique. La constipation est due en effet à la paralysie ischémique de l'intestin. Il ne faut pas oublier que la paralysie est un phénomène à peu près constant à la suite des embolies qui portent sur les artères des membres. La distinction de Deckart n'a qu'une valeur clinique. Il est probable que le segment intestinal ischémié est toujours plus ou moins paralysé. C'est la partie saine qui réagit plus ou moins, et surtout sans doute, les portions intermédiaires où la circulation hésite dans les voies anastomotiques.

Même dans les cas où la diarrhée a marqué le début, des symptômes d'iléus s'installent plus tard. La constipation devient complète, et les vomissements, après avoir passé par une phase hémorrhagique, deviennent fécaloïdes.

Il s'agit alors d'obstruction paralytique due non seulement à l'ischémie, mais à la péritonite. Celle-ci se produit sans perforation, ou plutôt avant la perforation, car les microorganismes traversent la paroi intestinale sphacélée.

Le ballonnement du ventre, qui survient d'ailleurs dès le début, devient alors énorme, et on trouve parfois une quantité de liquide considérable épanché dans la séreuse.

Dans les cas de Cohn et de Munro (4), on a pu sentir, par la

---

(1) Trübel, Jahresbericht der Wiener Krankenanstalten für das Jahr 1874.
(2) Gallavardin, Lyon médical, 1900; Gaz. des hôpitaux, 1901.
(3) Deckart, Mitteilungen a. d. Grenzgebiete d. Med. u. Chirurg., 1900.
(4) Munro, Cent. f. Chirurgie, 1894, p. 383.

palpation, des tumeurs que l'autopsie a montré être formées par des hématomes du mésentère.

Au point de vue de l'évolution, on peut distinguer des cas aigus et des cas chroniques. Dans les premiers, le drame évolue en quelques jours, voire même en quelques heures. Dès le début surviennent des manifestations générales effrayantes, convulsions, perte de connaissance, sans que l'étendue des lésions soit toujours en rapport avec l'acuité des symptômes.

Dans les cas chroniques sur lesquels insiste Wilhelm Neutra, il survient parfois des rémissions, et on a même signalé quelques cas de guérison. On peut se demander si dans ces cas le diagnostic était bien certain. Peut-être s'agissait-il d'embolie de fines branches de l'artère mésentérique et non d'obstruction du tronc lui-même.

Le diagnostic de l'obstruction des artères mésentériques est incontestablement très difficile. Kussmaul [1] et Gerhardt [2] attachent avec raison une grande importance à la notion étiologique. Il est certes précieux de savoir que le malade est atteint d'une affection qui l'expose à des embolies, mais cette notion elle-même peut devenir trompeuse. J'ai observé un malade qui au cours d'une crise d'asystolie fut pris d'accidents abdominaux graves. Laignel-Lavastine fit avec toute espèce de raison le diagnostic d'embolie de l'artère mésentérique. J'ai pratiqué la laparotomie, et constaté qu'il s'agissait d'un étranglement interne.

L'erreur inverse est plus souvent commise, qui consiste à prendre pour un étranglement interne une embolie mésentérique. Borszeky [3] est d'avis qu'on ne peut faire le diagnostic différentiel de ces deux affections. C'est peut-être excessif. La paralysie intestinale est rarement primitive dans les embolies. Et les vomissements hémorrhagiques ne s'observent guère dans les étranglements. Admettons cependant l'impossibilité du diagnostic. Le malade n'en souffrira pas si on croit à un étranglement et qu'on l'opère vite.

C'est à cela que je voulais en venir. Sans doute, il est bon que le diagnostic soit aussi complet que possible, et il faut chercher sans cesse les moyens de le perfectionner. Mais, dans les cas où l'on ne peut arriver à la certitude, on ne demande pas la

(1) Kussmaul, Würzburger med. Zeitschrift 1864 B. V.
(2) Gerhardt, Würzburger med. Zeitschrift 1863 B. IV.
(3) Borszeky, Beiträge zur klin. Chirurgie 1921.

même chose au diagnostic chirurgical qu'au diagnostic médical. On lui demande à la fois plus et moins.

On lui demande plus en rapidité. C'est bien souvent l'évolution de la maladie qui conduit le médecin au diagnostic exact. Mais dans les affections du genre de celle qui nous occupe, si on attend des éclaircissements de la durée, on laisse passer le moment où la chirurgie pourrait être utile. Et pour les embolies mésentériques, on se trouve réduit aux résections intestinales, qui ont donné de si mauvais résultats.

On lui demande moins en précision, car si l'on parvient à circonscrire l'incertitude entre deux ou trois hypothèses qui toutes conduisent à la laparotomie, le chirurgien peut en toute conscience ouvrir l'abdomen. C'est à quoi l'on doit arriver. Car c'est surtout avec l'invagination, avec l'étranglement interne que l'on a confondu les embolies des mésentériques. Il est vrai qu'on peut les confondre aussi avec les thrombo-phlébites du système porte, et que contre les thromboses mésentériques étendues le chirurgien est désarmé. Mais les thrombo-phlébites sont bien plus rares (32 cas) que les embolies des mésentériques (86 cas). Et puis, ne vaut-il pas mieux faire une laparotomie inutile que de laisser sans secours un malade que l'on pourrait peut-être guérir?

Pourrait-on le guérir? Je le crois. Le ventre ouvert, il est facile de reconnaître sur l'intestin les altérations qui indiquent l'arrêt du cours du sang et leur circonscription indique quelle est l'artère lésée.

J'estime qu'il faut alors examiner l'artère obstruée. Sans doute l'origine de la mésentérique supérieure n'est pas facile à explorer, sans doute dans un mésentère gros le tronc des deux mésentériques est difficile à suivre. Mais si on trouve une petite embolie qui se puisse enlever, on rendra un immense service.

On peut faire un reproche aux interventions précoces. C'est qu'au début, les lésions intestinales sont mal limitées et que, s'il est impossible de rendre à l'artère sa perméabilité, on ne sait quelle étendue il faut donner à la résection. Je ne pense pas qu'on doive s'arrêter à ce reproche ni se servir de cet argument pour retarder l'opération, car il est bien certain que les opérations tardives, sans doute en raison de la péritonite, ont donné des résultats déplorables. Et d'autre part, il n'y a pas grand mal à réséquer quelques centimètres d'intestin en plus de ce qui serait nécessaire.

Je ne veux pas prolonger cette discussion n'ayant aucun fait pour l'étayer. Et je termine en soumettant à mes collègues les conclusions suivantes:

Quand on soupçonne une embolie des artères mésentériques, il faut intervenir aussi rapidement que possible. Avant de réséquer l'intestin, je conseille d'explorer le vaisseau obstrué. Si on trouve une coagulation limitée, il est facile d'inciser l'artère et d'enlever le caillot. Comme on n'est pas sûr de rétablir par cette opération la perméabilité du vaisseau, il serait peut-être bon de ne faire à la paroi abdominale qu'une suture incomplète et d'extérioriser pendant quelques jours sous un pansement la portion d'intestin menacée.

Si on ne trouve pas de caillot, si la coagulation est trop étendue, il ne reste qu'à faire une large résection intestinale.

V — ANÉVRYSMES ARTÉRIELS

Le retour à l'action directe sur le sac a constitué un notable progrès sur la ligature à distance dans le traitement des anévrysmes. J'ai défendu chaudement l'extirpation dans plusieurs mémoires dont le plus ancien remonte à 1888 (¹). Je me suis appliqué à démontrer qu'elle est moins dangereuse, qu'elle expose moins à la gangrène, qu'elle donne des guérisons de meilleure qualité que ne fait la ligature.

Elle n'est cependant point complètement satisfaisante. Elle supprime une artère de la circulation et par là, elle amène parfois la gangrène. On se rapprocherait bien davantage de la restitution ad integrum, qui doit toujours être l'objectif du chirurgien, si l'anévrysme supprimé, on reconstituait un canal artériel perméable.

Cette reconstitution est certainement réalisable dans un certain nombre de cas. Il reste à savoir si elle est pratique. Quand j'ai commencé ce rapport, j'espérais bien arriver sur ce point à des notions précises. Malheureusement, je n'ai pu trouver qu'un très petit nombre d'observations et les rédactions que j'ai pu me procurer sont si incomplètes qu'on n'en peut tirer grand enseignement.

La question de la cure radicale des anévrysmes avec rétablissement d'une artère normalement calibrée est donc encore du

---

(¹) *Pierre Delbet*, Revue de Chirurgie, 1888 et Congrès de Chirurgie, 1896.

domaine de l'espérance. Mais c'est une espérance si prochaine que l'on peut chercher quelles devront être les conditions de cette cure idéale et comment on pourra les remplir.

Matas a fait une tentative dans cette voie et il a décrit sa technique dans les «Annals of Surgery» de Janvier 1893. Je vais l'exposer avec quelques détails, car il ne me semble pas qu'elle ait été toujours bien comprise.

Après avoir découvert le sac, il le dissèque dans une certaine étendue, mais non pas en totalité. «Dans aucun cas, dit-il, la dissection ne doit être poussée au-delà de la partie proéminente ou superficielle du sac.»

Après une dissection partielle, il l'incise d'un bout à l'autre suivant l'axe de l'artère. Le sang et les caillots sont enlevés, et l'on place des écarteurs qui permettent d'inspecter toute la cavité anévrysmale. On doit voir tous les orifices qu'elle présente.

Si l'anévrysme appartient au type fusiforme, on reconnaît deux larges orifices souvent reliés par une traînée d'un gris jaunâtre qui représente la partie intacte de l'artère. Si l'anévrysme est sacciforme, il n'existe qu'un seul orifice de dimensions variables. «Dans les anévrysmes spontanés du type fusiforme, l'artère est si complètement confondue avec les parois du sac que sa continuité ne peut être rétablie, du moins dans l'état actuel de nos connaissances. Dans ce cas, le but de la suture est simplement de fermer les orifices de l'artère pour faire l'hémostase et oblitérer le sac. Dans les anévrysmes sacciformes avec un orifice unique, il est souvent possible de fermer cet orifice sans empiéter sur la lumière du vaisseau et en conservant la continuité aussi bien fonctionnelle qu'anatomique de l'artère.»

Voyons d'abord la conduite que conseille Matas dans les anévrysmes fusiformes. Il faut chercher soigneusement tous les orifices qui existent sur la face interne, outre les deux principaux. Ces orifices qui sont ceux des collatérales doivent être soigneusement suturés. Il en existait dans trois des quatre cas opérés par l'auteur. Cela fait, on suture les deux orifices principaux. Les bords en sont épais, de telle sorte qu'un nombre restreint de sutures suffit à les fermer. Un second surjet peut consolider le premier plan de suture. Quelquefois, la rigidité du sac rend ce second plan difficile; il n'est pas indispensable.

Dans les anévrysmes sacciformes, la suture doit fermer l'orifice unique en conservant la continuité de l'artère. Il faut avoir soin de prendre une certaine épaisseur des lèvres de l'orifice, mais cependant sans rétrécir le calibre du vaisseau. Les fils, dit l'auteur, ne doivent pas être au contact du sang. Il est bon de commencer la suture à une certaine distance au-dessus de l'orifice et de la continuer à une certaine distance au-dessous.

On supprime ensuite l'hémostase provisoire et l'on s'assure que les sutures sont bien étanches.

Le dernier temps a pour but l'oblitération du sac que l'on ne réséque pas. Il s'exécute de même dans les deux types d'anévrysme. Quand la poche est vaste, on fait un second plan de suture, qui renforce la ligne des sutures occlusives. Ce second plan doit réduire considérablement la cavité du sac. C'est en somme une sorte de capitonnage. La fermeture de la cavité anévrysmale est enfin obtenue en déprimant la peau jusqu'au fond de la cavité. Matas compare ce temps au procédé de Neuber pour fermer les cavités osseuses avec des lambeaux cutanéo-périostiques. Les sutures qui dépriment ainsi la peau sont liées sur un coussinet de gaze. Il ne reste plus qu'à affronter les deux lèvres de l'incision cutanée.

Dans certains cas, il est impossible de se servir de la peau pour combler la cavité. Ainsi, dans les anévrysmes iliaques et dans les autres anévrysmes abdominaux, Matas conseille alors de remplacer la peau par le péritoine. Enfin, dans les anévrysmes des membres ou du cou, quand le sac est séparé de la peau par des muscles, l'auteur déclare qu'il faut se contenter de replier le sac sur lui-même.

Toutes ces manœuvres sont bien compliquées pour supprimer la cavité d'un sac qu'on laisse et qu'il serait si facile d'enlever.

Dans son article, Matas dit avoir employé quatre fois son procédé, mais il ne donne pas ses observations. Deux fois il s'agissait d'anévrysmes traumatiques siégeant sur l'humérale ; deux fois d'anévrysmes spontanés, l'un de la fémorale, l'autre de la poplitée. Si l'on en croit l'une des phrases de son article que j'ai citée, dans trois cas il s'agissait d'anévrysmes fusiformes. Il n'a donc pas cherché à conserver la perméabilité du vaisseau. Je n'ai pu réussir à trouver la relation détaillée de ces faits, sauf du premier qui a été publié dans le *Medical News*, le 27 Octobre 1888.

Il s'agissait d'un anévrysme traumatique de l'humérale consécutif à un coup de feu. La compression, la ligature, tout avait échoué. Matas ouvre le sac et constate l'abouchement dans sa cavité de collatérales importantes qui continuaient à donner même après la ligature de l'humérale au-dessous et au-dessus du sac. Ne pouvant extirper l'anévrysme en raison de ses adhérences, il eut l'idée de suturer les orifices artériels par l'intérieur du sac. Il en réséqua une partie et laissa le reste se combler par bourgeonnement.

Je n'ai pu trouver que trois observations d'anévrysmes traités par la méthode de Matas. Deux appartiennent à Danna (¹) et une à Gibbon (²).

Dans l'un des faits de Danna, il s'agissait d'un anévrysme de la fémorale rompu et qui avait été pris pour un abcès. Après avoir placé une ligature d'attente au-dessous du ligament de Fallope, Danna incise la poche qui est remplie de caillots et constate que le sac est rompu en deux points. Il suture les orifices artériels par des points séparés et fait par dessus un surjet de renforcement. Mais il constate une dilatation anévrysmale au niveau de la ligature d'attente et on lie au-dessus. La plaie a guéri par seconde intention.

Son second malade, âgé de 20 ans, portait depuis six ans un anévrysme poplité qui s'était rompu depuis quelques jours. Après avoir appliqué la bande d'Esmarch on incise la tumeur et on suture les orifices artériels. La guérison s'est faite par seconde intention et a laissé des raideurs dans le genou.

Gibbon a opéré un homme de 31 ans, d'un anévrysme poplité qui datait de 8 à 9 mois. Le sac incisé, il ne peut trouver l'orifice inférieur; il n'y avait pas de collatérale s'ouvrant dans la cavité. Gibbon a fait le capitonnage du sac avec du catgut. La plaie a suppuré: de petites plaques de gangrène ont apparu sur le pied et le malade a guéri avec des raideurs du genou.

Matas a décrit un autre procédé qu'il n'a jamais employé, mais qui pourrait être applicable à certains anévrysmes sacciformes. Il consiste à refaire avec la paroi du sac un canal artériel en se servant d'un tube de caoutchouc comme tuteur. Le sac ouvert, on introduit le tube dans les deux bouts de l'artère. Ce tube traverse donc le sac dont on suture les parois par dessus. On l'enlève avant de serrer les derniers fils.

Ce procédé a été employé par Robert Morris (³) le 16 Mai 1903. Le malade âgé de 58 ans avait un anévrysme volumineux

(¹) Danna, J. of Am. Med. Assoc., 1903, I at, p. 393
(²) Gibbon, Amer. Medicine, 1903, p. 309
(³) Morris, Annals of Surgery, Fev. 1903

de l'artère poplitée. Toute la jambe était œdémateuse. Après avoir appliqué la bande d'Esmarch, Morris incise le sac suivant son grand axe, et en retire deux poignées de caillots. Il constate alors que l'anévrysme appartient au type fusiforme, mais que le sac présente un diverticulum à parois minces qui constitue la plus grande partie de la tumeur. Avec du catgut n° 1, l'auteur pratique un surjet à travers les fissus du fond du sac, construisant sur cinq centimètres environ une artère nouvelle. Un second surjet consolida le premier. On ne réséqua rien du sac.

La nouvelle artère fut saisie entre mes doigts, dit l'opérateur, et on enleva la bande élastique. A ce moment, l'ondée sanguine bondit à travers le nouveau conduit et aucun point ne fut forcé par elle. Le pied du malade devint chaud, mais l'œdème ne permit pas de sentir les pulsations des artères du pied.

La plaie fut suturée sans drainage et réunie par première intention.

Les troubles sensitifs et moteurs qui existaient avant l'opération disparurent peu à peu. Le 22e jour, il persistait encore des troubles moteurs dans les muscles antéro-externes.

Ce jour même, on examina la poplitée pour la première fois et voici comment l'auteur décrit le résultat de cet examen: «La nouvelle artère donne l'impression d'être plus grosse (larger) que l'artère poplitée gauche. Il est difficile de dire si cela tient à ce que les parois de la nouvelle artère sont plus épaisses, ou si je n'ai pu me rendre compte très exactement du calibre de l'artère normale.»

L'interprétation de cette phrase n'est pas facile. L'artère battait-elle? Était-elle dilatée? Ou bien au contraire, est-ce d'un cordon fibreux qu'il s'agit. Il n'est pas fait mention de pulsation dans les artères de la jambe et du pied. L'auteur dit bien que le résultat fonctionnel était très satisfaisant. Mais cela ne prouve pas que l'artère soit restée perméable.

En somme, les huit faits que j'ai pu relever où la méthode de Matas a été employée sont très disparates. Il en est six où l'on n'a pas tenté de conserver la circulation dans l'artère malade. On l'a essayé dans les deux autres. Encore, ne puis-je être affirmatif sur le cas de Matas, dont je n'ai pu trouver la relation détaillée. Reste le fait de Morris, qui ne semble pas très encourageant, quelqu'interprétation que l'on donne à la phrase un peu énigmatique que j'ai citée. En effet, si l'artère ne battait pas, le but n'a pas été atteint. Si elle battait, comme elle était «larger» que l'artère du côté opposé, on peut craindre que l'anévrysme soit en train de se reformer.

En somme, les faits sont trop rares et trop insuffisamment rapportés pour qu'on puisse juger d'après eux la méthode de Matas. On ne peut l'apprécier qu'au point de vue théorique.

Il faut tout d'abord remarquer que Matas n'emploie pas les expressions fusiforme et sacciforme dans leur sens habituel. On désigne cliniquement sous le nom d'anévrysmes fusiformes ceux qui sont dus à la dilatation de toute la circonférence de l'artère.

Pour ceux-là, on ne peut songer à refaire un canal artériel de bonne qualité en rétrécissant simplement le sac. Mais il est évident que Matas n'a point entendu parler de ces anévrysmes, seuls véritablement fusiformes, puisqu'il déclare que dans ceux qu'il appelle fusiformes on voit souvent une traînée jaunâtre, allant d'un orifice à l'autre, qui représente le segment d'artère resté sain. Ainsi, ces anévrysmes fusiformes sont en réalité des anévrysmes sacciformes dans lesquels la paroi artérielle a cédé d'un seul côté, mais sur une longueur considérable. Dans de tels cas, l'artère paraît bien communiquer avec le sac par deux orifices, comme dans les anévrysmes fusiformes, mais, au point de vue de la réparation possible, la différence est énorme. Les anévrysmes vraiment fusiformes sont d'ailleurs rares partout et surtout aux membres.

Pour apprécier la méthode de Matas, il faut distinguer les faits où il suture les orifices de ceux où il tente de rétablir un canal artériel perméable.

Dans le premier cas, sa méthode rentre dans le groupe des incisions du sac. Elle ne diffère de l'antique méthode d'Antylus que par la manière de faire l'hémostase et par le capitonnage de la poche.

L'incision du sac présente un danger particulier, l'hémorrhagie secondaire. Les collatérales qui s'ouvrent dans le sac sont souvent oblitérées par des caillots. Elles passent inaperçues lorsqu'on vide la poche. Mais lorsque la circulation collatérale s'établit, les caillots peuvent céder et l'hémorrhagie survenir. Matas a bien senti ce danger, car il recommande de chercher attentivement l'orifice des collatérales. Il insiste sur la nécessité pour les trouver de ne pas employer la bande d'Esmarch qui suspend la circulation dans tout le membre. Il recommande de faire l'hémostase par la compression directe de l'artère, de telle sorte que la circulation collatérale fasse saigner les branches qui s'ouvrent dans le sac.

Quoiqu'on fasse, on ne peut être sûr de trouver toujours tous les orifices, puisque Gibbon n'a même pas pu découvrir l'orifice inférieur du vaisseau principal. En admettant même que le capitonnage de Matas mette sûrement à l'abri de l'hémorrhagie secondaire, on ne voit pas les avantages qu'il peut y avoir à conserver le sac, tandis que les inconvénients de cette pratique ne sont pas douteux. Il en est qui sont inhérents à sa conservation même, et d'autres qui tiennent à la manière dont Matas le traite.

D'abord le sac, surtout lorsqu'il est volumineux, forme une sorte de tumeur qui tient de la place, qui comprime les collatérales, qui gêne le rétablissement de la circulation. En outre, j'ai montré [1] en 1888 que les accidents nerveux qui accompagnent certains anévrysmes, impotence, paralysie, douleurs, troubles trophiques, sont dus non pas tant à la compression qu'à l'enserrement des nerfs par les tissus fibreux qui se forment autour de la tumeur. C'est pour cela que ces accidents peuvent persister, s'aggraver ou même débuter après guérison de l'anévrysme, au moment où le sac se rétracte. Dans ma première statistique [2] j'avais relevé douze cas où les troubles paralytiques ou trophiques ont persisté, et dans deux de ces cas, ils ont été assez graves pour nécessiter l'amputation. En 1896, dans ma seconde statistique [3], j'en ai relevé cinq autres. Deux fois, après la guérison d'anévrysmes axillaires traités par la ligature, le bras est resté impotent. Trois anévrysmes poplités, guéris de la même façon, ont laissé soit de l'impotence, soit des douleurs, douleurs qui ont été assez vives dans un cas pour nécessiter l'extirpation secondaire du sac.

En conservant le sac, Matas s'expose à ces accidents. Dans le cas de Morris, traité par sa méthode, il y avait encore des troubles moteurs dans les muscles de la région antéro-externe de la jambe, vingt-deux jours après l'opération. Que sont-ils devenus?

La manière particulière dont Matas traite le sac me paraît encore augmenter les inconvénients de sa conservation. En le capitonnant d'une manière compliquée et serrée, il en fait une sorte de tampon fibreux épais et rigide qui dans certaines régions, le creux poplité par exemple, doit être singulièrement gênant. Et en effet, l'un des malades de Danna et celui de Gibbon ont guéri avec des raideurs du genou.

---

[1] *Pierre Delbet*, Revue de Chirurgie, 1888.
[2] *Pierre Delbet*, Revue de Chirurgie, 1888, pag. 533.
[3] *Pierre Delbet*, Congrès de Chirurgie, 1896.

En outre, Matas fixe la peau à la plicature du sac. Il en résulte la formation d'un bloc fibreux qui va de l'artère à la peau adhérente. Ce résultat ne me semble pas heureux.

En somme, la conservation du sac à la manière de Matas me semble n'avoir que des inconvénients et j'estime qu'il est bien préférable de l'extirper.

Quant à la manière de faire l'hémostase en suturant les deux bouts de l'artère au lieu de les lier, il est possible qu'elle soit commode dans certains cas, mais elle n'a aucun avantage sur la ligature faite au ras des orifices.

Les tentatives de Matas pour refaire une artère perméable sont beaucoup plus intéressantes. Quand la communication avec l'artère se fait par un orifice unique, il le suture. En outre, il a proposé pour les cas où l'une des parois artérielles est effondrée sur une grande étendue, de refaire une artère en la calibrant sur un tube de caoutchouc. Morris a suivi son conseil, mais il est difficile, je l'ai déjà dit, de savoir quel résultat il a obtenu.

Je crois qu'à l'heure actuelle, quand les anévrysmes siègent sur des artères dont la ligature est dangereuse, il faut résolument chercher à les guérir en reconstituant un vaisseau perméable. Je ne m'illusionne pas au point de penser qu'on y réussira toujours, mais ce n'est qu'après l'avoir essayé qu'on saura dans quels cas on peut atteindre ce but idéal. La méthode de Matas ne me semble pas un très bon moyen d'y arriver. À mon avis, on devra toujours, pour les raisons que j'ai précédemment exposées, disséquer le sac et le réséquer.

Pour refaire un canal artériel perméable, divers artifices sont possibles: suturer l'orifice de communication comme Matas; réséquer le segment artériel malade et faire la suture bout à bout; remplacer le segment d'artère par un segment de veine.

Peut-on par la suture de l'orifice à la manière de Matas obtenir un résultat durable? La suture ne peut porter sur l'artère elle-même, car, si petit que soit l'orifice de communication, elle rétrécirait trop le calibre du vaisseau. Il faut qu'elle porte sur le sac. Ce sont donc des tissus malades qui seront étreints par le fil. Résisteront-ils suffisamment pour ne pas se dilater de nouveau? Quand le sac est mince, la question ne se pose même pas. Souvent il est épais, surtout au voisinage du point où il se continue avec l'artère. Mais que valent ces tissus, même épais, au point de vue de la résistance? Il est bien vrai qu'on peut les affronter sur une grande épaisseur et constituer une espèce de colonne. Mais sa solidité ne sera-t-elle pas plus apparente que réelle? Sa base, son point d'implantation sur l'artère, point sur lequel on ne peut agir, ne se laisserait-il pas distendre?

Il faut reconnaître que cette suture si simple, d'exécution si facile, est bien tentante et peut-être serait-on autorisé à y recourir quand l'orifice est très étroit.

Quand l'orifice est large, quand la paroi artérielle est effondrée sur une longueur telle que l'anévrysme sacciforme peut être confondu avec un anévrysme fusiforme, la reconstitution de l'artère par la suture du sac serait-elle prudente? Je ne crois pas que la coagulation soit à craindre, car au voisinage de l'orifice, le sac est revêtu d'endothélium et les caillots ne viennent pas jusque-là, à moins que l'anévrysme soit oblitéré; mais pourrait-on obtenir une paroi artérielle suffisamment résistante? Cela n'est pas probable, cependant il faut bien reconnaître que nous n'en savons rien.

Peut-être serait-il plus sage de réséquer un segment d'artère et de réunir les deux bouts par une suture circulaire. Nous avons vu qu'on peut réséquer plusieurs centimètres d'artère sans compromettre le rapprochement des deux extrémités, de sorte que, dans les anévrysmes des membres où la lésion artérielle est en général très localisée, la résection suivie de suture serait le plus souvent possible.

L'objection qui se présente tout de suite est celle de l'état de l'artère. On est tenté de se demander si au voisinage d'un anévrysme, la paroi des artères ne présente pas des altérations qui rendraient fatalement la suture inefficace. Avec les connaissances que nous avons sur la pathogénie des anévrysmes, avec ce que nous ont appris les nombreuses extirpations pratiquées depuis vingt ans, on peut répondre catégoriquement: Non, cette objection n'est pas fondée. Au voisinage d'un anévrysme, dans l'immense majorité des cas, l'artère est saine et la suture peut être exécutée dans de bonnes conditions.

Quant à l'artifice qui consisterait à remplacer le segment d'artère réséqué par un segment d'égale longueur de la veine correspondante, je ne crois pas qu'on puisse fonder sur lui grand espoir. Il semble très simple de sectionner l'artère en deux endroits et de suturer les deux bouts du segment ainsi détaché aux deux bouts de l'artère; mais nous avons vu dans la partie de ce rapport consacrée aux expériences que les tentatives de ce genre n'ont donné de résultats qu'entre les mains de Carrel qui les a mentionnés sans aucun détail. D'autre part, les veines sont souvent altérées, voire même oblitérées au voisinage des anévrysmes. Enfin, il ne serait pas sage de supprimer en tant que veines celles qui auraient conservé leur perméabilité. En effet, quand la ligature d'une artère est dangereuse, celle de la veine correspondante n'est pas indifférente. Et l'on ne peut songer à aller chercher une veine dans une autre région du corps pour la greffer sur l'artère, car les greffes artério-veineuses expérimentales n'ont pas donné de bons résultats.

L'intervention pour les anévrysmes des grosses artères doit se proposer un double but, l'un toujours réalisable, la suppression du sac, l'autre souvent impossible à atteindre, sorte d'idéal vers lequel il faut tendre, la reconstitution d'une artère perméable et bien calibrée.

Voici comment on pourrait, il me semble, conduire l'intervention.

J. L. Faure (1) a accusé la bande d'Esmarch d'être un facteur de gangrène. Il est possible que dans certains cas il vaille mieux ne pas s'en servir. D'ailleurs, il n'y a guère que pour les anévrysmes poplités qu'elle puisse être en question. Pour les anévrysmes de la fémorale commune, de l'axillaire, elle n'est pas applicable.

On commencera donc par découvrir l'artère au-dessus et au-dessous de la tumeur et on fera l'hémostase provisoire comme s'il s'agissait d'une plaie.

Faut-il ensuite inciser le sac avant de le disséquer ou le disséquer avant de l'inciser? Il est impossible de fixer une règle à cet égard. Dans certains cas, il peut être plus facile de disséquer la poche remplie et tendue; dans d'autres, il peut y avoir avantage à mettre le doigt dans la cavité pour se rendre compte de l'épaisseur de la paroi.

En tout cas, après ou avant la dissection, il faudrait ouvrir le sac pour étudier ses rapports avec l'artère. Si on arrive à bien voir l'orifice de communication, on se rend mieux compte de l'étendue de la lésion et on ne s'expose pas à sacrifier inutilement un segment trop considérable d'artère, ce qui pourrait arriver si l'on agissait par la périphérie de la poche. En effet, souvent le sac s'étale sur l'artère et la masque. Je crois que dans la très grande majorité des cas, on n'aura pas besoin de réséquer plus de deux

____

(1) J.-L. Faure, Soc. de Chirurgie 1906.

ou trois centimètres du vaisseau pour trouver une portion saine
capable de supporter les points de suture. On pourrait donc dans
bien des cas tenter la suture circulaire.

Il ne faut pas se faire des illusions exagérées sur ce que l'on
obtiendra de cette façon. Je pourrais répéter ici ce que je disais
à propos des plaies. La suture est bonne chez les gens jeunes dont les
artères sont saines et qui n'en ont pas besoin. Elle est mauvaise
ou inapplicable quand le système artériel est malade, alors qu'elle
serait utile. Et puis, dans certaines régions, par exemple au niveau du carrefour tibio-péronier si dangereux, elle se heurtera
à bien des difficultés. Cependant elle permettra peut-être d'éviter
quelques cas de gangrène.

Et si j'insiste sur le rétablissement de la circulation artérielle, ce n'est pas seulement pour les avantages que cette méthode
peut donner dans la cure des anévrysmes des membres, c'est
surtout parce qu'il doit permettre, me semble-t-il, d'étendre le domaine chirurgical.

Jusqu'ici les anévrysmes de l'aorte abdominale ont échappé
à l'action du chirurgien, puisque toutes les ligatures de cette portion de l'aorte se sont terminées par la mort. Tillaux et Riche [1]
en ont réuni 13 cas. Il faut y ajouter un cas de ligature temporaire qui appartient à Morris et qui a été publié depuis le mémoire des deux auteurs français.

Il s'agissait d'un nègre de 24 ans, syphilitique. L'opération
fut pratiquée le 1er Mai 1901. L'anévrysme sacciforme s'étendait
du tronc cœliaque à l'artère mésentérique. L'aorte fut liée au-dessus de l'anévrysme avec une sonde de caoutchouc mou fixée par
une pince. Neuf heures après l'opération, les membres inférieurs
sont chauds, mais la sensibilité y est abolie et ils sont le siège
de vives douleurs. Vingt-deux heures après, l'anévrysme diminue
et les pulsations deviennent moindres. A la vingt-septième heure,
on enlève la ligature. Le pouls devient perceptible dans les deux
fémorales. Le malade meurt au bout de cinquante-trois heures
par gangrène de l'intestin. Celle-ci est attribuée à la pression de
la pince. A l'autopsie, on trouva l'anévrysme rempli de caillots
avec l'aorte perméable, mais il y avait une embolie dans l'artère
iliaque gauche.

Le rétablissement de la circulation avait donc entraîné une
embolie dans l'iliaque.

---

[1] *Tillaux et Riche*, Revue de Chirurgie 1901.

De leur étude, Tillaux et Riche ont tiré les conclusions suivantes: «1.º La ligature de l'aorte abdominale chez l'homme n'a jamais amené de gangrène. 2.º Les phénomènes congestifs du côté de l'extrémité céphalique, sont rares et sans importance. 3.º Les phénomènes paraplégiques sont inconstants, variables et passagers. 4.º Les morts ne sont pas directement attribuables à l'opération.» D'où il résulte qu'on est autorisé à pratiquer la ligature de l'aorte abdominale. Mais comme tous les opérés sont morts, je pense que l'opération ne tentera personne.

Ne serait-il pas légitime d'essayer de faire la cure d'un anévrysme de l'aorte abdominale en conservant la perméabilité du vaisseau? Quand tous les moyens médicaux ont échoué et que l'anévrysme grossit, il me semble qu'on est autorisé à l'essayer. Mais quel procédé employer? La suture circulaire serait peut-être bien hasardeuse? La suture de l'orifice tiendrait-elle? Si elle mettait à l'abri de l'hémorrhagie secondaire, quand bien même la cicatrice devrait se distendre secondairement, elle pourrait encore rendre des services et prolonger la vie des malades. Il ne faut pas se montrer trop difficile pour une affection dont le pronostic est si grave. Mais mettrait-elle à l'abri de l'hémorrhagie secondaire? On peut en douter quand on voit que chez le malade de Keen (¹) une ligature aseptique de l'aorte a amené la section du vaisseau et une hémorrhagie mortelle au 48.º jour. Cette incertitude commande certes une extrême prudence, mais non pas l'abstention absolue. Il est d'ailleurs des cas où l'on a la main forcée. Ainsi, lorsque l'anévrysme se rompt, et qu'il se forme comme dans le cas de Keen un volumineux hématome sous-péritonéal, ne vaudrait-il pas mieux dans une telle occurrence faire une suture à plusieurs plans qu'une ligature? C'est par des faits de ce genre que nous apprendrons petit à petit, avec le temps, ce qu'on peut obtenir des conquêtes nouvelles de la chirurgie artérielle appliquée au traitement des anévrysmes de l'aorte abdominale.

Avec les appareils qui permettent d'assurer la respiration malgré l'ouverture large de la plèvre, l'aorte thoracique n'est plus inabordable. Elle n'est cependant pas d'un accès aisé, et je ne sais pas si l'audace qui peut être justifiée dans certains anévrysmes de l'aorte abdominale serait ici permise.

Mais c'est peut-être au niveau de la crosse de l'aorte que les

____

(¹) Keen. Ann. of Med. Sciences, Sept. 1900.

difficultés sont le plus insurmontables. On ne peut espérer faire une opération aussi compliquée que la cure radicale d'un anévrysme ni sur sa portion horizontale, ni sur sa portion descendante.

Sa portion ascendante est moins difficilement accessible, mais l'embarras est accru par l'impossibilité de faire l'hémostase provisoire. En effet, on ne peut suspendre le cours du sang dans la portion ascendante de la crosse aortique sans amener la mort immédiate par arrêt du cœur.

Tuffier (¹) a cependant tenté la cure opératoire d'un anévrysme de ce siège. Voici quelques extraits de la relation qu'il a donnée, à la Société de chirurgie de Paris, de cette intervention audacieuse.

«Pour aborder l'anévrysme, je taille un volet à convexité droite, à base attenant au bord droit du sternum et allant en hauteur depuis la deuxième côte jusqu'au cinquième espace intercostal droit, et, en largeur, du bord droit du sternum à quatre travers de doigt au dehors. Ce lambeau comprend à la fois la peau, le tissu cellulaire sous-cutané, les fibres du grand pectoral; celles du petit pectoral n'existent plus au niveau de l'anévrysme; leurs restes sont rabattus en dehors. Je tombe de suite sur l'anévrysme et je puis constater que la deuxième côte est luxée, incomplètement adhérente à la tumeur, et qu'elle adhère en outre à la face postérieure de la troisième côte et au cartilage costal correspondant, enfin à la plèvre médiastine. De ces adhérences, la moins intime me paraît celle de la troisième côte. Je la libère et je la résèque dans l'étendue de quatre travers de doigt. Je constate que le sac anévrysmal est d'une minceur extrême, sans trace d'induration; et le libère très prudemment en dehors... Pour éviter la rupture brusque de la poche anévrysmale, je sectionne la deuxième côte en dedans et en dehors et je laisse la partie médiane de cette côte adhérente à la face antéro-supérieure de la tumeur. Au cours de ces manœuvres, j'ouvre la plèvre médiastine, mais, à cause des adhérences, je n'ai qu'un pneumothorax très limité.» Tuffier poursuit lentement le décollement de la plèvre, du péricarde, du médiastin. «Je fais l'exploration de la poche anévrysmale, et, dans ce but, l'exprimant lentement et progressivement avec les doigts (après avoir constaté qu'elle ne contient pas de

---

(¹) *Tuffier*, Soc. de Chirurgie, 1902, pag. 326.

caillots, ce qui est facile, vu la minceur extrême et la souplesse
de la paroi, je cherche avec l'index, coiffé de la paroi anévrysmale, l'orifice de communication de la poche avec l'aorte. Je
trouve cet orifice relativement petit, admettant juste mon index et,
tout autour, une collerette d'adhérences entre la poche anévrysmale et la paroi aortique. Il semble donc possible de placer en
ce point une ligature sans courir trop de risque de rompre le pédicule du sac, puis d'enlever le sac et de refaire une suture aortique à la Lembert. Tout le sac étant disséqué, il ne me reste plus
qu'à placer une ligature sur son orifice. Je comprime le sac pour
débarrasser le champ opératoire qu'il gêne par son volume et par
ses pulsations, puis, faisant veiller sur le pouls et la respiration
de la malade, je pratique cette ligature à l'aide de deux fils de
catgut que je serre lentement, progressivement. Il ne se produisit
pas le moindre trouble de la respiration ni du pouls. C'est alors
que je commis une faute dont vous verrez plus loin l'importance:
je ne fis pas l'ablation du sac anévrysmal, maintenant vide et flasque. Je pensais que dans le cas où la ligature céderait, il pourrait encore servir à limiter l'hémorrhagie et, heureux, d'ailleurs,
d'avoir pu conduire l'opération jusque là sans accidents, je ra-
battis le volet thoracique et je le suturai après avoir assuré le
drainage du médiastin.»

La malade a succombé à une hémorrhagie dans le courant du
treizième jour.

L'autopsie a été faite et Tuffier en conclut: «que la malade a
succombé à une hémorrhagie secondaire par gangrène du sac.»

Malheureusement la pièce si intéressante, réclamée par divers
membres de la Société de chirurgie, n'a pu être présentée. Malgré
son énorme intérêt, elle a été perdue, perte d'autant plus regret-
table que des doutes ont été émis sur le siège de la ligature qui avait
été faite. Poirier (¹) a critiqué certaines obscurités de l'observation et conclu en ces termes:

«Telle quelle, elle prouve surabondamment que M. Tuffier n'a
point placé ni deux, ni un fil autour du collet aortique de l'anévrysme; la ligature a été placée sur la partie moyenne du sac, à
distance de l'orifice aortique, plus près du sommet que du collet
du sac; la lecture attentive de l'observation, celle surtout de l'autopsie, ne permettent aucun doute à cet égard; ainsi, sur les des-

---

(¹) *Poirier*, Soc. d. chirurgie 1903 p. 419

sins, le sac apparaît divisé sur la ligature en deux tumeurs jumelles,... et l'orifice aortique est libre de toute ligature.»

Il faut convenir que les dessins semblent donner raison à Poirier; mais en l'absence de la pièce, la question reste éternellement discutable.

Aussi je ne la discuterai pas. J'y suis d'autant moins enclin que, quand bien même le fil double aurait été placé sur l'orifice de communication de l'aorte avec l'anévrysme, l'opération de Tuffier n'aurait eu, à mon avis, aucune chance de succès. On n'oblitère pas une plaie artérielle comme une plaie veineuse par une simple ligature latérale. Et ce qu'a voulu faire Tuffier n'est même pas l'homologue d'une ligature latérale posée sur une veine, car les fils auraient été placés sur le sac, c'est-à-dire sur des tissus malades et de peu de résistance.

Tuffier croit que l'hémorrhagie a été causée par la gangrène du sac; je pense qu'elle se serait produite sans cela. Mais s'il avait été sûrement jusqu'à l'orifice aortique, s'il l'avait suturé, comme il en a eu l'intention, et non lié, peut-être aurait-il obtenu un beau succès.

En tout cas, son audace et son sang froid ont montré qu'il n'est pas impossible d'aborder chirurgicalement un anévrysme de la portion ascendante de la crosse de l'aorte. Mais il reconnaît lui-même que les anévrysmes de ce siège qui pourraient devenir justiciables d'une intervention chirurgicale sont infiniment rares. Ce n'est pas de ce côté que les nouvelles conquêtes de la chirurgie artérielle donneront une belle moisson.

VI — PLAIES DES VEINES

La ligature latérale des veines est depuis longtemps passée dans la pratique. Quand une veine présente une étroite déchirure, quand une petite collatérale est arrachée au ras de son insertion, on saisit l'orifice avec une pince à forcipressure et on applique une ligature en bourse.

Puis, la suture latérale est devenue une sorte de coquetterie chirurgicale. On suture des veines dont la ligature n'entraînerait aucun dommage. Rares d'ailleurs sont les veines dont la ligature est dangereuse.

Heinlein (1), Turazza (2), Koehler (3) ont suturé les saphènes,

---

(1) *Heinlein*, cité par Kay, Inaug. Dissertation, Kiel 1891, et Brachet, Th. de Bordeaux 1896.
(2) *Turazza*, cité par Kay, Inaug. Dissertation, Kiel 1891, et Brachet, Th. de Bordeaux 1896.
(3) *Koehler*, cité par Kay, Inaug. Dissertation, Kiel 1891, et Brachet, Th. de Bordeaux 1896.

et certainement il a été fait sur les veines petites ou moyennes un grand nombre de sutures qui n'ont pas été publiées et qui ne méritaient pas de l'être.

La suture des grosses veines a plus d'intérêt. Et dans tous les cas que j'ai pu relever où elle a porté sur des vaisseaux des membres, elle n'a donné que des succès.

Je parle de succès cliniques, car il est fort difficile d'être renseigné sur le résultat anatomique. Les veines ne battent pas, et bien souvent leur obstruction ne s'accuse par aucun symptôme. Aussi Lister [1] et Heinlein [2] ont suturé la veine axillaire, mais dans nombre de cas la ligature de ce vaisseau n'a amené aucun trouble circulatoire, pas même une minute d'œdème. Et cela n'est pas surprenant, car la veine axillaire n'est pas unique. Il y a toujours des canaux veineux collatéraux et particulièrement la collatérale externe, souvent presqu'aussi volumineuse que le tronc principal.

La sous-clavière est moins bien suppléée, et il peut y avoir intérêt à la suturer. Farino [3] l'a fait avec succès. La petite plaie due à un coup de couteau a été oblitérée par deux points à la soie.

C'est une suture du tronc brachio-céphalique que Ricard [4] a exécutée dans un cancer du corps thyroïde qui l'avait obligé à réséquer la jugulaire jusqu'à la terminaison. Il a fait deux plans.

Marin [5] a également suturé avec succès le tronc brachio-céphalique lésé par une balle de révolver.

La veine jugulaire a été suturée un certain nombre de fois. J'en ai relevé sept cas. Le premier est le seul qui se soit terminé par la mort. Il appartient à Czerny [6]. Ce n'est pas la suture qu'il faut incriminer, mais les conditions dans lesquelles elle a été faite. Le vaisseau avait été ulcéré par une suppuration consécutive à une œsophagotomie externe. Deux jours après la suture, il se produisait une hémorrhagie secondaire qui obligea à faire la ligature. Le malade succomba à la pyohémie. Ce cas montre que pas plus pour les artères que pour les veines, il ne faut faire de suture en milieu septique.

[1] [2] Cités par Brachet, Th. de Bordeaux 1895.
[3] Farino, Clinica Chirurgica, Milano 1902 T. 10 p. 361.
[4] Ricard, Congrès de Chirurgie 189?.
[5] Marin, New York Med. J. 1892 T. 68 p. 411.
[6] Czerny, in Brachet, T. de Bordeaux 1895.

Kay [1] a rapporté trois cas de suture de la jugulaire interne.
Pasca [2] et Clermont [3], chacun un.

Le fait de Schede [4] est le plus intéressant, parce qu'il a été
suivi d'une vérification nécropsique tardive. La veine avait été
blessée au cours de l'extirpation d'un ganglion tuberculeux du cou.
Le malade a bien guéri. Mais il succomba quatre mois après à
des accidents typhiques, et l'on put constater que la veine suturée ne présentait aucune altération.

Kay a rapporté une observation de suture de la poplitée, provenant de la clinique de Kiel, et où la perméabilité de la veine
semble avoir persisté.

En opérant un myxo-sarcome, il dut réséquer une lanière de
la veine adhérente à la tumeur. L'ouverture fut fermée par un
surjet à la soie. La plaie ayant été tamponnée, en changeant le
pansement le septième jour, on put reconnaître la veine, sous
forme d'un cordon grisâtre. Rien n'indiquait qu'elle fût thrombosée.

Schede [4], Heineke [5], Kummel [5], Tansini [5], Postemsky [5],
Lauge [5], Marin [6], ont fait avec un succès clinique la suture
latérale de la veine fémorale.

Dans le cas de Ricard [7], il s'agissait d'une dilatation ampul-
laire de la saphène qui se prolongeait sur la fémorale. On ne pouvait donc la réséquer sans lier la fémorale. Ricard fit la suture, et
sa malade a bien guéri.

Tous ces faits sont intéressants, car la ligature de la veine
fémorale n'est pas inoffensive.

Celui de Kummel [8] l'est davantage car il a fait une suture circulaire. Ce chirurgien avait dû réséquer sur une étendue de deux
centimètres la fémorale adhérente à une tumeur. Il ne restait qu'un
pont étroit de deux millimètres. La suture fut faite en surjets à
points perforants. Il ne se produisit aucun incident.

Tous les chirurgiens se rappellent l'émotion causée en 1892
par la publication du premier cas de suture de la veine cave.

---

[1] Kay, Inaug. Dissertatio, Kiel 1894.
[2] Pasca, Bull. della Soc. Lancisiana T. XVI 1896.
[3] Clermont, Presse Méd. 1901 n.° 40 p. 229.
[4] Schede, in Bruche, J. de Bordeaux 1893 obs. VII.
[5] Niebergall, Deutsch. Zeitschrift für Chirurg. T. XXIII.
[6] Marin, N. York Med. Journal 1893 T. 68 p. 411.
[7] Ricard, Congrès de chirurgie 1893.
[8] Kummel, Wien. med. Press. 1900 n.° 2.

Schede [1] ayant fait en extirpant un cancer du rein une plaie de deux centimètres à ce vaisseau, la ferma par un surjet au catgut. Les suites opératoires ne furent marquées d'aucun incident, et le malade ayant succombé, trois semaines après, à la dégénérescence graisseuse du cœur, on put constater que la veine était parfaitement perméable. Il n'y avait pas trace de caillot au niveau de la suture.

Bien que les anastomoses de la veine cave soient innombrables, le volume du vaisseau inspirait la crainte, et on ne pouvait croire qu'il pût être lié sans de graves inconvénients. Mais, voilà que Houzel [2], s'étant trouvé dans la nécessité de le lier, constate que la circulation se rétablit sans aucune difficulté. Il ne se produisit qu'un léger œdème malléolaire.

Héresco [3], qui connaissait le cas de Houzel, ayant déchiré la veine cave au cours d'une néphrectomie transpéritonéale pour pyonéphrose calculeuse, ne chercha pas à la suturer et fit une double ligature. Les suites de cette ligature furent aussi simples que possible: elle n'entraîna même pas le plus léger œdème des membres inférieurs.

Kuster [4], en examinant un volumineux cancer du rein qu'il venait d'extirper, s'aperçut qu'il avait enlevé un morceau de la veine cave. Celle-ci avait donc été liée. Le malade mourut d'embolie 16 heures après la fin de l'opération. Ce fait ne prouve pas que la circulation ne puisse se rétablir après la ligature du vaisseau.

D'autres sutures ont été faites au cours de néphrectomies. Le malade de Grohe [5] succomba au bout de 24 heures. Giordano [6] perdit également le sien. Mais Zoegé Manteuffel [7] obtint un beau succès. Il avait dû extirper une lanière de veine cave mesurant neuf centimètres de long sur deux centimètres et demi de large. Il ne put naturellement suturer cette brèche qu'au prix d'un notable rétrécissement. Le malade a bien guéri.

Dans cette question, on ne peut pas faire état de la mortalité, car la blessure de la veine cave n'est qu'un incident au cours

---

[1] Schede, Archiv. f. klin. Chirurg. 1891
[2] Houzel, Soc. Chirurgie 1901.
[3] Héresco.
[4] Kuster, cité par Albarran, Soc. Chirurgie 1902, p. 1397
[5] Grohe
[6] Giordano
[7] Zoegé Manteuffel, Cent. f. Chirurgie 1899

d'opérations considérables qui pourraient sans cela entraîner la mort. Ce qu'il faut retenir de ces faits, c'est que les troubles circulatoires entraînés par la ligature de la veine cave sont insignifiants ou même nuls. Quand on se trouve en présence d'une blessure de ce vaisseau, on a donc le choix entre la ligature et la suture. La suture est plus élégante, elle est plus physiologique, elle satisfait mieux l'esprit : il vaut mieux la pratiquer quand les circonstances sont favorables. Mais quand on opère en milieu septique, comme cela est arrivé à Héresco, la double ligature donne peut-être plus de sécurité.

Il est une autre veine pour laquelle la suppléance est à peu près impossible. C'est la veine porte. Si on venait à la blesser au cours d'opérations sur les voies biliaires, la suture serait naturellement indiquée. Dans les plaies accidentelles, elle serait possible, car la mort n'est pas immédiate. Le sang s'infiltre dans l'épiploon gastrohépatique ; l'hémorrhagie se fait en plusieurs temps, de telle sorte que dans bien des cas on pourrait intervenir avec des chances de succès.

VII.—ANÉVRYSMES ARTÉRIO-VEINEUX

On verra de moins en moins de ces vieux anévrysmes artério-veineux pourvus de sacs intermédiaires ou veineux qui rendent le traitement malaisé. On en verra de moins en moins parce qu'on les diagnostiquera plus tôt et qu'on fera des opérations plus précoces. Alors, on trouvera de simples fistules artério-veineuses, et il sera facile de suturer les deux orifices vasculaires.

Il ne me paraît donc pas douteux que la suture doive remplacer dans le traitement des anévrysmes artério-veineux la quadruple ligature que j'ai défendue il y a dix-sept ans [1].

Les faits de suture ne sont pas nombreux, ce qui n'a rien de surprenant, car les anévrysmes artério-veineux sont rares. Je n'en ai relevé que six cas.

Gérard-Marchant [2] et Peugneiz [3] ont lié la veine et suturé l'artère seule.

Dans le cas de Gérard-Marchant, la lésion portait sur les

[1] *Pierre Delbet.* Traitement des Anévrysmes artério-veineux. T. de Paris 1891.
[2] *Gérard-Marchant.* Soc. de Chirurgie 1898 p. 727.
[3] *Peugneiz.* Gazette Médicale de Picardie 1900.

vaisseaux huméraux. Il ne semble pas que la perméabilité de l'artère ait persisté.

Dans le fait de Peugniez, l'anévrysme occupait le pli du coude. Le chirurgien plaça sur l'artère sept points séparés. Le pouls radial se rétablit.

J'ai déjà rapporté au chapitre des plaies artérielles le cas très complet de Zoege Manteuffel [1]. L'artère fémorale profonde fut liée; l'artère et la veine fémorale commune, suturées. Le malade a guéri sans gangrène.

Je rappelle que Matas [2] a traité également par la suture et avec succès un anévrysme artério-veineux du triangle de Scarpa. Je n'ai pu trouver aucun détail sur ce cas.

Koerte [3] fit la suture de l'artère et de la veine. L'anévrysme portait sur les vaisseaux poplités. La guérison se fit sans incident, et les vaisseaux restèrent perméables.

Dans un cas d'anévrysme des vaisseaux sous-claviers droits, Matas [4] a suturé la veine et lié l'artère. Il a commencé par faire une résection ostéoplastique de la clavicule, puis il a été à la recherche du tronc brachio-céphalique. Ce dernier ne paraissant pas exister, il a mis un fil sur la sous-clavière près de l'aorte. Puis il a cherché à séparer l'artère de la veine. Cette séparation ayant amené une hémorrhagie assez abondante, l'auteur fit la ligature de l'artère au-dessus et au-dessous de la perforation, puis il sutura latéralement la veine. Le malade a guéri, mais il a perdu le pouce et le petit doigt qui se sont gangrénés. Il a eu une nécrose du cubitus. Les doigts subsistants et le poignet sont restés raides et insensibles.

VIII — GREFFES DE MEMBRES ET D'ORGANES

Tous les expérimentateurs qui ont étudié les sutures circulaires des vaisseaux ont rêvé de maintenir vivants des membres ou des organes complètement séparés de l'organisme pendant quelques instants.

Les greffes par simple juxtaposition ne réussissent que pour des fragments petits et à structure simple comme le bout du nez,

[1] *Zoege Manteuffel*. Berl. klin. Woch. 1891.
[2] *Matas*, cité par Hoepfner. Arch. f. klin. Chirurgie 1903 T. 70.
[3] *Koerte*, 33 Congrès de la Soc. Allemande de Chirurgie 1904 p. 430.
[4] *Rudolph Matas*, Journal of the American Association 1902. p. 103, 173, 243, 313.

la pulpe des doigts. Dès que le fragment détaché a une structure complexe, même s'il est de petites dimensions comme une phalange, la greffe échoue. Il semble que l'insuffisance de la circulation soit la seule cause de l'échec.

Les cellules supportent un certain temps l'ischémie totale sans succomber. Si par une suture circulaire des vaisseaux on ramenait le sang vivifiant à leur contact avant qu'elles ne soient gravement altérées, pourquoi ne continueraient-elles pas à vivre? Pourquoi ne pourrait-on pas maintenir vivants des membres entiers, des organes compliqués? Certains, qui sont infiniment précieux pour l'équilibre de la santé ou même la conservation de la vie, semblent particulièrement bien disposés pour la greffe. Ainsi la rate, ainsi le rein, dont la circulation est assurée par une artère et une veine uniques.

Mais le sang n'est pas tout, l'influx nerveux n'est-il point indispensable au fonctionnement normal de certaines cellules? Et s'il est possible de rétablir immédiatement la circulation par une bonne suture vasculaire, il n'y a pas de suture nerveuse qui puisse rétablir instantanément l'influx nerveux. Il n'est pas besoin de discuter ici la réparation autogène des nerfs, car il est bien évident qu'elle ne peut se produire dans un membre ou un organe complètement détaché de l'organisme.

A côté de la circulation, il y a donc une autre condition capitale pour le succès des greffes massives, c'est que les cellules des tissus à greffer résistent à l'énervation, et puissent attendre sans présenter d'irrémédiables altérations la régénération des nerfs.

A ce point de vue, il faut distinguer les membres et les parenchymes glandulaires. Cette distinction a été soigneusement faite par Hoepfner (1).

Dans les membres, tous les tissus peuvent vivre énervés. Ils ne présentent même pas de troubles trophiques lorsque les nerfs sont sectionnés. Ces troubles sont dus aux névrites, et non à la section des nerfs, c'est-à-dire aux perturbations quantitatives ou qualitatives de l'influx nerveux, et non à sa suppression. A la vérité, les muscles s'atrophient, mais ils ne disparaissent pas; ils restent longtemps susceptibles de se régénérer. Les résultats des sutures nerveuses tardives le prouvent surabondamment.

---

(1) *Hoepfner*, Arch. f. klin. Chirurgie 1903 t. 70, p. 417.

Il semble donc n'y avoir aucune raison pour que la greffe d'un membre complètement séparé pendant quelques instants du reste de l'organisme ne réussisse pas. Le rétablissement de la circulation par la suture des principaux vaisseaux permettra aux cellules de vivre. Insensibles et immobiles mais vivantes, elles attendront la régénération des nerfs.

L'entreprise présente incontestablement d'énormes difficultés, mais elle méritait d'être tentée. C'est ce qu'a fait Hoepfner et il a presque réussi. Ses belles expériences méritent d'être rapportées avec quelques détails.

Toutes les trois ont porté sur des chiens et sur les pattes de derrière.

Il a commencé par sectionner la peau de la face interne de la cuisse à trois travers de doigt au-dessous du pli de l'aine. L'artère et la veine fémorale sont soigneusement préparées pour éviter toute lésion accidentelle. Les muscles sont ensuite coupés circulairement, et tout ce qui saigne est pincé et lié. Les moignons musculaires, le nerf sciatique et les grosses branches du nerf crural sont repérés par des fils. C'est seulement quand toutes les parties molles sont coupées qu'il sectionne l'artère et la veine fémorale après avoir assuré l'hémostase par des pinces. Il termine en sciant le fémur en escalier ou très obliquement après avoir percé des trous qui serviront au passage des fils métalliques.

L'amputation ainsi terminée, il procède immédiatement à la greffe. L'os est d'abord fixé par des fils de bronze d'aluminium, puis il réunit les vaisseaux par la méthode de Payre. Les muscles et les nerfs sont suturés aussi exactement que possible avec du catgut, et la peau est affrontée par des surjets à la soie interrompus par place pour permettre le drainage. Par dessus le pansement, on applique un appareil plâtré muni d'attelles en aluminium qui a été préparé d'avance.

Dès que la circulation est rétablie par la suture, d'un seul coup, le membre reprend sa couleur normale. Il se réchauffe et les petits vaisseaux du côté amputé, dilatés sans doute par la paralysie, se mettent à saigner. La dilatation vasculaire persiste dans les jours suivants, et la température du membre au-dessous de la ligne d'amputation reste notablement plus élevée que celle du reste du corps.

Les deux grosses difficultés, dit Hoepfner, qui ne parle même pas de celles de l'opération, sont de maintenir l'asepsie du pansement et d'obtenir une bonne fixation du membre amputé. Le pansement est facilement souillé par les excréments. En outre, l'insensibilité du membre fait que l'animal ne prend aucune précaution. Ainsi, l'un des chiens sautait joyeusement au huitième jour en s'appuyant sur le membre greffé.

Voici le résultat de ces trois expériences. Dans le premier cas, les vaisseaux se thrombosèrent dès le premier jour. Le membre se gangréna, et l'animal fut tué le cinquième jour.

Dans le troisième cas, la circulation se maintint pendant six jours. Mais le cinquième jour étaient apparus des signes d'une inflammation phlegmoneuse, qui amena la thrombose.

C'est la seconde expérience qui faillit donner un succès complet. La circulation se maintint pendant onze jours. Le onzième jour, on endormit le chien pour changer le pansement, et il mourut pendant la narcose. Je ne puis penser sans émotion au crève-cœur qu'a dû être cet accident pour l'expérimentateur, qui par sa sage audace, par son habileté, par sa patience admirable, était arrivé si près du succès. En effet, l'autopsie a montré que toutes les conditions du succès complet étaient réalisées. La peau n'était désunie qu'à la face interne, et elle était en ce point recouverte de granulations rosées. Dans tout le reste de la circonférence du membre, la réunion par première intention était parfaite. Les muscles étaient solidement réunis, et il fallut une traction considérable pour les séparer. Les vaisseaux étaient perméables. Seul l'os dépouillé de son périoste sur une certaine étendue montrait peu de tendance à la réparation.

Il est vraiment impossible d'approcher plus près du succès. Toutes les constatations nécropsiques permettent de penser qu'il eût été complet sans ce malheureux accident chloroformique.

Ces tentatives ne sont pas d'ordre purement spéculatif. Les circonstances où l'on pourrait greffer un membre sur un homme, seront sans doute rares, mais il n'est pas impossible qu'on les rencontre. Les écrasements presque linéaires qui sont produits par les roues métalliques étroits des tramways pourraient en fournir l'occasion. Actuellement, quand les vaisseaux et les nerfs sont coupés, on ampute. Il y a des cas où l'on pourrait peut-être tenter la conservation en suturant nerfs et vaisseaux.

Certaines tumeurs malignes des os commandent l'amputation, voire même la désarticulation. Or, il est bien certain que ce n'est pas la partie du membre située au-dessous de la tumeur qui est dangereuse pour la récidive. Il n'y aurait donc pas d'inconvénient à la conserver. Il n'est pas impossible que l'on rencontre des dispositions telles que l'on puisse tenter l'amputation ou plutôt la résection d'une tranche de membre en conservant les parties sous-jacentes.

C'est pour les parenchymes glandulaires que se pose la question du rôle des nerfs. Les nerfs sécrétoires sont aujourd'hui bien connus, et l'on s'est habitué à cette idée qu'ils sont indispensables.

Si cette idée correspond à la réalité, il faut renoncer à greffer les organes glandulaires. En effet, à la suite de la greffe, seul le tissu de soutènement continuerait à vivre, tandis que les cellules sécrétoires succomberaient. On aurait greffé non pas une glande, mais un squelette de glande. Et quand bien même les cellules épithéliales pourraient attendre dans un demi-sommeil la régénération des nerfs, elles n'en étaient pas moins incapables de fonctionner immédiatement. Or, le principal intérêt pratique de la greffe glandulaire est d'obtenir le fonctionnement immédiat de l'organe greffé.

Mais les nerfs sont-ils aussi nécessaires à la sécrétion que l'on s'est habitué à le croire?

Dans les paralysies faciales d'origine infratemporale, on observe quelquefois la diminution de la sécrétion salivaire, mais non sa disparition complète. Après les sections même élevées de la moelle épinière, les reins continuent à sécréter. S'ils s'infectent facilement, ils suffisent cependant à l'élimination urinaire. Il est vrai que nous ne savons pas ce que devient dans ces cas le plexus solaire qui leur fournit de nombreux filets.

La question ne pouvait être tranchée que par la voie expérimentale. C'est ce que Floresco [1] s'est appliqué à faire dans une intéressante série de recherches.

Sur un chien anesthésié, il met à nu le rein gauche par la voie dorso-lombaire, dissèque avec de fines pinces tous les filets nerveux qu'il peut trouver dans le pédicule et les sectionne; puis le rein est remis à sa place et la plaie suturée. Quinze jours après, il enlève le rein droit (côté opposé), et l'animal reste en bonne santé. Le rein énervé fonctionnait donc; mais peut-être n'était-il pas énervé complètement. Les nerfs qui cheminent dans la paroi des vaisseaux n'avaient pas été touchés.

Aussi, Floresco a-t-il fait d'autres expériences.

[1] *Floresco*, Journal de Physiologie et de pathologie générale 1905 p. 27 et 47.

Il sectionne sur un chien la veine rénale et la suture, puis il coupe les filets nerveux et lymphatiques. Seule, l'artère n'a pas été sectionnée. Quelques jours après, on enlève le rein du côté opposé et le chien reste en bonne santé.

Dans une autre expérience, il sectionne tout sauf l'urétère. Mais voici comment il procède. Les filets nerveux sont coupés d'abord, puis, après avoir assuré l'hémostase provisoire, il sectionne la veine et la suture immédiatement. Enfin, il coupe et suture l'artère rénale. Quelques jours après le rein du côté opposé est enlevé. L'animal ne présente aucun trouble et l'urine a le même caractère chimique qu'avant l'opération.

Dans une dernière expérience, artère, veine, nerfs, urétère, tout a été sectionné et, après suture, le rein a continué à fonctionner normalement.

Ces belles expériences, auxquelles je ne vois rien à objecter, prouvent indiscutablement que le rein complètement énervé peut fonctionner normalement. C'est un résultat fort surprenant; mais il faut s'incliner devant la constance des succès expérimentaux de Floresco.

Les transplantations du rein n'en ont pas donné d'aussi bons. Ulmann [1], Exner [2], Carrel [3] avaient essayé de greffer le rein dans la région cervicale. Aucune de ces tentatives ne semble avoir été couronnée de succès.

Floresco a tenté des expériences de greffes homoplastiques dans la région inguinale, c'est-à-dire qu'il a enlevé le rein d'un chien et l'a greffé dans l'aine d'un autre chien en suturant l'artère et la veine rénale à l'artère et à la veine fémorale. Dans toutes ces expériences, le rein transplanté a commencé à se nécroser dès le lendemain de l'opération. Floresco attribue ces échecs à la région.

Il a ensuite essayé la transplantation dans la région cervicale en anastomosant la veine rénale avec la jugulaire et l'artère rénale avec la carotide. Il a toujours fait des greffes homoplastiques; toutes ont échoué. Le rein s'est nécrosé du deuxième au neuvième jour.

Enfin, il a fait des greffes dans la région lombaire, à la place normale du rein; c'est-à-dire qu'il a pris un rein à un chien et l'a

---

[1] *Ulmann*, Wiener klin. Woch. 1902.
[2] *Exner*, in Floresco, Journal de Physiologie et de Pathologie générale 1905 p. 17 et 47.
[3] *Carrel*, Lyon Médical 1902.

greffé sur un autre chien néphrectomisé en suturant l'artère et la veine rénale de l'un à l'artère et à la veine rénale de l'autre.

Un chien est mort le troisième jour: l'artère était nécrosée, le rein transformé en une bouillie puante.

Dans un autre cas, l'artère rénale du chien sur lequel on greffait le rein était si large, et le courant sanguin si fort, que le rein devint turgescent, au point que sa rupture semblait imminente. L'auteur dut réduire le calibre de l'artère par des sutures latérales.

Tous les animaux succombèrent du deuxième au cinquième jour. L'uretère avait été fixé à la peau, et l'on crut que l'infection s'était faite par lui.

Floresco tenta de nouvelles expériences en anastomosant l'uretère à l'uretère. Le résultat ne fut pas meilleur.

Dans ces expériences, le rein était privé de sang bien plus longtemps que dans celles qui avaient pour but d'étudier le rôle des nerfs. Dans celles-ci en effet, on ne sectionnait l'artère qu'après avoir déjà anastomosé la veine ou réciproquement. Aussi, Floresco fut-il conduit à se demander si les insuccès de la transplantation n'étaient pas dus à la faible vitalité du tissu rénal. Pour voir si le rein était en état de supporter l'ischémie pendant le temps nécessaire à la transplantation, il fit le pincement des vaisseaux rénaux pendant une heure. Un rein ainsi traité s'atrophia de moitié en deux jours. Dans un autre cas, la circulation ne fut suspendue que pendant une demi-heure, le rein ne présenta pas d'altération. Il semble donc que la stase sanguine prolongée soit une des causes des échecs de la transplantation.

Pour la supprimer, Floresco, après avoir pincé l'artère et la veine, introduit une aiguille dans l'artère au-delà de la compression et lave le rein avec la solution physiologique de chlorure de sodium (7,5 ‰). Une aiguille plantée dans la veine assure l'écoulement du liquide. On suture les deux piqûres et au bout d'une heure, on enlève les pinces hémostatiques. Le rein ne diminue pas de volume dans la suite. La même expérience faite avec la solution de Locke a donné le même résultat.

Fort de ses expériences, Floresco transplante un rein après en avoir chassé tout le sang par un lavage. Le chien meurt le troisième jour, et l'on constate à l'autopsie que le rein est nécrosé.

Pour empêcher le sang de se coaguler dans le rein, tout en l'y laissant, Floresco fait au chien auquel il emprunte le rein une injection intra-veineuse de peptone, d'extrait de tête de sangsue, ou d'hélicorubine. Le rein transplanté se sphacèle aussi du deuxième au quatrième jour.

Floresco arrive alors à se demander si la nécrose n'est pas due à l'air qui reste dans les vaisseaux entre les ligatures provisoires et qui, en embolisant les capillaires, empêche la circulation de se rétablir. Alors, avant de terminer la suture, il injecte de la solution physiologique ou de la solution de peptone dans le segment de l'artère et de la veine compris entre les ligatures provisoires de manière à en chasser l'air. Le rein se sphacèle encore dans le même laps de temps.

Enfin Floresco se sert de la vaseline qui a, comme on le sait, la propriété de retarder la coagulation du sang. Avant de terminer la suture, il introduit de la vaseline dans les bouts des vaisseaux. «Par ce procédé, dit-il, on obtient deux résultats; on chasse les bulles gazeuses, et une couche mince de vaseline adhérent aux parois vasculaires empêche la coagulation du sang».

Dans toutes les expériences faites avec cette technique où l'uretère fut abouché à l'extérieur, les animaux succombèrent par infection du rein.

Floresco refait les mêmes expériences en anastomosant les uretères bout à bout.

Un premier chien survit; l'opération avait été très rapide: elle n'avait duré qu'une demi-heure. Le seizième jour, on l'endort et on rouvre la plaie pour inspecter le rein transplanté: «Il ne présente aucune partie molle et est encastré dans les organes voisins. Le chien reste en bonne santé».

L'observation s'arrête au vingt-cinquième jour, et l'auteur déclare qu'il se propose de faire ultérieurement l'ablation du rein qui n'a pas été touché.

L'observation suivante est intitulée; «Rein transplanté avec uretère anastomosé à l'autre uretère. Résection du rein normal». Dans le détail de l'observation, il n'est pas dit à quel moment a été faite la néphrectomie. L'animal est mort le douzième jour.

Enfin, dans une dernière expérience, le rein est transplanté gorgé de peptone, et le rein normal est réséqué. L'observation s'arrête au huitième jour. L'animal se portait bien.

Floresco conclut de cette belle série de recherches que la transplantation du rein est très difficile, mais possible. La conclusion est excessive. Elle escompte l'avenir, car au moment où l'auteur a publié son mémoire (Janvier 1905), la preuve n'était pas faite qu'un rein transplanté pouvait sécréter d'une manière suffisante en quantité et en qualité. Elle était bien près de l'être, puisque deux chiens survivaient avec un rein provenant d'un autre animal de même espèce. Mais ils avaient encore le rein sain. Sans doute on le leur a depuis enlevé, et j'espère qu'ils ont survécu avec le rein transplanté.

Le rein est le seul organe glandulaire sur la transplantation duquel nous ayons des renseignements circonstanciés.

Floresco termine le travail que je viens d'analyser en disant qu'il a fait avec succès la transplantation de la rate, mais il ne donne aucun détail.

Carrel (1) a transplanté le cœur d'un petit chien dans la région cervicale d'un plus gros, en anastomosant la veine jugulaire et la carotide avec l'aorte, l'artère pulmonaire, une des veines caves, et une veine pulmonaire. Les détails manquent sur cette singulière opération qui d'ailleurs n'a pas réussi. Le sang s'est coagulé dans les artères cardiaques au bout de deux heures.

TABLE DES MATIÈRES

(1) Carrel, *American Medecine*, 30 déc. 1905.

THÈME 2 — **LES ANASTOMOSES GASTRO-INTESTINALES
ET INTESTINO-INTESTINALES**

(Les anastomoses intestinales et gastro-intestinales)

Par M. le Prof. HENRI HARTMANN (Paris)

Désirant, dans ce travail, envisager la question des anastomoses intestinales et gastro-intestinales spécialement au point de vue de la technique opératoire, nous ne nous limiterons pas à la description de l'anastomose, simple moyen de dérivation, comme le font les auteurs qui se placent au point de vue clinique exclusif, et, conformément au sens précis du mot *anastomose* (ανα, ensemble, στομα, bouche), nous parlerons de tous les cas où l'on est amené à aboucher l'un à l'autre deux segments du tube digestif.

L'opération peut se réduire à une simple anastomose entre

deux anses d'intestin, c'est l'ancienne *entéro-anastomose* de Maisonneuve, qui établit une communication latérale entre deux anses plus ou moins éloignées ; lorsque la communication latérale est établie entre l'estomac et une anse d'intestin, elle porte le nom de *gastro-entérostomie*, opération très couramment pratiquée aujourd'hui.

Dans d'autres cas on fait suivre l'entéro-anastomose de la section et de l'oblitération uni ou bilatérale d'un segment de l'anse intermédiaire aux points anastomosés, excluant ainsi une portion d'intestin de la circulation digestive ; c'est *l'exclusion uni* ou *bilatérale* de l'intestin.

Enfin l'anastomose intestinale ou gastro-intestinale peut constituer le *dernier temps d'une résection segmentaire du canal alimentaire* et n'a pour but que de rétablir le cours du contenu digestif.

Suivant la manière dont les portions d'intestin sont mises en rapports, on distingue les anastomoses en *latéro-latérales*, *termino-terminales* ou bout à bout, et *termino-latérales* ou par implantation.

Dans tous les cas, la technique de l'anastomose reste la même et donne lieu à des considérations générales identiques.

I. — TECHNIQUE GÉNÉRALE DES ANASTOMOSES

Il faut, lorsqu'on pratique une anastomose sur le tube digestif :

1° Éviter la contamination du péritoine pendant et après l'opération ;

2° Avoir un bon fonctionnement de la bouche que l'on vient de créer.

§ 1. — *Éviter la contamination du péritoine.*

Il faut *éviter la contamination du péritoine par le contenu septique du tube digestif*, sous peine de voir le malade succomber à des accidents péritonitiques. Comme cette contamination peut se produire à différents moments, il y a lieu d'étudier successivement les moyens qui permettent d'éviter la contamination : 1° au cours de l'opération ; 2° après l'opération.

A. — Moyens d'éviter la contamination du péritoine au cours de l'opération.

Pour éviter la contamination du péritoine au cours de l'opération, un certain nombre de chirurgiens ont imaginé des procédés dans lesquels l'ouverture du tube digestif ne se fait qu'une fois des adhérences établies entre les cavités à anastomoser.

Le premier temps, le seul opératoire, consiste dans l'accolement des deux anses d'intestin.

Le deuxième, consistant dans l'ouverture des cavités, a lieu sans intervention nouvelle du chirurgien, qui s'est placé dans des conditions telles que l'opération, commencée lors du premier temps, doit fatalement se terminer d'elle-même.

J. M. F. Gaston of Atlanta[1], Franz Bardenheuer[2], Theo. A. Mac Graw[3] employèrent dans ce but des ligatures élastiques. Dans le plus connu de ces procédés, celui de Mac Graw, on enserre un pouce et demi d'intestin dans une ligature faite avec un caoutchouc de 2 millimètres de diamètre. Comme on a soin d'amincir la portion de caoutchouc qui traverse le chas de l'aiguille et de le maintenir fortement étiré pendant son passage à travers les tuniques intestinales, le trou fait à la paroi est plus petit que le caoutchouc lui-même dans sa portion extérieure, et tout épanchement fécal est empêché. Graw prend du reste la précaution d'enfouir les parties étreintes par la ligature élastique entre un double rang de sutures non perforantes de Lembert.

Kaïe, Postnikow, Bastianelli, Paul Souligoux, Doyen, etc., sont arrivés au même résultat en employant des procédés différents.

Knie[4] résèque la séro-musculeuse des cavités à anastomoser sur une petite étendue; puis il suture entre elles les couches extra-muqueuses, interposant entre les muqueuses un peloton de soie non désinfectée pour empêcher leur adhérence. La perforation des muqueuses se fait secondairement.

Postnikow[5] opère de même, mais il place une ligature à la soie sur la muqueuse attirée.

Bastianelli[6] incise la séreuse et la musculaire avec le thermocautère, puis il cautérise à plat la muqueuse, allant lentement pour ne pas détruire cette dernière.

(1) Gaston, dans ses expériences sur des chiens, ne s'occupait que d'anastomoses entre la vésicule biliaire et l'intestin.

(2) Bardenheuer (Franz). Experimentelle Beiträge für Abdominal-Chirurgie. Inaug. Dissert, Bonn, 1882.

(3) Graw (Theo. A. Mac). Upon the use of elastic ligature in the surgery of the intestines. Journ. of the Americ. med. Association, Chicago, 16 mai 1891, t. XVI, p. 685. — The use and limitations of the elastic ligature in intestinal surgery. Medic. Record, New-York, 3 oct. 1903, t. IX, p. 511. — Carlo Porta. Di altro metodo di gastro-enterostomia. Atti della Società italiana di chirurgia, Roma, 1893. — Nuovo contributo clinico-sperimentale ad un altro metodo pratico di gastro-enterostomia. Boll. dell'Associazione sanitaria Milanese, nov.-déc. 1890. — Tout récemment Ochsner a réuni 112 gastro-enterostomies faites par ce procédé (A. J. Ochsner. The Mac Graw ligature. Journ. of the Americ. medic. Assoc. Chicago, 24 oct. 1903. — En Allemagne, Tiefenthal a fait une étude expérimentale du procédé (Georg Tiefenthal. Gastro-Enterostomie mittels elastischer Ligatur. Eine Experimentalstudie. Beitr. z. klin. Chir., Tübingen, 1904, t. XLIII, p. 748. — Dudley Tait. The ligature method. Annals of surgery, févr. 1903, p. 180 (Bibliogr.).

(4) Knie. Verhandl. d. X. internat. medic. Congress. Berlin, 1890, t. II, fasc. VII. Chir., p. 86.

(5) Postnikow. Die zweizeitige Gastro-Enterostomie. Centr.-Bl. f. Chir., Leipzig, 1903, p. 1018.

(6) Bastianelli. Un metodo semplice di gastro-enterostomia senza apertura della mucosa. Riforma medica, Napoli, 1894, t. III, p. 206.

Paul (1), après excision des tuniques séro-musculaires, cautérise l'ovale dénudé au chlorure de zinc.

Souligoux (2) procède d'une manière un peu différente. Après écrasement du bord libre de l'intestin entre les mors épais d'une pince puissante, qui détruit tout sauf la séreuse, il cautérise les surfaces broyées avec un morceau de potasse caustique et enfouit les parties sous un surjet non perforant.

Roazi (3) place, entre les surfaces à anastomoser, une tablette de la grandeur d'une pièce de 2 centimes, contenant un caustique solide, puis réunit tout autour de la tablette l'estomac à l'intestin par un surjet non perforant.

Se fondant sur ce fait qu'un point perforant placé sur l'estomac ou sur l'intestin donne naissance à une fistule dont les dimensions dépassent beaucoup celles du point primitif, Podres (4) place deux fils en croix prenant 2 centimètres des parois de l'estomac et de l'intestin.

Coffey (5) excise les tuniques externes, étreint les muqueuses, gastrique et intestinale, dans des liens de caoutchouc, puis enfouit ces parties muqueuses étranglées sous un surjet circulaire non perforant.

Ces divers procédés en deux temps, qui avaient été adoptés en France par Chaput, Gross, Picqué, Reclus, Schwartz, Weiss, etc., et contre lesquels nous nous étions élevé dès leur apparition (6), sont, croyons-nous, abandonnés aujourd'hui, même par leurs inventeurs.

Il suffit, pour éviter la contamination du péritoine au cours de l'opération, de prendre quelques précautions:

1.º *Opérer autant que possible en dehors du ventre*, sur un lit de compresses de toile stérilisée, limitant très exactement le champ opératoire. Il faut donc éviter, autant que possible, de pratiquer des anastomoses au niveau de portions fixes de l'intestin, les angles du côlon, par exemple, en particulier l'angle splénique, en général profondément situé. Lorsque le siège du mal met dans la nécessité d'opérer sur des portions fixes de l'intestin, comme le rectum, il y a lieu, comme nous le verrons plus loin, de recourir à des procédés spéciaux.

2.º *Éviter l'écoulement du contenu digestif dans la plaie.*

On a eu tout d'abord recours à la compression manuelle de l'anse intestinale, ou à son enserrement dans une anse de

(1) *Paul*, Surgical treatment of pyloric obstruction. *Brit. med.*, 1898, t. I, p. 1430.

(2) *Souligoux*, Gastro-entéro-anastomoses, entéro-anastomoses, etc., sans ouverture préalable des cavités à anastomoser. *Presse méd.*, Paris, 1898, p. 390.

(3) *Roazi*, Tabletta anastomotica. *Clinica chirurgica*, Milano, 1897, p. 260.

(4) *Podres*, Gastroenterostomie und Entero-Anastomose. *Arch. f. klin. Chir.*, Berlin, 1898, t. LVII, p. 358.

(5) *Coffey*, Extra-visceral rubber ligature in gastro-enterostomy. *Medical News*, N. Y., 4 septembre 1900, p. 386.

(6) *Hartmann*, Congrès français de chirurgie, Paris, 1896, p. 430.

caoutchouc, de soie épaisse, de gaze iodoformée. Aujourd'hui on se sert généralement de compresseurs spéciaux dont les modèles sont multiples (Hahn, Billroth, Wehr, Heinecke, Rydygier, Czerny, Lücke, Gussenbauer, Küster, A. Lane, Moynihan, etc.). Les meilleurs compresseurs sont, à notre avis, ceux qui sont construits sur le modèle des pinces à pression élastique de Doyen. Le modèle curviligne de ce chirurgien convient spécialement à la compression de l'estomac; pour les opérations sur l'intestin nous avons fait construire par Collin un modèle droit. L'important est que les pinces jouissent d'une élasticité suffisante pour que le doigt puisse en supporter la pression. Dans ces conditions il est inutile d'en garnir les mors de caoutchouc, ces pinces ne contusionnant nullement les parties, pourvu que l'on n'exagère pas leur serrement et qu'on se borne à assurer la fermeture des cavités sans écraser les tissus compris entre les mors.

En tous cas, quel que soit le procédé utilisé, il est bon, avant d'appliquer le compresseur, de vider, par des pressions, le segment sur lequel on opère. Sur l'estomac il est le plus souvent nécessaire de placer deux pinces, dont les extrémités doivent non seulement se rejoindre, mais encore se dépasser l'une l'autre pour assurer une occlusion parfaite.

Pour certaines anastomoses l'emploi de compresseurs est inutile. Nous ne nous en servons jamais dans une des opérations les plus communément pratiquées, la gastro-entérostomie. Lorsque le malade est bien endormi, qu'il est placé dans une position légèrement élevée du bassin, 20° environ, que l'estomac et l'intestin sont amenés à l'extérieur, les liquides stomacaux restent dans la partie déclive, au voisinage du diaphragme, et rien n'apparaît à l'extérieur au moment de l'ouverture de l'organe, d'autant que les champs opératoires, placés entre les parties extériorisées et les lèvres de la plaie abdominale, exercent déjà une certaine compression sur les parties.

B. — Moyens d'éviter la contamination du péritoine après l'opération

Pour éviter la contamination du péritoine après l'opération, il faut avoir une bonne réunion des parties anastomosées. Il faut que l'occlusion des cavités soit et reste hermétique pendant les jours qui suivent l'opération. Pour l'obtenir, on recourt soit à des *sutures*, soit à des appareils spéciaux connus sous le nom de *boutons*.

Sutures. — Nous ne ferons pas ici l'historique de la suture intestinale. Ceux que la question intéresse le trouveront très complet dans l'ouvrage de Terrier et Baudouin[1]. Les procédés se sont tellement multipliés que, même en nous limitant à la période moderne, celle des sutures perdues, il nous faudrait un volume si nous voulions en donner l'exposé. Deux grands principes dominent la question : *mettre les séreuses au contact*, en renversant en dedans les bords de la plaie [2], *passer les fils sans traverser toute l'épaisseur de la paroi*, de manière à ne pas avoir de sutures perforantes, fatalement infectées [3].

Le matériel employé peut varier (catgut, soie, fil de lin, fil de celloïdine, etc.), la manière d'appliquer les sutures peut différer, le nombre des plans de sutures peut être plus ou moins grand, peu importe : toujours nous retrouvons à un moment ces deux mêmes principes, posés par Jobert et par Lembert, isoler la cavité digestive de la cavité péritonéale par un rang de sutures non perforantes, affrontant les séreuses.

Personnellement nous avons recours à la *suture en surjet en deux plans.*

Un premier plan comprend toutes les tuniques : séreuse, musculaire et muqueuse ; les points de ce plan sont perforants. Cette première suture, en même temps qu'elle ferme les cavités, assure l'hémostase, supprimant ainsi toute ligature isolée des vaisseaux. C'est une *suture occlusive et hémostatique* ; mais, comme les points qui la constituent sont perforants, qu'elle exposerait, si elle était isolée, à l'infection du péritoine par suite de la possibilité d'une filtration microbienne le long des fils, je l'enfouis sous un deuxième rang de sutures, celles-ci non perforantes ; cette deuxième suture est *isolante* et prévient toute contamination du péritoine.

Cette suture, que nous employons depuis 1892, que nous avons pratiquée des centaines de fois, nous a toujours satisfait. Depuis que nous l'avons préconisée, nous l'avons vu adopter par un grand nombre de nos collègues en France, où elle semble en train de se généraliser. Il semble qu'à l'étranger beaucoup de chirurgiens y ont recours.

[1] F. Terrier et M. Baudouin, la Suture intestinale, Paris, 1898.

[2] Jobert de Lamballe, Mémoire sur les plaies du canal intestinal, Paris, 1826.

[3] Lembert (A.), Mémoire sur l'entérorraphie, Répertoire général d'anatomie et physiologie pathologiques et de clinique chirurgicale, Paris, 1826, n.° 2, p. 104.

Kocher l'utilise fréquemment, Mikulicz en était partisan, Moynihan l'emploie systématiquement, Rydygier, en Pologne, déclare s'y être rallié, etc.(¹).

Un certain nombre de chirurgiens croient utile de faire un plan spécial pour la muqueuse, de lier isolément les vaisseaux qui saignent sur la tranche, etc., ce sont là complications inutiles. Très rapidement l'occlusion est réalisée.

Sur la coupe d'une gastro-entérostomie, morte 20 heures après l'opération chez un cancéreux cachectique, on voit que les séreuses sont déjà intimement accolées, sous forme d'une mince ligne noire sans réaction leucocytaire marquée. Les deux tranches muqueuses de l'estomac et de l'intestin sont déjà réunies par une cicatrice conjonctive unissant les deux sous-muqueuses; les épithéliums sont encore séparés par une masse sombre, formée d'un magma de leucocytes, de fibrine et de sang coagulé; le glissement des épithéliums n'aura lieu qu'au bout de quelques jours.

Sur des pièces d'autopsie tardive, après des périodes de 4 mois à 2 ans, on voit que les bouches anastomotiques sont parfaites. Les muqueuses se continuent très exactement; les bords de l'orifice sont souples; il n'y a pas trace de formation fibreuse, pas la moindre rétraction cicatricielle.

Pour pratiquer cette suture, l'instrumentation nécessaire est des plus simples : une pince à griffes, une aiguille à coudre droite, de couturière, et de la soie fine. L'aiguille à couturière que j'emploie est celle du modèle Kirby, que l'on peut trouver partout, qui est très bon marché et qui possède, en dehors de ce premier avantage, une qualité importante : la partie de l'aiguille correspondant au chas est évidée latéralement, de sorte que le passage de l'aiguille enfilée n'agrandit pas le trou fait par la portion antérieure, que, par conséquent, elle n'expose pas à un arrêt au moment où l'anse de fil arrive au niveau du trou fait par l'aiguille.

Je commence par le plan non perforant postérieur, traversant avec l'aiguille les tuniques séreuse et musculaire, évitant de perforer la muqueuse, mais cherchant à charger la sous-muqueuse, qui, ainsi qu'Halsted l'a bien montré, est la plus résistante de toutes les tuniques de l'intestin. Partant du point le plus

---

(¹) Quelques auteurs confondent cette suture avec celle d'Albert ; c'est une erreur : la suture d'Albert est une suture à points séparés.

éloigné de l'opérateur, on fait rapidement avec cette aiguille un plan de sutures non perforantes en surjet. La ligne de suture terminée, le fil est arrêté, conservé long et placé entre des compresses stérilisées. Une deuxième aiguille charge les parties situées immédiatement en dehors du point initial de la ligne de suture, et l'extrémité du fil qu'elle porte est nouée avec le chef initial du premier. Cette aiguille et son fil sont placés dans une compresse stérilisée. Cette aiguille servira tout à l'heure à faire le rang de sutures antérieures lorsque le plan de suture totale aura été terminé.

Cette suture en surjet non perforant n'est, en somme, que la vieille suture préconisée par Dupuytren[1].

J'incise alors par transfixion toutes les tuniques de l'intestin et j'agrandis avec des ciseaux fins la petite incision faite jusqu'à ce qu'elle présente des dimensions suffisantes pour l'établissement de la bouche anastomotique, plaçant sur les points qui saignent des pinces de Kocher de très petites dimensions, ce qui a le double avantage d'assurer l'hémostase et d'empêcher le glissement des diverses tuniques les unes sur les autres. Ce glissement est toutefois impossible à empêcher complètement pour la muqueuse de l'intestin qui fait hernie et dont il y a intérêt à réséquer la partie exubérante.

Avec une nouvelle aiguille je fais le surjet total, arrêtant le fil au niveau des points qui saignent et aux angles de l'incision, là où la suture tourne pour passer en avant de l'orifice. Lorsque tout l'orifice anastomotique est encerclé dans la suture, l'aiguille est revenue à son point de départ et les deux extrémités du fil sont nouées l'une à l'autre.

Nous désinfectons avec soin la suture ainsi faite avec un tampon de gaze trempée dans une solution de sublimé, ébarbant, si c'est nécessaire, les parties de la muqueuse herniée; puis, reprenant l'aiguille du surjet non perforant, nous enfouissons en avant la suture totale perforante.

Cette suture a l'avantage d'être rapide, d'assurer un affrontement large et solide des parties, et de supprimer en même temps toute ligature au niveau des tranches de section, le surjet total suffisant pour assurer l'hémostase, en étreignant les vaisseaux lors du passage des anses successives du surjet.

---

[1] Dupuytren, Leçons orales de clinique chirurgicale, Paris, 1839, 2e éd., t. V, p. 185.

SUTURE D'HALSTED. — Halsted [1] a préconisé la suture en capiton, à points séparés. Il passe d'abord tout un rang de points sans les nouer, de manière à pouvoir bien les placer en ligne droite. Il les noue alors et les coupe court.

À chaque extrémité de cette ligne postérieure de sutures, il place, suivant deux lignes faisant avec la première un angle de 135°, deux points également en capiton qu'il noue et coupe.

Les sutures antérieures sont alors placées mais non serrées, les deux extrémités de chaque fil étant tenues dans une pince à pression.

Alors seulement on ouvre les cavités à anastomoser liant les points qui saignent, puis on serre et l'on noue les sutures antérieures.

Ce procédé a l'avantage de placer toutes les sutures avant d'ouvrir l'intestin, ce qui diminue les risques d'extravasation fécale.

SUTURE DE TERRIER. — Pendant des années, Terrier, pour éviter la contamination du péritoine, a de même placé toutes ses sutures avant d'ouvrir les cavités. Un premier rang de sutures séro-musculaires était placé en arrière et les fils coupés court. Un deuxième rang de sutures presque parallèle au premier, mais convergeant vers lui à ses extrémités, était ensuite placé en avant de l'endroit que l'on allait inciser. Mais, comme les fils maintenus longitudinaux auraient gêné pour l'incision, on tirait la partie moyenne de chaque fil pour en faire une anse qu'on rejetait sur le côté. Une pince était fixée à l'extrémité de chaque fil, une troisième sur la convexité de l'anse formée. Chaque fil et les trois pinces qui le maintenaient étaient séparés du suivant par une compresse stérilisée, qui isolait chaque ensemble de fils et de pinces et évitait toute confusion.

Les cavités étaient alors ouvertes, les muqueuses suturées en arrière, puis en avant. Cette suture muqueuse terminée, on serrait et on réunissait les fils séro-séreux antérieurs déjà placés.

SUTURE DE MAUNSELL. — Après une résection segmentaire du canal alimentaire, Maunsell réunit les bords, mésentérique et convexe, de chaque bout par deux sutures, comprenant toute l'épaisseur des tuniques. Il incise ensuite le bord convexe du bout inférieur à environ 4 centimètres de la section intestinale, sur une longueur égale au diamètre de l'intestin. Avec une pince il attire dans cette incision les chefs des sutures préalablement placées, invaginant le bout supérieur dans le bout inférieur et amenant ainsi les deux cylindres, l'invaginant et l'invaginé, dans la boutonnière faite à l'intestin. Un rang de sutures comprenant toutes les tuniques de l'intestin réunit les deux bouts l'un à l'autre. Lorsque cette suture est terminée, on remet les parties en place et l'on referme la boutonnière faite à l'intestin au-dessous de l'anastomose.

Quelques chirurgiens complètent l'opération par la pose, au niveau de l'anastomose, d'un rang de sutures de Lembert, de manière à être plus sûrs d'éviter toute extravasation de liquide.

EMPLOI DE SUPPORTS. — Pour faciliter la suture, un grand nombre de chirurgiens ont préconisé des supports. Le procédé n'est pas nouveau. Dès 1544, les chirurgiens de l'école de Salerne, Roger de Parme et Roland, faisaient leur

<hr>

[1] Halsted (W. S.), Circular suture of intestines, an experimental study. *Amer. J. of med. sc.*, Philad., 1887, t. XCIV, p. 436 ; et *Bull. of the John Hopkins Hosp.*, Baltimore, 1891, t. II, p. 1.

suture sur une canule de sureau. Il y a près d'un siècle, Choisy conseillait de prendre un morceau de trachée [1].

Plus récemment, Hohenhausen [2], s'est servi d'un cylindre de farine de froment évidé; Jennings [3], d'un tube de beurre de cacao; Halsted [4] et Treves [5], d'un petit sac de caoutchouc gonflé d'air; Neuber [6], d'un tube en os décalcifié; Landerer [7], d'un support en pomme de terre.

Actuellement encore, en Angleterre, on se sert beaucoup des bobines en os décalcifié de Mayo Robson [8], d'Allingham [9], et de Ch. Ball [10].

En Amérique, on s'est ingénié à construire des pinces destinées à faciliter la suture. Nous citerons, entre autres, la pince de O'Hara et celle de Laplace.

E. Lambotte en Belgique, a de même imaginé une série de petits instruments pour réaliser rapidement les anastomoses.

Toute cette instrumentation est inutile et ne nous semble présenter qu'un intérêt historique.

Plaques ou boutons. — Trouvant le procédé des sutures trop long, Senn eut l'idée de maintenir les surfaces à anastomoser en contact, au moyen de plaques résorbables en os décalcifié [11]. Vulgarisé en Angleterre par Jessett, son procédé est actuellement abandonné, il en est de même de tous les appareils similaires, plaques en chou-rave de Baracz [12], anneaux de catgut de Abbe [13], etc.

Le bouton, imaginé et vulgarisé par Murphy, a rapidement conquis la faveur de tous ceux qui n'étaient pas satisfaits des sutures [14].

---

[1] *Choisy (G. L.)*, Dissertation et proposition sur quelques points de pathologie, Th. de Paris, 1834, n° 13.

[2] *Hohenhausen*, Experimenteller Beitrag zur Darmnaht, *Deutsche med. Woch.*, Leipzig, 1883, p. 329.

[3] *Jennings*, d'après le *Jahresbericht*, 1884, t. II, p. 426.

[4] *Halsted, loc. cit.*

[5] *Treves*, On resection of portions of intestine, *Med. Chir. Trans.*, London, 1883, t. LXVI, p. 53.

[6] *Neuber*, Zur Technik der circulären Darmnaht, *Verhandl. d. deutsch. Gesellsch. f. Chir.*, Berlin, 1884, t. XIII, p. 53.

[7] *Landerer*, Zur Technik der Darmnaht, *Centr.-Bl. f. Chir.*, Leipzig, 1895, p. 521.

[8] *Mayo Robson*, A method of performing intestinal anastomosis by means of decalcified bone bodies, *Brit. med. J.*, 1893, t. I, p. 688.

[9] *Allingham (H. W.)*, A new bobin for intestinal anastomosis, *Lancet*, 1895, t. II, p. 518.

[10] *Ball (Charles B.)*, A new pattern of decalcified bone ring, *Brit. med. J.*, 24 avril 1897, t. I, p. 1001.

[11] *Senn (N.)*, An experimental contribution to intestinal surgery, *Annals of surgery*, Saint-Louis, 1888, t. VII, pp. 1, 99, 171, 264, 337 et 421. — Intestinal surgery, Chicago, 1889.

[12] *Roman von Baracz*, Kohlrabienplatten als Ersatz für decalcinirte Knochenplatten bei der Senn'schen Platten-Darmnaht, *Arch. f. klin. Chir.*, Berlin, 1892, t. XLIV, p. 580.

[13] *Abbe (R.)*, Intestinal anastomosis, *Medical News*, Philad., 1889, t. LIV, p. 389.

[14] *Murphy (J. B.)*, Cholecysto-intestinal, gastro-intestinal, entero-intestinal anastomosis and approximation without sutures, *Medical Record*, N.-Y., 1892, t. XLII, p. 665; *Ibidem*, 1894, t. XLV, pp. 650, 684, 721. — *Murphy et Hartmann*, lieus, XIIIe *Congrès internat. de médecine*, Paris, 1900, section de chirurgie générale, p. 777.

Deux idées ont guidé Murphy dans la conception de son procédé :

1° Obtenir sans sutures une adhésion rapide, solide et permanente des surfaces séreuses, à l'aide d'un instrument capable d'amener, par une pression douce et continue, le sphacèle des tuniques au contact ;

2° Créer une ouverture suffisamment large pour permettre le passage des divers liquides physiologiques ou nutritifs, et aussi peu que possible susceptible de subir plus tard le rétrécissement cicatriciel.

Description du bouton. — Le bouton de Murphy se compose de deux pièces, qui ont été comparées, avec assez de justesse, à un champignon. Chacune de ces pièces est constituée par une sorte de cupule surmontant une tige creuse qui vient se fixer à son centre, et dont le diamètre a été calculé de telle façon que l'une, dite mâle, pénètre exactement dans l'autre, dite femelle. La première de ces pièces présente à son intérieur deux petits ressorts, fixés par une extrémité à la circonférence intérieure, près de la cupule, et saillant sur sa face externe sous forme de crochet sur leur extrémité libre, à travers une fenêtre ménagée dans la paroi de la tige, près de sa partie terminale. La tige femelle porte à son intérieur un pas de vis creux.

Si l'on introduit la tige mâle dans la femelle, les deux petits crochets des ressorts de la tige mâle viennent se loger successivement dans les rainures du pas de vis de la tige femelle.

Le crochet d'arrêt rend impossible l'écartement des deux moitiés du bouton, du moins par traction directe. Pour les séparer de nouveau, il faut dévisser la tige mâle.

Avec un bouton ainsi constitué, la pression, exercée par les deux cupules sur les tissus qu'elles étreignent, risquerait d'être trop forte ou trop faible ; leurs bords trop étroits pourraient couper les parties. Aussi Murphy a-t-il eu soin : 1° de donner à son bouton des bords mousses très épais ; 2° d'annexer à la partie mâle une troisième pièce destinée à régulariser les pressions. C'est une sorte de bague à bords très mousses, qui est supportée par un ressort de laiton.

Quand les deux pièces du bouton sont séparées, la bague déborde la cupule de 2 à 3 millimètres ; mais si l'on vient à les rapprocher fortement, elle rentre à l'intérieur de la cupule et met en jeu l'élasticité du ressort qui la supporte.

Il est facile de comprendre que ce ressort, cherchant toujours à satisfaire son élasticité, entretiendra une pression continue, mesurée, de l'anneau contre le bord de la cupule femelle, si bien que les tuniques intestinales, placées entre les deux, se sphacèleront peu à peu.

Mode d'application. — L'application de ce bouton est simple et rapide. Deux anses de soie sont faufilées à travers les deux anses d'intestin à anastomoser, *perforant toutes les tuniques de l'intestin* et entourant la partie sur laquelle va porter l'incision ; elles permettront, lorsqu'on les serrera, de ramener les bords des incisions intestinales à l'intérieur des cupules du bouton.

On fait alors l'incision de l'intestin. Cette incision doit avoir une longueur égale aux deux tiers du diamètre du bouton.

Les deux moitiés du bouton, portées sur des pinces, sont mises en place et fixées par la striction des soies qui entourent les incisions, la pièce mâle plus lourde étant placée dans le bout inférieur de l'intestin, de manière à amener, si possible, la chute du bouton de ce côté.

Il suffit, pour terminer l'opération, d'enlever les pinces qui portent ces deux moitiés, et de rapprocher progressivement ces dernières, saisies avec les doigts à travers les tuniques de l'intestin. La pression doit être suffisante pour amener les surfaces intestinales solidement au contact et pour comprimer les tissus.

L'application du bouton de Murphy peut être simplifiée dans un certain nombre de cas, en procédant comme l'a récemment conseillé Pauchet (¹).

Après une résection de l'intestin ou de l'estomac, comme aussi dans l'entéro-anastomose complémentaire d'une gastro-entérostomie, en un mot, toutes les fois que l'intestin, pour une raison quelconque, a été ouvert en un endroit voisin de celui où l'on veut établir une anastomose, il y a lieu de jeter dans les deux anses à anastomoser les deux pièces métalliques du bouton avant de refermer la cavité digestive (intestin ou estomac).

Les deux anses à anastomoser sont amenées au contact, puis, à travers les tuniques intestinales, on fait saisir la tige de chaque moitié du bouton. Au centre de la lumière de la tige, on perce l'intestin au thermocautère.

La tige fait hernie au travers de l'étroit orifice. Les deux pièces sont alors emboîtées et serrées à fond.

De nombreux modèles de boutons ont été construits depuis

(¹) *Pauchet* (V.). Technique du bouton de Murphy dans quelques opérations gastro-intestinales. *Arch. provinc. de chirurgie.* Paris, janvier 1906, p. 52.

que Murphy a fait connaître son procédé: Boari [1], F. de
Beulé [2], Chaput [3], Watson Cheyne [4], Destot [5], Duplay et
Cazin [6], J. Frank [7], Garampazzi [8], Garbarini [9], Hagopoff [10],
Jaboulay [11], Juvara [12], Martin Gil [13], Ramaugé [14], Sachs [15],
Villard [16], etc.

Le modèle initial de Murphy reste toujours le plus employé.
Il compte encore un grand nombre de partisans, particulièrement
en Amérique et en Allemagne.

Personnellement, à part des cas spéciaux, nous n'y avons
plus recours, ayant du reste abandonné tous les appareils imaginés
pour faciliter les anastomoses digestives. En dehors des re-
proches qu'on leur a adressés, accidents résultant d'une mauvaise
application (déchirure de l'orifice pendant l'introduction d'une
des pièces, pincement d'un lambeau de muqueuse entre les bour-
relets séreux, défaut de serrage du bouton, etc.), difficultés de
l'introduction du bouton dans un bout d'intestin rétracté, oblitération du cylindre central par des concrétions fécales, occlusion
intestinale, difficulté d'élimination, et même séjour permanent
dans l'estomac, etc., il y a tout au moins une raison qui doit
en faire rejeter l'emploi d'une manière générale, c'est que tous
ces appareils sont inutiles et qu'on obtient beaucoup plus simplement des résultats excellents en se servant d'une simple aiguille

---

[1] *Boari (A.)*, Modificazione al metodo anastomico di Murphy. *Clinica chirurgica*, Milano, 30 avril 1897, p. 144.

[2] *F. de Beulé*, Meine Methode der Gastro-Enterostomie. *Zent.-Bl. f. Chir.*, Leipzig, 1903, p. 1409.

[3] *Chaput*, Nouveau bouton anastomotique. *Bull. et Mém. de la Soc. de Chir.*, Paris, 1895, p. 746.

[4] *Watson Cheyne*, Manual of surgical treatment, London, 1900, t. VI, p. 267.

[5] *Destot*, Modification du bouton de Murphy. *Arch. provinc. de chir.*, Paris, 1894, p. 736.

[6] *Duplay et Cazin*, Sur un nouveau procédé de suture intestinale. *Congrès français de chir.*, Paris, 1895, p. 251.

[7] *Frank (J.)*, A New contrivance for intestinal end to end anastomosis. *Med. Rec.*, N. Y., 1896, t. I, p. 469.

[8] *Garampazzi*, Un nuovo bottone (alla Murphy) scomponibile. *Riforma medica*, Napoli, 4, 5 et 6 oct. 1897, pp. 17, 37 et 50.

[9] *Garbarini*, Delle anastomosi intestinali col bottone Murphy. *Clinica chirurgica*, Milano, 1894, t. IV, p. 49.

[10] *Hagopoff*, Bouton et instrument dit tire-bouton. *Presse médicale*, Paris, 7 déc. 1898, p. 652.

[11] *Jaboulay*, *Lyon médical*, 1903, p. 94.

[12] *Juvara*, Un nouveau bouton anastomotique. *Archives des sciences médic.*, Paris, 1895, p. 255.

[13] *Martin Gil*, Decalcified ivory discs for end to end and lateral anastomosis, 1897, *Lancet*, Londres, t. II, p. 512.

[14] *Ramaugé*, Enteroplaxie, Buenos-Ayres, 1893.

[15] *Sachs (W.)*, Modification der Darmnaht. *Cent.-Bl. f. Chir.*, Leipzig, 1890, p. 733.

[16] *Villard*, Bouton de Murphy modifié. *Ga; zette hebdom. de méd.*, Paris, 1895, pp. 157 et 149.

et d'un fil. Ces appareils, en particulier le bouton de Murphy, ont marqué une époque dans l'évolution de la chirurgie intestinale; mais aujourd'hui, avec les procédés simples des sutures que nous employons, les boutons n'ont plus leur raison d'être comme moyen général d'anastomose; ils ne conservent leur utilité que pour des cas spéciaux.

§ 2 — *Obtenir une circulation régulière du contenu digestif après l'anastomose.*

Lorsqu'une anastomose a été établie entre deux segments du tube digestif, il ne suffit pas que le malade soit à l'abri des accidents opératoires immédiats résultant de l'infection de la cavité péritonéale, il faut que l'anastomose fonctionne régulièrement et que le cours du contenu digestif se fasse normalement.

On n'arrivera à ce résultat qu'en observant certaines précautions.

La première est de *veiller à ce que*, l'anastomose établie, *les contractions des deux segments anastomosés se fassent dans le même sens*, qu'elles soient, comme l'on dit, *isopéristaltiques*. Il faut donc, avant de réunir les parties, préciser le sens du courant intestinal. Le procédé de Nothnagel, qui consiste à placer sur l'intestin un grain de sel et à regarder dans quel sens se font les mouvements péristaltiques, est insuffisant (¹). Il faut préciser la situation de l'anse considérée et ses rapports avec des points fixes, facilement reconnaissables, de l'intestin, l'angle duodéno-jéjunal pour la partie initiale, la région iléo-cæcale pour la partie terminale de l'intestin grêle.

Il est toujours possible d'arriver aisément et rapidement sur ces points, puis de descendre ou de remonter l'intestin jusqu'à l'endroit où l'on désire établir l'anastomose.

Une deuxième précaution à prendre est de chercher, autant que possible, à *ne pas supprimer une trop grande étendue du canal intestinal*, pour ne pas laisser entre le point malade du conduit digestif et l'anastomose une anse flottante, dans laquelle peuvent s'accumuler des liquides, et aussi pour ne pas diminuer, dans des proportions trop considérables, la surface de la muqueuse absorbante. On a vu, au début de la pratique de la gastro-entérostomie, des malades, opératoirement guéris,

---

(¹) Nothnagel a constaté qu'en pareil cas il se fait des contractions péristaltiques ascendantes.

succomber à une inanition progressive, parce qu'on avait fixé à l'estomac un point de l'intestin voisin du cæcum (Lauenstein, Angerer, Roux) ou même le cæcum (Obalinski).

Il ne faut toutefois pas aller trop loin dans ce sens et ne pas prendre, pour faire une anastomose, deux anses trop voisines d'un néoplasme, sous peine de risquer de voir la bouche anastomotique envahie par le processus cancéreux, comme le fait est survenu chez une de nos opérées.

Il y a là une question de mesure qu'il est facile d'apprécier. Dans certains cas même on aura avantage à prendre des points assez éloignés, par suite de considérations spéciales, comme nous le verrons en étudiant les points particuliers à chacune des anastomoses que nous allons décrire en particulier.

II. — TECHNIQUE SPÉCIALE DES ANASTOMOSES

Suivant le siège et la variété d'anastomose que l'on établit, il y a des particularités sur lesquelles il est utile que nous insistions.

D'une manière générale, dans les anastomoses bout à bout, ce qui est à craindre, c'est une mauvaise réunion, celle-ci pouvant être insuffisante soit immédiatement, soit secondairement par suite d'une mortification partielle à son niveau, mortification secondaire à une irrigation sanguine insuffisante ; dans les anastomoses latérales, ce que l'on a à craindre, c'est une circulation imparfaite du contenu digestif.

§ 1. — *Anastomoses termino-terminales.*

La suture est quelquefois imparfaite dans les anastomoses bout à bout et, dans tous les cas, présente quelques difficultés techniques, parce que le calibre des deux segments à anastomoser n'est quelquefois pas identique, qu'il s'agisse d'une réunion de l'estomac à l'intestin, de l'intestin grêle au gros intestin, ou même de deux anses du même intestin ensemble, parce que le plus souvent l'anse sus-jacente à l'obstacle qui a motivé l'intervention est dilatée d'une manière anormale.

Pour remédier à l'inégalité de calibre des deux bouts, on a opéré de manière différentes : on a rétréci le bout trop large ou, par un débridement longitudinal, dont les lèvres sont écartées en V, on a élargi le bout trop étroit.

Résections pyloriques. — D'une manière générale, c'est la première manière de procéder qui est suivie dans les anastomoses bout à bout de l'estomac avec le duodénum[1]. Billroth, dans son premier procédé de pylorectomie, suturait partiellement la section stomacale jusqu'à ce que la partie laissée béante eût un calibre égal à celui du duodénum. Le danger de cette manière de procéder est la perforation de la ligne de suture au point de rencontre de la suture d'occlusion et de la suture d'abouchement. Aussi beaucoup de chirurgiens ont-ils pour cette raison renoncé, après la résection gastrique, à l'abouchement bout à bout. Notre collègue Ricard, à Paris, a cependant obtenu de nombreux succès par ce procédé, prenant simplement la précaution de multiplier les sutures au point de réunion des trois branches de l'Y.

Résections intestinales. — Lorsqu'après une résection intestinale on veut pratiquer une anastomose bout à bout, dite entérorraphie circulaire, il faut : 1° que l'on ne crée pas de rétrécissement à son niveau ; 2° que la réunion soit immédiatement bonne et le reste consécutivement.

Pour éviter le rétrécissement consécutif, le moyen le plus simple est de fendre la paroi de chacun des bouts d'intestin, sur son bord convexe et parallèlement à son axe, excisant ensuite les quatre pointes des lambeaux pour faciliter la réunion. Si, préalablement à l'opération, un des bouts de l'intestin est dilaté, l'autre au contraire étant rétréci, on ne fait porter le débridement que sur le bout le plus étroit, lui donnant une étendue suffisante pour avoir, au moment de l'application de la suture, deux sections de calibre à peu près égal à affronter. C'est ce que nous avons fait plusieurs fois avec succès.

Chaput a imaginé un procédé d'entérorraphie longitudinale avec fente. Dans un premier temps il place les deux bouts encore intacts côte à côte parallèlement ; à égale distance du mésentère et du bord convexe, il fait deux rangs de sutures non perforantes pour adosser, sur une étendue de 6 à 7 centimètres, les deux bouts de l'intestin en canon de fusil. Dans un deuxième temps il fait sur chaque bout une fente longitudinale, immédiatement en avant de la suture d'adossement.

---

[1] Rutherford Morison a cependant fendu le duodénum sur son bord convexe, puis adapté l'ouverture de l'intestin ainsi élargi à la section gastrique, sans avoir besoin de rétrécir cette dernière (Rutherford Morison, Remarks on pylorectomy, *Brit. med. Journ.*, London, 1898, t. I, p. 291). Ce procédé ne permet de remédier qu'à de petites différences de calibre entre les deux surfaces de section et n'a pour cette raison été qu'exceptionnellement appliqué aux anastomoses gastro-intestinales.

Il réunit les deux fentes ainsi produites, fait une suture non perforante antérieure semblable à la suture postérieure d'adossement et enfin ferme l'orifice terminal.

Jeannel commence par faire des sections circulaires perpendiculaires à l'axe du canal intestinal, puis il taille une ellipse sur le flanc antérieur du bout supérieur et une deuxième ellipse sur le flanc postérieur du bout inférieur. Il réunit ensuite bord à bord les deux ellipses ainsi taillées; les mésentères croisés sont fixés par quelques points de suture qui les font adhérer l'un à l'autre.

Un autre procédé encore assez employé consiste dans la section oblique de l'intestin aux dépens du bord opposé à l'insertion mésentérique, de manière à ménager les connexions vasculaires. C'est un procédé simple, mais qui a l'inconvénient de laisser, une fois la suture faite, un canal angulaire, formant un angle rentrant au niveau du mésentère.

Pour assurer une bonne réunion, il faut:

1° Bien fermer les cavités;

2° Veiller à ce que les parties suturées soient suffisamment irriguées, pour qu'il n'y ait pas de mortification secondaire au niveau de la ligne de réunion.

1° La *fermeture des cavités* est obtenue à l'aide des procédés habituels de réunion. Pour avoir une suture étanche, il faut en particulier surveiller le point qui correspond à l'insertion mésentérique. On sait qu'au niveau de ce point, qui correspond à l'arrivée des vaisseaux, la tunique péritonéale manque et que les deux feuillets séreux, constituant le méso, s'écartent quelque peu au point où ils abordent l'intestin. Au niveau des côlons, ascendant et descendant, l'écartement est même tel que l'intestin est directement en rapport avec le tissu cellulaire rétro-péritonéal et que la réunion bout à bout doit être abandonnée. Sur le reste de l'intestin, en particulier sur l'intestin grêle, l'écartement est minime et permet un affrontement séro-séreux. Il y a toutefois là un point à surveiller et il faut s'attacher à très bien faire la suture à ce niveau.

C'est par l'attache mésentérique qu'il faut la commencer, chargeant dans les premiers points de suture non perforante le feuillet séreux du mésentère. Le premier plan de sutures non perforantes, commencé au niveau de l'insertion mésentérique, est continué jusqu'au niveau du bord convexe de l'intestin; en ce point le fil est arrêté et son chef conservé long.

On fait alors le surjet total, soignant toujours particulièrement l'insertion mésentérique, point où se produisent le plus facilement les infiltrations intestinales, chargeant, en même temps que les tuniques intestinales, la portion de mésentère intermédiaire aux deux feuillets séreux, et l'on termine par l'enfouissement antérieur de ce surjet perforant en reprenant le surjet séromusculaire déjà placé en arrière.

2° La *suture ne restera étanche* que si les parties anastomosées sont bien irriguées. Aussi, dans les anastomoses après résection de hernies gangrenées, est-il nécessaire de faire porter la section sur des parties certainement saines de l'intestin, loin de la partie gangrenée, en particulier sur le bout supérieur, plus malade que l'inférieur. Si les veines sont thrombosées, si les artères ont cessé de battre, il ne faut pas hésiter à faire porter loin la résection, même si l'intestin a repris sa couleur une fois l'étranglement levé. Il importe peu d'enlever une grande longueur d'intestin, cela ne complique pas l'acte opératoire, et cela assure une bonne coaptation des parties qu'on va réunir. C'est le cas de dire que «trop» vaut mieux que «pas assez».

Roux ne redoute pas de mettre hors cours plusieurs mètres d'intestin grêle, par exemple, pour opérer sur des anses saines; il a vu des malades vivre avec la seule fonction d'un mètre et demi d'intestin grêle et la moitié du gros intestin.

Pour qu'il n'y ait pas de mortification secondaire, il faut aussi que la résection mésentérique ait été faite d'une manière telle que l'irrigation des tranches de section soit assurée. Il faut, en particulier, ménager l'arcade vasculaire qui borde immédiatement l'intestin et ne jamais réséquer qu'un coin mésentérique dont la base corresponde exactement à la portion d'intestin enlevée, sans jamais la dépasser; il est même bon de faire une résection du mésentère moins étendue que celle de l'intestin.

Madelung a conseillé, pour ménager l'arcade vasculaire du bord de l'intestin, la résection losangique du mésentère.

Quand cela est possible, dans les plaies ou les ruptures, par exemple, on peut sectionner le mésentère parallèlement à l'anse que l'on va enlever et presque à son contact, liant les points qui saignent. Lorsque l'anastomose est terminée, il reste un pli redondant de mésentère, que l'on suture à lui-même pour éviter la persistance d'un trou, dans lequel pourrait s'engager une anse d'intestin.

Lorsqu'au contraire, par suite de la présence d'une tumeur mésentérique ou de lésions gangréneuses, on est obligé de réséquer une certaine étendue de ce repli, on est amené à faire l'ablation d'une grande longueur d'intestin.

De toutes façons, qu'elle soit grande ou petite, la brèche

mésentérique doit être refermée par des sutures. Pour éviter la piqûre de petits vaisseaux et la formation secondaire d'hématomes, Littlewood et Moynihan conseillent de lier les points qui saignent et de repasser l'extrémité des fils à ligatures conservés longs à travers la lèvre opposée du méso, de manière à fermer avec eux la perte de substance.

§ 2. — *Anastomoses termino-latérales.*

Dans les anastomoses termino-latérales on fixe un des bouts du canal sectionné dans une boutonnière faite sur l'autre bout préalablement oblitéré à sa partie terminale. Le plus souvent, on implante l'extrémité du bout supérieur dans une incision faite sur le bout inférieur (iléo-colostomie par exemple); d'autres fois, on implante l'extrémité supérieure du bout inférieur dans le bout supérieur (implantation duodéno-gastrique).

Cette implantation peut être réalisée avec le bouton de Murphy, dont on place une des moitiés sur une des sections comme dans les anastomoses bout à bout, dont on place l'autre dans une incision latérale comme dans les anastomoses latérales.

Personnellement nous préférons la suture. Après avoir déterminé le point sur lequel nous allons faire l'implantation, nous commençons par fixer la lèvre postérieure du bout sectionné sur la partie latérale de l'autre bout par un surjet non perforant, que nous arrêtons à ses deux extrémités.

Nous incisons alors, en avant de cette ligne de sutures, la région sur laquelle doit se faire l'implantation, sur une longueur à peu près égale au diamètre de l'intestin; nous réunissons par un surjet total, arrêté de place en place, particulièrement au niveau des points qui saignent, le bout sectionné à tout le pourtour de l'incision latérale faite, puis nous reprenons le fil du surjet non perforant déjà placé en arrière du siège de l'implantation et nous enfouissons en avant le surjet total déjà terminé.

Au niveau de la région iléo-cæcale, on a quelquefois cherché à réaliser une nouvelle valvule; dans ce but, après résection iléo-cæcale, Chavie fait sur le côlon, aussi loin que possible du mésocôlon, une incision verticale, ayant comme longueur le diamètre de l'iléon; il engage dans cette incision l'extrémité de l'iléon sectionné de manière à le faire saillir de 1 centimètre et demi à 2 centimètres dans la cavité du côlon. Retroussant le bout coupé du côlon, de manière à rendre plus accessible l'invagination ainsi faite, il fixe la séro-musculaire de l'iléon à la muqueuse et à la musculaire du côlon; il ferme le côlon, puis par un rang de sutures non perforantes réunit le bout de l'iléon invaginé à la paroi du côlon.

Ces anastomoses par implantation termino-latérales, d'une exécution un peu moins simple que celle des anastomoses latérales, que nous allons décrire, ont sur ces dernières l'avantage de faciliter la circulation des matières.

§ 3. — *Anastomoses latérales.*

Les anastomoses latérales entre l'estomac et l'intestin ou entre deux anses intestinales présentent sur les autres variétés d'anastomoses un certain nombre d'avantages.

L'anastomose peut être établie sans qu'on ait à se préoccuper du calibre des anses à réunir. Comme on la fait sur le bord convexe de l'intestin, en un point où le revêtement péritonéal est complet, elle se trouve dans les meilleures conditions de solidité et de rapidité des adhérences. Comme rien ne limite l'étendue de la bouche anastomotique, on peut la faire aussi grande que l'on veut et, par conséquent, n'avoir pas à se préoccuper du rétrécissement ultérieur. Ses bords peuvent être longuement accolés, sans qu'on ait à se préoccuper de la formation d'un diaphragme, les contractions de l'intestin ne pouvant avoir comme effet que d'ouvrir la bouche anastomotique. Enfin, par le fait que l'incision siège au bord opposé à l'insertion mésentérique, elle n'intéresse que peu de vaisseaux et l'on n'a pas à s'occuper de l'écoulement sanguin toujours minime.

La technique en est des plus simples. Après avoir amené au contact les deux anses à anastomoser, les avoir vidées, avoir réalisé la coprostase, on affronte d'abord par un surjet non perforant les surfaces en arrière de la ligne d'incision projetée. On ouvre les cavités, on les circonscrit par un surjet total perforant, occlusif et hémostatique; puis, reprenant le fil du surjet postérieur non perforant, on enfonit en avant la suture totale.

Lorsque l'anastomose porte sur le gros intestin, il est bon, croyons-nous, de la faire porter sur une bande longitudinale du canal, ces bandes fournissant au fil de suture un point d'appui plus solide que le reste de l'intestin.

Cette anastomose latérale peut être pratiquée aussi simplement avec le bouton de Murphy. C'est même le seul mode d'anastomose qui convienne à quelques cas spéciaux, à ceux où l'on est dans la nécessité de réduire considérablement la surface anastomosée et à ceux où la situation trop profonde des parties à accoler empêche de placer facilement des sutures.

C'est ainsi qu'après certaines résections étendues de l'estomac, dans quelques gastro-entérostomies pour cancer occupant la plus grande partie de l'organe ou le fixant d'une manière telle qu'il est à peu près impossible d'extérioriser les parties, il y a intérêt à recourir au bouton.

Il en est de même pour la technique de l'anastomose colo- ou iléo-rectale. Les petites dimensions de la face antérieure du rectum, seule portion pourvue de revêtement péritonéal, et sa fixité font que la méthode des sutures est à peu près impossible à appliquer dans cette région [1].

Le mieux est alors de recourir au bouton de Murphy, appliqué suivant la technique imaginée par Lardennois (de Reims) [2]. Nous l'avons employée plusieurs fois avec succès.

L'introduction de la pièce femelle ne présente rien de particulier ; pour éviter que du liquide intestinal s'écoule au moment où l'on porte cette moitié de bouton dans l'excavation pour la coapter à la pièce rectale, on peut oblitérer sa lumière avec du beurre de cacao qui, fondant à 25°, sera rapidement liquéfié une fois l'opération terminée. Pour placer la branche mâle, Lardennois se sert d'une pince longue et courbe, qui permet de l'introduire par l'anus et de l'appliquer contre la face antérieure du rectum. L'articulation des branches de cette pièce est exécutée comme celle des dilatateurs utérins ; en rapprochant les anneaux on écarte les mors. Ceux-ci pénètrent dans le cylindre mâle ; il faut les placer suivant le diamètre perpendiculaire à celui qui réunit les deux petits crochets à ressort de manière à ne pas gêner l'articulation des deux pièces.

Un petit arrêt, en saillie, a été ménagé, pour supporter le bouton et l'empêcher de s'enfoncer plus avant.

Les anneaux sont alors serrés et les mors s'écartent, fixant et maintenant le cylindre par une pression excentrique.

Un aide introduit doucement dans l'anus la pince portant le bouton ; abaissant les anneaux entre les jambes du malade, il soulève avec le cylindre du bouton la paroi antérieure du rectum. Sur la saillie ainsi produite, le chirurgien incise plan par plan les tuniques rectales jusqu'à ce que l'aide poussant le bouton fasse apparaître à travers la muqueuse, qui cède sous la pression, la tige mâle qu'il suffit alors d'articuler avec la branche femelle. La pince est enlevée, l'opération terminée.

Pour faciliter l'abaissement du manche de la pince, il est bon de placer un coussin sous le sacrum du malade, de manière à ce que la main de l'aide ne vienne pas heurter le plan de la table sur laquelle est couché le malade.

---

[1] Un certain nombre des anastomoses dites iléo en colo-rectales faites avec les sutures portaient certainement sur cette partie de l'ancien rectum qu'on rattache aujourd'hui au côlon pelvien, mais ne portaient certainement pas sur le rectum proprement dit, sur la portion de l'intestin dépourvue de méso.

[2] Lardennois, L'anastomose entéro-rectale par le procédé de la pince porte-bouton. *Congrès français de chirurgie*, Paris, 1905, p. 708.

D'une exécution en général facile, les anastomoses latérales sont celles qui exposent le moins aux accidents opératoires immédiats, à la condition cependant d'observer certaines précautions, dont la principale est de faire porter l'opération sur des parties saines des viscères à anastomoser.

Il est bon de ne pas supprimer, au point de vue fonctionnel, une trop grande étendue du canal digestif; mais il ne faut pas cependant exagérer et sacrifier, au désir de conserver la plus grande surface possible de muqueuse absorbante, la sécurité que donne l'établissement d'une bouche en tissu sain; c'est dire que, dans les anastomoses pour obstruction chronique, cause la plus ordinaire de l'établissement des anastomoses latérales, il ne faut pas hésiter à faire porter l'opération sur un point assez éloigné du siège du rétrécissement pour peu que le bout supérieur présente des lésions inflammatoires manifestes dans une certaine étendue, ce qui est fréquent.

Même en l'absence des lésions inflammatoires manifestes du bout supérieur, il est bon, dans les cancers, de ne pas faire porter la bouche trop près du néoplasme, celui-ci pouvant, par suite de son extension, envahir secondairement l'anastomose.

Au contraire, dans les anastomoses faites après résection et fermeture des deux bouts, il y a lieu de ne pas s'éloigner du bout oblitéré pour éviter la formation de cul-de-sac au delà de l'anastomose [1].

Ces diverses précautions sont faciles à observer et ne compliquent pas l'opération. Ce qui rend l'anastomose latérale inférieure, à certains points de vue, aux autres variétés d'anastomoses, c'est qu'elle expose, si elle n'est pas établie suivant certaines règles, à un mauvais fonctionnement secondaire.

Cet écueil de l'anastomose latérale a été surtout observé au niveau des bouches gastro-intestinales, qui ont été quelquefois suivies d'un reflux bilieux dans l'estomac, connu sous le nom de *circulus viciosus*.

Pour l'éviter, on a conseillé divers procédés :

---

[1] (*Frey E.*) admet qu'avec le temps les culs-de-sac disparaissent (Ueber Technik der Darmanast. *Beitr. z. klin. Chir.*, Tübingen, 1898, t. XIV, p. 1), ce que contestent *Frussa* et *Poterake*, qui ont vu dans plusieurs expériences sur le chien se former, au niveau du bout supérieur, un cœcum artificiel dans lequel s'accumulaient des débris alimentaires (*Comptes rendus de la Société de biologie*, 1902).

PROCÉDÉ DE KOCHER. — Kocher [1], qui pratique la gastro-entérostomie antérieure précolique, dispose l'anse grêle perpendiculairement à l'estomac, ayant soin que son bout afférent soit à gauche, son bout efférent à droite. Il ouvre l'intestin transversalement sur la moitié opposée au mésentère et fixe l'anse de telle façon que le bout afférent soit au contact immédiat de l'estomac, tandis que le bout efférent repose sur l'afférent. On obtient ainsi une disposition telle que l'anse afférente, quand elle est distendue, peut comprimer l'afférente, mais que l'inverse est impossible.

Pour assurer encore mieux le passage dans le bout efférent, Kocher fait une valvule, en incisant l'intestin non pas au niveau de la suture, mais suivant une ligne à convexité antérieure. Il unit alors la face péritonéale de cette valvule à l'estomac en laissant son bord libre. Par contre, la lèvre supérieure de l'incision stomacale est suturée suivant le procédé habituel à la partie concave de l'incision intestinale.

Procédé de Sonnenburg. — Sonnenburg, une fois l'incision de l'intestin grêle faite, borde l'incision par des points séparés au catgut, ourlant l'orifice avec la muqueuse qu'il suture à la séreuse, et il coupe les fils courts. Il fait de même au niveau de l'estomac, mais ne coupe qu'un des chefs de chacun des fils, laissant l'autre chef long, puis il réunit par un nœud l'extrémité de tous ces fils laissés longs.

Sonnenburg fait alors, à 2 centimètres au-dessous de la première ouverture de l'intestin, une deuxième incision, par laquelle il sort le paquet des fils stomacaux. Une traction exercée sur eux invagine l'estomac dans l'intestin et crée une valvule.

Il fixe l'estomac à l'intestin, dans cette situation, par des points de Lembert, coupe le paquet de fils qui sort par la petite incision secondaire de l'intestin et termine l'opération en suturant cette dernière [2].

J.-L. Faure est arrivé à un résultat analogue en procédant d'une manière un peu différente [3].

ENTÉRO-ANASTOMOSE. — Lauenstein eut le premier l'idée, pour assurer l'évacuation du bout duodénal, d'anastomoser à l'anse afférente une autre anse jéjunale. Braun fit très justement remarquer qu'il était plus simple d'unir l'une à l'autre les deux branches, afférente et efférente, de l'anse anastomosée à l'estomac [4].

GASTRO-ENTÉROSTOMIE EN Y. — Proposée par Wölfler [5] dès 1883, la gastro-entérostomie en Y est couramment pratiquée par Roux [6] à Lausanne, par Mongrofit à Angers, par Rotgans à Amsterdam.

Après avoir reconnu le jéjunum, Roux le sectionne, à 20 centimètres environ du pli duodéno-jéjunal, et prolonge l'incision dans le mésentère jusqu'à la première bifurcation artérielle, choisissant de préférence pour cette section un endroit

---

[1] *Kocher*, Chirurgische Operationslehre, 3e éd., Iéna, 1907, p. 174.

[2] *Schlatter*, Ueber Gastro-Enterostomie. *Deutsche Zeitschr. f. Chir.*, Leipzig, 1894, t. XXXVIII, p. 476.

[3] *Faure* (J.-L.), Sur un nouveau procédé de gastro-entérostomie: la gastro-entérostomie par invagination. XIe *Congrès français de chirurgie*, Paris, 1897, p. 425; Sur une modification de la gastro-entérostomie par invagination. *Revue de gynécologie et de chirurgie abdominale*, Paris, 1903, t. III, p. 81.

[4] *Braun* (H.), Ueber Gastro-enterostomie und gleichzeitig ausgeführte Entero-anastomose. *Arch. f. klin. Chir.*, Berlin, 1893, t. XLV, p. 361.

[5] *Wölfler*, Verhandl. d. deutsch. Gesellsch. f. Chir., 1883, p. 23.

[6] *Roux*, De la gastro-entérostomie. *Rev. de gynéc. et de chir. abdomin.*, Paris, 1897, t. I, p. 67.

où elle puisse être la plus longue possible, sans dépasser l'arcade du premier rang.

Le bout supérieur du jéjunum, fermé par une pince, est alors coiffé d'une compresse de gaze et mis de côté sur la lèvre gauche de l'incision abdominale. Le bout inférieur est saisi par l'aide, qui tient l'estomac hors de la brèche mésocolique, et approché mollement au moyen de la pince, pendant que le chirurgien place le premier plan de suture séro-séreuse continue sur ce qui sera le bord postérieur de l'ouverture.

Incision de la séro-musculaire stomacale et intestinale, seconde suture continue séro-musculaire.

Ouverture de la muqueuse stomacale, abrasion de la muqueuse intestinale, troisième suture continue sur la muqueuse faisant tout le tour. Suture séro-musculaire profonde antérieure, puis suture séro-séreuse.

L'estomac est lâché et le mésocôlon fixé sur les bords de la brèche, autour de la collerette gastro-intestinale, par quelques points au catgut.

L'implantation jéjuno-jéjunale se fait de la même manière; on choisit, autant que possible, le bord opposé au mésentère et on a soin de faire l'incision beaucoup plus courte, de manière à avoir une communication ressemblant à une grosse ampoule de Vater, plutôt qu'à un abouchement ordinaire. Cette manœuvre est facilitée par l'existence des plis transversaux de la muqueuse, qui donnent à ses bords ectropionnés plus d'ampleur. L'anastomose terminée, il est bon de fixer les bords de l'incision mésentérique par deux ou trois points au catgut (1).

Nous nous sommes toujours bien trouvés d'opérer de la manière suivante:

Après avoir déterminé le point déclive de l'estomac encore en place dans le ventre, nous le relevons, le rabattons sur l'angle supérieur de l'incision abdominale avec le côlon transverse et le mésocôlon. Nous faisons à ce dernier un trou, par lequel nous attirons le point déclive de l'estomac préalablement déterminé, et nous fixons aux bords du trou l'estomac ainsi hernié. Puis, prenant à partir du pli duodéno-jéjunal une longueur d'intestin strictement suffisante pour atteindre la portion d'estomac sur laquelle doit porter l'anastomose, nous fixons l'intestin à l'estomac suivant une ligne oblique en bas et à droite, se terminant au niveau de la grande courbure. Cette fixation est assez longue; les cavités ne sont ouvertes que dans la partie voisine de la grande courbure, si bien qu'au-dessus de la bouche se trouve une zone où intestin et estomac sont simplement accolés. Une fois les parties remises dans le ventre, comme le pli duodéno-jéjunal est situé à un ni-

---

(1) Tricomi, qui a adopté la gastro-entérostomie en Y, la pratique avec deux boutons de Murphy (Tricomi. Contributo clinico al metodo Roux nella gastro-enterostomia. *Riforma medica*, Napoli, 1899, t. I, pp. 20 et 39).

veau plus élevé que la grande courbure, l'estomac se trouve
réuni à un point de l'intestin qui normalement se trouve en rapport avec lui. Il n'y a pas de couture : le bout afférent se continue directement avec le bout afférent. C'est là un point qu'a
bien indiqué Petersen[1].

Si, cependant, l'estomac est petit, comme cela peut arriver
au cours d'une gastro-entérostomie après résection pylorique,
ou si le pli duodéno-jéjunal est anormalement bas situé, la portion
en amont de la bouche peut devenir descendante ; aussi est-il bon,
comme l'ont conseillé Ricard et Chevrier, d'accoler l'intestin à
peu près verticalement sur toute la face postérieure de l'estomac
et de n'ouvrir la bouche qu'au voisinage de la grande courbure.
Dans ces conditions, quels que soient les rapports respectifs du
pli duodéno-jéjunal et de la grande courbure, l'intestin, au niveau de la bouche anastomotique, descend toujours verticalement[2].

En opérant ainsi, nous n'avons jamais eu le moindre trouble
dans le fonctionnement de la bouche dans un nombre considérable de gastro-entérostomies.

Malheureusement, il n'est pas toujours possible de pratiquer
ainsi la gastro-entérostomie. Par suite de l'étendue des lésions,
de la fixité de l'estomac, on peut être obligé de recourir à la
gastro-entérostomie antérieure et se trouver dans la nécessité de
la faire sur une portion d'estomac située très à gauche ; en pareil
cas nous n'hésitons pas à établir immédiatement une entéro-anastomose entre les branches ascendante et descendante de l'anse,
faisant cette bouche au point le plus déclive de l'anse ascendante. Il est de même utile de faire cette entéro-anastomose complémentaire lorsqu'après une gastro-entérostomie postérieure, au
lieu d'avoir un bout afférent obliquement descendant, on a une
anse intermédiaire au pli duodéno-jéjunal et à la bouche, comme
cela peut arriver dans des cas où, après pylorectomie, la petite
portion d'estomac restante se trouve plus haut située que le pli
duodéno-jéjunal. Faute d'avoir pris garde à ce point un peu spécial, nous avons, après une pylorectomie étendue avec fermeture des deux bouts et gastro-entérostomie, observé un cas de
circulus viciosus.

---

[1] *Petersen* (M.), Anatomische und chirurgische Beiträge zur Gastro-Enterostomie. *Beitr.
z. klin. Chir.*, Tübingen, 1901, t. XXIX, p. 597.
[2] *Ricard et Chevrier*, De la gastro-entérostomie. *Gaz. des hôp.*, Paris, 1906, p. 96.

Dans les anastomoses latérales intestinales on a moins à
s'occuper des conditions de circulation au niveau de la bouche,
la circulation se faisant en général assez bien, si l'on a pris la
précaution élémentaire de veiller à ce que les contractions des
deux anses soient isopéristaltiques. Quelquefois il est utile de
combiner à l'anastomose une ou deux sections de l'intestin, de
manière à exclure plus ou moins complètement un segment de
l'intestin de la circulation des matières. Nous nous contenterons
d'une simple mention pour ces faits qui rentrent dans l'étude de
l'exclusion de l'intestin.

III. — INDICATIONS GÉNÉRALES DES ANASTOMOSES GASTRO-INTESTINALES ET INTESTINALES

Si nous laissons de côté les quelques cas exceptionnels où,
en présence de plaies intestinales, on a fait l'anastomose de ces
plaies, nous pouvons dire que, d'une manière générale, l'établissement d'une anastomose est indiqué toutes les fois qu'il y a lieu
de rétablir la circulation du contenu digestif, que celle-ci soit
interrompue par le fait d'une résection segmentaire préalable
ou qu'elle soit simplement gênée par suite de l'existence d'un
rétrécissement du canal.

Nous n'énumérerons pas tous les cas où l'on rétablit la circulation digestive par anastomose des deux bouts après une résection; ce serait faire l'histoire des résections du tube digestif.
Nous nous bornerons à la recherche de ceux où l'on pratique une
anastomose sans s'attaquer directement au point malade.

Indications dans les maladies aiguës. — Dans les obstructions
aiguës de l'intestin, l'entéro-anastomose est le plus souvent contre-
indiquée, soit par les conditions générales où se trouve le malade, soit par l'état local de l'intestin.

Lorsque le malade arrive au chirurgien dans un état tel
qu'il ne peut supporter que l'entérotomie, il faut aller au plus
pressé et se contenter d'ouvrir l'intestin pour faire cesser des
accidents menaçants. Il n'y a pas lieu de discuter l'indication
d'une entéro-anastomose, pas plus que dans les cas où l'intestin
est gangrené et où la mort peut survenir par suite de la continuation de l'évolution des lésions locales; dans ces derniers la
résection immédiate des parties malades s'impose.

Toutefois, dit Roux, l'anastomose peut être combinée quelquefois avec l'extra-péritonéalisation des anses suspectes, dont

on fait la résection un ou deux jours après, quand le malade s'est remis du choc nerveux abdominal ; c'est une pratique recommandable dans la hernie étranglée du haut de l'intestin grêle, pour laquelle un anus contre nature peut être suivi d'une dénutrition trop rapide[1].

Indications dans les maladies chroniques. — Dans les affections chroniques l'indication de l'anastomose se présente, au contraire, fréquemment. Il est bien évident que le plus souvent, en particulier lorsqu'il s'agit de néoplasmes, l'anastomose n'est indiquée que si l'on ne peut recourir à l'opération radicale, à l'excision, soit par suite de l'extension des lésions, soit par suite de la faiblesse du malade qui ne supporterait pas une intervention trop laborieuse.

L'anastomose doit céder le pas à la résection toutes les fois que celle-ci est possible, mais est très supérieure à l'anus artificiel, seule opération pratiquée autrefois. Elle occupe le milieu entre ces deux opérations.

Dans quelques cas, l'*anastomose* n'est que le temps *préliminaire* d'une opération plus radicale.

Deux fois, chez des malades porteurs de cancers pyloriques, en état d'inanition absolue, avec cyanose des extrémités, j'ai rapidement établi une gastro-entérostomie, puis, quinze jours plus tard, j'ai pu, avec succès, pratiquer une pylorectomie.

L'anastomose, en permettant au malade de s'alimenter, avait rendu possible une opération d'exérèse, à laquelle on ne pouvait songer au début.

Elle rend de même possibles certaines ablations de tumeurs intestinales, en faisant disparaître la gangue inflammatoire qui les enveloppe.

L'*anastomose définitive*, dans les cancers inopérables accompagnés de phénomènes d'obstruction, pylorique ou intestinale, rend les plus grands services. Elle prolonge l'existence, et surtout elle supprime les phénomènes si douloureux et si pénibles de la rétention, procurant bien souvent au malade une mort douce par affaiblissement progressif et sans douleurs vives.

Dans les lésions autres que les néoplasmes, l'anastomose suffit souvent pour amener la guérison, tout au moins la guérison symptomatique. On ne compte plus aujourd'hui les malades por-

---

[1] Roux, Anastomoses intestinales. XIII° Congrès international de médecine, Paris, 1900, section de Chirurgie générale, p. 736.

leurs d'une sténose pylorique ou d'un ulcère rebelle au traitement médical qui ont vu tous les troubles disparaître à la suite d'une gastro-entérostomie. Dans les fistules pyostercorales, dans certaines affections péricœcales, l'anastomose, surtout combinée avec l'exclusion unilatérale, rend de grands services. Elle guérit quelquefois complètement les malades, elle permet d'autres fois une opération secondaire qui eût été primitivement impossible.

Nous n'insisterons pas plus longtemps sur les indications de ces opérations d'anastomose, qui se sont vulgarisées dans ces vingt dernières années et qui constituent, avec les perfectionnements successifs de leur technique, un des plus grands progrès de la chirurgie moderne.

TABLE DES MATIÈRES

THÈME 9 — ANASTOMOSES GASTRO-INTESTINALES ET INTESTINO-INTESTINALES

Par M. le Prof. AUGUSTO DE VASCONCELLOS, Lisbonne

1) *Anastomoses gastro-intestinales*

Je limiterai mon rapport à l'étude de la gastro-entérostomie, sans parler de la gastro-duodénostomie et d'autres opérations, d'indications tellement rares qu'on a fini presque par les abandonner.

Gastro-entérostomie. Dans la gastro-entérostomie on fait en règle l'union d'une anse du jéjunum à l'estomac, soit à la paroi antérieure, soit à la postérieure.

La gastro-entérostomie constitue aujourd'hui une des opérations les mieux réglées et fournissant les plus éclatants succès de la chirurgie contemporaine. Je l'étudierai en retenant surtout et en discutant les procédés classiques, sans me perdre dans le monde infini des modifications plus ou moins originales, même avec sacrifice du nom de leurs plus ou moins glorieux auteurs.

Indications. Il y en a qui sont absolument admises par tous les chirurgiens; d'autres se voient encore aujourd'hui vivement discutées.

On peut dire, sous une formule générale, que la gastro-entérostomie est l'opération contre la sténose pylorique. En effet, même dans les cas où elle ne se dirige pas contre la sténose, comme dans certains cas d'ulcères, ou dans la dilatation, c'est tout de même contre des symptômes qui sont communs aux sténoses et à ces autres affections que la gastro-entérostomie s'applique avec succès.

La gastro-entérostomie est l'opération de choix dans les *sténoses bénignes du pylore*, soit que le rétrécissement vienne d'un ancien ulcère cicatrisé, soit d'une brûlure par caustique, c'est à l'unanimité des chirurgiens qu'on pourrait voter cette proposition. Car les partisans de la pyloroplastie ou de la divulsion digitale (Loreta) se sont effacés, en sorte qu'on ne parle plus de leurs exploits. Et la pylorectomie se voit réservée pour des rétrécissements d'un autre genre, n'étant pas raisonnable d'appliquer une opération d'une bien plus haute gravité, là où une intervention plus simple suffit au plus souhaitable succès.

Dans les *rétrécissements néoplasiques* du pylore la gastro-entérostomie trouve son indication toutes les fois que le néoplasme n'est plus extirpable. Dès qu'il y a des adhérences, et surtout des adhérences postérieures d'une certaine importance, dès qu'il y a des signes manifestes d'une extension de la néoplasie à des tissus, ganglionnaires ou autres, qu'on ne peut pas atteindre, la gastro-entérostomie est absolument indiquée comme le moyen le plus sûr de prolonger la vie des malades, en même temps qu'elle leur épargne des souffrances intolérables. Et si dans cet ordre d'idées je suis presque avec Roux, lorsqu'il proclame que dans ces cas «la seule contre-indication c'est la mort», il faut bien se garder d'exagérer l'intervention de la gastro-entérostomie dans les cas de sténoses néoplasiques, et de l'appliquer aux cas encore susceptibles d'une bonne extirpation.

C'est une formule malheureuse, ce'le d'appliquer une opération purement palliative à des cas où la chirurgie possède des moyens qui visent à la guérison et qui quelquefois l'ont indéniablement obtenue.

Dans les *sténoses spasmodiques* les succès de la gastro-entérostomie sont déjà discutés. Et cependant je crois que les cas de guérison opératoire de la supposée *maladie de Reichmann* ne sont que des cas de sténose, ou spasmodique, ou fibreuse, que la gastro-entérostomie avait le devoir de guérir et a [en] effet guérie. Dans les cas d'hystérie et en d'autres semblables, on a opposé à la gastro-entérostomie la pyloroplastie, peut-être plus simple et aussi efficace. Les tendances modernes vont encore à la préférence de la gastro-entérostomie, même dans ces cas. Et ce sont les insuccès assez nombreux de la pyloroplastie, obligeant à des gastro-entérostomies secondaires, qui ont assuré la préférence d'une opération très sûre comme résultat, qui n'est pas beaucoup plus compliquée que la première et qui pourtant n'expose pas les malades aux désagréments d'une deuxième intervention.

Dans les *gastroptoses* ou dans les énormes *dilatations* la gastro-entérostomie a le beau nom de Roux comme défenseur. Malgré la grande autorité d'un si éminent maître, j'avoue mon peu de sympathie pour l'anastomose gastro-intestinale dans ces cas. Cependant, si les accidents provoqués par ces affections deviennent d'une acuité dangereuse, je n'hésiterai pas à me ranger à l'opinion de Roux. En dehors des symptômes aigus mettant en jeu la vie du malade, ce qui est vraiment exceptionnel, je ne crois pas que la gastro-entérostomie devienne une opération courante chez les dilatés de l'estomac, sans sténose, s'il c'est vrai qu'il puisse y avoir de grandes dilatations sans sténose.

Je citerai comme hors-d'œuvre l'indication de la gastro-entérostomie associée à la gastrostomie dans les sténoses de l'œsophage (Lindner), pour permettre l'évacuation rapide de l'estomac.

Choix de l'opération. A moins d'impossibilité pour adhérences ou invasion néoplasique, je préfère toujours la *gastro-entérostomie postérieure transmésocolique* (van Hacker). Évidemment je ne discuterai pas la gastro-entérostomie antérieure rétro-colique (Billroth-Brenner), qu'on ne fait plus. Mais il y aurait toujours quelque chose à dire sur les avantages ou inconvénients de la gastro-entérostomie antérieure, ou de la gastro-entérostomie en Y. Je me suis, ailleurs, largement occupé de la question, alors (1898) vivement discutée, et je ne viendrai pas remettre en cause toute une vieille argumentation, sans doute surannée. Seulement, j'insisterai sur une conclusion de 1898, préférant toujours l'opération de van Hacker, à moins de contre-indication anatomo-pathologique. Depuis lors, la gastro-entérostomie postérieure a presque partout été préférée à l'opération de Wölfler, évidemment en déchéance. Et toute ma pratique, assez étendue, et tout ce que j'ai lu et vu après n'ont fait qu'affermir l'opinion que je soutenais dès l'abord, accordant la préférence à la voie postérieure dans la gastro-entérostomie. Je suis chaque fois plus convaincu que le succès fonctionnel de l'opération dépend de la parfaite et totale évacuation de l'estomac et je ne crois pas que celle-ci puisse être toujours complète, avec une bouche à la paroi antérieure de l'organe, surtout si la musculature gastrique est par l'effet de la maladie quelque peu affaiblie. Tandis qu'à la paroi postérieure, sous le haut patronage de la gravité, je pense au contraire qu'il devient difficile de ne pas obtenir une bonne évacuation avec une technique raisonnablement correcte. Des cas d'insuccès de la gastro-entérostomie antérieure dans les formes spasmodiques sont d'ailleurs venus confirmer ce qui n'était, au début de la discussion, qu'une simple vue théorique, quoique solidement fondée, puisqu'elle s'appuyait sur la physiologie.

La gravité des inconvénients de la gastro-entérostomie antérieure a été si éloquemment démontrée par les faits que la plupart des chirurgiens qui l'emp'oient encore aujourd'hui lui associent une entéro-anastomose. Avec cette correction, disparaissent en effet les plus lourdes charges contre la vicieuse mécanique gastro-intestinal et surtout la facilité de *formation* du *circulus vitiosus*, la plus grave de toutes. Mais il ne faut pas oublier que là où la gastro-entérostomie postérieure se tire d'affaire avec une seule opération, l'antérieure en exige deux.

Avec le procédé de Roux, en Y, on obtient sans doute une très correcte situation relative de l'estomac et de l'anse jéjunale. Et ce serait un procédé à préférer, s'il ne forçait à une beaucoup plus grande complication technique, d'ailleurs inutile, puisque avec le procédé de van Hacker on arrive aux mêmes résultats, sans d'encombrantes manœuvres. Je comprends que pour un chirurgien avec l'habilité et la pratique de Roux l'argument perde de sa force; il la garde néanmoins pour la plupart des opérateurs, qui n'osent pas se mesurer avec le maître de Lausanne.

C'est donc à la gastro-entérostomie postérieure que je recourrai, à moins de *veto* anatomo-pathologique; c'est donc sur la technique de cette opération que j'ajouterai quelques remarques.

S'il est une opération en chirurgie, dont la technique soit tout à fait réglée dans ses grandes lignes, c'est certainement la gastro-entérostomie. Il y a cependant des détails qu'on discute encore et qui ont une grande importance pour la réussite immédiat de l'opération. D'après les intéressants travaux de Petersen, la mensuration de la distance de la bouche intestinale à l'angle duodéno-jéjunal et de sa corrélation avec l'ouverture stomacale est un détail auquel ce chirurgien attache une grande valeur. J'ai eu l'occasion de confirmer dans mes opérations la justesse de vues de Petersen; c'est à l'exacte application de ses conseils, combinée avec une modification dans la direction de la suture d'anastomose—que je vais de suite vous exposer—que j'attribue l'heureux fait de n'avoir presque plus de vomissements bilieux après mes gastro-entérostomies.

Je suis tout à fait classique dans les différents temps de l'opération, jusqu'à l'isolement de l'anse jéjunale, à la mensuration de la distance de la bouche intestinale à l'angle duodéno-jéjunal et à sa transposition sur la paroi de l'estomac, en sorte que l'orifice d'anastomose soit toujours dans une situation plus déclive que l'angle sus-mentionné. Je fais toujours la coprostose avec les clamps élastiques de Doyen et de même j'isole toujours avec ces clamps le pli de la paroi de l'estomac, où sera faite l'anastomose. Dans la suture j'emploie les deux plans, séro-séreux et suture des trois tuniques bord à bord, d'après la technique de Hartmann, que je défendais chaleureusement en 1898, même avant les publications de cet éminent chirurgien. Seulement ces sutures et l'incision intestinale qu'elles bordent, je les fais en sorte qu'elles tombent complètement sur la paroi antérieure de l'anse intestinale, en les dirigeant un peu obliquement et à partir d'un point tout à fait opposé à l'insertion du mésentère. La moitié postérieure de celle anse intestinale devient donc, après l'anastomose, plutôt inférieure; et c'est de cette situation, qui difficulte évidemment le reflux de la bile dans l'estomac, que je crois obtenir les excellents résultats que je tiens à vous signaler. Dans les autres temps je reprends les procédés classiques, sans modifications sensibles.

De cette description vous pouvez déjà conclure que j'emploie les sutures, mais il faut que je vous dise que je les emploie toujours, étant un *suturiste* aussi enragé que convaincu. Voyons toutefois s'il y a des cas où l'on doive employer comme moyen d'anastomose le bouton de Murphy, ou n'importe quel autre des appareils qui ont été inventés à la suite du fameux et ingénieux bouton américain.

La rapidité, voilà son succès. C'est entendu; le bouton de Murphy et presque tous les sous-boutons épargnent de 15 à 20 minutes dans la durée d'une gastro-entérostomie. Et pour moi, c'est tout ce qu'on doit leur accorder. Tous les autres avantages cités ont été démentis par la pratique, notamment l'absence de rétrécissement secondaire de l'orifice d'anastomose et l'impossibilité de la formation d'un éperon avec toutes les graves conséquences du *circulus vitiosus*. Après les intéressantes recherches de Ettlinger, de Francfort, et de Neuweiler, de Happerswéiler, toutes ces hypothèses de miracle s'évanouissent; on arrive à la conclusion que les boutons sont des instruments de rapidité plus aléatoires que les sutures, en tout ce qui se rapporte à la sûreté de l'anastomose et à la prophylaxie des accidents éventuels.

Neuweiler, que je viens de citer, est un défenseur du bouton de Murphy et malgré son plaidoyer, malgré ses nombreuses expériences, on arrive à la conclusion que la péritonite par perforation est assez fréquente avec l'emploi du bouton de Murphy dans certaines conditions d'application et malgré une technique correcte. Or, je conteste absolument que cette péritonite puisse se faire avec les sutures, à moins que celles-ci ne soient mal faites. Je n'en ai jamais eu; je crois que tout chirurgien un peu rompu à la pratique de la chirurgie abdominale a le devoir de ne pas en avoir. Donc, je suture au lieu d'employer l'ingénieux instrument qui faisait dire avec justice à un chirurgien italien: «Il suo buon funzionamento è sempre nelle mani di Dio». Tant que nous n'aurons pas des créances de Divinité, il faudra suturer. D'autant plus, et comme raison finale, que même en admettant que tout se passe dans le meilleur des mondes au point de vue opératoire, je n'arriverai jamais à me convaincre que la présence d'un bouton dans l'estomac d'un malade puisse être un détail insignifiant. Je vois même qu'il y a des chirurgiens qui limitent l'emploi du bouton dans les gastro-entérostomies aux cas de cancer de l'estomac, en vue de la rapidité opératoire. Et je me demande si dans un estomac cancéreux—et qui sera demain ulcéré, s'il ne l'est pas encore—un bouton qui se balade n'est pas un hôte dangereux au dernier degré. Évidemment le bouton peut abandonner l'estomac et avoir la bonté de sortir; mais il peut rester, il aime souvent le séjour de l'estomac et s'il y reste, je crains beaucoup plus ses aventures ambulatoires que les 15 à 20 minutes opératoires exigées par les bonnes sutures.

Et les statistiques? Est-ce que les chiffres des opérations réalisées avec le bouton de Murphy ne sont pas bien plus favorables que ceux de toutes les autres méthodes? Je n'en sais rien. En matière de chiffres, on sait qu'il est facile de leur faire dire tout ce qui nous plaît, et les boutonnistes le savent tout aussi bien que moi. Ainsi, quand on fait la comparaison d'une série de gastro-murphy-entérostomies réalisées en 1905, avec une vieille série de gastro-entérostomies par sutures, exécutées en 1895, il n'y a pas à dire, la série moderne est absolument merveilleuse. Mais si l'on prend des séries de la même année, exécutées par des chirurgiens rompus à la chirurgie abdominale, alors il faut en rabattre des premières impressions. On arrive à des résultats qui ne s'éloignent pas sensiblement et qui sont tout à fait favorables aux suturistes, si l'on pense que les fameux boutons fournissent bien des ennuis et des résultats éloignés malheureux, sans que les statistiques opératoires s'en occupent. Je vous épargnerai une longue énumération de chiffres, que je devrais choisir en Portugal; d'autant plus que les chirurgiens portugais sont, à de rares exceptions, boutonnophobes, et de ce fait les chiffres boutonniens seraient plutôt maigres, n'autorisant pas de conclusions bien positives.

Si, au lieu des boutons, nous nous tournons du côté des méthodes d'écrasement, qui ont eu leur moment d'auréole dans les anastomoses viscérales, nous arrivons à peu près à de semblables conclusions. Pour moi, le procédé idéal d'anastomose sera toujours celui qui permettra l'union primaire des tissus en contact par coaptation des tuniques identiques, avec le ma-

ximum de vitalité. C'est entendu que je ne nie pas le rôle capital
joué dans l'union par la séreuse et les adhérences qu'elle sait
créer autour des surfaces juxtaposées. Mais si le rôle principal
échoit à la séreuse quand on juxtapose des bords cruentés des
musculeires et des muqueuses, si ces bords gardent toute leur
vitalité, l'union se fera avec d'autant plus de solidité que cette
juxtaposition sera exacte et cette vitalité intégrale. Si on l'a-
moindrit par un écrasement, qui épargnera seulement la séreuse,
on diminuera d'autant les chances d'une parfaite et solide union.
Qu'on se réserve ces procédés pour l'occlusion d'un bout intestinal, où il n'y a pas danger, ni même besoin d'obtenir une
exacte cicatrice linéaire, qui ne rétrécisse la lumière du tube
par son irrégularité, ça se comprend; c'est de la bonne chirurgie que je défendrai à sa place. Seulement cette place n'est
pas ici, où, sous couleur de ne pas ouvrir les viscères pour une
anastomose, on risque de se lancer dans l'aventure d'une union
imparfaite, ou d'une cicatrice vicieuse.

Comme conclusions: dans l'anastomose gastro-intestinale
j'adopte toujours le procédé de van Hacker, à moins de contre-
indication anatomo-pathologique. Je fais les sutures en deux
étages (surjets séro-séreux et des trois tuniques). Et j'applique
l'anastomose obliquement sur la moitié antérieure de l'anse
intestinale. Dans la gastro-entérostomie antérieure, quand je suis
forcé de la faire, j'adapte l'anse jéjunale, assez longue pour
m'éviter la compression du côlon, à l'estomac dans la direction
du péristaltisme intestinal, en la fixant à l'estomac au-dessus
et au-dessous de la bouche anastomotique, en sorte que la
formation d'un éperon devienne invraisemblable. Je rejette tous
les procédés à valvule, tous les appareils à anastomose, tous
les procédés à écrasement.

2) Anastomoses intestino-intestinales

Il faut distinguer dans les anastomoses intestinales:
a) les anastomoses entre anses différentes de l'intestin grêle;
b) les anastomoses entre l'intestin grêle et le gros intestin;
c) les anastomoses entre deux segments du gros intestin.
Tous ces groupes possèdent une individualité chirurgicale
bien marquée, et ce serait une grosse erreur d'appliquer, sans
critique, aux interventions d'un des groupes, ce que l'on aura
comme vrai et sûr pour les autres.

Sur les *indications*, peut-être on pourra trouver un terrain neutre, en sorte qu'il soit possible d'appliquer des principes généraux. Voyons.

De même que la gastro-entérostomie est essentiellement l'opération de la sténose du pylore, l'entéro-anastomose est l'opération de la sténose de l'intestin. Il est certain qu'on l'applique aussi quelquefois dans certains cas de fistules intestinales; mais il n'est pas moins certain que l'entéro-anastomose n'est pas une opération qui guérisse les fistules intestinales. Elle leur diminue la sécrétion, mais c'est tout ce qu'on peut lui demander; elle restera toujours dans ces cas une opération incomplète.

Dans les *sténoses malignes* évidemment on ne doit pas même penser à l'entéro-anastomose, tant qu'il sera légitime de tenter l'extirpation totale de la néoplasie. Mais si l'extirpation est devenue impossible deux opérations se présentent, presque à égales chances de rendre les derniers jours du malade un peu plus tolérables: l'entéro-anastomose et l'exclusion totale. Je préférerai l'entéro-anastomose au cas où la situation de la néoplasie permettra un facile drainage naturel de la partie sténosée. Mais si, au contraire, le drainage naturel n'est pas facile—côlon ascendant, cæcum, par ex.,—et si l'état général du malade n'est pas trop déchu je ferai l'exclusion. Car, avec l'entéro-anastomose, les produits éminemment septiques et toxiques, qui viennent de la tumeur, tomberont dans un cul-de-sac, comme le cæcum, et aggraveront rapidement l'état d'ailleurs précaire du malade.

Dans les *sténoses tuberculeuses*, si on ne peut pas les enlever, il faut en faire plutôt l'exclusion totale.

Les *sténoses cicatricielles* ou *par procès inflammatoires* autour du tube intestinal (appendicite) fournissent une excelente indication pour l'entéro-anastomose. Sans oublier cependant que l'exclusion totale trouvera aussi, mais bien plus rarement, l'occasion de succès éventuels, que l'entéro-anastomose peut-être n'obtiendrait pas.

Je passerai à vol d'oiseau sur les *sténoses spasmodiques* ou *syphilitiques*, qui pourront sans doute indiquer une entéro-anastomose, pour finir avec les sténoses extrinsèques (compression par tumeurs, coudure d'une anse, etc.) où cette opération trouve sa meilleure indication, puisqu'elle devient la seule ressource à prendre.

Pour la technique revenons à nos groupes.

a) *Anastomose d'anses d'intestin grêle.* Pour la simple anastomose latérale après les soins et les temps classiques, avec une coprostase obtenue par les excellents clamps élastiques de Doyen, je fais la suture, comme dans une gastro-entérostomie, à deux plans, un surjet séro-séreux qui prend un peu de la musculaire et un surjet sur les trois tuniques, avec juxtaposition des bords, aussi exacte que possible. Si la muqueuse a une trop grande tendance à la hernie, je la résèque partiellement, ayant toujours le plus grand soin qu'elle soit complètement réduite après la suture des trois tuniques. J'emploie toujours la soie très fine pour mes sutures. Et j'arrête les sutures correspondantes à chaque bord près des angles de l'incision, pour les réunir respectivement par des nœuds indépendants. Détails auxquels j'attribue la plus haute importance en ce qui regarde à la sûreté du résultat.

Comme pour la gastro-entérostomie, je n'emploie jamais de boutons anastomotiques, je ne me sers pas des procédés à écrasement. Je préfère toujours l'adaptation directe des bords des deux plaies intestinales dans l'intention d'obtenir la réunion primaire. Cependant je comprends qu'on puisse se servir d'un bouton de Murphy pour les anastomoses entre anses de l'intestin grêle, ce sont des parois de la même épaisseur, de la même structure, très facilement *écrasable*, si vous me permettez l'adjectif. En outre, il n'y a pas de gros danger de rétention du bouton, car à l'intestin grêle il se détachera forcément; seulement, il pourra s'arrêter dans le gros intestin. Je ne fais pas à votre érudition l'injure de vous citer des accidents de ce genre. En tenant compte de la rapidité de son application, je comprends qu'en présence d'un malade très affaibli, très déprimé, par n'importe quelle cause, on puisse penser au bouton de Murphy et même aller jusqu'à son emploi. C'est le maximum de concessions, que je puisse accorder à ma boutonnophobie raisonnée.

Et puisque me voilà dans le terrain des concessions, je vous parlerai d'un procédé d'entéro-anastomose qui tient le milieu entre cette opération et l'exclusion de l'intestin. En effet, l'entéro-anastomose classique, que je viens de vous décrire rapidement, s'exécute avec la continuité intégrale du tube digestif. Mais on voit bien qu'elle pourra se faire avec section de l'intestin au-dessus de la sténose, occlusion du bout inférieur et implantation du supérieur au-dessous de la sténose, ou entéro-anastomose latérale après occlusion des deux bouts. Ce n'est pas encore une exclusion, au vrai sens du terme, ce n'est plus une entéro-anastomose cissaque. Eh bien! cette opération ajoute une nouvelle page à mes faiblesses chirurgicales; car je crois de bonne pratique faire l'occlusion des bouts intestinaux par écrasement. On applique donc un des modèles de pinces écrasantes à toute la largeur de l'intestin à sectionner, au point dûment choisi, et on pousse à fond toutes les forces écrasantes. Quand c'est bien fini, on sectionne l'intestin par la partie écrasée, sans ouvrir la cavité du tube intestinal; on fait la ligature des segments écrasés et puis on enfouit les moignons par une suture en surjet Lembert. Il ne reste qu'à faire l'entéro-anastomose; ou, si l'on préfère l'implantation, à traiter le bout à implanter selon les conseils de Roux, de Lausanne, pour sa gastro-entérostomie en Y.

Voici une opération qui, quoique un peu plus longue, méritera la préférence toutes les fois que le segment sténosé aura une muqueuse malade et pourra donner lieu à des absorptions de produits toxiques. Évidemment elle trouve son indication précise dans les sténoses malignes, si l'état général n'est pas trop affaibli. Quant au choix entre l'implantation et l'anastomose latérale, je crois aujourd'hui que c'est la dernière qui doit être préférée, modifiant ainsi mes anciennes idées.

C'est que, avec l'écrasement, là où il n'y a pas des adaptations exactes de bords cruentés à faire, on n'ouvre la cavité intestinale qu'au moment de l'incision pour l'anastomose, tandis qu'avec l'implantation il faut tenir un des bouts plus longtemps ouvert. Et encore ce bout qu'on implante est lui-même un bout écrasé, c'est-à-dire un tissu de résistance et de vitalité amoindries. On pourrait ne pas faire l'écrasement, mais alors on se priverait d'un procédé qui, dans ces cas spéciaux d'occlusions terminales, me semble d'une heureuse application.

En conclusion: dans les anastomoses intestino-intestinales d'intestin grêle, je ferai selon l'indication, ou l'entéro anastomose latérale, a sutures ou la section de l'intestin après écrasement et occlusion des deux bouts, suivie d'entéro-anastomose latérale.

b) *Anastomoses entre l'intestin grêle et le gros intestin.* En nous rappelant la pathologie de la région iléo-cæcale, nous serons. forcés de dire que cette variété d'anastomoses doit être des plus fréquentes soit à cause de lésions inflammatoires (appendicite), soit par néoplasies.

Dans les lignes générales, ce que nous avons établi pour le groupe précédent s'applique aussi à cette classe d'anastomoses. Seulement, on ne l'oubliera pas: le gros intestin limite une cavité éminemment septique. Donc, l'ouverture de cette cavité doit être si soigneusement exécutée qu'elle ne puisse être l'origine d'une infection de la cavité abdominale. La coprostase, surtout du côté du gros intestin, doit être la plus énergique qu'on doive obtenir sans lésions du côté de l'intestin.

Dans la technique je ne vous conseillerai rien de particulier. Ici moins qu'à l'intestin grêle, je n'emploierai les boutons: la différence d'épaisseur des parois intestinales rendrait l'adaptation, non seulement difficile, mais dangereuse.

c) *Anastomoses de segments du gros intestin.* Il faut dire qu'en vérité les indications de ces anastomoses sont assez limitées. Il n'y a qu'au côlon transverse, ou peut-être à l'anse sigmoïde, qu'on puisse rapprocher deux segments, assez voisins pour pouvoir s'anastomoser et assez éloignés pour que l'indication de l'intervention soit remplie. En tout cas, si l'opération est admise en principe, il n'y a pas de doute que le procédé de section et d'occlusion des bouts suivie d'anastomose doit être la méthode de choix. Et la technique au fond ne variera pas. Mais c'est le pronostic qui varie, car ces opérations sur le gros intestin sont d'une gravité beaucoup plus élevée que les interventions sur l'intestin grêle.

Voilà, messieurs, très rapidement exposée, mon opinion sur la question; l'autorité réduite du rapporteur, vous la tiendrez en compte dans votre critique. Elle n'aura qu'un mérite, cette opinion: la sincérité et la conviction; elle ne trouvera qu'une justification à la hardiesse de se présenter devant vous: la certitude de votre bienveillance.

THÈME 5—ANASTOMOSES DES VAISSEAUX SANGUINS

(Une nouvelle méthode d'anastomose vasculaire et ses applications à la replantation et à la transplantation des veines, des artères, des membres et des organes)

Par MM. les Drs. ALEXIS CARREL et C. C. GUTHRIE (Chicago)

Une condition indispensable à la réussite des opérations nouvelles que nous étudions en ce moment consiste dans le rétablissement parfait de la circulation des vaisseaux transplantés. Nous savons dû chercher le moyen d'obtenir, *de façon constante,* de anastomoses sans rétrécissement ni thrombose. Nous nous sommes arrêtés à une méthode qui, exécutée correctement, donne pratiquement toujours des résultats positifs. Elle convient également aux anastomoses termino-terminales, termino-latérales, et latéro-latérales, et aux variétés artério-artérielles, veino-veineuses, et artério-veineuses de ces anastomoses.

I. CONDITIONS NÉCESSAIRES AU SUCCÈS D'UNE ANASTOMOSE VASCULAIRE

Les deux principales conditions de la réussite d'une anastomose vasculaire sont une asepsie rigoureuse, et le rétablissement exact de la continuité de l'endothélium, dont la délicatesse doit, d'autre part, être soigneusement respectée.

Une asepsie rigide est absolument indispensable. Le degré d'asepsie, qui suffit au succès d'une opération abdominale, peut être incapable d'assurer la réussite d'une intervention sur les vaisseaux. En effet, l'asepsie clinique est bien loin d'être l'asepsie absolue. Entre l'asepsie absolue et le degré d'infection qui se traduit par une réaction thermique et par les signes classiques de l'inflammation, il y a un grand nombre d'états intermédiaires d'infection. Ces infections atténuées n'empêchent pas la réunion de la plaie par première intention, mais il est probable qu'elles peuvent provoquer dans les vaisseaux la formation d'une thrombose. Pour éviter sûrement cet accident, l'asepsie opératoire doit se rapprocher autant que possible de l'asepsie absolue.

Le rétablissement exact de la continuité de l'endothélium et son intégrité ont une importance capitale. Une blessure, même légère, de l'endothélium provoque la formation d'un dépôt de fibrine. D'autre part, tous les tissus, à l'exception de l'endothélium, possèdent un pouvoir de coagulation plus ou moins considérable.

Ils ne doivent donc jamais être au contact du courant sanguin. Par contre, les corps étrangers à surface lisse peuvent, dans certaines conditions, ne provoquer aucune coagulation.

Chacune de nos manœuvres opératoires est calculée de manière à être inoffensive pour l'endothélium vasculaire. Les vaisseaux sont disséqués à l'aide d'un bistouri bien tranchant, et pour les saisir, on ne se sert jamais de pinces. Ils sont maniés exclusivement avec les doigts. L'emploi de pinces ou de clamps pour l'hémostase temporaire est dangereux, car la pression est trop dure et altère la nutrition de l'endothélium. Nous nous ser-

vous pour cet usage de petites bandes de toile. Pendant la suture,
les extrémités vasculaires sont saisies avec de petites pinces, qui
ne mordent que l'extrême bord de la surface de section. La
seule blessure de l'endothélium, impossible à éviter, est produite
par les points de suture. Des points de suture perforants doivent
toujours être employés.

Par un artifice très simple, ces blessures sont rendues inof-
fensives. Elles sont, d'abord, réduites au minimum par l'usage
d'aiguilles rondes et extrêmement fines. Puis, les fils sont appliqués chargés de vaseline. Cette substance se dépose dans les petites plaies faites par l'aiguille, et prévient la coagulation du sang
à leur niveau. L'endothélium peut donc être considéré comme
pratiquement intact.

Lorsque, au niveau de la suture, la continuité de l'endothélium n'est pas exactement rétablie, la fibrine se dépose sur le tissu étranger, qu'il s'agisse d'un fragment de la tunique externe,
ou de la surface de section de la paroi vasculaire. La gaine conjonctive externe a un très grand pouvoir de coagulation. Le suc
des muscles et des organes est également très dangereux. L'union
des vaisseaux doit être établie de telle sorte que les surfaces endothéliales soient exactement juxtaposées. Pour ce motif, il ne
faut pas employer les méthodes par invagination, qui, par suite
de la présence de la surface de section de la paroi artérielle dans
la lumière du vaisseau, rendent impossible l'approximation
exacte de l'endothélium.

En un mot, les conditions nécessaires au succès de l'anastomose sont réalisées, quand le vaisseau se trouve dans un état
aussi voisin que possible de la *restitutio ad integrum* et que
toutes les manœuvres opératoires ont été aseptiques.

II — TECHNIQUE

Nous décrirons la technique en prenant comme type l'anastomose termino-terminale, puis nous indiquerons ses modifications
dans les anastomoses termino-latérales et latéro-latérales, et dans
leurs variétés artério-artérielle, veino-veineuse et artério-veineuse.

A. *Anastomose termino-terminale*

Les ciseaux et les bistouris, usés en chirurgie vasculaire, sont
semblables sous le rapport du tranchant et de la précision aux

instruments employés pour la chirurgie oculaire. Les pinces à disséquer, clamps, ou pinces pour l'hémostase temporaire ne sont plus employées.

De très petites pinces, à mors aigus, servent à saisir le bord des vaisseaux. Des bandelettes de toile, larges de 1 ou 2 cent., sont préparées, ainsi que de petites *serre-fines*, pour l'hémostase. De fines canules de verre, munies d'une poire en caoutchouc ou d'un long tube conduisant à un bock, sont employées pour le lavage des vaisseaux.

La suture est pratiquée à l'aide d'aiguilles Kirby rondes, droites, très acérées, n.° 15 et 16. Pour les gros vaisseaux, nous employons de la soie de Chine n.° 1. Pour les petits vaisseaux, un fil de soie à trois brins d'une extrême finesse. Les fils sont stérilisés dans de la vaseline à 117° pendant une demi-heure, et appliqués chargés de vaseline.

L'opération elle-même est d'une grande simplicité. Sa partie essentielle consiste dans l'application de trois fils d'appui en trois points équidistants de la circonférence du vaisseau. Par *une traction exercée sur chacun des fils, on transforme la circonférence en triangle*, et on peut alors dilater aussi largement qu'on veut le périmètre de ce triangle. En faisant un surjet le long de chacun des côtés du triangle pendant qu'ils sont fortement tendus, *on évite sûrement la sténose du vaisseau au point de l'anastomose*.

L'opération comprend plusieurs temps:

1° *Hémostase temporaire et préparation des bouts vasculaires.*

A quelques centimètres au-dessus et au-dessous de la future anastomose, on place sous le vaisseau une petite bandelette de toile. Les deux chefs sont tendus et fixés par une serre-fine. Les extrémités vasculaires sont coupées franchement d'un coup de ciseau. La tunique externe est réséquée.

La lumière du vaisseau est lavée avec la solution isotonique de chlorure de sodium. Puis elle est remplie de vaseline stérilisée.

2° *Application de trois fils d'appui en trois points équidistants de la circonférence du vaisseau.*

Les extrémités vasculaires sont réunies par trois fils perforants, placés en trois points équidistants de leur circonférence. Une traction excentrique est exercée sur chacun d'eux et transforme la circonférence en triangle.

3° *Suture des trois côtés du triangle.*

Chacun des côtés du triangle est tendu à l'aide des fils d'appui et suturé par un surjet. Avant de fermer le dernier côté, on chasse par pression toute la vaseline contenue dans le vaisseau. On peut faire ensuite une suture de la gaine tunique externe, mais cela n'est pas nécessaire.

4° Rétablissement de la circulation.

Les bandelettes sont enlevées et la circulation se rétablit. Si une hémorrhagie se produit en un point de la ligne de suture, elle est arrêtée par compression ou par un point de suture complémentaire.

B. Anastomose termino-latérale

Dans l'anastomose termino-latérale, l'extrémité du plus petit vaisseau est implantée sur la paroi du plus gros. L'extrémité du petit vaisseau est préparée pour l'anastomose de la manière habituelle. L'hémostase est assurée dans un segment du gros vaisseau et un lambeau triangulaire de sa paroi est réséqué en deux coups de ciseaux. La gaine conjonctive est extirpée sur une petite étendue autour de l'orifice. Trois fils fixent alors trois points équidistants de la circonférence du petit vaisseau aux trois angles de l'ouverture triangulaire du gros vaisseau. On tend les fils et ou termine l'opération par un surjet conduit le long de chacun des côtés du triangle.

C. Anastomose latéro-latérale

L'hémostase temporaire étant assurée, les deux vaisseaux sont placés parallèlement. Une ouverture est pratiquée dans la paroi de chacun d'eux. Cette ouverture est obtenue par une simple incision longitudinale ou par la résection d'un lambeau elliptique ou d'un lambeau triangulaire à large base postérieure.

Les extrémités de l'incision longitudinale ou du grand axe de l'ellipse ou de la base du triangle sont unies par deux fils dont les nœuds sont sur la face extérieure des vaisseaux. On conduit alors un surjet le long de ce bord.

Les points médians de la lèvre antérieure des incisions longitudinales ou des ouvertures elliptiques ou les sommets des ouvertures triangulaires sont unis par un troisième fil d'appui. Une traction sur les fils tend les côtés antérieurs du triangle et l'opération est achevée par un surjet.

D. Variétés artério-artérielle, veino-veineuse et artério-veineuse des anastomoses

Quelques manœuvres spéciales sont employées suivant la nature des vaisseaux qu'il s'agit de réunir.

1° Variété artério-artérielle.

Les surfaces de section des extrémités de la paroi artérielle sont juxtaposées aussi exactement que possible. Nous ne pratiquons jamais l'éversion des bords en dehors, car cette manœuvre produit une sténose du vaisseau. Les parois artérielles doivent se trouver en continuité l'une de l'autre de telle sorte que la surface externe du vaisseau soit aussi lisse et régulière que la surface interne.

Si les artères sont de très gros volume, il est possible de faire la suture sans intéresser l'endothélium.

Lorsque les artères sont de calibre égal, l'anastomose est facile et rapide, quatre minutes environ pour l'anastomose bout à bout de la carotide du chien.

Si elles sont de calibre différent, on réduit le calibre de la plus grosse en faisant chaque point un peu plus large sur le gros vaisseau que sur le petit, ou bien par une opération plastique spéciale.

2° Variété veino-veineuse.

Il est naturellement impossible de juxtaposer les surfaces de section de la paroi de deux veines. L'union est pratiquée par l'éversement en dehors de la paroi veineuse, de telle sorte que les surfaces endothéliales soient appliquées l'une contre l'autre.

La surface interne du vaisseau après la suture est parfaitement lisse, tandis que sur la surface externe la suture forme un bourrelet circulaire.

L'élasticité et la minceur de la paroi veineuse permettent l'anastomose de vaisseaux de calibre très différent. Après le passage des trois fils d'appui, chacun des côtés du périmètre triangulaire du gros vaisseau est beaucoup plus long que le côté correspondant du petit. La réunion se fait cependant sans difficulté en plissant longitudinalement la paroi du gros vaisseau à chaque point de suture. La circulation se rétablit ordinairement sans la moindre hémorrhagie, si les plis sont réguliers.

3° Variété artério-veineuse.

Elle est la plus difficile des anastomoses vasculaires.

Cette difficulté est produite par la différence du calibre et de l'épaisseur de la paroi des vaisseaux.

La réunion se fait, comme dans la variété veino-veineuse, par l'éversion en dehors de la paroi vasculaire, de telle sorte que l'endothélium veineux soit appliqué contre l'endothélium artériel. La circonférence de la veine est diminuée par une série de plis longitudinaux.

Si les vaisseaux sont de calibre très différent, une hémorrhagie se produit fréquemment au moment du rétablissement de la circulation par la base de l'un des plis longitudinaux.

Il faut alors placer un point complémentaire, autant que possible, sans interrompre la circulation.

Si les plis sont réguliers, et l'union de l'endothélium exacte, la variété artério-veineuse donne d'aussi bons résultats que les deux autres.

III — Applications

Nous employons cette méthode d'anastomose dans les transplantations uniterminales et biterminales des artères et des veines, et dans les replantations et les transplantations des membres et des organes. Sa technique ordinaire peut s'adapter facilement à ces différentes opérations par l'addition de quelques détails opératoires que nous allons exposer.

A. *Les transplantations veineuses*

La transplantation veineuse consiste à disséquer, à sectionner, ou à extirper une veine et à la greffer sur un autre point de l'appareil circulatoire.

1° La transplantation est *uniterminale* quand la veine ayant été disséquée dans la totalité ou dans une partie seulement de son étendue est unie par une de ses extrémités à une artère ou à une autre veine. La transplantation d'une veine sur une artère comprend plusieurs variétés suivant que le bout central ou le bout périphérique de la veine est uni au bout central, au bout périphérique ou à la paroi de l'artère. Ses applications sont très nombreuses. La transplantation d'une veine sur une veine est employée pour anastomoser deux parties du système veineux. La transplantation d'une veine sur une artère est la base des opérations qui ont pour but de modifier la circulation d'un organe ou d'une partie de l'appareil circulatoire. Par différentes combinaisons d'anastomoses, par la transformation de veines en artères, ou d'artères en veines, il est possible d'augmenter ou de diminuer la circulation d'un organe, d'y établir une circulation de sang noir, ou encore de modifier profondément la constitution anatomique des vaisseaux d'une région, etc.

La transplantation d'une veine comprend deux temps, la dissection de la veine et l'anastomose artério-veineuse. La dissection peut être très exacte et étendue sans produire la thrombose, si on

prend le soin de ne pas blesser la paroi veineuse en la maniant
brutalement avec les doigts ou une pince. Lorsque la transplantation a pour but la reversion complète de la circulation dans un
organe, il est utile de laver l'appareil circulatoire de cet organe
et d'y interrompre ensuite la circulation pendant toute la durée
de l'opération. Si cette précaution n'est pas prise, des infarctus
peuvent se produire.

2° La transplantation est *biterminale* quand un segment de
veine est uni par ses deux extrémités aux extrémités sectionnées
d'une artère ou d'une autre veine. Elle est *incomplète* lorsque la
partie moyenne du segment veineux garde ses connexions normales
avec les tissus et les organes voisins. Elle est complète quand on
extirpe complètement le segment veineux avant de le transplanter.
Nous pratiquons la transplantation autoplastique ou hémoplastique. Ces transplantations sont employées pour rétablir la continuité d'une artère dont un segment a été réséqué. Elles pourraient ainsi devenir une méthode de traitement radical des anévrysmes. Elles sont aussi employées dans la *transplantation en
masse* des organes.

La dissection du segment veineux peut être indifféremment
immédiate ou médiate. Chaque petite collatérale doit être liée
avec le plus grand soin, car elle peut donner lieu à une hémorrhagie abondante lorsque la veine se trouve distendue par le sang
artériel. Dès que le segment veineux est enlevé, il est lavé dans
la solution isotonique de chlorure de sodium et conservé dans
cette solution ou enfoui dans une masse de vaseline. Il faut faire,
d'ailleurs, la transplantation aussitôt que possible après l'extirpation. La suture se fait par la méthode habituelle. Auparavant,
la longueur du segment doit être réglée avec soin. S'il est trop
court une tension dangereuse se produit sur les sutures. S'il est
trop long, il en résulte des coudures nuisibles à la circulation.
En résumé, le segment veineux doit être adapté aussi exactement
que possible au calibre des extrémités artérielles et à la distance
qui les séparent.

B. La transplantation artérielle

La transplantation des artères peut être, de même que la transplantation des veines, uniterminale ou biterminale. La transplantation uniterminale possède comme la transplantation uniterminale des veines de nombreuses applications. Quant à la transplan-

lation biterminale, elle est ordinairement une transplantation hémoplastique et sert à la transplantation en masse des organes.

Il est nécessaire dans les transplantations artérielles de choisir des artères de calibre aussi semblable que possible. On ne peut pas unir bout à bout dans de bonnes conditions des artères de volume très inégal. Dans les cas où il existe une grande différence dans le diamètre de chacune des artères, il vaut mieux recourir à une implantation latérale qu'à une anastomose termino-terminale.

C. La replantation et la transplantation des membres

Nous avons pratiqué la replantation de la patte antérieure, de la patte postérieure, et de la cuisse. La replantation de la patte avec une moitié de l'avant-bras ou de la jambe est d'une extrême difficulté, à cause du faible calibre des vaisseaux. Nous avons opéré des chiens de volume moyen, sans arriver à rétablir une circulation normale. Cette opération ne peut être réalisée dans de bonnes conditions que sur des animaux de grande taille.

La replantation de la cuisse, au contraire, est d'une exécution relativement facile sur des chiens de taille moyenne, même de petite taille. Elle est suivie du rétablissement d'une circulation excellente, exagérée par le fait de la vaso-dilatation paralytique.

Les vaisseaux fémoraux sont découverts par une incision longitudinale s'étendant de la partie moyenne de la cuisse à la partie moyenne du triangle de Scarpa. Les vaisseaux fémoraux, et la veine saphène et l'artère qui l'accompagne sont disséqués. La dissection doit être médiate. La veine saphène surtout doit rester enfouie dans le tissu conjonctif environnant. Puis les vaisseaux sont sectionnés immédiatement au-dessus de l'embouchure de la saphène et rabattus du côté de la partie inférieure de la cuisse. La cuisse est alors amputée transversalement, un peu au-dessous de sa partie moyenne. On réséque ensuite environ deux ou trois centimètres du fémur. Une petite canule de verre est doucement introduite dans le bout périphérique de l'artère fémorale. On y injecte de la solution isotonique de chlorure de sodium jusqu'à ce que le liquide sorte clair par la veine fémorale. Le membre est alors enveloppé de compresses humides, en attendant la replantation. Celle-ci doit être pratiquée aussi rapidement que possible après l'amputation. Une heure et demie de suppression de la circulation ne paraît pas nuisible, lorsque les vaisseaux ont été exactement lavés,

La replantation est commencée par une suture solide des extrémités osseuses. On suture ensuite le quadriceps et le grand adducteur. Puis les vaisseaux sont anastomosés ainsi que le nerf crural. La circulation est immédiatement rétablie et on fait l'hémostase de la surface de section périphérique de la cuisse. Puis on suture l'aponévrose fémorale au-dessus des vaisseaux, puis les autres muscles, le sciatique, et la peau, et on immobilise le membre dans un solide appareil plâtré. L'animal lui-même n'est pas immobilisé. On lui permet de se promener le soir même de l'opération.

La transplantation de la cuisse d'un chien à un autre chien s'opère de la même façon. Il faut avoir soin de conserver de longs segments musculaires afin de ne pas avoir de tension dans la suture. Cette opération est longue, mais plus facile que la simple replantation. Elle n'a été pratiquée qu'une seule fois.

Dans les replantations et transplantations de la cuisse, le facteur le plus important est l'asepsie. Chez le chien, il est dangereux d'établir un drainage. Il vaut mieux fermer exactement la plaie, et essayer d'obtenir une rapide guérison par première intention, si la plaie est aseptique, en risquant la chance d'un phlegmon diffus mortel si elle ne l'est pas.

D. La replantation et la transplantation des organes

1° La replantation d'un organe consiste, après l'avoir extirpé complètement avec ses vaisseaux, à le remettre à sa place et à rétablir la circulation par des anastomoses vasculaires. La circulation peut être normale ou revertie.

Dans ce cas le sang rouge passe par les veines et le sang noir par les artères. Il est très important de laver complètement l'appareil circulatoire de l'organe, immédiatement après son extirpation. Cette précaution permet le rétablissement d'une circulation excellente. Depuis que nous l'employons, nous n'avons jamais observé d'infarctus. Les replantations du sein et du corps thyroïde seules ont été pratiquées.

2° La transplantation des organes peut être autoplastique, homoplastique, ou hétéroplastique. Le manuel opératoire est à peu près identique dans ces différents cas. Au point de vue de la technique, il y a deux catégories de transplantation, la *transplantation simple* et la *transplantation en masse*.

a) *La transplantation simple* consiste à disséquer les vaisseaux d'un organe, à les sectionner, puis à extirper cet organe, et à le transplanter sur un autre animal ou en un autre point du corps du même animal. Par exemple, on résèque une anse intestinale avec ses vaisseaux. On la place dans le cou de l'animal et on y rétablit la circulation en implantant l'artère et la veine intestinales sur la paroi de la carotide et de la jugulaire. Au bout de 20 minutes, on observe des mouvements péristaltiques normaux. La transplantation du rein ou du corps thyroïde s'exécute de la même manière. La transplantation simple a l'inconvénient de détruire les connexions de l'organe avec ses centres nerveux sympathiques. D'autre part, les fautes de technique dans la suture sont faciles à commettre lorsqu'il s'agit de petits vaisseaux tels que les vaisseaux thyroïdiens ou rénaux de chiens de taille petite ou moyenne. Une simple sténose produite par un fil trop serré peut troubler beaucoup la circulation. C'est pour éliminer ces inconvénients que nous employons la méthode suivante:

b) La transplantation en masse consiste à transplanter en un seul bloc un ou plusieurs organes avec leurs vaisseaux et les segments correspondants des gros vaisseaux sur lesquels ils s'implantent, leurs nerfs et ganglions nerveux, et leur atmosphère conjonctive. Cette méthode permet la transplantation simultanée des deux reins et des capsules surrénales. Elle rend possible la transplantation avec leurs vaisseaux d'organes tels que l'ovaire ou la glande thyroïde de petits animaux. Nous avons pu même transplanter en un seul bloc tous les organes abdominaux.

La transplantation des reins est l'exemple le plus typique de cette sorte de transplantation. Les deux reins d'un chien ou d'un chat sont extirpés avec leurs uretères, leurs nerfs, leurs vaisseaux et les segments correspondants de l'aorte et de la veine cave, leur tissu conjonctif et leur tunique péritonéale. Ils sont placés dans la cavité abdominale d'un autre chien ou d'un autre chat, dont l'aorte et la veine cave sont coupées transversalement. La circulation est alors rétablie dans les organes par une simple transplantation biterminale des segments d'aorte et de veine cave, entre les bouts sectionnés de l'aorte et de la veine cave du second animal. Puis les uretères sont anastomosés.

La transplantation en masse est un procédé bien supérieur à la transplantation simple, et permet de réaliser sans grande difficulté la transplantation de presque tous les organes.

Conclusions

1.° La méthode ci-dessus décrite permet de réaliser facilement toutes les variétés d'anastomoses vasculaires.

2.° Elle rend possible une série d'opérations nouvelles telles que la transplantation des vaisseaux et les opérations qui en dérivent, et les replantations et transplantations de membres et d'organes.

THÈME 3. — **LES ANASTOMOSES GASTRO-INTESTINALES ET INTESTINO-INTESTINALES**

(Die Anastomosen am Magen-Darm-Canale)

Par M. le Prof. SCHLOFFER (Innsbruck)

Die vielfach unklare Nomenclatur auf dem Gebiete der Magen-Darmoperationen bringt es mit sich, dass das auf diesem Congress zur Discussion bestimmte Thema «Les anastomoses gastro-intestinales et intestino-intestinales» zwei verschiedene Auffassungen erfahren kann. Auf der einen Seite kann man dabei die rein *technische* Frage der Vereinigung offener Lumina im Auge haben, vor allem in Bezug auf die Herstellung *seitlicher* Anastomosenöffnungen, dann auch in Bezug auf die circuläre Vereinigung, also ungefähr jenes Gebiet, welches man sonst auch mit der Bezeichnung «Darmnaht» oder «Darmvereinigung» zu versehen pflegt. Auf der andern Seite kann das vorliegende Thema zur Abhandlung zweier streng umschriebener Gebiete aus der Magen-Darmchirurgie veranlassen, der Gastro-Enterostomie (*Wölfler*) und der Enteroanastomose (*Maisonneuve*).

Diese letztere Auffassung habe ich meinem Referate zu Grunde gelegt, da sie die weitaus breitere Basis abgibt und da überdies das Interesse an der *rein technischen* Frage der Anastomosenbildung in der letzten Zeit sehr gesunken ist. Denn heute haben sich auf technischem Gebiete nicht nur die Anschauungen der einzelnen Chirurgen geklärt und ihr Können verbessert, sondern es ist auch über fast alle principiellen Fragen eine recht vollkommene Einigung zustande gekommen. Nur in Bezug auf wenige Punkte herrschen noch principielle Meinungsverschiedenheiten; und vor Allem wissen wir, dass man mit mehreren *verschiedenen* Methoden ziemlich gleich gute Resultate erzielen kann.

Auch über die Gastroenterostomie und Enteroanastomose
haben sich, was deren Indicationen und Leistungsfähigkeit betrifft, in den letzten Jahren ziemlich einheitliche Anschauungen
herausgebildet. Diese heute giltigen Anschauungen ohne viele
Rücksicht auf ihre historische Entwicklung in ihren Hauptzügen
darzustellen, will ich im Folgenden versuchen.

Die *Gastroenterostomie* ist stets sowie im ersten Falle, bei
dem *Wölfler* (¹) diese Operation ausgeführt hat, vor Allem bestimmt gewesen, die Passagestörung bei der Pylorusverengerung
zu beseitigen. Trotz aller Erweiterungen der Indicationen für
die Gastroenterostomie, stellen die Stenosenfälle doch das haupt-
sächliche und wichtigste Contingent für diese Operation. Es
kommen dabei in erster Linie die organischen Verengerungen
in Betracht: Das *Pyloruscarcinom* und die Verengerung des
Pylorus infolge *Geschwürs oder Narbenbildung*.

Es ist aber unverkennbar, dass das Bestreben, der Resection beim *Magencarcinom* ein möglichst weites Geltungsgebiet
zu verschaffen, die Gastroenterostomie bei dieser Erkrankung
zurückgedrängt hat; vor Allem, seitdem die Fortschritte in der
Diagnostik die Fälle im Allgemeinen früher dem Chirurgen zu-
führen als ehedem, und technische Fortschritte die Mortalität
selbst nach ausgedehnten Magenresectionen wesentlich herabge-
setzt haben. Aerzte, in deren Händen die Magenresection besonders wenig Gefahr brachte, haben sogar zu dieser gegriffen,
wenn sie dabei auf eine *radicale* Heilung ihrer Kranken nicht
rechnen zu dürfen glaubten (*Mikulicz*). Dennoch möchte ich
mich *Mikulicz* (²) nicht anschliessen, wenn er ausspricht, dass
der Gastroenterostomie beim Magencarcinom der Wert überhaupt
nicht zukomme, der ihr früher beigemessen wurde. Der Erfolg
der Gastroenterostomie beim Magencarcinom ist eben in hervor-
ragenden Masse von der Art der Fälle abhängig, bei denen
sie verwendet wird. Bei ausgesprochen stenosierenden Carcinomen am Pylorus, die nicht von beträchtlicher Grösse sind
und an sich nicht schmerzhaft, pflegt die Gastroenterostomie
einen Zustand so gut wie völliger Gesundheit herbeizuführen,
der verschieden lange dauert, je nach der Schnelligkeit mit der
das Carcinom wächst und die Gastroenterostomie-Oeffnung erreicht
bezw. verlegt. Gar nicht wenige solche Fälle gehen an ihrem

(¹) Zntbl. f. Chir. 1881, p. 705.
(²) 73. Versammlung deut. Naturforscher und Aerzte in Hamburg. Zbl. f. Chir. 1901, p. 1097.

Carcinom und seinen Metastasen zu Grunde, ohne dass überhaupt noch schwerere Erscheinungen seitens des Magens auftreten. Dass man bei ausgedehntem Carcinom durch die Gastroenterostomie so gut wie nichts erreicht, oder die geringfügigen Erfolge nur von kurzer Dauer sind, ist allgemein bekannt und deshalb mag auch in solchen Fällen ausnahmsweise die Jejunostomie verwendet werden, die sonst als der Gastroenterostomie in jeder Hinsicht nachstehend beim Magencarcinom zu verwerfen ist.

Was die *nicht am Pylorus sitzenden Carcinome* des Magens betrifft, so möchte ich die Gastroenterostomie ausnahmsweise auch bei Fällen von Carcinom in Anwendung gezogen wissen, wo keine ausgesprochene Pylorusstenose und keine Ectasie des Magens vorliegt; denn auch ich verfüge über mehrere Beobachtungen, bei denen nicht sehr ausgebreitete Carcinome an der kleinen Curvatur, bei welchen sich die Radicaloperation verbot, durch die glatt functionierende Gastroenterostomie wesentlich gebessert wurden. Ich glaube, wir müssen berücksichtigen, dass solche Fälle insofern sehr grosse Verschiedenheiten in ihren Symptomen aufweisen, als die einen bei sehr beträchtlichem Tumor geringe subjective Beschwerden, die anderen bei geringer Grösse der Geschwulst schwere Gastralgien zeigen. Aehnliche Verschiedenheiten finden wir ja auch beim Ulcus, bei dem oft erst ein hoher Grad von Stenosierung des Pylorus dem Patienten sein Geschwür zum Bewusstsein bringt, während andere Male schon ganz kleine Geschwüre beträchtliche subjective Erscheinungen herbeiführen. Offenbar hängen alle diese Dinge von schwer controllierbaren Factoren ab, von der Schmerzhaftigkeit des Geschwüres oder Krebses und seiner Verwachsungen bei Zerrung durch die Peristaltik und dergleichen. So wird wohl verständlich, dass auch manchmal bei nicht am Pylorus sitzenden Carcinomen die Gastroenterostomie, die die Entleerung des Magens erleichtert und deshalb den Tumor mehr oder weniger ruhig stellt, die subjectiven Symptome ganz oder teilweise zum Schwinden bringt.

Auch sonst haben wir ja überhaupt die Vorteile der Gastroenterostomie beim Carcinom vor Allem in der wesentlichen Besserung des subjectiven Befindens der Kranken zu erblicken, da die Verlängerung des Lebens, die die Gastroenterostomie bewirkt, bei richtiger Indicationsstellung nur ausnahmsweise Jahre, meist weit kürzere Zeit beträgt. Es ist ja die durchschnittliche Lebensdauer der Carcinomkranken nach der Gastroenterostomie nur ein halbes oder drei viertel Jahre.

Leider ist die *directe operative Mortalität* der Gastroenterostomie beim Carcinom noch immer eine sehr beträchtliche. *Wölffler* (¹) hat im Jahre 1896 eine solche von 33 % berechnet, und die Statistiken aus neuester Zeit geben nur zum Teile wesentliche bessere Ziffern.

Ich habe aus einer Reihe von casuistischen Mitteilungen der letzten Jahre mit Berichten über eine grössere Zahl von Operationen eines und desselben Operateurs 1208 (²) Fälle gesammelt, die noch immer 28 % Mortalität ergaben; dabei ist allerdings zu bedenken, dass jene Operateure, die über grössere Zahlen berichten, auch ältere Fälle mit einbeziehen. Berücksichtigt man lediglich die Operationen der letzten Jahre, so sinkt die Mortalität im Allgemeinen auf 25 %, selbst 20 %. Allerdings weisen die einschlägigen Ziffern grosse Verschiedenheiten auf. Dies rührt, wie wir seit langem wissen, hauptsächlich davon her, dass die Fälle, die zur Gastroenterostomie herangezogen werden, bei den verschiedenen Chirurgen keineswegs gleichwertig sind, indem z. B. Mancher, der eine hohe Mortalität bei seinen Gastroenterostomien wegen Carcinom aufweist, für die Gastroenterostomie nur die schlechten Fälle aufspart und dafür seine Indication zur Resektion viel weiter ausdehnt als Andere.

(¹) Ueber Magen-Darm-Chirurgie. Festvortrag am 25. Congress der deut. Ges. f. Chir. Berl. klin. Wchschr. 1896, N.° 23.

(²) Die Fälle stammen von:

Rydygier, Deut. Zeitschr. f. Chir. 1900, Bd. 56.
Merkens, Freie Vereinig. d. Chir. Berlins, Zentrbl. f. Chir. 1900, p. 276.
Permann, Hygiea LXI, p. 593, ref., Zentr. f. Chir. 1900, p. 447.
Chlumsky-Mikulicz, Beitr. z. klin. Chir., Bd. 27, 1900.
Weber-Lindner, Beitr. z. klin. Chir., Bd. 31, 1901.
Kolbe-Roux, Le cancer de l'estomac etc., Thèse, Lausanne, 1901.
Pauchet, Congr. fr. de Chir. 1903, Rev. de Chir. 1904, II, p. 635.
Schönholzer-Kronlein, Beitr. z. klin. Chir., Bd. 39, 1903.
Stich-Garrè, Beitr. z. klin. Chir., Bd. 40, 1903.
Klapp-Kümmel, Beitr. z. klin. Chir., Bd. 35, 1903.
Ranzhof-Steinthal, Mediz. Korrespbl. des würt. ärztl. Landesver. 1904, ref. Zentr. f. Chir., 1904, p. 947.
Jaboulay, Rev. de Chir., 1904, I., p. 9.
Maraglianu-Krause, Beitr. z. klin. Chir., Bd. 41, 1904.
Nordmann-Körte, Arch. f. klin. Chir., Bd. 73, 1904.
Clairmont-v. Eiselsberg, Arch. f. klin. Chir., Bd. 70, 1905.
Hercst, I. Internat. Chir. Kongr., Rev. de Chir., 1905, II, p. 590.
Montprofit, I. Internat. Chir. Kongr., Rev. de Chir., 1905, II, p. 576.
Czerny, Jahresberichte der Heidelberger chir. Klinik 1897—1904, Beitr. z. klin. Chirurgie, Bd. 34—46.

(³) Die Zahlen differieren ein wenig von jenen der Referate in den Wochenschriften, da ich nachträglich noch einige Statistiken einbezogen habe.

Bei *nicht malignen Prozessen* ist die Gastroenterostomie zunächst für das stenosierende Ulcus am Pylorus sowie die Pylorusnarbe bestimmt. Daneben aber geben zahlreiche andere Prozesse mit und ohne Ulcus ventriculi hin und wieder die Indication zur Gastroenterostomie ab, wobei die Grenzen für die Operation seitens einzelner Chirurgen sehr weit ausgedehnt werden. Die bekannten Wechselwirkungen zwischen Pylorospasmus und Hyperacidität, zu denen sich nicht selten das Ulcus ventriculi hinzugesellt, geben auch bei nicht am Pylorus sitzendem Ulcus, das der inneren Therapie trotzt, Veranlassung zur Gastroenterostomie, welche dabei umso günstigere Heilungsresultate zu ergeben pflegt, je näher das Geschwür dem Pylorus sitzt.

Da man aber manches Ulcus ohne Eröffnung des Magens nicht nachweisen kann, liegt die Versuchung nahe, bei Kranken, bei denen man ein Ulcus vermutet, dasselbe aber nach Eröffnung der Bauchhöhle nicht tastet, dennoch die Gastroenterostomie zu machen, in der Annahme, das Ulcus werde gewiss vorhanden sein. Diese Annahme hat aber im Allgemeinen nur dann Berechtigung, wenn die Anamnese von Blutungen und anderen deutlichen Ulcussymptomen berichtet und auch die Magensaftuntersuchung ziemlich regelmässig Hyperacidität ergibt. Freilich wurden auch bei anderen, unklaren Prozessen ausnahmsweise günstige Resultate erzielt (*Czerny-Petersen-Macholl* [1]). Bei nervösen Erkrankungen ohne nachweisbare anatomische Läsion sollte nicht operiert werden (*Brün* [2], *v. Eiselsberg* [3], *Pantaloni* [4]). Der Prozess kann durch die Operation sogar verschlimmert werden (*Herczel* [5]). Ob bei chronischer Gastritis, schwerer Dyspepsie die Gastroenterostomie (*Defontaine* [6], *Jonnesco* [7]) gerechtfertigt und zweckmässig ist, müssten erst weitere Erfahrungen lehren. Bei einfacher atonischer Dilatation scheint

[1] Beitr. zur Pathol. und Therapie d. gutart. Magenerkrankungen, Beitr. z. klin. Chir., Bd. 33, 1902, p. 297.

[2] De la gastro-entérostomie dans les troubles gastriques des névropathes, Congr. fr. de Chir., 1904, Rev. de Chir., 1904, II, p. 937.

[3] Intervent. chir. dans les mal. non cancéreuses de l'estomac, I. Internat. Chir. Kongr., Rev. de Chir., 1905, II, p. 573.

[4] La valeur de la gastro-entérostomie en Y pour les affect. non canc. de l'estomac, Congr. fr. de Chir., Rev. de Chir., 1904, II, p. 357.

[5] I. Intern. Chir. Kongr., Rev. de Chir., 1905, p. 561.

[6] De la gastro-entérostomie pour dyspepsies ou gastrites rebelles, Arch. prov. de Chir., Bd. 6, 3, ref. Ztrbl. f. Chir., 1898, p. 310.

[7] I. Internat. Chir. Kongress, Rev. de Chir., 1905, II, p. 581.

aber die Gastroenterostomie zur Beseitigung der Störungen wohl in Betracht zu kommen (*Mayo Robson* [1], *Kausch* [2]).

Auch bei der *Gastroptose* wird die Gastroenterostomie statt der Gastropexie empfohlen (*Mattoli* [3]), während von anderer Seite doch wieder der Gastropexie das Wort geredet wird (*Roesing* [4]). Von anderen Indicationen, die bei gutartigen Processen für die Gastroenterostomie bestehen, seien noch erwähnt: die congenitale Pylorusatresie bzw. -Stenose (*Lorthioir* [5], *Trautenroth* [6] u. A.), das Geschwür und die Narbe nach Verätzung (*v. Eiselsberg* [7], *Quénu et Petit* [8]), die Tuberculose des Pylorus (*v. Eiselsberg-Clairmont* [9], *Ricard und Chevrier* [10] u. A.).

Ebenso wie das Ulcus ventriculi giebt auch das *Ulcus duodeni* eine Indication für die Gastroenterostomie ab, nur mit dem Unterschiede, dass hier die Gastroenterostomie fast die einzige in Frage kommende Operation darstellt.

Unter Umständen erheischen *Adhaesionen* des Magens oder Duodenums mit der Umgebung die Gastroenterostomie. Beachtenswert scheint mir in dieser Richtung ein Vorschlag *Clairmont's* [11], in Fällen mit hochgradigen Magenbeschwerden, bei denen sich Adhaesionen in der Bauchhöhle finden, die auf andere Weise keine naheliegende Erklärung finden, ein ulcus duoden. anzunehmen und der *Gastrolyse die Gastroenterostomie folgen zu lassen*.

Eine wichtige Frage, die in letzter Zeit viele Chirurgen beschäftigt, ist die: wie weit reicht die Wirksamkeit der Gastroenterostomie beim Ileus und in welchen Fällen ist dieselbe durch die Resection zu ersetzen? Gelegentliche Beobachtungen von nach der Gastroenterostomie nicht ausheilenden oder recidivierenden Geschwüren, von schwerer Blutung oder Perforation nach

[1] 1. Internat. Chir. Kongr., Rev. de Chir., 1905, II, p. [illegible].

[2] Ueber [späte] Ergebnisse nach Gastro[enterostomie bei Magen]senkung und gutartigen Erkrankungen, Mittheilungen a. d. Grenzgeb. etc. Bd. IV, p. [illegible].

[3] La gastroenterostomia, Roma, Società editrice Dante Alighieri, 1905.

[4] 1. Internat. Chir. Kongr., Rev. de Chir., 1905, II, p. 593.

[5] 1. Internat. Chir. Kongr., Rev. de Chir., 1905, II, p. [illegible].

[6] Ueber die Pylorusatresie der Säuglinge, Mittheilungen a. d. Grenzgeb. etc., Bd. IX, 1901, p. 72[illegible].

[7] 1. Internat. Chir. Kongr., Rev. de Chir., 1905, II, p. [illegible].

[8] Les ulcères cicatriciels du pylore consécutifs à l'ingestion de liquides caustiques, Rev. de Chir., 1905, I, p. 51.

[9] Arch. f. klin. Chir., Bd. 78, 1905, p. 18[illegible].

[10] Tuberculose du pylore, Rev. de Chir., 1905, II, p. [illegible].

[11] Bericht über 158 von Prof. v. Eiselsberg ausgeführte Magenoperationen, Arch. f. klin. Chir., 1905, Bd. 78, p. 18[illegible].

der Gastroenterostomie aus dem zurückgelassenen Ulcus, schliesslich die erwiesene Möglichkeit des Hervorgehens eines Carcinoms
aus dem Ulcus bzw. der Narbe, haben diese Frage angeregt.

Speziell jene Geschwüre, auf deren chirurgische Bedeutung
zuerst *Hofmeister* aufmerksam gemacht hat, bei denen Verwachsungen und ein Uebergreifen des Geschwüres auf die Umgebung
statthaben, die *penetrierenden, callösen* Geschwüre nach *Brenner* [1], haben seiner Zeit Brenner stets zur Resektion veranlasst.

Auch von anderer Seite (*Ali Krogius* [2], *Jedlička* [3] u. A.)
ist die Resection des Magengeschwüres der Gastroenterostomie
vorgezogen worden. Aber es hat sich gezeigt, dass nicht nur
die Mortalität der Magenresection bei Geschwüren, speziell bei
verwachsenen Geschwüren eine wesentlich höhere ist, als die
der Gastroenterostomie (*Waracke's* [4] Statistik 39%: 18,8%, *Brenner* 28,6%: 13,3% [5], sondern dass auch die Möglichkeit des
Ausbleibens der Heilung, beziehungsweise des Eintrittes eines
Recidivs bei beiden Operationen vorhanden ist, so dass auch
Brenner [6] wieder zur Gastroenterostomie zurückgekehrt ist.
Schwierig ist für jeden die Entscheidung in solchen Fällen, bei
denen der Befund bei der Operation eine sichere Diagnose nicht
ergibt, wo die harten Ränder des Geschwüres ein Carcinom
nicht ausschliessen und Verwachsungen vorliegen, die ebenso
gut für Ulcus als für Carcinom sprechen können. Der Vorschlag, in solchen Fällen erst ein Stückchen der Geschwulst zu
excidieren, sofort mikroskopisch zu untersuchen und, falls Carcinom gefunden wird, zu resecieren, wird gelegentlich befolgt werden können. Aber im Allgemeinen wird man bei derartigen verwachsenen Tumoren, die unter allen Umständen die Resection
schlecht vertragen und, wenn Carcinom vorliegt, eine Radicalheilung ohnehin kaum erwarten lassen, doch lieber von vorneherein nur die Gastroenterostomie ausführen. Aber auch bei

---

[1] Ueber die chirurgische Behandlung des callösen Magengeschwüres. Arch. f. klin. Chir., Bd. 69.

[2] Ein Wort für die radikale operat. Behandlung d. chron. Magengeschwürs. Arch. f. klin. Chir., Bd. 75, 1905.

[3] Zur operat. Behandlg. d. chron. Magengeschwüres etc., Sborník klinický, Bd. VI, 1904, ref. in Zentbl. f. Chir., 1905, p. 494.

[4] Ueber die Indikationen zur operat. Behandlung des Ulcus ventriculi etc., Göttingen, 1904. Dieterichsche Univer. Buchdruckerei.

[5] Umgekehrt hat Ali Krogius in ... 25%, was sich wohl durch das ungewöhnliche Vorkommen von 3 Todesfällen an Blutung nach G. E. erklärt.

[6] Archiv f. klin. Chir., 1905, Bd. 78.

anderen Fällen haben wir in der Resection stets einen schweren, in der Gastroenterostomie einen ungleich leichteren Eingriff zu erblicken, dessen curativen Effect wir erst abzuwarten haben, bevor wir an die Resection herangehen. Eine Ausnahme bilden in dieser Hinsicht nur solche Geschwüre, die einen für die (segmentäre) Resection ungewöhnlich günstigen Sitz aufweisen.

Ich glaube, dass die Erfolge der Gastroenterostomie speciell beim sog. ulcus callosum nicht unterschätzt werden dürfen. Es existiert in der Literatur eine grosse Reihe von Fällen von ulcus ventriculi mit Tumorbildung, bei denen die Erscheinungen, auch der Tumor, nach der Gastroenterostomie vollkommen und dauernd zurückgegangen sind (*Mayo Robson* [1], *Stick-Garré* [2], *Wölfler-Schloffer* [3], *Ringel-Kümmel* [4], *Clairmont-Eiselsberg* [5] u. A).

Die günstige Wirkung der Gastroenterostomie beim ulcus ventriculi im Allgemeinen ist vor allem bedingt durch die Ermöglichung eines raschen, oft im Vergleiche zur Norm beschleunigten Abflusses des Mageninhaltes in den Darm. Es kommt dadurch die Hyperacidität zum Schwinden, die Zersetzung des Mageninhaltes fällt weg und vor allem hört die stürmische Peristaltik des Magens auf, die vordem bei bestehendem Passage-Hindernis vorhanden war und durch welche das Geschwür immer wieder Insulte erfuhr. Es finden also die Geschwüre vom Momente der vorgenommenen Gastroenterostomie an Bedingungen, wie sie zur Heilung nothwendig sind. Damit hängt es wohl auch zusammen, dass die Gastroenterostomie gerade auch auf die *Blutungen* des Magengeschwüres, namentlich jene Form der Blutungen, die man als chronisch recidivierende bezeichnet, den segensreichsten Einfluss ausübt, auch ohne dass das ulcus selbst in irgend einer Weise angegriffen würde (*Staudel* [6], *Petersen-Macholl* [7] u. A.), sodass wir heute in der Gastroenterostomie das Normalverfahren für solche Blutungen zu erblicken haben. Wird aber einmal das Ulcus direct angegriffen, dann kommt daneben im Sinne *Kösters* [8] immer auch

[1] I. Internat. Chir. Kongr., l.c.
[2] Beitr. zum Magengeschw., Beitr. z. klin. Chir., Bd. XL, 1903.
[3] Beitr. zur klin. Chir., Bd. 32, 1904.
[4] Beitr. zur klin. Chir., Bd. 39, 1903.
[5] l.c.
[6] Die in den letzten Jahren an der Czerny'schen Klinik ausgeführten Magenoperationen, etc. Beitr. z. klin. Chir., Bd. 23, 1899.
[7] Beitr. z. Pathol. u. Therap. d. gutart. Magenerkrankungen, Beitr. z. klin. Chir., Bd. 33, 1902.
[8] 33. Kongr. d. deutsch. Gesellsch. f. Chir., Zntbl. f. Chir., 1894, 48.

noch die Ausführung der Gastroenterostomie in Betracht; ausnahmsweise kann auch an eine Combination der Gastroenterostomie mit der Jejunostomie gedacht werden (*Moynihan, Burge, Lieblein* [1]).

Nach der Gastroenterostomie heilt also der grösste Teil der Magengeschwüre dauernd aus. *Warnecke's* ( ) Statistik zeigt fast 90 % Dauererfolge. *Lieblein* ( ) hat die bis zum Jahre 1903 bekannten Fälle von uncompliciertem nicht stenosierendem Magengeschwür gesammelt. Von den 43 derartigen mit Gastroenterostomie behandelten Fällen liegen von 15 die Spätresultate vor. Nur einmal gab es ein Recidiv, sonst waren die Erfolge durchweg gut, nur 3 mal persistierten leichte Störungen.

Dass in einem Theile der Fälle (ich glaube in durchschnittlich 10 %) die Erfolge der Gastroenterostomie beim ulcus ventriculi und seinen Folgeerscheinungen schlechte oder unvollkommene sind, entspricht auch heute noch den Thatsachen.

Auch einer Folgekrankheit der Gastroenterostomie haben wir zu gedenken. Der directe Uebertritt des sauren Magensaftes nach der Gastrojejunostomie bringt es nämlich mit sich, dass in einem Bruchteile der Fälle s. g. peptische Jejunalgeschwüre entstehen, die wie die Zusammenstellungen von *Tiegel* [1], *Lieblein* [2], und *Gosset* [3] lehren, doch glücklicherweise so selten sind, dass sie die Chancen des Einzelfalles kaum verschlechtern. Nach Gosset, von dem die jüngste Statistik über das ulcus peptic. jejuni vorliegt, sind bisher 31 Fälle bekannt.

Wesentlich günstiger als beim Carcinom ist die *Mortalität der Gastroenterostomie bei gutartigen Erkrankungen.*

Wir verfügen über eine ziemlich umfangreiche Sammel-statistik über die Gastroenterostomie beim ulcus ventriculi von *Warnecke* [1] aus dem Jahre 1901 über 398 Fälle mit einer Mortalität von 18.8 %. Ausserdem liegt eine grosse Statistik von *Mattioli* [2] aus dem Jahre 1903 vor, in welcher im ganzen 1028 Gastroenterostomien wegen gut- und bösartiger Magenerkran-

---

[1] *Lieblein u. Hilgenreiner* — Die Geschwüre und die erworbenen Fisteln des Magendarm kanals. Deutsche Chirurgie, Lieferg. 46 c. 1905.
[2] Loc. cit.
[3] Loc. cit.
[4] Ueber das peptische Geschwür des Duodenum nach Gastroenterostomie, Mittlg. aus d. Grenzgebieten d. Med. u. Chir., 1904. Bd 15.
[5] Deutsche Chirurgie. Lieferg. 46 c. 1905.
[6] L'ulcère peptique du jejunum après gastro-enterostomie. Rev. d. Chir., 1910. t. 35. p. 54.
[7] Loc. cit.
[8] Loc. cit.

kung aus der italienischen Litteratur zusammengestellt sind. Ich habe aus dieser Statistik nur jene Fälle herausgezogen, die zu wenigstens zwanzig von ein und demselben Operateur herrühren. Es kommen so 543 Fälle heraus, 152 Gastroenterostomien wegen Carcinom mit 68 Todesfällen (45 %), 298 Gastroenterostomien wegen gutartiger Processe mit 25 Todesfällen 8,4 %). Conform der oben angeführten Berechnung für das Carcinom habe ich auch hier mehrere Statistiken von Operateuren mit grösserem Materiale aus neuerer Zeit zusammen gezogen und bei 1233 gutartigen Fällen [1] eine Mortalität von 9,6 % berechnet.

Wenn man aber die einzelnen Statistiken vergleicht, so fällt noch mehr als beim Carcinom die Verschiedenheit der Mortalitätsziffern auf, was in der grösseren Verschiedenheit in der Indicationsstellung seine vorwiegende Begründung finden dürfte. Es wäre wohl wünschenswert, wenn auf irgend eine Weise eine wenigstens beiläufige Vorstellung über die Grenzen der Indicationsstellung zur Gastroenterostomie bei gutartigen Processen seitens der betreffenden Operateure gewonnen werden könnte. Vielleicht gelänge dies dadurch, dass, falls nicht die

[1] Die Fälle stammen von:

Merkens — Loc. cit.
Germann — Loc. cit.
Ublinsky-Mikulicz — Loc. cit.
Weber-Lindner — Loc. cit.
Pantaloni — Congr. fr. d. Chir., 1901. Rev. d. Chir., 1904, II, p. 357.
Herzfeld-Korte — Arch. f. klin. Chir., Bd. 67, 1901.
Dalziel — Lancet, 1903, II, p. 458.
Fauchet — Loc. cit.
Dollinger — Orvosi Hetilap, 1902, n° 9, ref. Zbl. f. Chir., 1903, p. [illegible].
Moynihan — Brit. Med. Journal, 1903, II, p. 526.
Hamphof-Steinthal — Loc. cit.
Ukas — Brit. Med. Journal, 1902, II, p. [illegible].
Muraglione-Krause — Loc. cit.
Alt-Krogius — Arch. f. klin. Chir., Bd. 73, 1903.
Brenner — Arch. f. klin. Chir., Bd. 78, 1902.
v. Eiselsberg — I. Internat. Chir. Kongr., Rev. d. Chir., 1903, II, p. 575.
Anderson — Lancet, 1903, II, p. 914.
Guère — I. Internat. Chir. Kongr., Rev. d. Chir., 1903, II, p. 500.
Graham a. Mayo — Transact. of the Americ. Med. Assoc., 1903, ref. Zbl. f. Chir., 1903, pag. 639.
Hartmann — Congr. fr. de Chir., Rev. de Chir., 1901, p. [illegible] und Rev. de Chir., 1903, II, p. 555.
Herczl — I. Internat. Chir. Kongr., Rev. d. Chir., 1903, II, p. [illegible].
Jonnesco — I. Internat. Chir. Kongr., Rev. d. Chir., 1903, II, p. 551.
Mayo Robson — I. Internat. Chir. Kongr., Rev. d. Chir., 1903, II, p. [illegible].
Montprofit — I. Internat. Chir. Kongr., Rev. d. Chir., 1903, II, p. [illegible].
Maunsell Moullin — Med. Soc. of London, Lancet, 1903, II, p. 1225.
Cypros — I. Internat. Chir. Kongr., Rev. d. Chir., 1903, II, p. [illegible].

Carcinomoperationen separat publiciert werden, in den einschlägigen Publicationen neben der Zahl der ausgeführten Gastroenterostomien wegen gutartiger Erkrankungen auch die Zahl der in denselben Zeitraum fallenden Magenoperationen wegen Carcinom, angegeben würde.

Denn wenn sich auch in neuerer Zeit die Operationen wegen gutartiger Magenerkrankungen dem Carcinom gegenüber entschieden häufen, so scheinen mir doch Verhältniszahlen wie sie z. B. *Czerny* [*Steudel*] (1), 103 Carcinomoperationen zu 38 Operationen bei gutartigen Affectionen, *Garrè-Stich* (2), 109 : 55; *Moullprofit* (3), 63 : 37; *v. Eiselsberg* (4), 134 : 97; *Heresel* (5), 83 : 59, angeben, dafür zu sprechen, dass im Allgemeinen bei nicht zu weit gehender Indicationsstellung die Zahl der Carcinomoperationen, zum mindesten nicht kleiner zu sein pflegt, als die der Operationen wegen gutartigen Affectionen. Natürlich mögen örtliche und andere Momente, welche die Zusammensetzung des Materiales der einzelnen Chirurgen beeinflussen, zu gewissen Schwankungen der einschlägigen Ziffern führen, aber man wird doch sagen können, dass, wenn jemand ebensoviele oder mehr Ulcusoperationen macht als Carcinomoperationen, die Vermutung nahe liegt, er sei mit der Operation bei gutartigen Erkrankungen sehr freigebig gewesen und habe deshalb auch viele leichte Fälle operiert.

Was die *Technik der Gastroenterostomie* betrifft, so sind es vor Allem 2 Methoden, die neben einander das Feld beherrschen. Die alte Gastroenterostomia *antecolica anterior*, wie sie zuerst *Wölfler* (6) ausgeführt hat, und die von *v. Hacker* (7) empfohlene Gastroenterostomie *retrocolica posterior*. Beide Methoden geben gute Resultate. Die Gastroenterostomia antecol. ant. macht es allerdings nötig, dass man, um einen circulus vitiosus mit Sicherheit zu vermeiden, eine Anastomose zwischen zu- und abführendem Schenkel anlegt, die *Braun* (8) empfohlen hat.

Es lässt sich aber nicht verkennen, dass im Laufe der letz-

(1) Loc. cit.
(2) Loc. cit.
(3) La gastroentérostomie, Paris, Institut Internat. de Biblogr., 1903.
(4) Clairmont, loc. cit.
(5) I Internat. Chir. Kongr., Rev. de Chir., 1905, p. 371.
(6) Loc. cit.
(7) z. Kongr. d. deutsch. Gesellsch. f. Chir.; Zntbl. f. Chir. 1883, p. 64.
(8) Arch. f. klin. Chir., Bd. 45, 1893.

ten Jahre die Gastroenterostomia post. eine immer grössere Zahl von Anhängern gefunden hat, namentlich seitdem *Petersen* [1] an der Hand einer grossen Casuistik aus der *Czerny*'schen Klinik genaue Directiven über die zur Anastomisierung zu wählende Stelle am Darm gegeben und darauf hingewiesen hat, dass man bei der Gastroenterostomia post. nicht eine »Darmschlinge« verwenden dürfe, sondern eben jene Partie des obersten Jejunums, welche schon normaler Weise der hinteren Magenwand, nur getrennt durch das Mesocolon, anliegt. Dass man dies vorher nicht immer getan bzw. methodisch geübt hat, geht schon daraus hervor, dass in vielen Publicationen von der »Darmschlinge« die Rede ist, die zur Gastroenterostomia post. verwendet wird. In der von *Petersen* beschriebenen Weise ergiebt die *v. Hacker*'sche Gastroenterostomia post. so gut wie immer einen glatten Ablauf der Magendarm-Passage und es wird bei ihr wohl auch die *Braun*'sche Anastomose entbehrlich, die einzelne Chirurgen ausnahmsweise auch bei der posterior für nötig erachten (*Körte-Herzfeld* [2] und *Körte-Nordmann* [3]).

Ich möchte bei diesem Anlasse nicht unerwähnt lassen, dass auch an der *Wölfler*'schen Klinik schon seit 1902 neben der anterior die posterior häufiger als früher Verwendung gefunden hat, und dass ich, durch die guten Resultate der letzteren veranlasst, nun probeweise seit Jahren ziemlich regelmässig die posterior verwende und, von geringfügigen Störungen abgesehen, dabei fast stets eine tadellose und sofortige Wiederherstellung der Passage beobachten konnte. Die anterior habe ich dagegen in jenen Fällen herangezogen, bei denen bestimmte anatomische Gründe sie erforderten. Verbunden mit der *Braun*'schen Anastomose zwischen zu- und abführendem Schenkel giebt auch sie eine prompte Function.

Was die Methodik der Gastroenterostomie anbetrifft, sei hier noch der s. Z. von *v. Mikulicz* [4] verwendeten und neuerdings von *Kocher* [5] empfohlenen Gastroenterostomia inferior gedacht, einer Form der anterior, bei welcher die Anastomose in die Grosse Curvatur verlegt wird. Wie *v. Mikulicz* aber selbst schon erkannt hat, bietet die Anlegung der Oeffnung an

[1] Anat. u. chir. Beiträge zur Gastroenterostomie, Beitr. z. klin. Chir. 1901, Bd. 32.
[2] Ueber die chir. Behandlg. d. Magengeschwürs, etc., Arch. f. klin. Chir. 1901, Bd. 64.
[3] Zur Chirurgie der Magengeschwülste, Arch. f. klin. Chir. 1904, Bd. 73.
[4] Handbuch d. prakt. Chir., von Bergmann, Bruns u. Mikulicz, Aufl., Bd. III, p.
[5] Chir. Operationslehre, 4. Auflage, 1902, p. 309.

einem «tiefsten Punkte» des Magens, wie sie durch die Gastroenterostomia inferior bewirkt wird, doch nur theoretische Vorzüge; überdies kommt man dabei mit den Gefässen der grossen Curvatur in unliebsamen Conflict.

Dem gegenüber hat sich aber eine andere Methode einen
kleinen und überzeugten Kreis von Anhängern geschaffen, die
Y-Gastroenterostomie von *Wölfl'r-Roux*, und zwar besonders in
ihrer von *Roux* angegebenen Ausführung als Gastroenterostomia
posterior. Dass dadurch die anatomischen Verhältnisse weit besser nachgeahmt werden, als bei den anderen Methoden, ist
richtig, aber sie ist um so viel complicierter, als die sonst üblichen, dass sie trotz der guten Resultate, die *Roux* [1], *Mont
profil* [2], *Pantaloni* [3], *Tavel* [4] u. A. aufweisen, dennoch nicht
im Stande war, eine grössere Zahl von Chirurgen für sich zu
gewinnen.

Das Bestreben einer möglichst genauen Wiederherstellung
der anatomischen Verhältnisse liegt auch der *Gastroduodenostomie*, die in verschiedener Form von *Jaboulay* [5], *Villard* [6],
Heule-Miculicz [7], *Kocher* [8] angegeben wurde, sowie der *Fin-
ney'schen* [9] Operation, einer Abart der alten Pyloroplastik, zu
Grunde.

Aber naturgemäss ist die Gastroduodenostomie nur in einer
beschränkten Zahl von Fällen anwendbar, nämlich dann, wenn
der Process auf den Pylorus beschränkt ist, und beim Carcinom
überhaupt nicht.

Was das ulcus ventriculi betrifft, so ist aber gerade zu
bedenken, dass der curative Effect der Gastrojejunostomie nicht
nur in der raschen Entleerung des Magens begründet zu sein
scheint, sondern dass dabei auch unter Umständen die Alka-
lisierung des Magensaftes durch das Einfliessen von Galle und

[1] *Kübe* — La cancer de l'estomac et son traitement chirurgical. Inaug. Diss., Lausanne, 1901,
ref. Zrbl. f. Chir. 1898, p. 368.

Roux — De la gastroenterostomie. Rev. de Gynécologie et de Chir., abd. 1893, ref. Zrbl. f.
Chir. 1902, p. 212.

[2] Loc. cit.

[3] La valeur de la gastroenterostomie en Y pour les affections non cancéreuses de l'estomac.
II. Internat. Chir. Kongress, Rev. de Chir. 1901, II., p. 557.

[4] Le reflux dans la gastroenterostomie. Rev. de Chir. 1901, II, p. 708.

[5] Archives prov. de Chir., 1892, p. 365, und Lyon medical, 1892, t. 77, p. 454, cit. nach
Matani, loc. cit., p. 81.

[6] De la gastroduodénostomie sous-pylorique. Rev. de Chir., 1910, XXII, p. 321.

[7] *Heule* — Ein Fall von Gastroduodenostomie, Zrbl. f. Chir., 1896.

[8] Mobilisierung des Duodenum und Gastroduodenostomie. Zrbl. f. Chir., 1903, p. 33.

[9] Eine gute Beschreibung dieser Operation findet sich in Brit. Med. Journ., 1903, t. p. 122.

Pancreassaft mitwirkt. In jenen Fällen würde also der Gastroduodenostomie ein wichtiger heilender Factor abgehen.

Andererseits darf nicht vergessen werden, dass sich nach
der *Gastrojejunostomie* der Magen etwas schneller entleert als
normaler Weise und der prompte Zufluss von Galle und Pancreassaft gewisse Störungen erleidet; deshalb werden bestimmte
Nahrungsmittel unvollständig verdaut, ein Zustand, dem sich
Erwachsene allerdings gewöhnlich ohne Schwierigkeit accomo-
dieren.

Zur *Herstellung der Anastomosenöffnung* bei der Gastroenterostomie stehen vor Allem 2 Verfahren zur Verfügung, die
Naht und der *Murphy-Knopf*. Die erstere wird allgemein in
Form der doppelreihigen fortlaufenden Naht geübt, aber bei der
Gastroenterostomie—namentlich bei der posterior—wird ihr von
vielen Seiten der Murphy-Knopf noch vorgezogen. Vor Allem
war es *Czerny* (¹), der hiebei seiner Anwendung das Wort geredet hat. Ich glaube nicht, dass die Frage ob Knopf oder Naht
für die Erfolge der Gastroenterostomie post. von hoher Bedeutung ist. Aber dennoch bin ich der Meinung, dass die Verwendung des Knopfes manche Vorteile bietet, die durch die Nachteile
desselben nicht aufgewogen werden. Ich mache jetzt grundsätzlich alle hinteren Gastroenterostomien mit dem Knopf und habe
keine Ursache zur Naht zurückzukehren.

Ich will hier auf die zahlreichen Argumente, die für und
wider den Knopf geltend gemacht werden, nicht näher eingehen,
sondern nur kurz erwähnen, dass die theoretisch möglichen,
nachteiligen Eventualitäten bei demselben zwar alle praktisch
vorkommen, aber doch so selten, dass die Chancen des Einzelfalles dadurch nicht im ungünstigen Sinne beeinflusst werden. Vor allem wissen wir, dass der Knopf, wenn er nach einer
Gastroenterostomie in den Magen fällt, dort keine nennenswer-
ten Störungen herbeizuführen braucht. Im Uebrigen fällt er nach
der Gastroenterostomia post. fast niemals in den Magen zurück.
Die Naht bringt immerhin den Nachteil der längeren Dauer
der Anastomosenbildung. Der Magen muss länger vorgezogen
bleiben, was die Gefahr einer traumatischen Laesion des Geschwüres erhöht. Dieser Umstand erscheint mir aber mit Rück-

(¹) *Rubin* — Beitr. zur Anwendung des Murphyknopfes, Diss. Karlsruhe, 1901.

Czerny — Jahresbericht der Heidelberger chir. Klinik für 1902. Beitr. zur klin. Chir., Bd. 39, 1903.

Czerny — I. Internat. Chir. Kongr., Rev. de Chir., 1905, II, p. 528.

sicht auf die *postoperative Blutung oder Perforation nicht gleich-gültig zu sein*.

Von den zahlreichen *Modificationen des Murphyknopfes* be-deutet keine eine wirkliche Verbesserung, wenn auch damit ebenfalls gelegentlich günstige Resultate erzielt werden können, (z. B. *Jaboulay* [1], 10 Gastroenterostomien wegen Carcinom mit 18 Todesfällen).

In England spielen seit jeher einfache *decalcinierte Knoche-röhren* als Mittel zur Darmvereinigung eine gewisse Rolle und neuerdings werden dieselben von *Mayo Robson* [2] für die Gas-troenterostomie empfohlen. Sie haben den Vorzug, dass sie ähnlich wie der Murphyknopf die Fistel von Anfang an weit offen hal-ten, vielleicht auch die Anlegung der Naht erleichtern. Sie sind aber natürlich keine s. g. Darmschliesser. Die Resultate, die *Mayo Robson* damit erzielt hat, sind gewiss sehr gute zu nennen (186 Gastroenterostomien 3 % Mortalität).

Ich möchte Ihnen nun in Kürze über 119 Gastroentero-stomien berichten, die ich wegen Carcinom und wegen gutartiger Processe teils an der *Wölfler*'schen Klinik in Prag, teils seit 2 1/2 Jahren an der Innsbrucker Klinik ausgeführt habe. Es handelt sich um 66 Gastroenterostomien wegen Carcinom, 53 Gastroenterostomien wegen anderer Processe. Mit den Resectio-nen und Probelaparatomien, etc., sind es 105 Operationen we-gen Carcinom, gegenüber 67 wegen gutartiger Affectionen.

	Prag bis 1903		Innsbruck 1903–1906		Summe		
		Todes-fälle		Todes-fälle		Todes-fälle	
Benigne Processe							
Explor. Lap.			1	1	1	1	
Resect.	1	0	2	0	3	0	66
G. E.	21	1	29	1	53	2	
Andere Op.	4	0	5	0	9	0	
Carcinom							
Explor. Lap.	19	0	7	2	26	2	
Resect.	5	4	8	2	13	6	105
G. E.	37	12	29	2	66	14	

[1] Garrè — Le traitement du cancer de l'estomac par la gastroenterostomie au bouton de Ja-boulay — Lumière, Rev. d. Chir. 1904, I, p. 9.

[2] Gastroenterostomy and its use, etc. Lancet, 1905, I, p. 570.

The operation of Gastroenterostomy etc., Archives internat. de Chir., vol. I, fasc. I; ref. Zbl. f. Chir., 1904, p. 43.

I. Internat. Chir. Kongr., Rev. de Chir., 1905, II, p. 570.

Die 66 Carcinom-Gastroenterostomien ergaben 14 Todesfälle (21 %), die 29 letzten (innsbrucker) Fälle 2 Todesfälle (7 %).

Bei 53 Gastroenterostomien wegen gutartiger Affectionen handelte es sich 44 mal um eine anatomisch nachweisbare Veränderung am Pylorus: Geschwüre oder entzündliche Tumoren (23 Fälle), Narben bzw. «Verengerungen» (21 Fälle). In 8 von den übrigen 9 Fällen lagen Ulcus-Symptome, wie Bluterbrechen (6 Fälle), vor. 17 mal wurde die Gastroenterostomie anterior, davon 15 mal mit *Braun*'scher Anastomose ausgeführt, 36 mal die posterior, davon 34 mal mit Knopf.

Meine Fälle in blutende und nicht blutende Geschwüre zu sondern, vermeine ich, weil darüber in den Krankengeschichten bzw. Anamnesen oft nur unsichere Angaben enthalten sind, und meistens die Blutung ein nebensächliches Symptom darstellte. Die *vorwiegende Indication* zur Operation gaben *Blutungen* nur in 4 oder 5 Fällen ab. In diesen Fällen haben sie durchwegs nach der Operation sistiert, und auch sonst habe ich im postoperativen Verlauf nie störende Blutungen beobachtet. Hingegen habe ich einen Fall nach einer Probelaparatomie (der Fall wurde für ein Carcinom gehalten) an einer Arrosionsblutung der Arteria lienalis verloren.

Im Ganzen kamen nach 53 Gastroenterostomien bei gutartigen Processen 2 Todesfälle vor (3.8 %). Von den übrigen 51 Patienten habe ich bei 36 Nachrichten über das spätere Befinden, 4 sind inzwischen gestorben, bleiben noch 32. Von diesen sind 24 durch die Operation geheilt, 2 gebessert. In 5 Fällen hat die Operation keinen oder nur einen vorübergehenden Erfolg gehabt. Es erscheint mir sehr bemerkenswert, dass einer dieser Fälle eine ausgesprochene organische Pylorusstenose war. 2 der 5 Misserfolge aber waren Fälle mit fast völlig negativem anatomischen Befund, die ich heute nicht mehr der Gastroenterostomie unterziehen würde. Diese beiden Misserfolge wären also bei besserer Indicationsstellung zu vermeiden gewesen.

In 9 Fällen wurde die Gastroenterostomie bei entzündlichen *Magen-Tumoren*, die in das Gebiet des ulcus callosum gehören, vorgenommen. Von 7 derselben habe ich Nachricht; allen geht es gut, nur sind bei zweien einige Zeit nach der Operation die alten Beschwerden wiedergekommen, um dann in einem Falle von selbst dauernd zu sistieren, im anderen Falle nach Vornahme einer neuerlichen Gastroenterostomie.

ENTEROANASTOMOSE

Ein weit geringeres Anwendungsgebiet als die Gastroenterostomie hat die *Enteroanastomose*. Sie ist vielfach zu Gunsten
der vollkommeneren Methoden der Darmausschaltung zurückgedrängt worden, wenngleich sie auch heute nicht nur zum Zwecke der Umgehung von Passage-Hindernissen, wie dies s. Z.
Maisonneuve [1], dann *Billroth* [2] und *v. Hacker* [3] getan haben, sondern auch in der Absicht ausgeführt wird, den Darminhalt von einer bestimmten Strecke des Darmes ferne zu halten.

In Bezug auf die Nomenclatur dieser Operationen herrscht
so grosse Uneinigkeit und Unklarheit, dass ich kurz auf Wesen
und Namen derselben eingehen möchte.

Durch jede einfache Enteroanastomose, eine seitliche Communicationsöffnung zwischen zwei Darmschlingen, wird eine *unvollkommene* Darmausschaltung bewirkt. Doch ist dasselbe auch
bei der sogenannten unilateralen Darmausschaltung (*Haken*
[4]) der Fall, die in neuerer Zeit gelegentlich als Ersatz der bilateralen Ausschaltung verwendet wird.

Nennt man also die einfache Enteroanastomose eine «incomplete Darmausschaltung» so gibt dies zu Verwechslungen
mit der unilateralen Ausschaltung Anlass. In Frankreich hat
man sich dadurch geholfen, dass man jene Ausschaltungen, welche durch die einfache Anastomose bewirkt werden, nicht als
Ausschaltungen bezeichnet, sondern als *Maisonneure*'sche Anastomosen. Dieser Ausweg wäre—allgemein acceptiert—praktisch
recht brauchbar, jedenfalls besser als die ganz unzulängliche
Bezeichnung «incomplete Darmausschaltung». Dennoch entspricht es dem Wesen der Sache mehr, wenn wir auch die *Maisonneure*'sche Anastomose zu den «Darmausschaltungen» rechnen,
aber dann hinzufügen: «durch einfache Anastomose».

Von einzelnen Autoren werden umgekehrt auch manche unilaterale Darmausschaltungen zu den Enteroanastomosen gerechnet. Und in der Tat stehen manche solche Operationen, bei
denen die Durchtrennung des zuführenden Darmes unterhalb

[1] Soc. de Chir. de Paris, séance du 1er février 1894, n° 16.

[2] Hauser. — Darmresectionen und Enterorrhaphien in der Klinik Billroth, Ztschr. f. Heilkunde
Bd. V, 1885.

[3] Ueber die Bedeutung der Anastomosenbildung am Darm für die operative Behandlung der
Verengerungen desselben. Wiener klin. Wochenschr., 1888, n° 17.

[4] Allg. Bemerkungen zu den Hernien u. Laparotomie mit Darmimplantation, Inaug. Diss.,
Dorpat 1891, cit. nach v. Frey, Beitr. z. kl. Chir. Bd. 14, 1895.

der Anastomose lediglich aus technischen Gründen geschieht, wie zum Beispiel bei der Verbindung des Ileums mit dem tiefsten Dickdarmabschnitt, den *Maisonneuve*'schen Anastomosen sehr nahe. Es kommt eben bei allen diesen Operationen bis zu einem gewissen Grade darauf an, welche Absicht der Operation zu Grunde liegt. Will man bei einem Carcinom durch eine Ileo-Sigmoideostomie eine neue Passage herstellen, und durchtrennt man dabei aus irgendwelchem Grunde das Ileum, so liegt dieser Operation trotz der Durchtrennung eigentlich keine richtige Ausschaltungstendenz zu Grunde. Macht man aber wegen einer Colitis ulcerosa, oder um Darminhalt von einer bestehenden äusseren Fistel abzuhalten, auch nur eine einfache seitliche Ileo-Sigmoideostomie, so steht die (auf diesem Wege freilich nur teilweise erreichbare) Absicht der Ausschaltung so sehr im Vordergrund, dass man begreift, wenn solche Operationen den Ausschaltungen zugezählt werden.

So lange eine einheitliche kurze Bezeichnung für die verschiedenen einschlägigen Operationen nicht erzielt werden kann, müssen wir uns also entschliessen, bei der Benennung etwas ausführlicher vorzugehen, wenn Missverständnisse vermieden werden sollen. Es schiene mir, wie bemerkt, in dieser Hinsicht am zweckmässigsten, wenn wir von «Darmausschaltungen durch einfache, eventuell *Maisonneuve*'sche, Anastomosen» sprechen würden. Diese sind im folgenden gemeint, wenn von Enteroanastomosen die Rede ist.

Jede Enteroanastomose bewirkt eine Teilung des Kotstromes. Ein Teil des Inhaltes aus dem zuführenden Darm tritt durch die Anastomosenöffnung in den abführenden Darm, ein anderer Teil in die ausgeschaltete Schlinge. Das Verhältnis, in dem diese Teilung des Kotstromes eintritt, ist sehr verschieden. Handelt es sich z. B. am ausgeschalteten Teile knapp unterhalb der Anastomose um eine hochgradige Stenose, die keinen Darminhalt passieren lässt, so wird sogar der ganze Kotstrom in den abführenden Darm geleitet. In diesen Fällen ist das funktionelle Resultat der Enteroanastomose gewöhnlich ein vollkommenes; denn eine Anstauung in dem ausgeschalteten Teile des *abführenden* Darmes hat wenig zu bedeuten. Findet sich aber an dem ausgeschalteten Darm keine Striktur, dann kann natürlich auch in diesem Kot circulieren; liegt dann überdies noch eine äussere Fistel an demselben vor, so kann dieser Kot durch die Fistel nach aussen treten.

Je grösser die Anastomosenöffnung angelegt wurde, desto leichter wird im Allgemeinen die Passage zum abführenden Darm gefunden werden. Daneben spielt noch eine Reihe von anderen, zum Teile uncontrolierbaren Momenten mit, die Lagerung der Schenkel, etwaige Knickung der Schlinge u. dgl. So kommt es, dass z. B. unter Umständen bei Fällen von Darmfisteln oder anus praeter naturalis, die Enteroanastomose zur Beseitigung der Fistel genügt, während sie in anderen Fällen fast wirkungslos bleibt.

Um das Hinzutreten des Kotstromes in die auszuschaltende Partie mit grösserer oder voller Sicherheit hintanzuhalten, hat man bekanntlich die vollkommeneren Methoden der Ausschaltung: die «unilaterale» und «bilaterale» eingeführt. Leider sind diese Methoden gewöhnlich beträchtlich eingreifender als die einfache Anastomosenbildung. Und deshalb hatte es gewiss Berechtigung, wenn man versuchte, die einfachen Anastomosen durch bestimmte Massnahmen leistungsfähiger zu machen, und am zuführenden Darm knapp unter der Enteroanastomose ein Passagehindernis einzuschalten (v. *Hacker* [1], *Cou-te* [2], *Le Dentu* [3], *Chaput* [4] v. *Moseltig-Moorhof* [5] u. A.). Aber alle diese Massnahmen halten, ob sie jetzt in Umschnürungen, Knickungen, Faltenbildungen oder dergleichen bestehen, immer nur für kurze Zeit dem andrängenden Darminhalt stand, und richtige organische Stricturen zu erzeugen ist bisher unmöglich gewesen. Vielleicht zeigen in dieser Hinsicht die Ergebnisse meiner Tierversuche einen richtigen Weg, bei denen es mir am Kaninchendarm durch Mesenterialablösung öfter gelungen ist, echte Narbenstricturen herbeizuführen. Natürlich müsste die betreffende in ihrer Ernährung gefährdete Darmstelle durch Serosanähte eingestülpt werden.

Was wir von der Enteroanastomose bei den verschiedenen Processen, bei denen sie in Anwendung kommt, zu erwarten haben, geht schon aus den obigen Bemerkungen über den functionellen Effect dieser Operation hervor. Nichts oder wenig dort, wo wir *allen* Darminhalt von einer bestimmten Darmpartie ab-

---

[1] Wiener klin. Wochenschr., 1898, n° 17-18.
[2] Rev. méd. de la Suisse Romande, 1890, n° 6, cit. nach *Lance*, Thèse de Paris, 1903.
[3] Congrès français de Chir., 1894, cit. nach *Lance*, Thèse de Paris, 1903.
[4] Soc. de Chir., 1894, 6 Juin, Rev. de Chir., 1894, p. 600
[5] Rev. de Gyn. et de Chir. abdom., 1897, p. 1054, cit. nach *Gosinella*, Thèse de Paris, 1903

halten wollen, viel, wo es uns genügt, wenn die Hauptmasse des Kotstromes durch die Anastomosenöffnung streicht.

Eine Radicalheilung bringt die Enteroanastomose deshalb nur in sehr wenigen Fällen, bei nicht specifischen Stricturen (traumatischen, nach Invagination, etc., bei ausgeheilten tuberculösen Stricturen). In allen übrigen Fällen ist sie als Notbehelf zu betrachten, und wird nur ausgeführt, wenn eine leistungsfähigere Operation nicht gemacht werden kann.

Die grösste Bedeutung hat die Enteroanastomose beim *Carcinom* des Darmes und zwar in erster Linie beim Dünndarmcarcinom, namentlich wenn der Tumor hoch am Darm sitzt. Denn in solchen Fällen bringt die *Enterostomie*, abgesehen von dem qualvollen Zustand, den sie wegen des dünnflüssigen Darminhaltes schafft, auch die Gefahr der Inanition mit sich. Beim stenosierenden, inoperablen Dünndarmcarcinom wird also die Enteroanastomose als das normale Verfahren zu gelten haben und die Enterostomie nur in schweren Ausnahmsfällen herangezogen werden dürfen.

Dass man aber in neuerer Zeit darauf hinausgeht, auch beim Dickdarmcarcinom, selbst bei tiefem Sitze desselben die Entero- beziehungsweise Colostomie durch die Enteroanastomose zu ersetzen, bedeutete einen wichtigen Fortschritt auf dem Gebiet der Palliativoperationen. Denn dass der durch die Enteroanastomose bedingte Zustand dem Kranken ein ungleich freundlicheres Ableben sichert, fällt so schwer ins Gewicht, dass dadurch viele wirkliche und vermeintliche Nachteile derselben aufgewogen werden. Leider hat die Enteroanastomose dann ihre Grenzen, wenn sie als lebensrettende Operation der Enterostomie bzw. der Colostomie nachsteht, nämlich bei stürmischen Erscheinungen des Darmverschlusses, namentlich, wenn dieselben längere Zeit angedauert haben. In solchen Fällen, in denen die Ableitung des Darminhaltes das erste Erfordernis darstellt, leistet zweifellos die Anlegung einer äusseren Fistel mehr. Die Vorteile der Enterostomie liegen zunächst darin, dass der zuführende dilatierte Darm bei seiner Entleerung nicht mehr den Widerstand zu überwinden hat, den der abführende Darm abgibt, dann in dem Wegfall der Resorption von Giftstoffen während der Passage des Darminhaltes durch den abführenden Darm. Schliesslich ist auch die Gefahr der Peritonitis in Fällen von acuten oder lang andauernden Stenosen bei der Enteroanastomose wesentlich grösser als bei der Enterostomie. So hat

z. B. v. *Eiselsberg* [1] bei im Stadium des acuten Verschlusses vorgenommenen Enteroanastomosen von 13 Fällen 6 verloren, eine Mortalität, die jene der Enterostomie bei solchen Fällen gewiss übersteigt.

Der Zustand der Patienten, bei denen wegen Darmcarcinoms eine Enteroanastomose ausgeführt wurde, ist gewöhnlich ein günstiger, wenigstens was die Darmpassage betrifft. Nur ausnahmsweise kommt es durch Stauung im ausgeschalteten Darm zu Beschwerden. Die Lebenszeit nach der Enteroanastomose beträgt dabei gewöhnlich 6-9 Monate, manchmal 1-2 Jahre (*Prutz* [2], *Haberer* [3] u. A.). Dass die Colostomie eine längere Lebensdauer ergibt als die Enteroanastomose, ist aus theoretischer Erwägungen nicht von der Hand zu weisen, kann aber nicht als erwiesen betrachtet werden. Keinesfalls scheint es jedoch von grosser Bedeutung zu sein, ob die Secrete des erkrankten Darmes direct nach aussen abgeleitet werden oder in den abführenden Darm gelangen; nur ausnahmsweise, bei stark verjauchten Carcinomen dürfte darin ein merklich schädigendes Moment für den Kranken liegen.

Was die *Darmabschnitte betrifft*, zwischen denen die Anastomisierung vorgenommen zu werden pflegt, so sei gleich hier vorweggenommen, dass nicht nur beim Carcinom sondern überhaupt die häufigste Enteroanastomose die Ileocolostomie ist, sie gibt eine anerkannt günstige Function. Auch die Ileosigmoideostomie gibt functionell zufriedenstellende Resultate; vor Allem kommt das Hauptbedenken gegen die letztere Operation, die Ausschaltung des ganzen Dickdarmes, praktisch nicht, oder nur wenig in Betracht, da nur ein geringer Teil solcher Fälle dauernd an Diarrhoen zu leiden pflegt, die man a priori erwarten sollte (v. *Eiselsberg* [4], *Drachert* [5], *Crespin* [6], *Lanec* [7]). Es scheint im Gegenteile der Dickdarm knapp oberhalb der Ileosigmoideostomie die Function eines Reservoirs zu übernehmen, in wel-

[1] *Haberer*, Anwendung und Resultate der seit ... an v. Eiselsbergs Klinik in Wien ausgeführten Enteroanastomosen etc., Arch. f. klin. Chir., 1904, Bd. 72.
Prutz, Ueber die Enteroanastomosen etc., Arch. f. klin. Chir., 1903, Bd. 70.
[2] Loc. cit.
[3] Loc. cit.
[4] XIII° Congr. int. de Méd., Paris, 1900, Rev. d. Chir., 1900, II, p. ...
[5] Echo méd. du Nord, 1898, p. 325, cit. nach *Lanec*, Thèse de Paris, 1903.
[6] Etude sur les anastomoses de l'iléon etc., Thèse de Paris 1903.
[7] L'exclusion de l'intestin, Thèse de Paris, 1903.

chem der rückläufig eintretende Dünndarminhalt eingedickt wird, natürlich nur dann, wenn nicht gerade oberhalb der Ileosigmoideostomie ein stenosierender Tumor sich befindet.

Anders als beim Carcinom steht es mit der Wirkung der Enteroanastomose, die wir bei der stenosierenden *Darmtuberculose* anstreben. Bei dieser handelt es sich nicht nur um die Wiederherstellung der Passage, sondern auch um die *curative Entlastung* des Darmes. Seit *Conrath*'s Zusammenstellungen [1] über die Coecumtuberculose wissen wir, dass nach der einfachen Enteroanastomose ein guter Teil dieser Fälle ausheilen kann. Leider ist die Wirkung aber ganz inconstant und deshalb vermeidet man die Anastomose zu Gunsten der Resection, wo immer es angeht. So kommt es, dass auch in der neueren Zeit, wo die Resultate der Resection so viel bessere geworden sind, die Fälle von wirklicher Heilung der Darmtuberculose durch die Enteroanastomose (c. *Eiselsberg* [2], *Sörensen-Hahn* [3] u. A.) noch immer selten genug vorkommen. Es werden eben für die Enteroanastomose nur jene traurigen Fälle reserviert, bei denen der bessere Eingriff, die Resection, von vornherein aussichtslos ist.

Ein besonders schwieriges Capitel, das bei der Behandlung der stenosierenden Darmtuberculose oft in Betracht kommt, sind die *multiplen Stricturen*, die bekanntlich bei dieser Erkrankung häufig vorkommen und dann gar nicht selten über sehr grosse Strecken des Darmes verstreut sind. Die Resection der gesammten erkrankten Partien ist dabei in der Regel nicht vorzunehmen, und eine einfache Enteroanastomose, welche die ganze erkrankte Darmpartie ausschalten würde, pflegt mit Rücksicht auf die Ausdehnung der letzteren die Ernährung zu gefährden; dazu kommt noch, dass in solchen Fällen die einfache Enteroanastomose überhaupt nur ausnahmsweise (*Deppe* [4], *Erdheim-Mosetig* [5]) zur Beseitigung der Beschwerden genügt, weil trotz derselben Darminhalt in den ausgeschalteten Teil gelangt und sich zwischen den einzelnen Stricturen anstaut, was auch wei-

[1] Ueber die locale chron. Coecumtuberculose etc., Beitr. z. klin. Chir., 1898, Bd. 21.
[2] Pratt, loc. cit.
[3] Ueber stenosierende Darmtuberculose, Deut. Ztschr. f. Chir., Bd. 79, p. 169.
[4] Ueber multiple tubers. Darmstenose, In. Diss., Tübingen, 1899, ref. Zbl. f. Chir., 1899, pag. 1093.
[5] Ueber multiple Dünndarmstenosen, Wiener klin. Wochenschr., 1900, n.º 4, p. 79.

terhin zu den schwersten Koliken Veranlassung geben kann.

In solchen Fällen müssen entweder *mehrere Anastomosen* angelegt werden, oder man muss sich durch eine *Combination von Enteroanastomose u. d. Resection* helfen.

Ausnahmsweise kann sogar eine *Combination von Entero-anastomose u. d. Enterostomie* nötig sein, wie folgendes Beispiel beweist:

Ich selbst war einmal bei multiplen (allerdings carcinomatösen) Darmstricturen nach resectio recti carcinomatosa bei einem 25 jährigen Mädchen vor die Notwendigkeit eines neuerlichen Eingriffes gestellt. — Ich führte die einfache Enteroanastomose unter Ausschaltung der 3 oder 4 Stricturen tragenden erkrankten Darmpartien aus. Darauf besserte sich die Darmfunction insofern, als die Nahrungsaufnahme möglich wurde und wieder Stuhlgang kam; aber die Patientin war von beständigen Kolikschmerzen im Bauche gequält; eine geblähte Schlinge war durch die Bauchdecken zu fühlen. Bei der 3. Operation zeigte sich, dass eine mächtige ampullenförmige Erweiterung zwischen zwei ausgeschalteten Stenosen vorlag; erst eine dort angelegte Enterostomie beseitigte die Qualen, ohne übrigens nachher sehr lästig zu fallen. Die engen Stricturen liessen keinen Darminhalt durch die Fistel austreten.

Bei der *Darmfistel* und dem *anus praeter aturalis* gilt die Enteroanastomose als eine recht unzuverlässige Operation. Sie ist deshalb trotz ihrer Einfachheit bei diesen Processen sehr selten ausgeführt worden. *Hilgenreiner* konnte vor Kurzem erst 27 Fälle dieser Art sammeln mit 55 % Heilungen. Manche Autoren urteilen aber über den Wert der Enteroanastomose bei Kotfisteln sehr ungünstig (v. *Eiselsberg*), wenngleich auch in neuerer Zeit einzelne gute Erfolge bekannt wurden (*Sarariaud und Demoulin* [¹]). Nach *Hilgenreiner* ist die Enteroanastomose der unilateralen oder bilateralen Darmausschaltung bei Kotfisteln nur vorzuziehen, wenn man sich über zu- und abführenden Darmschenkel bei der Operation im Unklaren befindet, wenn man fürchtet, durch eine ausgedehntere Operation einen Abscess zu eröffnen, wenn der Kranke sehr herabgekommen ist und endlich wenn man glaubt, mit der Enteroanastomose auszukommen (*Hochenegg*).

Auch beim *Volvulus des Coecum* und der *Flexura sigm.* kommt nach der Detorsion zur Sicherung der Darmpassage die Enteroanastomose in Betracht. *A. v. Bergmann* [²] u. A. haben eine Reihe solcher Operationen ausgeführt.

[¹] Des. an. d'entero-anastomose etc., Rev. d. Chir., 1905. II, p. 831.
[²] Kongressbericht d. deut. Gesellsch. f. Chir., 1906. Zdbl. f. Chir., 1906, p. 75.

Seltenere Indicationen zur Enteroanastomose sind: *nicht exstirpierbare chronische Invaginationen*, gewisse *Appendicitisfälle* mit Erkrankungen des Coecums (*Morris* [1], *Jaffé* [2], *v. Eiselsberg* [3]) und die *Colitis ulcerosa* (*Glord* (?) [4], *v. Beck* [5]), bei welch letzterer übrigens der Fistelbildung von den meisten Autoren der Vorrang eingeräumt wird (*Nehrkorn* [6]).

Was die Technik betrifft, so ist dem bei der Gastroenterostomie Gesagten bezüglich des Murphyknopfes hinzuzufügen, dass bei der Enteroanastomose der Knopf nicht oder nur mehr ausnahmsweise Verwendung finden sollte. Denn in jenen Fällen, in denen eine sehr rasche Vollendung der Operation unerlässlich ist, tritt doch die Enterostomie in ihre Rechte und in anderen Fällen wird gewöhnlich die Anlegung der Anastomose in bequemer Weise vor den Bauchdecken vorgenommen, also ohne Bedenken zur Naht gegriffen werden können. Das wichtigste Bedenken gegen Knopf bei Enteroanastomose bildet sein Hineinfallen in den ausgeschalteten Darmabschnitt.

Die Aufstellung einer Statistik über die Enteroanastomose bietet wenig Aussicht ein brauchbares Bild über die Chancen dieser Operation zu gewinnen. Selbst nur verglichen mit der Gastroenterostomie bei malignen Tumoren ist die Casuistik eine verschwindend kleine und über einen grossen Zeitraum verstreute. Eine nennenswerte Zahl aus den letzten Jahren liegt nicht vor. *De Bovis* [7] hat im Jahre 1900 aus der Literatur 44 Fälle mit 12 Todesfällen zusammengestellt. Seither sind von verschiedenen Autoren meist in Verbindung mit Berichten über Darmresectionen wegen Tumoren und Tuberculose einzelne Fälle von Enteroanastomose mitgeteilt worden, grössere Zahlen nur von wenigen, so von *Zimmermann*, *Kröntein* [8], *Pribt u. Haberer* (*v. Eiselsberg* [9]), *Mikulicz* [10] u. A.

---

[1] Wien. f. Chir., 1901, p. 363.

[2] Zbl. f. Chir., 1901, p. 577.

[3] Haberer, loc. cit.

[4] cit. nach *Nehrkorn* s. unten.

[5] Die spastische Colitis und ihre Behandlung. Deut. Chir. Kongr., 1901, II, p. 376.

[6] Die chir. Behandlg. der Colitis als chron. Mittheilungen a. d. Grenzgebieten etc., Bd. XII. 1904, p. 322, ferner
Nehrkorn, Congr. d. d. Gesellsch. f. Chir., 1901, II, p. 230.

[7] Le cancer du gros intestin, rectum excepté. Rev. d. Chir., 1900 I, p. 695.

[8] Ueber Operat. u. Erfolge der Dickdärme wegen Carcinom. Beitr. z. klin. Chir., Bd. 49. 1906, p. 303.

[9] Loc. cit.

[10] Chir. Erfahrungen über das Dickdarmcarcinom. Arch. f. klin. Chir., Bd. 69, 1903.

Die weitaus grösste eigene Statistik hat *v. Eiselsberg* (¹),
57 Enteroanastomosen, 14 gestorben. Durch Herbeiziehen der Fälle
aus einigen neueren einschlägigen Arbeiten unter Ausschluss
von Einzelfällen habe ich 144 Enteroanastomosen zusammengestellt mit einer Mortalität von 25,8 °/₀ (²). Unter Ausschluss
der Fälle mit schweren Occlusionserscheinungen kommen wir zu
einer Mortalität von circa 20 °/₀, also etwas weniger als die durchschnittliche Mortalität der Gastroenterostomie wegen Carcinom.

Fasse ich die *wesentlichsten Ergebnisse meines Referates*
zusammen, so ergeben sich folgende Punkte:

Die Gastroenterostomie und die Enteroanastomose leisten
wertvolle Dienste in allen jenen Fällen, bei denen ein bestehendes
Passage-Hindernis am Magendarmkanal umgangen werden soll.
Sie gewinnen den Charakter einer *radical* heilenden Operation
bei den *nicht specifischen Stricturen* des Pylorus, bzw. Magens
und Duodenums und den viel selteneren Fällen von nicht specifischen Darmstricturen.

Daneben ist die Gastroenterostomie in einem grossen Teile
der Fälle von *Ulcus ventriculi*, vor Allem beim Ulcus pylori
im Stande, die *Heilung* solcher Geschwüre und das *Sistieren
chronischer, recidivierender* Blutungen derselben zu bewirken.

Die Gastroenterostomie soll beim Ulcus ventriculi nur in
Ausnahmsfällen durch die *Resection* des Geschwüres ersetzt

(¹) *Haberer*, loc. cit.

(²) Die Fälle sind entnommen den Statistiken von:

Sörensen (Hahn). Ueber 28 Fälle von Carcinom des Ileum und Colon. Diss. Leipzig u. Deut.
Ztschr. f. Chir., loc. cit.

Erdheim (Moritz). Ueber multiple Dünndarmstenosen tubercul. Ursprungs. Wiener klin.
Wochenschr., 1901, n.º 4, ru. Ztrbl. f. Chir., 1906, p. 612.

Deppe. Ueber multiple tubercul. Dünndarmstenosen. Diss. Tübingen, 1899, cit. Ztrbl. f. Chir.,
1899, p. 1059.

v. Eiselsberg (Haberer), loc. cit.

Mauriaud. Deux cas d'entéro-anastomose pour cancer du gros intestin. Rev. d. Chir. 1905,
II, p. 384.

Terrier. Des anastomoses iléo-rectales. Rev. d. Chir., 1905, I, p. 133.

Gerard. Des anastomoses iléo-rectales. Rev. d. Chir., 1906, I, p. 152.

Schloffer (Weibel). Zur operat. Behandg. des Dickdarmcarcin., Beitr. zur klin. Chir.
Bd. 38, 1903.

Lauers (Poppert). Ueber 5 operat. behandelte Fälle von Darmstenose in d. Beurcoalgegend.
Diss. Giessen, 1902.

Mikulicz. Chir. Erfahrungen über das Darmcarcinom. Arch. f. klin. Chir., Bd. 69, 1903.

Pollack (Mikulicz). Beiträge zur Kenntnis des tuberculösen Ileocoecaltumors. Diss.
Breslau, 1905.

Körte. Die operative Behandlung der malignen Dickdarmgeschwülste. Arch. f. klin. Chir.,
Bd. 61, 1901.

M. v. Bergmann, loc. cit.

werden, und dann stets die Methode *Billroth II* zur Ausführung kommen.

Beim *Carcinom des Magens u. d. Darmes* sind die Gastroenterostomie und die Enteroanastomose segensreiche *Palliativ-Operationen* und es ist dabei die Gastroenterostomie der Jejunostomie, die Enteroanastomose der Entero- bzw. Colostomie, wenn irgend möglich vorzuziehen.

Bei der *Darmtuberculose* hat die Enteroanastomose zunächst die Bedeutung einer *Palliativ-Operation* zur Beseitigung der Stenosen-Erscheinungen. Daneben begünstigt sie in nicht zu schlechten Fällen *manchmal* die *Heilung* der Erkrankung.

In allen jenen Fällen, in denen wir *von der Enteroanastomose eine richtige Darmausschaltung* erwarten, also vor allem beim anus praeternaturalis und der Darmfistel, dann bei multiplen Stricturen sind die *Resultate* der Enteroanastomose äusserst *unzuverlässig.*

Comptes Rendus des Séances

SÉANCE D'OUVERTURE (20 AVRIL)

Présidence: M. OLIVEIRA FEIJÃO

M. OLIVEIRA FEIJÃO: Le plus noble et en même temps le plus utile des buts des Congrès internationaux est de faire connaître les pays, leurs avancements au point de vue scientifique et de reserrer les liens qui doivent à tout jamais, depuis que la civilisation nous a faits, — à tous, frères, comme fils d'un même idéal, le progrès, — unir dans le monde entier ceux qui pensent, ceux qui ont voué leur vie au bonheur de l'humanité, et dont le travail, appartenant au présent, est un legs précieux pour le bien-être des générations de l'avenir.

Connaître les pays, connaître l'état où ils se trouvent sous le rapport des sciences! Comme sous ce double point de vue le petit Portugal est mal connu! Placé à une extrémité de l'Europe, où l'on parle une langue, à présent très peu connue, il faut qu'on y vienne exprès pour qu'on puisse bien le connaître, car, malheureusement, les descriptions qu'on en fait ne sont pas, bien souvent, l'expression de la vérité.

Trois siècles se sont écoulés depuis l'époque à laquelle le Portugal fit connaître son nom au monde entier, et par ses travaux, plus qu'aucune autre nation, fit avancer le monde.

C'était alors le temps des découvertes, le temps des aventures et des guerres; mais les temps sont changés. Aujourd'hui ce n'est plus par la découverte des pays inconnus, mais par la découverte des grandes vérités de la science, qu'on donne au monde l'impulsion qui le fait marcher.

Le Portugal du quinzième et seizième siècles tint le premier rang parmi les nations, et si le Portugal d'aujourd'hui ne peut pas réclamer une place à l'avant-garde des peuples, il peut, heureusement, leur montrer qu'il sait les accompagner dans le mouvement évolutif et progressif qu'ils font faire à l'humanité.

Sous ce rapport et comme démonstration de ce fait, l'histoire de la chirurgie en Portugal est un exemple probant.

Ce ne fut fut qu'au quinzième, ou plutôt au seizième siècle, que la chirurgie prit dans mon pays un certain développement; jusqu'alors l'instruction, entièrement dans les mains des moines, auxquels la religion défendait de les tremper dans le sang humain, ne pouvait pas faire des progrès en matière chirurgicale.

Ce fut au seizième siècle que furent établis les cours réguliers d'anatomie et de chirurgie à l'Université de Coïmbre, et dans le même siècle, avec la fondation de l'Hôpital de Todos os Santos à Lisbonne, les études anatomiques et de chirurgie prirent un remarquable développement, qui dut se continuer dans les siècles futurs et jusqu'à nos jours.

Alors quelques professeurs étrangers vinrent, à l'invitation du roi, enseigner l'anatomie et la chirurgie à l'Hôpital de Todos os Santos; un cours régulier y fut établi et, au XVIII siècle, il y avait sept professeurs des matières chirurgicales.

Là est née l'Ecole Royale de Chirurgie, qui, dans la première moitié du XIX siècle, après la chute des barrières qui jusqu'alors avaient séparé la médecine et la chirurgie, fut transformée en un institut où les sciences médicales seraient enseignées en toutes leurs branches.

C'est sans doute dans le dernier siècle que la chirurgie ont dans le monde un plus remarquable progrès; mais, déjà bien avant, au XVII et XVIII siècles on trouve des noms de chirurgiens portugais, dignes d'être placés à côté des premiers de ces époques, qu'il suffise de citer Antonio da Cruz et Antonio Ferreira, dont l'œuvre monumentale égale les meilleures de son temps.

Sous l'influence des grands chirurgiens du commencement du XIX siècle, la chirurgie fit partout d'énormes progrès, et dans l'Ecole de Lisbonne ces progrès s'accentuèrent bientôt. L'étude de l'anatomie, qui attirait déjà toute l'attention grâce aux travaux de Constancio, est faite avec le plus grand soin, et des chirurgiens tels que Teixeira, Santos et Lourenço da Luz, l'opérateur élégant, dont la renommée est arrivée jusqu'à nous, donnent à la chirurgie portugaise un éclat nouveau, et les ligatures des grandes artères, les opérations pour les hernies, les résections, etc., sont pratiquées en Portugal. Les élèves des grands chirurgiens d'alors poursuivent l'œuvre commencée et accompagnent pas à pas les progrès de la science dans les pays les plus avancés, et

Barbosa, Magalhães Coutinho, Thomaz de Carvalho, Ribeiro Vianna, Alves Branco et bien d'autres furent des chirurgiens et des opérateurs éminents de la seconde moitié du dernier siècle, et, même avant l'avènement de l'antisepsie, les chirurgiens portugais exerçaient la gynécologie et la statistique des ovariotomies, antérieure à l'antisepsie, est des plus brillantes.

Ce fut assurément après la pratique de l'antisepsie que la médecine opératoire prit sa plus étonnante impulsion. Libres des affreuses complications des plaies opératoires, pouvant compter avec la réunion immédiate des plaies, les chirurgiens acquirent une hardiesse qui, auparavant, aurait été jugée comme de vraies folies, et les actes opératoires les plus extraordinaires devinrent des moyens de sauver des vies jusqu'alors condamnées.

En Portugal, la méthode de Lister fut mise en pratique très peu de temps après sa publication et, avant 1880, on opérait déjà suivant la méthode listérienne.

J'ai eu le bonheur d'être en Portugal le divulgateur des procédés de Lister et de faire devant mes élèves l'application de la méthode. J'ai pu instruire ainsi bien des jeunes chirurgiens pendant plus de 28 ans à la pratique de l'antisepsie et de l'asepsie et j'ai eu aussi le plaisir de voir la chirurgie portugaise, pratiquée par mes élèves, monter à la hauteur où elle se trouve aujourd'hui.

Dans la pratique de la médecine opératoire, mon pays accompagne les autres nations. Toutes les opérations nouvelles sont pratiquées.

Les opérations dans la cavité abdominale, les sutures du diaphragme, du foie, de la rate, les opérations pour des tumeurs de l'abdomen, la chirurgie des voies biliaires, du foie, des résections d'estomac et de grandes portions des intestins, des néphropexies et néphrotomies, la splénectomie, les opérations sur la vessie et la prostate, sur les organes sexuels, la chirurgie du poumon et du cœur, l'extirpation du larynx, les opérations sur le système nerveux, la laminectomie, la résection des nerfs, du ganglion de Gasser, les opérations sur le cerveau, le sympathique, tout a été fait, tout est aujourd'hui chirurgie courante dans les hôpitaux de Lisbonne.

Tel est l'état où nous nous trouvons sous le rapport de la médecine opératoire et quant aux résultats nous avons des succès opératoires qui ne sont point inférieurs à ceux obtenus à l'étranger. Je peux donc hardiment dire que, si le Portugal a prêté

son concours au progrès du monde au XV siècle et a fait alors
connaître l'inconnu, il travaille au XX siècle et, soldat du progrès, il accompagne les autres travailleurs dans le mouvement
scientifique, qui fait aujourd'hui marcher le monde.

A chaque siècle son rôle, et le siècle actuel, de science et de paix,
portera plus de bonheur et de bien-être a l'humanité. Ouvriers
du bien, nous, les chirurgiens, nous donnons à nos concitoyens le
bénéfice de leurs vies. Liés, tous, par les liens de la science et
par la sainteté du sacerdoce, nous travaillons pour le bien-être
général, et à ces liens qui nous unissent, les congrès internationaux viennent joindre un autre lien, tout personnel mais éminemment agréable, l'établissement des relations amicales, qui seront
pour moi un des plus agréables souvenirs de ce Congrès.

Mesdames et messieurs,

L'œuvre du bureau est accomplie, ses travaux sont finis. Je
vous prie de procéder à l'élection du nouveau bureau, qui doit
continuer nos travaux.

M. GARRÈ propose que le bureau provisoire soit maintenu,
proposition qui est approuvée.

M. OLIVEIRA FEIJÃO: Je vous remercie pour l'honneur que
vous venez de m'accorder en me nommant à la présidence de la
neuvième Section du Congrès International de Médecine de Lisbonne. Votre vote m'est cher, car il signifie non pas l'hommage
fait à un vieux chirurgien qui n'en est pas digne, mais la publique démonstration de vos bons sentiments, de la plus exquise
cordialité envers mon pays, que vous avez honoré de votre présence, et envers la science portughise que vous avez voulu honorer
encore en nommant président de cette section un chirurgien portugais. Encore une fois, au nom du Portugal, mes remerciements
et ma plus profonde gratitude.

Sont nommés présidents d'honneur de la section MM. Bardenheuer, Cologne; Salvador Cardenal, Barcelone; Marcos B. Cavalcanti, Rio de Janeiro; Ladislas de Farkas, Budapest; Davide Giordano, Venise; A. W. Mayo Robson, Londres; J. B. Murphy, Chicago; Paul Reclus, Paris; Jean Sabaneeff, Odessa; Ch. Willems,
Gand.

Chirurgie du grand sympathique

Par MM. Thomas Jonnesco, Bucarest (1)
et Salazar de Souza, Lisbonne (v. page 30)

Discussion

M. L. Bruhn : Ich muss Protest erheben gegen die Ausführungen des Herrn Jonnesco. Der Mb. Basedow zeigt grosse Schwankungen, und kann nach einigen Jahren spontan ausheilen. Deshalb ist eine Photographie ohne Weiteres kein Beweis für die Wirksamkeit einer Operationsmethode. Wir in Deutschland, Oesterreich und die Schweiz verwerfen die Resection des Halssympathicus als ganz unsicher und schwierig.

Diese Operation kann keinen Vergleich aushalten mit dem normalen Vorgehen der Resection des Kropfes. Gefährlich wird diese letztere Operation erst bei Myodegeneration cordis. Dann ist überhaupt ein jeder Eingriff gefährlich. Die Resection des Kropfes bei Mb. Basedow giebt gute Resultate. Wir operieren ohne Narkose.

M. Garré : Die bei Glaucom erzielten Resultate entsprechen doch nicht ganz den Erwartungen die man an die von Jonnesco empfohlene Operation geknüpft hat. In 4 Fällen, bei denen ich die Exstirpation des obern und mittleren Ganglion gemacht habe, war das Resultat gleich null. Es sind Fälle die von Prof. Axenfeld mir zur Operation überwiesen worden sind. Im Hinblick auf die Häufigkeit der Erkrankung will eine Statistik von 80 Fällen nichts sagen : sie beweist nur dass da und dort die Operation versucht worden ist mit mehr oder weniger befriedigendem Resultat.

M. Jonnesco : Je répondrai, à propos du glaucome, ce qui suit :

En 1905, M. Abadie publie des cas guéris par la sympathectomie, depuis 7, 5, et 1 an. Hof, de Lyon, publie en 1905 un cas où la resection du sympathique a été pratiquée d'un côté et l'iridectomie de l'autre. L'œil sympathectomisé a été beaucoup plus amélioré, et cette amélioration de la vue se maintient depuis 5 ans.

Introduction to the study of the fundamental cause of splanchnoptosis — Abdominal incompetence : A developmental factor

Par Mᵐᵉ Agnes C. Victor, Boston

PRÉSENTATION

In 1892, while teaching physical diagnosis at the Woman's Medical College of the New York Infirmary, the writer demonstrated to her students several cases of girls and women who had never worn corsets nor sufficiently constricting clothing, and who yet presented what has been called the corset figure retraction of the lower thorax, with more or less marked lumbo-sacro-thoracic anterior convexity.

(1) M. Jonnesco n'a lu qu'un résumé de son rapport ; le travail entier sera imprimé à la fin de ce volume, si l'auteur nous le remet à temps, ainsi que nous le lui avons demandé.

Directing her attention to this point, an increasing number of such patients continued to come under observation. These patients grouped themselves into three sub-classes: (1) Girls and women who had absolutely never worn corsets or sufficiently constricting clothing; (2) girls and women who, while wearing corsets or other constricting clothing, yet did not wear these garments, and had never worn them, sufficiently tight to make it appear reasonable that such garments could produce such marked anatomical changes; (3) girls and women wearing definitely constricting clothing.

Gradually, it appeared evident that all girls and women could be classified as conforming to one or the other of two types, which types appeared to develop spontaneously and in accordance with natural laws.

These types may be called as to the lower thorax «broad» or «retracted», though it will be shown later that they can be also classified according to the spinal column.

The writer next observed that while a large number of girls and women with retracted lower thorax presented a displacement of one or more of the abdominal viscera, yet apparently an equally large number of abdominal visceral displacements occurred in patients who had the broad lower thorax. These visceral displacements seemed sometimes to be most easily demonstrable in the retracted thorax class; and this at first made it appear as if they were more frequent in this class. Further study showed that many of them are as frequent in the broad thorax class, but that they occur along somewhat different lines, and at times require somewhat different methods for demonstration.

In endeavoring to discover the time of onset and original course of these changes, they were found already begun in childhood.

In the study of children, these changes were found to develop spontaneously in boys as well as in girls, but at first they seemed to be a transient phase in boys, tending to disappear towards puberty, while tending to persist in girls.

Extending the field of her observations, the writer next noted that the transiency of these changes in boys was not uniform: that they persisted in many boys beyond the age of puberty, and, further, that they existed in many men.

Eventually, it became evident that boys and men grouped themselves under the same two types as girls and women, i. e., the broad and the retracted lower thorax types.

As the study of these cases proceeded, the problem developed complications in many directions. The spinal column, the pelvis, the lower extremities, and even the upper extremities and head, all seemed to be contributing factors that could not be eliminated.

By slow degrees during the ensuing years the clinical observations made appeared to correlate themselves along certain lines, but the practical difficulties in studying these correlations were for a long time insurmountable.

A series of clinical studies culminating in 1900-01 in that of Case LX. showed that of the two types, one, the broad lower thorax, is basic and physiological; while the other, the retracted lower thorax, is secondary and tends toward the pathological. This case not only gave the key to the path followed in the spontaneous evolution of the retracted from the broad lower thorax, but it also gave the key to the later evolution of the abdomen. This case seemed to show that the evolution of the abdomen and lumbo-sacral spine was especially correlated with the evolution of the lower extremities, and, though to a less extent, also with that of the upper extremity. This was followed by the clinical demonstration that the evolution of the thoracic cage depends largely on the evolution of the abdomen. At the same time, evolution of the abdomen was observed largely to modify and determine the mechanics of respiration.

In 1901-02, the writer was able to go to Europe, to have access to many of the originals of the historical records of the race, as expressed in mural drawings, sculpture and painting. She studied the records of older Asia, of Egypt, of Greece, of Rome, of medieval Europe, of more modern Asia, and of modern and contemporary civilizations, as found in the museums and art galleries of Paris, Dresden, Leipzig, Berlin, Holland, Belgium and London. The intervention of a serious illness prevented her visiting the south of Europe, and compelled her to return home.

The study of these records showed that her clinical observations and deductions were correct, and, further, that the two types of development which she finds existing to-day are the two main types along which the race has been developing since the date of the earliest records she has yet found. Further, at the *Musée d'Anthropologie*, at the *Jardin des Plantes*, in Paris, she found photographs and other records of contemporary peoples of more primitive civilization, showing development along the same two main lines. Through the courtesy of Professor Halmy, she is able to show copies of some of the photographs of these peoples.

In 1903-04, through the granting of a fellowship by the Medical Board of the Hospital of the Society of the Lying-In, in New York, she was able to study in the newborn the anatomical paths predisposing to the evolution of these types. To some extent, she was also able to follow these paths backward in the fetus. At the same time she was able to begin the study of the postnatal evolution of the abdomen in the young infant, and to study some of the modifications presented in the pregnant woman.

In 1904, through the courtesy of Prof. Emmet L. Holt, she was able to make some studies of the young child at the New York Foundling Hospital.

SUMMARY.

(a) RÉSUMÉ

General argument leading to conclusion that question is one of evolution.

Outline of evolution of human abdomen.

A — Prenatal.

A' — Status at term.

B — Postnatal.

Study of evolution of human abdomen leads back to earlier vertebrate series and forward to postnatal development.

Outline of evolution of vertebrate abdomen, including man, showing continuity and correlations.

Outline of evolution of specific human abdomen. Correlated with evolution of spine, pelvis, thorax and extremities; especially with extension, adduction and forward rotation of the lower extremities, so that the patella and toes point forward. Effects of abdominal incompetence on the mechanics of respiration. Anatomical and physiological variations predisposing some of the viscera to displacement, and relation of this predisposition to certain frequent pathological conditions. Spontaneous tendencies of the trunk and extremities towards such structural variations as are called pathological *(developmental deformities)*. These developmental deformities include round shoulders, lateral and antero-posterior curvatures of the spine, modifications of weak foot, including *pes planus*; retracted lower thorax; marked lumbar or lumbo-thoracic anterior convexity; marked forward rotation of the pelvis;

abdominal incompetence, and visceral ptosis—*en masse* and *individual*.

Evolution towards two main types of human figures, depending upon variations in these correlations.

Type 1. Broad lower thorax; slight lumbo-sacral anterior convexity; slight forward rotation of pelvis.

Type 2. Retracted lower thorax; marked lumbo-sacral anterior convexity; marked forward rotation of pelvis. (This type must be considered pathological—a variety of developmental deformity).

Correlations towards which each type tends: In abdomen, thorax, lower extremities, respiratory mechanics, and specialized activities.

(b) Main Lines of Argument.

General argument leading to conclusion that question is one of evolution.

In their highest development, the abdominal walls not only contain the abdominal viscera, but also retain them in position against gravity and other opposing forces.

The abdomen may then be said to be competent.

A failure in the retaining power of the abdominal walls leads to visceral displacement as a result of the action of gravity and other displacing factors.

Such an abdomen may be said to be incompetent.

An incompetent abdominal wall is largely compensated for in the supine position, for then it is not called upon to share in the support of the viscera and the rest of trunk; gravity in this position causes the viscera to rest on the back, which, in turn, rests upon the bed or other supporting surface. As soon as the sitting or standing position (or even the lateral supine) is assumed, an incompetent abdominal wall yields to gravity and other displacing factors and it becomes displaced.

Given a cavity which contains no free space, and whose contents are movable; whenever the walls of the cavity are displaced, in whole or in part, its contents are displaced, in whole or in part.

Hence, incompetence of the abdominal wall always leads to some displacement of one or more of the abdominal viscera; and, in itself, is sufficient to cause all stages of visceral ptosis, up to the complete dislocation of all the abdominal viscera.

Illustrations of this law as manifested in areas of partial incompetence [active or potential] of the abdominal walls—both physiological and pathological.

The viscera retain their «normal» positions as the result of an equilibrium between gravity and other displacing factors, on the one side, and certain counterbalancing forces on the other side.

The essential factors in visceral displacement are gravity and altered respiratory equilibrium, including unantagonized downward and forward excursion of the diaphragm and lungs in inspiration.

Unsupported abdominal viscera tend to travel downward, forward and towards the median line. After traveling in this direction for a certain distance, the hollow viscera tend to travel also upward and forward, this latter movement being increased in portion to the amount of gas in their contents.

The downward course is the result of the direct action of gravity, which is constantly at work in this direction, in the sitting and standing positions. It acts upon the abdominal wall as well as upon the contained viscera.

The upward and forward course is due to the distention of the hollow viscera by gaseous, liquid, or solid contents. When these viscera are empty and collapsed, they follow the influence of gravity alone and travel downward.

Part of the downward course and of the ventrad and medad modification of the entire downward course are due to the unantagonized downward and forward excursion of the diaphragm and inspiring lungs, which are in action fourteen to eighteen times every minute; and this displacing action is active in the supine as well as in the sitting and standing positions.

Part of the ventrad and medad modification of the entire downward course is also due to the greater relative development, and the greater bony content, of the posterior and postero-lateral abdominal and pelvic walls, as compared with the anterior and antero-lateral walls.

The diaphragm is set obliquely from above downward and from before backward, between the thorax and the abdomen. When passive and relaxed, it domes upward towards the thorax; when active and contracting, it descends into the abdomen. Whatever variations in activity may occur in different parts of the diaphragm, the oblique plane of its attachment makes its unmodified descent favor enlargement of the base of the thoracic cavity, from above downward and from behind forward, and diminution of the abdominal cavity in the same direction, *i. e.*, from above downwards and from behind forwards.

This action would make towards excursion of the inspiring lungs downward and forward, and towards excursion of the abdominal viscera downward and forward.

Clinical observation shows that this excursion is also towards the median line; this latter modification is explained by the observation of the writer that the sides of the diaphragm descend more than the center.

The great counterbalancing factor against these two forces which make for movement of the viscera downward, forward, and towards the median line of the abdomen, is the abdominal walls: (1) The anterior and antero-lateral muscles of these walls, which make towards antagonizing the descent of the diaphragm and lungs, and towards pushing the abdominal viscera backward, upward and laterally; and (2) the posterior and postero-lateral muscles and bones of these walls and of the posterior wall of the whole trunk, which make *(a)* for stability of the region which furnishes a point of departure for the action of all the abdominal muscles, as well as for all the large extensor activities of the trunk and lower and upper extremities; and which make *(b)* for enlargement of the thoracic cage in its posterior and postero-lateral planes. This favors backward and outward expansion of the lungs during inspiration; and this action lessens the downward and forward excursion of the diaphragm and lungs (with consequent *en masse* displacement of the viscera), decreases stress on the weaker anterior abdominal walls, and favors the development and conservation in them of the condition of reflex activity which the writer designates as competence.

Exposure of the viscera to the action of gravity is caused directly by incompetence of the abdominal walls, and, indirectly, by this incompetence of the abdominal walls modifying other body conditions, and being in turn modified by them, so that these body conditions themselves still further expose the viscera to the action of gravity and other displacing factors.

These body conditions are as follows:

(1) Erect (vertical) position of the trunk.

(2) Extension of the lower extremities in the plane of the trunk; this extension being, in its highest form, accompanied by adduction and forward rotation, so that the patella and toes point forward.

(3) Altered respiratory equilibrium, including unantagonized downward and forward excursion of the diaphragm and inspiring lungs.

(4) Retarded or uncompleted evolution of the abdominal viscera.

(5) Retarded or uncompleted evolution of the trunk and extremities (and even the head) in the direction of mutual independence for the release of specialized activities.

These conditions can all be studied in their earlier manifestations through comparative anatomy and physiology. In their advanced development, their study becomes exceedingly involved and intricate, because it enters the stage of evolution with which the human race is at present struggling.

Hence, the conclusion that abdominal competence is a developmental factor. This conclusion is verified by finding that its earlier phases can be traced backward through the vertebrate series and in human prenatal life;—while the evolution of its later phases can be observed and studied throughout human postnatal life.

Outline of evolution of human abdomen.

(A) Prenatal.

(A') Status at term.

(B) Postnatal.

Viscera appear before body walls.

Body walls at first merely enclose the viscera. This enclosure at first imperfect; later, the enclosure, as a whole, becomes complete, but certain localized areas of incompleteness (actual or potential) remain.

Viscera withdraw within the walls, and, by an orderly progression, take up within the body cavity certain positions which occur with sufficient predominance to be called "normal". These normal positions are antagonized by the unbalanced downward and forward excursion of the diaphragm and inspiring lungs, in the supine as well as the sitting and standing positions; by extension of the lower extremities in the plane of the trunk, in the supine or standing positions; and by gravity as soon as the individual assumes a sitting or standing position.

Coincident with the progression of the viscera toward such positions and relative size and volume as are called normal, the abdominal walls, as a whole, pass through a series of developmental changes, as a result of which they not only enclose the viscera, but also, by counteracting the displacing action of the diaphragm and inspiring lungs, of extension of the lower extremities and of gravity, they retain the viscera in their normal positions.

From the point of view of this retention of the viscera in position, the abdomen, as a whole, may be said to proceed in an orderly development from incompetence to competence.

When a competent abdomen is studied, its principal characteristic is seen to be the intimate and exact correspondence existing between the viscera and the muscle walls, by which the latter always move in the direction required to retain and support the former. The muscle reflex is so active that when the body is in motion, there is a constant play of the muscles of the anterior, lateral and posterior walls of the abdomen, adapting the latter to the changed conditions of pressure and stress which would otherwise reach the viscera; and *against gravity*, protecting these viscera from such conditions by interposing a firm muscle plane.

The abdominal wall is neither a rigid nor a flaccid structure, but one which is elastic and contractile; and this elasticity and contractility is constantly controlled by visceral and other reflexes. These reflexes are so co-ordinated that a relaxation of one part of the wall is controlled by the adjacent parts of the wall. In a perfectly passive condition, the wall may relax in part or as a whole; but in a competent abdomen the reflexes are also competent, and as soon as an active factor is introduced into relationship with the abdominal wall, its muscle reflexes are immediately aroused. Even during sleep, the muscular response of the abdominal walls to the visceral and other reflexes may be observed and studied. The earliest characteristic of an incompetent abdomen is a change in this muscle reflex, which becomes erratic, irregular, or partly or entirely absent. Later, structural changes occur, and portions of the abdominal walls may hang as more or less flaccid pouches whose reflex activity, under ordinary circumstances, has diminished almost, or quite, to a vanishing point.

One of the earliest characteristics of an incompetent abdomen is seen in the respiratory reflex. The incompetent portion of the abdomen is relaxed during expiration, as well as during inspiration; and upon forced expiration, as in coughing, is protruded (as in the case of hernia) downward and forward, as well as upward and forward. In advanced cases the whole abdomen acts in this manner.

Again, the portion of the abdomen which tends towards competence tends, in these cases, to overaction or even spasm. This tendency is seen in inspiration as well as in expiration. It affects most strongly the upper abdominal zone; and clinical observation indicates that this is one of the most potent factors in producing the retracted lower thorax.

The same tendency to spasm is seen in the extensor muscles of the back, and is an important factor in increasing the sacro-lumbo-thoracic anterior convexity.

In proportion as the abdomen fails to develop, or loses after development, its competence, the viscera tend to be displaced, downward, forward and towards the median line; and the hollow viscera also upward and forward; in proportion as the abdomen develops competency the viscera tend to be held upward, backward and laterally.

Every abdomen is, as a whole, competent or incompetent. This competence may vary greatly in degree.

Every abdomen possesses areas of localized incompetence; this localized incompetence may be only potential, or it may be actual.

General incompetence of the abdomen is physiological only in early prenatal life.

Development of general competence of the abdomen begins in later prenatal life; but its further development can be observed and studied from the moment of birth, through infancy and childhood to, in selected cases, its completion before the age of puberty.

Clinical observation shows that in the majority of cases this evolution is not completed at the age of puberty; that incompetence of the abdomen, with more or less visceral ptosis, persists through adolescence and early adult life — proceeding, at times, towards greater competence, or remaining stationary, or retrograding towards greater incompetence and more pronounced visceral ptosis, according to the activity of the concomitant factors to be enumerated. And, finally, that in the neighborhood of the fourth decade and beyond there is marked tendency in all individuals towards increased incompetence of the abdomen, with increased visceral ptosis.

Competence of the abdominal walls is, then, evolutionary; and while related to evolution of the abdominal viscera, is a later stage of development, and thus appears as to some extent independent of this latter; so that the abdominal viscera may proceed to the attainment of their normal position, although the walls are insufficiently developed towards competence; and it is, at least, possible that competent walls might be developed around viscera that had not entirely attained their normal position.

Nevertheless, bearing in mind the law that, given a cavity which contains no free space, and whose contents are movable, whenever the walls of the cavity are displaced, in whole or part, its contents are displaced in whole or part, and as it can be demonstrated that the abdominal wall is under the constant control of visceral and other reflexes, and is competent or incompetent according as these reflexes are active or in abeyance, it is rational to think that abdominal walls which have not attained competence must always affect the relative size and volume, and hence the relative or actual position of the contained viscera. And, conversely, that viscera which have not attained their normal size and volume, and hence their relative or actual position, must affect the attainment of competency by the containing walls.

Hence the study of visceral ptosis requires the study of the development of both viscera and walls.

STUDY OF EVOLUTION OF THE HUMAN ABDOMEN LEADS BACK TO EARLIER VERTEBRATE SERIES, AND FORWARD TO POSTNATAL DEVELOPMENT

Evolution of human abdominal walls and viscera closely related to evolution of mammalian, or even vertebrate, abdominal walls and viscera.

Prenatal human development so closely resembles prenatal vertebrate development that failures in evolution of the human abdominal walls and viscera would most naturally be expected along lines suggesting the varying vertebrate paths.

Study of the evolution of the vertebrate abdominal walls and viscera, taken in connection with the fact that a progressive postnatal evolution of the human abdominal walls and viscera is constantly present in every individual, show that so-called congenital variations in either the abdominal walls or viscera should not necessarily be regarded as end results. These congenital variations may be merely retarded steps of the still ascending ladder; and, in such cases, their normal evolution may be accelerated or assisted by a knowledge of the normal postnatal development.

OUTLINE OF EVOLUTION OF VERTEBRATE ABDOMEN, INCLUDING MAN, SHOWING CONTINUITY AND CORRELATIONS

(A) Prenatal. (A) Status at term.

For details, see Report of Research Fellowship of the Society of the Lying-In Hospital of New York, 1903-04, by Agnes C. Victor, M.D. *(In press.)*

(B) Postnatal.

In the supine position of infancy, the postnatal evolution of the abdomen proceeds. This evolution differs from the prenatal in that there are added the reactions of a new environment.

(1) Beginning of two new forms of visceral reflex activity with birth: *(a)* respiratory (absolutely new), and *(b)* digestive; this latter is new in regard to the presence in the stomach and bowels of food derived from the outside world, and the new activities set in motion by this factor in the liver, pancreas, kidneys, etc., setting free numerous new reflex stimuli to the muscles of the abdominal wall.

(2) Beginning of new surface stimuli from changed environment (thermal, tactile, etc.).

(3) Increased and new activity of the muscles of the lower extremities, spine, pelvis, thorax, upper extremities, and even the neck and head. Activity of all these regions can be shown to have direct connection with the activity and development of the abdominal walls—the lower extremities, pelvis, lumbar spine and thoracic cage being most immediately and powerfully related though the upper extremities are also of great importance.

Such a large number of contributing factors sufficiently indicate the complexities of the process of evolution of the abdominal walls.

Clinical observations of the writer during fourteen years show that this complex process is still in progress; that the human race is still struggling towards the attainment of a competent abdomen and the retention of the abdominal viscera against gravity and other displacing forces; that only a minority of the race attain this higher development, and that though attained, it is an unstable possession and may be lost at any subsequent age.

This instability of the abdomen exists at the present day in the most primitive as well as the most civilized peoples; and its existence can be traced among all peoples as far back as pictorial history extends. Illustrations.

Incompetence of the abdominal walls with the consequent displacement of the abdominal viscera, continually struggling towards competence of the abdominal walls with the consequent retention of the viscera in position is, therefore, a generic condition, or even a vertebrate condition.

Seeking the anatomical basis for this generic condition, one is carried backward to the vertebrate series, and one notes that competence of the abdominal walls is correlated successively with:

(1) The ascent of the trunk from a horizontal to a vertical plane; an ascent in which the dorsal surface or back leads, the ventral surface lagging. This ascent begins at the cephalic extremity of the body and proceeds caudad.

(2) The tendency of the ventral and dorsal surfaces of this vertical trunk to approach each other in approximately parallel planes.

(3) The affiliation of the pelvis with the spine, and its consequent association with the trunk rather than with the lower extremities—the pelvis becoming virtually an expanded sacrum, following this latter bone in all its positions: a transference of affinities from the position of proximal division of the lower extremity to that of distal division of the trunk.

(4) The gradual transference of the weight-bearing function which, beginning with the body wall itself, is transferred to four specialized out-growths of this wall, the two fore and two hind limbs. These limbs combine the function of weight-bearing (a more or less passive process) with various specialized functions (active processes), prehension, locomotion, etc.; and in proportion as one of these classes of functions predominates, the other is impaired, and conversely. Thus, exercise of the weight-bearing function impairs the exercise of the higher specializing functions; and exercise of the higher specializing functions impairs the exercise of the weight-bearing function.

(5) The gradual transference of the weight-bearing function from the cephalic towards the caudal extremity of the trunk, and the consequent development of the cephalic division and out-growths of the trunk, so set free, towards independence and more highly specialized functionating.

These processes may be seen epitomized studying the ascent of the infant from the prone to the creeping position.

(6) The assumption along this path of the weight-bearing function by the pelvis, which is now the lowest division of a more

or less vertical trunk. The pelvis is more or less erect, resting on the *tuber ischii* or on the oblique plane posterior to these processes, more rarely on the oblique plane anterior to these processes. It acts as a containing basin and assists the abdominal walls and back in the support of the viscera. In this position, the hind limbs are freed from weight-bearing, but the thighs remain flexed, abducted and rotated outward, in a position well suited to that variation of their weight-bearing function which leads to their supplementing the pelvis and abdominal walls in supporting the weight of the viscera, but also a position favoring earlier specialized functions.

This is an occasional position of many mammals, especially of the anthropoids and of the sitting child. Its evolution may be shown in the study of ascent of the infant from the supine to the sitting position.

(7) The further transference caudad of the weight-bearing function to the two lower extremities, which become, for the first time in the animal series, fully extended in the plane of the vertical trunk.

The expanded, weight-bearing base of the trunk, the pelvis, is suddenly contracted to the small area of contact between the acetabula and the heads of the femora, in connection with the bony portions of the pelvis which act as a medium of weight transference between the spine and the acetabula.

This bony support is supplemented by fibrous and muscular tissues, but the weight of the trunk walls and viscera is so great that until these walls have adapted themselves to the new position by transitional changes, the lower extremities are still called upon to assist in weight-bearing in the older mammalian way. This is done by the femora continuing flexed, abducted and rotated outward, with corresponding positions of the leg and foot.

This is a frequent position of many mammals, and these processes may be shown in development in studying the change from the horizontal to the vertical trunk in one of the higher mammalia, as the dog or bear.

As the trunk is erected and the weight-bearing is transferred to the lower extremities, the pelvis follows the sacrum, which, in turn, follows the main spine in its vertical ascent. As a result, the pelvis is no longer erect, resting on the *tuber ischii* or on the oblique plane posterior or anterior to these processes, and assisting the abdominal walls and back in the support of the viscera. Instead, the pelvis becomes inclined obliquely to the vertical plane, so that the crests of the ilii tend to fall forward and downward, and the *tuber ischii* rise backward and upward. Instead of a containing basin, acting as a receptacle for the viscera, the pelvis becomes a tilted basin, throwing the viscera forward and downward against the abdominal walls.

This forward inclination of the pelvis follows the extension of the lower extremities (thigh) in the plane of the trunk. It may be studied in the stillborn, in the supine position, by changing the lower extremities (thigh) from the position of spontaneous flexion, abduction and outward rotation, present at term, to that of extension, adduction and forward rotation.

These processes may be shown in studying the young infant, in the supine position, as it spontaneously develops this extension of the lower extremity, with forward rotation of the pelvis; and in the child, as it progresses from the sitting to the standing position.

(8) And, finally, the concentration of the caudad transference of weight-bearing along each lower extremity, independently, so that, in its highest form, each lower extremity is in itself able to support the weight of the entire body, leaving the other lower extremity free to exercise its specialized function of locomotion, etc., in the vertical plane.

Illustrations of (1) to (7) in studying the changes produced in passing from the horizontal to the vertical trunk in one of the higher mammals, as the dog or the bear.

Similar changes observed in studying the newborn and infant.

Study of the newborn, the infant and the child illustrates similar changes, and also the evolution of (8).

Mechanism of this evolution as observed in the study of attitudes and spontaneous movements of newborn and infants, and the creeping, sitting and standing child.

Illustration of this mechanism by diagrams, measurements and photographs of stillborn, and by photographs of infants and children.

Illustrations of continuity of this mechanism in the adolescent and adult by diagrams, measurements and photographs.

OUTLINE OF EVOLUTION OF SPECIFIC HUMAN ABDOMEN

Correlated with evolution of pelvis, thorax and extremities; especially with extension, adduction and forward rotation of the lower extremities, so that the patella and toes point forward.

The final distinguishing characteristic of the human genus is the full extension of the lower extremities in the plane of the vertical trunk, the dorsal and ventral surfaces of which tend constantly to approach each other in approximately parallel planes.

This extension of the lower extremities upon the vertical trunk

(a) Removes the support of the erect (sitting) pelvis from the abdominal viscera.

(b) Removes the support of the flexed thighs which supplement the erect pelvis in supporting the abdomen.

(c) Adds forward rotation of the pelvis and anterior convexity of the lumbar spine; both of these conditions throwing the viscera forward and so facilitating their descent, directly through gravity, indirectly by increasing the stress on the supporting anterior and posterior abdominal walls, and so impairing the supporting power of these walls.

(d) Alters the conditions of respiratory equilibrium, because whatever affects the supporting power of the walls of the abdomen affects the action of the diaphragm, which latter is only another abdominal wall — the superior wall or roof.

If these various changes are not counterbalanced by compensatory changes in the anterior and posterior abdominal walls, they lead to further visceral displacement.

Soon after the enclosure of the viscera by the body walls, the four extremities appear. Whether viewed as outgrowths of, or additions to, the body wall, these extremities are, throughout the vertebrate series, more or less bound to this body wall by muscles and integuments. This connection of the extremities with the body wall decreases as one rises in the animal series till in their highest development these extremities become specialized to nearly complete independence of the trunk; the latter serving only as a fixed point upon which all the more highly specialized movements of the extremities are based. This fixed point is utilized through the large muscles which pass from the trunk to the extremity. And these connecting muscles require a certain amount of trunk stability to furnish a point of departure for their activities.

In proportion as the evolution of the extremity is imperfect or incomplete, clinical observation shows that stress upon it is carried backward to its attachment to the trunk; and if this attachment is deficient in strength or coördination, the stress is carried still further backward, and the body wall itself strives to make up for the insufficiency of the extremity to the demand made upon it. In this manner may be produced abdominal incompetence, visceral ptosis and deformities of the spine, pelvis, thorax, and even of the other extremities, since insufficiency of the body wall may be further conveyed to these.

Examples of this will be given later. It is mentioned here because it is a manifestation of a law which seems to explain the action which insufficiently developed (in strength or coördination) extremities, both upper and lower, but especially the lower, have in causing visceral ptosis; this being one of the most common causes of this affection.

The converse of this is also observed. The circle of insufficiency and deformity may begin with abdominal incompetence or visceral ptosis, causing inefficiency of the trunk as a point of departure for developing activities of the extremities, leading to inefficiency or imperfect development of these extremities.

Those portions of the body wall which make up the abdomen are easily and early involved in attempts to compensate for weakness of the extremities.

If the abdominal walls have developed competence, they aid the body wall in meeting these demands, and the stress is met.

If the abdominal walls have not developed competence, they share in the stress, and are, by so much, diverted from their function of supporting and retaining the viscera. In this way, varying degrees of visceral ptosis are due to weakness of the extremities or of other portions of the body wall. The converse of this is also observed, as already noted.

EFFECT OF ABDOMINAL INCOMPETENCE ON THE MECHANICS OF RESPIRATION

Clinical observation shows two main types of respiration:

(1) This may be called the *anterior* type. The abdomen is incompetent; the diaphragm and inspiring lungs make marked downward and forward excursion into the abdomen, displacing the viscera downward and forward, the viscera are also displaced upward and forward; the sternum rotates on its superior extremity, upward and forward, carrying with it its attached ribs; the bony thorax grows shorter and broader in the anterior plane, its anterior wall moving upward and forward towards the horizontal; backward expansion of the trunk is diminished or may be absent; the ribs move forward and upward, they move outward very

slightly, except in their anterior third or half; expiration becomes increasingly inefficient.

These changes in the thorax anteriorly lead to two main types of changes posteriorly: (a) The posterior wall of the thorax attempts to parallel the anterior wall; the ribs retract posteriorly, and an increased lumbo-thoracic anterior convexity appears. In the supine position, this forward and upward rotation of the whole thorax may be seen with each inspiration. This type of respiration is favored by the conformation of the trunk, especially when the lower extremities are extended, since the anatomical paths leading to it may be developed at term. (b) The tendency towards (a) is antagonized by a slight lumbar anterior convexity and a slight forward rotation of the pelvis; and in such patients the attempts of the posterior wall of the thorax to parallel the anterior, leads to hyperextension of the thoracic spine, or lumbo-thoracic junction, or upper lumbar spine.

This change appears to be the physiological one, developing spontaneously in the healthy child beginning to stand and walk alone.

(2) This may be called the *posterior* type. The abdomen is competent; the whole posterior wall of the trunk moves backward in inspiration, backward and upward, and backward and downward; the lateral walls move backward and outward, as well as upward and downward; there is relatively slight excursion of the diaphragm and inspiring lungs downward and forward into the abdomen, and this occurs mainly in the upper zone or epigastrium; the sternum and ribs tend to rotate upward and forward, but this tendency is antagonized by the downward and outward pull of the abdominal muscles, and by the backward as well as the outward, and upward and downward pull of the posterior and postero-lateral walls; this tends to make the anterior wall approach a plane more or less parallel with the posterior.

The predominant forward and upward and forward and downward movement of the anterior type is now translated into a backward and upward, and backward and downward movement. The outward movement of the antero-lateral planes has become translated into an outward movement of the postero-lateral planes.

In the anterior type the anterior wall models the trunk; in the posterior type, the posterior wall models it.

At birth, respiration is modified by all the factors enumerated and by many others. It is therefore struggling and incoördinated.

On the whole, it most nearly approaches the anterior type; but the advanced stage of development of the back muscles, and the supine position strongly favor the efforts towards the posterior type which steadily gains.

As soon as the sitting position is assumed, the pull of the viscera and the stress on the back, which is struggling to support the trunk in the vertical plane, again favor the anterior type.

When the sitting is changed to the standing position the stress is still greater, and the anterior type becomes increasingly easier. Nevertheless the struggle towards the evolution of the posterior type is always present. The result is the development of many variations of combinations of both types.

ANATOMICAL AND PHYSIOLOGICAL VARIATIONS PREDISPOSING SOME OF THE VISCERA TO DISPLACEMENT; AND THE RELATION OF THIS PREDISPOSITION TO CERTAIN FREQUENT PATHOLOGICAL CONDITIONS

Experiments and dissections show that abdominal incompetence opens the anatomical paths for the production of displacements of the abdominal viscera, leading to conditions making for repeated traumatisms, through the action of gravity, and of traction of the viscera on each other and on the connecting peritoneal folds which contain the nerves and blood and lymph vessels.

The observations support the clinical hypothesis that abdominal incompetence is the primary factor in the development of the common surgical diseases of the upper abdomen — the stomach, duodenum, gall bladder and bile ducts, jejuno-ileum, pancreas and kidneys (especially the right), being the most important viscera affected.

SPONTANEOUS TENDENCY OF THE TRUNK AND EXTREMITIES TOWARDS THE DEVELOPMENT OF SUCH STRUCTURAL VARIATIONS AS ARE CALLED PATHOLOGICAL; DEVELOPMENTAL DEFORMITIES

Dissections show that at birth a lumbo-sacral anterior convexity is present; that an anatomical condition of spontaneous flexion, adduction and outward rotation of the lower extremities (thighs) is present; that the lower extremities and the pelvis are united at such an angle that in proportion as the lower extremities (thighs) are flexed, etc., the lumbo-sacral anterior convexity is reduced to a minimum or successively obliterated and converted into an anterior concavity; that in proportion as the lower extremities (thighs) are extended, adducted and rotated forward, the lumbo-sacral anterior convexity is increased and extended through (1) forward rotation of the united pelvic bones and sacrum, and (2) through the attachment of the fifth lumbar vertebra to the sacrum and ilia, the supra-incumbent lumbar (or even the thoracic) vertebræ are carried into anterior convexity, proportionate to their mobility.

For the relation of the postnatal modification of these conditions to the evolution of the trunk and the developmental deformities enumerated, as well as the details of the above-mentioned visceral experiments, dissections and clinical observations, the reader is referred to the following articles by the writer.

(1) Introduction to the study of the prenatal evolution of the abdomen, with special reference to the status at term. Report of Research Fellowship of the Society of Lying-In Hospital of New York, 1903-04 (in press).

(2) Introduction to the study of the postnatal evolution of the abdomen (in preparation).

(3) Clinical study of abdominal incompetence and visceral ptosis (in preparation).

EVOLUTION TOWARDS TWO MAIN TYPES OF HUMAN FIGURES, DEPENDING UPON VARIATIONS IN THESE CORRELATIONS.

Type 1. Broad lower thorax; slight lumbo-sacral anterior convexity; slight forward rotation of pelvis.

Type 2. Retracted lower thorax; marked lumbo-sacral anterior convexity; marked forward rotation of pelvis.

This type must be considered pathological — a variety of developmental deformity. It presents a retraction of the trunk walls, with a proportionate degree of visceral ptosis en masse — a condition which predisposes to various forms of individual visceral ptosis.

Correlations towards which each type tends: In abdomen, thorax, lower extremities, respiratory mechanics and specialized activities.

According as an equilibrium among the factors enumerated is reached by one or other varying paths of compensation, study of the ascent of the trunk to the vertical plane, and the extension of the lower extremities in the plane of this trunk, shows a spontaneous development of two main types of the human figure.

These types are suggested in the higher mammalia, but they are fully developed in the human being.

The fundamental difference between these two types appears in that portion of the trunk between the thoracic cavity and the heads of the femora—the abdomen and pelvis. In this region the prominent points of differentiation between the two types are the lower thorax; the lumbo-sacral spine, including its sacral expansion, the pelvis; and the posterior, lateral and anterior muscle walls of the abdomen and pelvis.

Broadly speaking, what may be called the basic or primary type of figure is represented by a broad lower thorax, a slight anterior convexity of the lumbar spine, a slight anterior inclination of the pelvis, and in selected cases, a competent abdominal wall. The simplest variant of this type has the abdomen incompetent but the back unaffected. The next simplest variant shows an incompetent abdomen, with hyperextension of the lower thoracic spine, of the lumbo-thoracic junction, or of the upper lumbar spine.

Again, broadly speaking, what may be called the second type of figure is represented by a more or less retracted lower thorax, a more pronounced anterior convexity of the lumbar spine, extending up into the thoracic spine, an increased anterior inclination of the pelvis, and usually a more or less well-developed incompetence of the abdominal walls.

All grades of variations of these two types of figures are observed, including exaggerations of the tendencies of both; including also transitional figures showing passage from one type to the other.

These variations all resemble each other in that the equilibrium attained is very unstable, and, therefore, these variations are constantly interchanging details to a greater or less extent.

The first mentioned type appears to be basic or primary because it is always present at birth and in early life; because it is the type towards which the greatest number of figures tend; because it is found most often in strong and robust individuals; and because the equilibrium of this type is, as a whole, the most stable.

The second type appears to be the variant, secondary, aberrant type, because it is never present at birth or in early life;

because it is produced from the basic type at a subsequent age;
because it is most often found in individuals with a weak musculature or presenting other evidences of weakened or poor nutrition. Furthermore, it tends spontaneously to approach the basic type whenever nutrition is improved, general muscular activity increased, and when certain arbitrary conditions are removed, leaving the figure to the spontaneous modeling of all the muscles. On the other hand, the equilibrium of this type is very unstable; it tends constantly to vary under slight variations in the correlative factors mentioned, and to pass readily into such pathological variations as result in what are called deformities.

Clinical observation shows that competence of the abdominal walls increases throughout childhood, and in selected cases is complete before the age of puberty. It also shows the relation of competence of the abdomen to the development of the rest of the body walls and the extremities. It is well-established that during this period of development deformities of the spine, thorax, pelvis and extremities appear, and the evidence at present accumulated seems to show that these deformities develop along the lines just described.

Further, this evidence seems to the writer to justify the addition to the list of developmental deformities of the added ones of round shoulders; modifications of weak foot, including *pes planus*; antero-posterior and lateral curvatures of the spine; retracted lower thorax; marked lumbar anterior convexity; marked forward rotation of the pelvis; abdominal incompetence and visceral ptosis—both *en masse* and *individual*.

These are developmental deformities because, within physiological limits, there is a spontaneous tendency to their occurrence in the efforts of the individual to correlate the varying factors enumerated.

To sum up:

The body of the individual at any given time represents a moment of equilibrium in the struggle towards attaining competence of the abdomen, with the consequent retention of the viscera in position, in a vertical trunk whose dorsal and ventral surfaces tend constantly to approach each other in approximately parallel planes; this trunk being supported on two lower extremities which are extended in the same vertical plane, this extension being accompanied by adduction and forward rotation, so that the patella and toes point forward.

This struggle may be tending, along the paths indicated, towards the attainment of an equilibrium which makes for relative stability and the release of energy in the form of specialized activities of the various regions of the body.

Or, it may be tending, also along the paths indicated, towards compensations for failures to reach this relatively stable equilibrium. These compensations result in types of figures which may be merely unstable variants of the basic generic type; or the structural variations may be so pronounced as to be called deformities.

The existence of so many separate factors and the number of natural laws simultaneously at work make it impossible to trace the origin of a given deformity in each case without having a detailed life record of the individual. Many of the deformities are, when first observed, of the nature of cicatrices, their initial cause having disappeared in the presence of growth changes, or being obscured by later growth changes. But the further back into childhood one carries one's studies and the greater the number of observations which one accumulates, the more the evidence points to the existence of the fundamental laws already formulated.

On the whole, type (1), the broad lower thorax type, tends towards the development of the following correlations:

(a) Increasing competence of the abdomen.

(b) Predominance of backward and upward, and backward and downward, as well as outward expansion of the trunk, during inspiration, with increasing inspiratory capacity and increasing expiratory efficiency.

(c) Greater proportionate increase of transverse than antero-posterior diameters of trunk.

(d) Pelvis maintains its affiliations with the trunk. Lumbo-sacral anterior convexity tends towards a minimum and the pelvis shows slight anterior rotation. During weight-bearing, lower extremities tend to maintain extension at hip and knee, and feet tend to maintain such an angle of dorsal flexion as leads to ascent of the forefoot to the horizontal plane of the heel.

(e) Independence of action of trunk and extremities; trunk tends to such stability that it furnishes only a point of departure for developing the activities of the extremities, with a minimum participation in such activities; extremities tend to develop such independence of action that their call upon the trunk is minimized.

(*f*) The conservation of energy following the foregoing increases the power of resistance of the individual, and favors growth and development. Hence, as this type is approached, the individual displays vigor and stability.

On the whole, type (2), the retracted lower thorax type, tends towards the development of the following correlations:

(*a*) Retarded or uncompleted competence of the abdomen.

(*b*) Predominance of forward expansion of the trunk during inspiration, forward and upward, and forward and downward, with decreasing inspiratory capacity and decreasing expiratory efficiency.

(*c*) Less proportionate increase of transverse over antero-posterior diameters, and tendency to proportionate increase of antero-posterior over transverse, especially in the abdomen.

(*d*) Pelvis tends to increased forward rotation. Lumbo-sacral anterior convexity tends to increase. During weight bearing, lower extremities tend toward flexion at hip and knee, and feet tend toward extension so that the plane of the heel is higher than that of the forefoot.

(*e*) Trunk and extremities tend toward interdependence. Trunk is in condition of unstable equilibrium, and shares largely in the activities of the extremities. There is retarded or unattained independence of the extremities; the activities of the extremities are hampered by the lack of the stable point of departure required by voluntary muscles.

(*f*) The unnecessary expenditure of energy following the foregoing decreases the power of resistance of the individual, and favors a condition of habitual overstrain which depreciates powers of growth and development. Hence, as this type is approached, the individual displays weakness and instability.

CONCLUSIONS

Fundamental cause of splanchnoptosis is abdominal incompetence.

In their highest development, the abdominal walls not only contain the viscera, but also retain them in position, against gravity and other displacing forces. The abdomen may then be said to be competent. Competence of the abdomen is a developmental factor; stage of evolution with which human race is at present struggling; earlier phases can be traced backward through vertebrate series and in human prenatal life.

Distinctive characteristic of human genus not the erect trunk, nor even the erection of the trunk on two hinder or lower extremities, but distinctive human characteristic is the full extension of the lower extremities in the plane of a vertical trunk, the dorsal and ventral surfaces of which tend constantly to approach each other in parallel planes; this extension being accompanied by adduction and forward rotation, so that the patella and toes point forward.

Development of abdominal competence correlated with evolution of this extension, adduction and forward rotation of the lower extremities. At birth, abdomen is incompetent, and lower extremities (thighs) are flexed, abducted and rotated outward. Postnatal evolution of lower extremities in direction of extension, adduction and forward rotation tends to be completed in early childhood, but is an unstable possession, and in a large number of cases never fully attained; in another large number of cases is attained but after varying periods of time, more or less reversion to the condition found at birth occurs; tendency to this reversion always present, but becomes more pronounced with approach of fourth decade and beyond. Postnatal evolution of abdomen in direction of competence proceeds throughout infancy and childhood, and, in selected cases, is complete at or before puberty. Very unstable possession; in majority of cases never fully attained; even when attained, tendency to reversion to condition of more or less incompetence constantly present; tendency becomes more pronounced with approach of fourth decade and beyond.

This instability of abdomen and lower extremities exists at the present day in the most primitive as well as the most civilized peoples, and its existence can be traced among all peoples as far back as pictorial history extends.

Development of abdominal competence also correlated with postnatal evolution of abdominal viscera. Evolution of viscera always incomplete at birth; considerable evidence to show that in many cases never completed.

Development of spine, lower extremities, thoracic cage, and even upper extremities and head, correlated with development of abdominal competence, and *vice versa*. Variations in these correlations result in spontaneous grouping of body forms along two main paths: (1) Basic or primary type of figure, represented by broad lower thorax, slight anterior convexity of lumbar spine, slight anterior inclination of pelvis. (2) Secondary or aberrant type of figure, represented by retracted lower thorax, pronounced anterior convexity of lumbo-thoracic spine, increased anterior inclination of pelvis. Abdominal incompetence and visceral ptosis in both types. Variations in the correlations enumerated show a spontaneous tendency of the trunk and extremities towards the developmental deformities: round shoulders, lateral and antero-posterior curvatures of the spine; modifications of weak foot, including *pes planus*; retracted lower thorax, marked lumbar or lumbo-thoracic anterior convexity; marked forward rotation of the pelvis; abdominal incompetence, and visceral ptosis — both *en masse* and *individual*.

Experiments and dissections support the clinical hypothesis that abdominal incompetence is the primary factor in the development not only of splanchnoptosis, but also of the common surgical diseases of the upper abdomen, the stomach, duodenum, gall bladder and bile ducts, jejuno-ileum, pancreas and kidneys (especially the right) being the most important viscera affected.

Cause probable des fièvres après la splénectomie

(A propos de cinq cas examinés)

Par M. E. DE HERCZEL, Budapest.

Les publications littéraires, de même que l'observation exacte de la marche de la guérison en cinq cas de splénectomies, exécutées depuis un an et demi, nous ont fourni des données importantes et d'un intérêt incontestable pour la meilleure connaissance de la nature des accès de fièvre survenant après les splénectomies, et d'origine inconnue.

On sait bien depuis longtemps que dans un grand nombre de cas la convalescence, qui suit la splénectomie, est troublée par des élévations de température qu'on ne pourrait attribuer, ni à une infection quelconque ni à une exsudation au niveau du moignon ni à quelque autre complication, par exemple à la pneumonie. Nous croyons être autorisés à assurer presque avec certitude que les accès de fièvre et les exsudations, qu'on peut observer, sont des *effets des lésions du pancréas. En effet, à cause de la situation* spéciale de la rate, la face intérieure de cet organe est si près de la queue du pancréas qu'on ne peut lier que bien rarement ses artères ou couper sa tige sans causer une lésion à la queue du pancréas; il y a même beaucoup d'opérateurs qui, pour s'assurer de l'efficacité de la ligature, obéissent à un conseil exprimé par Billroth, portant qu'il faut lier exprès aussi le pancréas. Mais les expériences de Katz et Winkler ont prouvé que seule la simple ligature ou le perçage du pancréas suffit pour en faire sortir le contenu qui, en sa qualité de ferment, digère la graisse et cause autour de lui des nécroses des tissus adipeux. Ces nécroses se manifestent ensuite comme dans notre 2e et 3e cas — par des accès de fièvre et par une infiltration. La rémission et l'exacerbation réitérée de la fièvre s'expliquent par le fait que l'entassement et l'absorption des produits de dissolution des tissus en nécrose se font périodiquement; si les intervalles sont réguliers, c'est que l'exacerbation aussi apparaît régulièrement, comme dans notre 3e cas.

Donc, si l'on prend soin pendant l'opération de ne pas léser le pancréas, on est bien fondé d'espérer que les accès de fièvre ne surviennent pas au cours de la convalescence. Cela a été ainsi dans nos cas 4 et 5.

Il est évident, par conséquent, que, pour éviter la fièvre post-opératoire, il faut prendre garde de ne pas léser le pancréas. Et pour arriver à ce résultat il ne faut que lier les artères de la rate tout près du hilus et encore une à une avec deux fils de soie. Pour avoir plus de place il faut éviter de se servir des pinces de gros calibre et de la ligature en masse, d'autant plus que, pour entraver les hémorrhagies, la ligature en masse n'est pas aussi efficace que la ligature faite séparément sur tous les vaisseaux.

Entre les cinq cas suivants, des accès de fièvre ont été occasionnés dans l'un par une broncho-pneumonie catarrhale et dans deux par une nécrose du tissu adipeux provoquée par la lésion du pancréas. Quant au 4e et au 5e cas, dans lesquels le pancréas est resté intact, la convalescence se faisait tout à fait sans fièvre.

Le premier cas était une malade de trente-deux ans, chez laquelle la splénomégalie, combinée avec une hypertrophie du foie, une ascite et une anémie, s'est déclarée à la suite d'un accès de paludisme. Après la splénectomie, faite le 15 juin 1904, elle a eu à souffrir pendant 6 semaines de la convalescence d'une broncho-pneumonie catarrhale; cet inconvénient étant passé, la malade se rétablit complètement.

Dans le second cas, la splénectomie fut exécutée à cause d'une splénomégalie d'origine suppurative compliquée avec motilité de cet organe et anémie secondaire de moindre degré. Au cours de l'opération, faite le 14 juin 1904, une partie de la queue du pancréas a été liée avec la tige de la rate. Après l'opération, le terrain entamé ne montre aucune réaction, la plaie de laparotomie guérit promptement *per primam*, mais la température ne reste néanmoins subfébrile que pour monter le 27e jour après l'opération jusqu'à 39-40° C. A partir de ce temps, tous les trois jours et le plus souvent précédée d'un accès de frisson, la température monte au-dessus de 40° C. ; dans les deux jours qui séparent les accès, le malade n'est pas fébrile. L'examen microscopique du sang pour déceler des plasmodiums du paludisme, donna des résultats négatifs. Pendant la durée des accès de fièvre l'examen du ventre montre au niveau de la rate une résistance douloureuse, qui s'étend à droite jusqu'à la ligne parasternale droite, se termine en bas deux doigts au-dessus du *ligament inguinal gauche dans le prolongement de la ligne mammillaire*, tandis qu'en haut elle se perd sous l'arc costal gauche. La fièvre a cessé au cours d'un traitement résorptif ; la résistance disparut peu à peu et le malade se rétablit rapidement.

Dans le 3e cas, concernant un malade de 36 ans, la splénectomie fut exécutée à cause d'une splénomégalie anémique, qui s'est développée sur base paludéenne. Pendant l'opération de 7 juillet 1905 le *ligamentum gastrolienale* étant trop court, en tranchant la tige de la rate, on s'approcha de trop près de l'estomac et surtout du pancréas. Ici encore la plaie n'offrit aucune réaction, mais le 4e jour une élévation de température à 39° C. survint néanmoins, qu'on ne put s'expliquer qu'en partie par une bronchite aiguë. On trouva à l'endroit de la tige, à gauche de l'échine, dans la profondeur, une résistance dure, douloureuse et grosse comme le creux de la main.

A partir du 38e jour après l'opération, la température devient normale et la résistance, après traitement correspondant, a été résorbée. Le 18 avril, le malade quitte l'hôpital, en bonne condition, mais après deux semaines il revient au service des maladies internes, où il reste à peu près 8 semaines à cause des accès fiévreux. Il quitte l'hôpital guéri.

Le quatrième cas était une malade âgée de 37 ans chez qui on a procédé à la splénectomie, le 27 septembre 1905, à cause d'une splénomégalie combinée avec une hypertrophie du foie. Pendant l'opération, on a pris grand soin de lier les artères de la rate de telle façon que le pancréas ne soit pas lésé. Sans compter de petites élévations de températures, qui durèrent jusqu'au 4e jour après l'opération et furent causées, sans doute, par une bronchite, la guérison se fit tout à fait sans fièvre et la malade fut vite rétablie.

Dans le cinquième cas enfin chez une malade de 33 ans, l'extirpation de la rate d'une longueur de 25 cm. et d'une largeur de 17 cm., fut exécutée le 7 mars 1906, à cause d'un kyste d'échinocoeus, gros comme la tête d'un homme et enfoncé dans le parenchyme de la rate. Renseigné par les cas précédents et surtout par le 4e cas, on a fait les ligatures des artères avec un soin plus grand encore, afin que le pancréas n'attrappe aucune blessure. Le cours de la reconvalescence a bien justifié ces précautions, car la température de la malade est restée continuellement normale.

SÉANCE DU 21 AVRIL

(Matin)

(Sections de Chirurgie, de Médecine, et de Médecine et chirurgie
des voies urinaires, réunies).

Président: M. OLIVEIRA FEIJÃO

La catastrophe de Californie — La mort de Curie

M. NUNO PORTO: Messieurs.

Vraiment ému par les deux grands malheurs, qui viennent de frapper le monde, j'ai l'honneur de vous proposer, en l'énonçant dans notre procès verbal, de signifier notre grande douleur à nos confrères Américains qui se trouvent ici, nous faisant l'honneur de nous accompagner dans la lutte contre la douleur et contre la mort, leur exprimant les plus vifs sentiments de condoléance pour la terrible catastrophe qui a blessé le cœur de leur grande nation, maintenant couverte de deuil; et, en même temps, à nos confrères français, au monde scientifique, qui a perdu une de ses plus éclatantes lumières par la mort du grand Curie. Je vous propose aussi d'adresser l'hommage de nos plus profonds et douloureux regrets, demandant à nos illustres présidents de présenter de notre part, dans une lettre, à la savante Mme Curie, sa compagne du cœur et de l'esprit, l'expression de nos plus respectueux sentiments de douleur.

Diagnostic fonctionnel des reins

Par M. G. KAPSAMMER, (Vienne (V, page 209 du volume de la Section
de Médecine et chirurgie des voies urinaires).

DISCUSSION

M. O. PASTEAU: Pendant longtemps les chirurgiens qui étaient amenés à opérer sur le rein se sont contentés de l'exploration extérieure de l'organe; les différentes méthodes de palpation ont été étudiées en particulier par Guyon, Israël, Glénard. Mais les résultats obtenus étaient bien incomplets, alors même que l'examen histo-bactériologique et chimique de l'urine recueillie dans la vessie était fait aussi complètement que possible. L'exploration de la surface du rein mise à nu et la néphrotomie étaient considérées non pas seulement comme de simples temps opératoires, mais comme des moyens d'arriver au diagnostic de l'état du rein.

Quand Nitze, Casper et Albarran apportèrent l'instrumentation nécessaire pour le cathétérisme urétéral, la question fit un pas décisif; l'examen séparé de l'urine de chaque rein donna des renseignements précis sur le côté atteint, le degré des lésions, l'état du côté opposé. Les différents diviseurs qu'on présenta ensuite ne changèrent pas la face des choses. Le but poursuivi était toujours le même: recueillir séparément l'urine de chaque rein. Dès 1897, avec Albarran, on n'opérait plus à Necker sans avoir fait un examen comparé de l'urine de chaque rein, examen histo-bactériologique et chimique; puis on y ajouta en 1898 la recherche de l'élimination du bleu de méthylène.

Actuellement les méthodes de recherche se sont multipliées: la cystoscopie, le cathétérisme urétéral, la recherche du bleu, la cryoscopie, l'élimination du sucre après l'injection de phlorhydzine, et surtout l'étude de la polyurie expérimentale donnent les résultats les plus complets. On arrive maintenant couramment à établir un diagnostic précis de l'état fonctionnel du rein et à réduire au minimum la mortalité opératoire due à l'insuffisance rénale.

M. CATHELIN, après avoir décrit son cystoscope à vision directe et à air et montré les caractères qui le différencient des autres, employés à l'étranger, reconnaît à cette méthode de cystoscopie les indications suivantes: *a)* utilisation dans *l'ablation des corps étrangers vésicaux,* d'origine endo-exogène (petits calculs, épingles à cheveux, sondes ou conducteurs laissés dans la vessie); *b)* utilisation dans *la thérapeutique des lésions vésicales,* en particulier dans les ulcérations et les points enflammés des cystites tuberculeuses ou non spécifiques.

Il conserve le cystoscope simple de Nitze pour l'examen de la paroi vésicale et le cathétérisme des uretères avec les instruments de Nitze ou d'Albarran. Il a recours à son diviseur des urines pour l'étude séparée de la sécrétion et de l'excrétion des reins malades, associée ou non au cathétérisme et à l'épreuve du bleu.

M. Cathelin apporte ensuite les résultats de 37 interventions sur le rein et l'uretère se décomposant ainsi: 2 néphrostomies, 14 néphrectomies, dont 9 primitives et 5 secondaires, 5 néphrolithotomies, 4 néphrorraphies, 3 abcès périnéphrétiques, 1 pyélotomie postérieure et 1 urétérostomie (statistique arrêtée au 1er avril 1904). L'étude du fonctionnement séparé des deux reins a été obtenue 16 fois avec la division intra-vésicale des urines, réalisée avec l'instrument de l'auteur, 3 fois avec le cathétérisme urétéral, 2 fois avec la division et le cathétérisme, 2 fois avec le cathétérisme par vision directe. Dans 14 des cas, aucun de ces procédés n'avait pu être réalisé, mais on eut recours, pour justifier l'intervention, à l'examen clinique, à la radiographie et à la cystoscopie simple. Grâce aux précautions prises, on n'eut à déplorer que 5 morts, ainsi réparties: une d'hémorragie au cours d'une néphrectomie transpéritonéale pour cancer, une le lendemain de l'opération par septicémie dans une tuberculose rénale, une le quinzième jour après néphrectomie pour énorme calcul caralté, une de méningite tuberculeuse après une néphrectomie secondaire et enfin une de péritonite le septième jour après urétérectomie par voie péritonéo-iliaque.

Il n'y eut aucune mort d'insuffisance rénale.

M. KÜMMELL: En se servant des anciennes manières éprouvées depuis longtemps et en y réunissant les nouvelles méthodes du cathétérisme des uretères et les différents moyens pour s'assurer de la fonction des reins, nous sommes pour ainsi dire sûrs de la diagnose et de la prognose des maladies rénales. Une seule méthode ne nous donnerait guère la sûreté de la diagnose dans des cas si graves, et nous sommes obligés de nous servir de tous les moyens à notre disposition pour parvenir à de parfaits résultats. Hors du cathétérisme urétéral, indispensable dans chaque cas, où il faut s'assurer de la fonction des reins, c'est la cryoscopie qui, selon notre idée, tient la première place et qui dans bien plus de 1000 cas ne nous a jamais trompés. J'espère de tout mon cœur que bientôt cette excellente méthode sera plus répandue dans la chirurgie moderne et que par un travail mutuel et en comparant les valeurs nous trouverons la cause de la différence des chiffres entre les observations de quelques uns de nos chirurgiens les plus éminents et mes résultats.

Dans 5 cas, où nous fîmes la nephrectomie, quoique nous n'eussions qu'un point de congélation de $\delta = 0{,}6$ et moins, les malades sont morts après peu de temps par suite d'urémie.

Entre 404 opérations rénales, il y avait 189 néphrectomies, dont 15 sont morts avant de nous servir de cette nouvelle méthode $= 36{,}5$ %, tandis que de 148 cas de néphrectomies faites en nous servant du cathétérisme urétéral, de la cryoscopie, etc., nous n'avions que 10 cas de mort $= 6{,}7$ %. Si dans 3 cas, où nous avions constaté un point de congélation de $\delta = 0{,}6$ et 0,65, nous n'avions pas opéré suivant notre méthode, nous n'aurions pas eu ces 3 cas de mort et notre mortalité entière n'aurait pas surpassé 4,7 %. Dans quelques groupes, p. ex. dans les néphrectomies des reins tuberculeux, la mortalité était seulement de 3 %.

M. KASSASOWER: Ein wesentlicher Erfolg der heutigen Discussion liegt darin, dass die Frage bezüglich der Gewinnung des Harnes von jeder Niere endgültig und übereinstimmend zu Gunsten des Ureterenkatheterismus entschieden ist. Albarran gegenüber ist darauf aufmerksam zu machen, dass uns die Zuckerbestimmung mit Berücksichtigung der Zeit des Auftretens auch aus dem Gesammtharne innerhalb gewisser Grenzen wichtige Aufschlüsse zu geben vermag. Finden wir 15 Minuten nach der Injektion im Gesammtharne Zucker, so ist mindestens eine Niere funktionsfähig; finden wir 15 Minuten nach der Injektion noch keinen Zucker, so sind beide Nieren derart geschädigt, dass eine Nephrektomie von vorneherein ausgeschlossen erscheint. Diese Orientierung gewinnt eine besondere Wichtigkeit, wenn z. B. bei Tuberkulose die Blase derart erkrankt ist, dass die instrumentelle Untersuchung auf Schwierigkeiten stösst. Die Untersuchungen über die normale Nierenfunktion hat Redner unabhängig von Albarran, gleichzeitig mit diesem gemacht und ist zu dem gleichen Resultate gekommen. Die Thatsache, dass beide Nieren gleichzeitig nicht vollkommen gleichmässig secerniren, hat bezüglich der Zeit des Auftretens keine ausschlaggebende Bedeutung; die Differenzen sind zu gering, als dass sie praktisch in Betracht kommen könnten. Bezüglich der geringen Verspätungen, welche Albarran ausnahmsweise auch bei anscheinend gesunden Nieren gesehen hat, ist zu bedenken, dass manchmal auch eine etwas verspätete Resorption bei starkem panniculus adiposus unwesentliche Verspätung bedingen kann. Redner hat bei mehr als 250 Beobachtungen niemals Abweichungen von der Norm ohne anatomische Laesion gesehen. Die Prüfungsmethode von Albarran sei ja vom theoretischen Standpunkte aus ausgezeichnet, doch erscheine sie dem Redner für die Praxis zu umständlich. Man müsse dem allgemeinen Chirurgen möglichst einfache Methoden zur Nierenfunktionsprüfung an die Hand geben. Die Methode Albarrans erfordere 2 bis 3 Stunden, die Methode des Redners 1/2 bis 3/4 Stunden. Wenn die kryoskopische Untersuchung wegen der Schwierigkeit der Technik eine derart grosse Uebung und Erfahrung erfordere, wie die Kümmells ist, so spricht dieser Umstand auch gegen ihre Anwendung für die Praxis.

Was die probeweise Freilegung der Nieren betrifft, geht aus den Mittheilungen von Albarran und des Redners hervor, dass auch auf diesem Wege eine

Tuberkulose, ja selbst ein Tumor der Niere vollkommen verborgen bleiben können. Man müsste also auch die Niere spalten und Giordano hat auf dem I. internationalen Chirurgencongress in Brüssel auch die probeweise Spaltung beider Nieren verlangt. Ganz abgesehen von der Gefährlichkeit eines solchen Eingriffes gibt er uns aber auch keinen verlässlichen Aufschluss. Allen ist bekannt, dass bei Obduktionen oft der pathologische Anatome, bevor er eine Diagnose stellt, den Kliniker über das Vorhandensein von Cylindern oder Albumen fragt. Es genügt also auch der probeweise Sektionsschnitt nicht um eine exakte Diagnose zu stellen; es genügt nur die histologische Untersuchung der Niere. Denselben Zweck erreichen wir aber auch mit den neuen Methoden der Nierendiagnostik.

(Après-midi)

Présidence: M. BARDENHEUER

The symptoms, treatment and sequelae of non-malignant duodenal ulcer

Par M. D'ARCY POWER, Londres

The symptoms, treatment and sequelae of non-malignant ulcer of the duodenum have hardly received the attention they deserve owing to their frequency and severity. Until about the year 1892 duodenal ulcers were of purely academic interest. They were recognised post mortem and their occurrence was occasionally suspected during life, but no attempt was made to treat them surgically or to differentiate them from gastric ulcer. Increasing familiarity with the surgery of the stomach led naturally to a better acquaintance with abnormal conditions in the duodenum. Surgeons dealt first with duodenal ulcers which had perforated acutely: they were then led to interfere in cases where haemorrhage was the chief symptom; more recently they have concerned themselves with the results of duodenal constriction due to cicatrisation of ulcers in this part of the alimentary canal.

My position as a hospital surgeon has given me numerous opportunities of seeing and treating various cases of duodenal ulcer and I have thought this a fitting opportunity of communicating what I have learnt about them and the opinions at which I have arrived.

Frequency. Duodenal ulcer occurs in a much smaller proportion of persons than gastric ulcer. Sir E. C. Perry and Dr. L. E. Shaw ([1]) investigated the records of 17.652 post mortem examina-

---

([1]) Guy's Hospital Reports, 1893, p. 171.

tions made at Guy's Hospital, and amongst these were seventy
cases of ulcer of the duodenum either open or healed. It appears,
therefore, that duodenal ulcer occurs in 0.4 per cent of persons
dying from all causes as against gastric ulcer which is observed
either open or cicatrised in about five per cent of all autopsies. It
is further worthy of remark that ulcer of the duodenum is three
times as frequent in males as in females, whereas gastric ulcer is
twice as common in females as in males. It is interesting, too, to
note that of the seventy cases of duodenal ulcer found post mortem, nine were fatal by hæmorrhage, eight by perforation and three
as the result of cicatrisation either of the bowel or common bile-
duct. Hæmorrhage or perforation is equally likely to cause death
in those affected with duodenal ulceration, but only in about thir-
teen per cent of the cases, whilst cicatrisation and constriction to
a dangerous extent takes place in about eleven per cent of the
cured cases.

Situation. Sir Edwin Perry and Dr. Shaw [1] state that in
149 cases of duodenal ulcer collected from various sources 123
were situated in the first part of the duodenum, 16 were in the
second part and only two were in the third part. The ulcers were
multiple and were scattered throughout the whole length of the
duodenum in eight cases. Duodenal ulcers are often associated
with chronic gastric ulcers, and in many cases the ulcer is situated so near the pylorus as to make it appear during an operation
that the perforation has taken place in the stomach.

Causes. Nothing is known with certainty as to the causes of
ulcer of the duodenum. It is often associated with ulcer of the stomach and the causes which produce gastric ulcer probably play a
part in causing ulcer of the duodenum. The duodenum, too, is liable to the same inflammatory conditions as other parts of the alimentary canal. Tuberculous and typhoid ulceration are therefore
not uncommon. There is no doubt that general septic and pyæ-
mic conditions may be associated with duodenal ulcer and to these
causes, perhaps is to be assigned the duodenal ulceration found
in a certain proportion of patients who have been burnt especially
when there has been much suppuration. The experiments made by
Dr. William Hunter [2] point in the same direction, for he showed that
the subcutaneous injection of toluene-diamine into dogs was followed

---

[1] Loc. cit.
[2] Pathological Society's Transactions, vol. 41, p. 208.

by marked duodenal ulceration, the drug being destructive to the red blood corpuscles and being eliminated by the liver. There seems to be an ill-defined relation between duodenal ulceration and some cases of interstitial and tubal nephritis, whilst the stress of anthrax infection may fall upon this part of the alimentary canal.

Symptoms. I do not want to weary you with lengthy and uninteresting details of cases of duodenal ulcer so that I will detail the symptoms by a composite picture, premising that every case of duodenal ulcer which has come under my notice with acute symptoms of perforation or haemorrhage has been in a man. Women suffer in a smaller proportion of cases and in them I have repeatedly performed a gastro-jejunostomy on account of adhesions and constriction owing to the cicatrisation of an ulcer.

(A) PERFORATING DUODENAL ULCER

Perforation. The subject of a perforating duodenal ulcer is usually a man in the prime of life who assures you that he has either never suffered from any dyspeptic symptoms up to the moment of his sudden illness or has had so little indigestion that he has taken no account of it. Without warning he is suddenly seized with a stomach-ache of such severity that he becomes collapsed at once and sends immediately for assistance. He may vomit, but from the onset he passes neither flatus nor faeces. Examination within an hour or two of the attack shows him lying on his back, afraid to move, his breathing shallow and rapid, his pulse small, regular and quick, but not nearly so much accelerated as his respirations. He looks pinched and haggard but his temperature is normal. The patient cannot localise the pain but complains that it is worse along the upper half and down the right side of the abdomen. The abdomen is not distended and is not motionless, though it moves less freely during respiration than it should do. At first it is held rigid and the muscles on the right side are somewhat more tonically contracted than those on the left. It is everywhere tender and tympanitic. The area of liver dulness may not be altered and there is sometimes a point of maximum tenderness in the right hypocondrium. If no operation be performed, the pain becomes less acute and more generalised than it was at first. The patient rallies from the initial shock and may fall asleep; he loses his pinched appearance, and though the abdomen is still rigid it moves slightly during respiration. If unfortunately the patient is still left untreated, either because an incorrect diagnosis has been made or because he does not apply for relief, the pain again becomes urgent, but is now felt in the right iliac fossa which becomes especially tender, full and motionless. The patient shows the ordinary signs of peritonitis, he again becomes collapsed, his pulse quickens, his temperature rises and he dies usually with a diagnosis of appendicitis.

The errors in diagnosis are quite excusable in those who have not already had to treat a case of perforated duodenal ulcer and in those who are only called in to see a patient in the later stages. The initial shock caused by the sudden perforation is generally sufficient to indicate that some grave catastrophe has occurred and has overwhelmed the peritoneum. The symptoms are not quite like those of a perforated gastric ulcer, because the duodenal contents are more digested and less acid than those of the stomach and there is consequently less irritation. The symptoms subside therefore for a time and the fluid poured out by the duodenum slowly accumulates in the iliac fossae and more in the right than in the left. The onset of peritonitis demands an examination of the abdomen and as the patient now locates his symptoms to the lower part of his abdomen it is easy to treat the case as one of appendicitis. Here are two cases illustrating these mistakes: —

A porter aged 41 was admitted into St. Bartholomew's Hospital saying that he was at work and quite well until 11 a. m. when he was suddenly attacked with pain in his epigastrium. The pain continued and he vomited several times before coming to the hospital. He had passed no flatus since the pain began; his bowels had been well open on the previous day. He was a temperate man and was sure that he had never suffered from indigestion. At 2 p. m. the patient was reported to be a well-nourished man in obvious pain. His tongue was clean and moist; his respirations were very shallow and 60 in the minute; his pulse was of fair volume and tension, regular and 100 a minute. In the chest the percussion note was impaired at the right base and the entry of air at the base of the right lung was weaker than at the left. No additional sounds were heard by auscultation. The abdominal pain was not localised but the patient complained of it chiefly over the upper half and down the right side. The abdomen was not distended but moved very little during respiration. The movement, however, was equal all over, though the abdomen was held somewhat rigid. It was tender and tympanitic everywhere except that the liver dulness was present. Nothing abnormal could be felt. It was impossible at this time to make any definite diagnosis and the surgeon left directions that the patient should be carefully watched on the assumption that he was suffering from pulmonary rather than abdominal trouble and most likely from pneumonia. There was no definit change at 6 p. m., an enema sapenis had been retained, but in spite of fomentations the pain was unrelieved. The temperature was 99°.8

F., the pulse was 120, the respirations 60. At 12 midnight there was still no material change in the condition of the patient, whose temperature was 99°.8 F., pulse 120, respirations 60-70. A little liquid had been vomited. At 1 a. m. the abdomen was distended and the patient was slightly collapsed with a pulse of 144 almost running. At 2 a. m. the patient was still more collapsed. I then saw him for the first time and at once determined to open his abdomen. Liquid escaped as soon as the peritoneal cavity was opened and on drawing the stomach into the wound a hole was found in the duodenum large enough to admit a full sized probe; there was a considerable deposit of lymph all round the margins of the aperture. An attempt was made to close the opening with Lembert's sutures, but the operation was very difficult, owing partly to the awkward position of the ulcer and partly to the rotten state of the tissues in the neighbourhood. Four sutures were passed and it seemed as though the opening had been successfully closed. During the suturing large quantities of a thin liquid kept welling up from the perforation until the last suture had been inserted. The peritoneal cavity was then cleansed and afterwards closed. The patient bore the operation badly and his pulse at the end was hardly perceptible. He died at 7.30 a. m.

A post mortem examination at three p. m. on the same day showed that the peritoneum was acutely inflamed, its endothelial aspect being covered with a layer of fibrino-purulent lymph. There were collections of purulent matter at the bottom of the pouch of Douglas, in the lumbar region and in the right subphrenic space which was almost completely shut off from the rest of the peritoneal cavity. The beginning of the duodenum at the upper and posterior part was the seat of a conical ulcer which measured half an inch in diameter. It had sharply cut edges but there was no infiltration at the margin. The floor of the ulcer had perforated but the sutures were not accurately applied as water and intestinal contents easily passed through.

The particular interest of this case lay in the fact that the localised peritonitis must have lasted a much longer time than the sudden onset of the symptoms would have led one to suppose, whilst the symptoms when they appeared were so obscure as to make it seem that the patient was suffering from pneumonia rather than from peritonitis. It is farther interesting because it is a record of the course taken by a case of perforated duodenal ulcer which though carefully watched was practically untreated.

The following case illustrates how easy it is to mistake a perforated duodenal ulcer for an acute attack of appendicitis:

A bookstall keeper, aged 26, was admitted into St. Bartholomew's Hospital under my care suffering from abdominal pain and sickness. He said that he had suffered from other attacks of similar pain, but this was much more severe, and had begun suddenly at 7 p. m. on the previous day. The abdomen when I saw him at 10 a. m. the next morning was hard, tense and painful. The temperature was 97°.2 F. and the pulse 112. He localised his pain over the right iliac region which was tender and full, the rest of the abdomen moving during respiration. I thought that he was suffering from acute appendicitis which had ended in perforation and

I therefore opened the abdomen in the right iliac region and found the appendix normal. Gas issued from the abdominal cavity as soon as the peritoneum was incised and there was gush of alkaline fluid which did not smell but was clearly bile stained. The end of the ileum was inflamed in patches which seemed to correspond with Peyer's patches. The clear alkaline fluid which escaped from the peritoneal cavity told me that the perforation had occurred much higher up the alimentary canal. I therefore plugged the iliac wound and opened the abdomen in the middle line above the umbilicus. The stomach was found to be normal, but a perforation was discovered in the duodenum and on its superior surface, measuring about an eight of an inch across. The hole was closed with two layers of Lembert's sutures. Drainage tubes were inserted at the upper and lower ends of the median incision as well as in the iliac wound. The patient bore the operation well, making a steady and uneventful recovery. He left the hospital on the 48th day after the operation. It is now three years since he was under my care. I have seen him at intervals of a year and he always says that he is a healthy man with unimpaired digestion and able to follow his original occupation.

Hæmorrhage. The hæmorrhage in some cases of duodenal ulcer is a characteristic symptom. It is sudden, painless and very considerable in quantity. It seems to be due to erosion of the large arterial trunks which lie outside the duodenum — the superior pancreatico-duodenal artery being the most commonly affected, though the gastro-duodenal, the pyloric, the gastric and the pancreatica magna as well as the superior pancreatico-duodenal vein have been found ulcerated. The hæmorrhage may be so severe as to be fatal at once, more often the patient is blanched or he may become faint without knowing the cause. This may happen on more than one occasion and as the hæmorrhage is concealed the cause is only recognised by the subsequent passage of large tarry motions. In other cases the patient may have hæmatemesis instead of melæna or both may be present.

Here is an example of such a case:

A man aged 31, a printer's labourer, was admitted into St. Bartholomew's Hospital under my care on May 18th, 1904, and was discharged on June 17th. The patient had been treated in Luke ward by my colleague dr. Herringham since April 22nd, for pain in the lower part of his abdomen and vomiting. The pain had first been felt six months previously and had gradually become worse until on getting out of bed one morning nine weeks since he had felt faint and vomited a quart of dark blood all in lumps. He was at home for five weeks after this and was then in the infirmary for three weeks. On April 19th he retched after food and on April 20th he vomited a pint of blood after food. There was no history of melæna and the patient said that he had never had any illness of importance. Two years ago he was in Australia and Canada. He drinks one or two pints of beer a day and smokes a little. He has never had venereal disease; is married and has two children living; the last two were stillborn. His father died of acute alcoholism at the age of 45, his mother in childbed.

The patient is a pale man with a temperature of 97° F., pulse 92, soft, and respirations 28. His abdomen moves evenly during respiration and there is a point of maximum tenderness in each iliac fossa. There is also a tender spot one inch to the right of the umbilicus, but this point varies somewhat in position.

So long as the patient was in the hospital he had neither pain, vomiting nor melæna; but in view of his history, of the large quantity of blood he had brought up and the situation of the pain I had no difficulty in making a diagnosis of duodenal ulcer. I performed a posterior gastro-jejunostomy upon him, with the concurrence of Dr. Herringham, on 19th May. The patient made an absolutely uneventful recovery; the wound was healed and the stitches were removed on May 28th, and when he was discharged to the Convalescent Home at Swanley on June 17th he had suffered neither indigestion, stomach ache or pain since the day after the operation.

The attacks of pain and vomiting recommenced about five weeks after the patient left the hospital and a fortnight after he had been at home and had returned to his ordinary diet. When he reported himself to me four months later, they were often as severe as they used to be before the operation. The attacks bear no relation to the taking of food which he says he limits to fish, stews milk and a very little meat, though his wife affirms that he denies himself nothing and she is sure he is the worse for it.

The patient was readmitted to the Hospital on January 6th, 1905 on account of sickness and pain after food. He vomited from time to time, vomit containing clots of blood, but the patient said that he did not feel ill in himself. He was placed on low diet, no solids, and was given a little essence. On January 10th, he suddenly became collapsed in the morning as he was lying in bed. He felt faint and became very cold. A few minutes later he vomited a little dark blood. His bowels were open involuntarily whilst he was collapsed and the motion seemed to contain a little blood. At 2.30 on the same day he vomited twenty ounces of dark coloured blood. At 4 a. m. on January 12th, he again became collapsed without any warning and at 8.30 a. m. on the same day he vomited twenty-five ounces of blood in clots, but he had no melæna on this or any subsequent day. He was collapsed for a third time on January 24th, the attack being quite sudden and his pulse becoming imperceptible, but he had neither hæmatemesis or melæna afterwards and was without further bad symptoms during the remainder of his stay in the Hospital. He was discharged on March 8th, 1905 and has not since been heard of.

Diagnosis. The diagnosis of a perforated duodenal ulcer should be easy but in practice it is often a matter of great difficulty as is shown by the cases I have just quoted. The patient is suffering acute abdominal pain and the attack began suddenly. The history of previous good health, the fact that the abdomen is moving during respiration, the absence of any great amount of rigidity in the abdominal muscles or of any point of maximum tenderness, are all misleading and make it difficult for the surgeon to believe that the patient is suffering from such a dangerous condition as a perforated ulcer of the duodenum. He may think of a perforating or leaking gastric ulcer, but the symptoms are much less characteristic than he is accustomed to find in this condition and it is not until he has seen one or two similar cases that the occurrence of a perforated duodenal ulcer is called to mind. The diagnosis, therefore, is too often left in abeyance in the hope that a few hours' delay will render the signs and symptoms more definite. Such advice is likely to prove fatal for instead of making the diagnosis clearer time only renders it more obscure. The slight clues which could be picked up shortly after the onset when the peritoneum was only affected at the point of perforation are soon masked by the general peritonitis produced by the diffusion of the duodenal contents throughout the abdominal cavity. Delay thus allows the extravasated fluid to gain access to the innermost recesses of the peritoneal folds so that a subphrenic, pelvic or iliac abscess may still further complicate a condition which is well-nigh desperate from the beginning.

When I am called to a patient who has been seized suddenly with intense abdominal pain, without much history of previous indigestion, I ask that he shall not be given morphia and that his pulse shall be counted carefully and accurately recorded by the same person every half hour. If on my arrival the pulse-rate has increased although the patient has been kept at rest and free from disturbing influences, I have no hesitation in advising an immediate exploratory operation, even though the objective signs be very slight.

The escape of gas and liquid as soon as the abdomen is opened prove that a perforation has occurred and the first thought of a surgeon will then be that he is dealing with a ruptured gastric ulcer. The character of the fluid often gives the first indication as to the seat of the perforation. When it comes from the duodenum it is limpid or bile-stained, free from smell, alkaline and thus wholly different from the extravasated contents of the stomach which often contain undigested portions of food. The fluid from the duodenum is the succus entericus and is, I suppose, the secretion of Brunner's glands. It is very abundant and comes welling up from the perforated intestine in quite a characteristic manner. The perforation is usually small, close to the pylorus and often rather at the back of the duodenum so that is very awkwardly placed for suture. It is however possible to close it completely as in the case which I have already quoted.

If the patient be left without operation, the diagnosis, as I have said, becomes still more obscure and my experience tells me that a perforated duodenal ulcer may be mistaken for pneumonia, for appendicitis or for suppurative peritonitis from any other cause.

(B) NON-PERFORATING ULCER

The second group of cases where there is a duodenal ulcer without perforation is even more interesting than the perforating variety which has just been considered. The diagnosis is more difficult and the sequelæ demanding surgical treatment are no less urgent though they may be more remote. As may be gathered from what has been said of perforated ulcers, the signs of a duodenal ulcer may be absent or wholly inconspicuous and in such cases no diagnosis is possible. In some cases the patient complains of a continued pain in the abdomen which he can neither localise nor account for. He keeps his bed for a few days and then feeling better goes about again saying that he has had a bad bilious attack. If he is nervous about himself or should the pain have been severe, he seeks medical advice and is treated for gallstones, renal colic or appendicitis. But the exact nature of his illness is probably not recognised unless he vomits a considerable quantity of blood or has a sharp attack of melæna. Even then the case is thought to be one of gastric ulcer, unless an abdominal section is performed and the stomach is found to be healthy.

I do not know how a diagnosis can be established in the present state of our knowledge, but it is of no practical importance, for in the majority of cases the patient recovers from the attack unaided by art or if the bleeding be sufficient to need an exploration the surgeon performs a gastro-jejunostomy, whether the ulcer be situated in the stomach or in the duodenum. I have tried to recognise the condition by the character of the bleeding, by the time of the occurrence of pain after taking food, by the character of the material vomited and in many other ways, but always without success, for what is true and seems a valuable sign in one patient is worthless in another. I believe, therefore, that there is no pathognomonic sign of a non-perforating ulcer of the duodenum whilst the ulceration is in progress.

Constriction of the duodenum. —But if a non-perforating duodenal ulcer offers very few signs by which its presence may be detected, it may have sequelæ of the gravest character. The ulcer is usually single, and is situated in the first part of the duodenum, but like a gastric ulcer it is very chronic and may cause extensive inflammation in the submucous and muscular coats of the intestine. The inflammatory changes may extend to the serous coat and to the under surface of the liver. In process of time the ulcer heals and by the subsequent cicatrisation of the inflammatory products the duodenum is either narrowed or it is constricted by the surrounding adhesions. The adhesions may not only affect the duodenum but they may also involve the liver, the gall bladder, the pancreas and such large blood vessels as the abdominal aorta, the hepatic artery and the portal vein. Such a patient presents himself as a man between 40 and 60, looking older than his years. Thin and haggard he tells you that he is a martyr to indigestion and that for months past he has suffered atrocious pain in his stomach which is relieved by vomiting. He has dieted himself in every possible manner, he has made all kinds of local applications to his stomach, he has visited all sorts of watering places and he has gone in vain from one physician to another seeking a cure. Examination shows him to be a mere bag of bones, badly constipated with cold extremities and a listless, dejected aspect. His abdomen is loose, the subcutaneous veins may be enlarged and there is visible peristalsis from left to right in the epigastric region. Palpation and percussion tell of a greatly dilated stomach and a tumour may sometimes be felt in the neighbourhood of the pylorus. For a moment you think of cancer of the pylorus or gall-bladder and you question the patient a little more closely. He is sure that he has been suffering for years, for so long, in fact, that he hardly recollects the beginning of his trouble. A few well-directed enquiries may elicit that 25 or 30 years ago, when he was a young man, he once or twice brought up a large quantity of blood without serious pain or discomfort or that he had an illness which no one seemed to know much about. He was treated for gallstones or for appendicitis or simply for «liver.» The attack was abdominal, was painful and kept him in bed, but the exact details have long since passed from his mind and for some years he was as healthy a man as ever.

This is a case of duodenal obstruction resulting from cicatrisation of an old ulcer, the irritation of which caused inflammatory thickening of the surrounding parts or of the duodenal walls. How many patients have been allowed to die of such a condition in the belief that they had malignant disease of the stomach no one can tell, but every pathological Museum contains several specimens of simple duodenal constriction. Here is such a case in detail:

A man, aged 69, was admitted into the hospital on August 15th, 1902 with a history that he had suffered severely from dyspepsia for the past five years and that for the last two years he had pain after his food and vomiting. During the six or seven months preceding his admission to the hospital there had been occasional streaks of blood in the material vomited. The attacks of vomiting usually took place once in two days and he would then bring up as much as two pints at a time. For the last two months he had rapidly lost flesh. It was noted on admission that he was a thin and wasted man with a flaccid abdomen, which moved freely during respiration. The stomach was greatly dilated as the lesser curvature lay about three inches below the costal margin and the viscus occupied the greater part of the epigastric, all the umbilical, a great part of the hypogastric and some of the iliac regions of the abdomen. A succussion splash was very distinct and a hard rounded tumour about the size of a Tangerine orange could be felt in the middle line, sometimes above and sometimes below the umbilicus. The liver was not enlarged. A test meal showed the presence of free hydrochloric, lactic and butyric acids with albumoses.

The patient was kept under observation and was dieted carefully until August 19th, when I performed a gastro-jejunostomy upon him as he was getting worse instead of better and I felt sure that he had a cancer of the stomach. When the peritoneum was opened, the pylorus was found to be thickened but the swelling which had been felt through the abdominal walls was a mass of adhesions surrounding the duodenum and attacking the whole of the first part to the neighbouring tissues.

The patient slept badly after the operation and was repeatedly sick suffering much pain until he left the hospital on September 19th. From the hospital he went to a nursing home at Reading and afterwards to Devonshire where he is still living.

He wrote to me under the date October 28th, 1903 — fourteen months after the operation: "I hardly know where to begin, so presume I had better start from our first interview which was on July 23rd, 1902. Went into Bart's August 1st. Operation performed on me August 19th, left September 19th, at my own request; went direct to a home at Reading; left there November 1st, for Ilfracombe direct; bore the journey well. Out in a bathchair November 5th, for an hour and so every day, when fine until December 11th, when the chair was dismissed and I walked. I can eat and digest my food. I occasionally take a glass of mild ale — no spirits or wine. I retire to bed about 10 o'clock, previously eating an apple. I rise at 6, make myself a cup of cocoa — half milk — and after washing, smoke a pipe and read till 8.30, then breakfast, — my best meal; — lunch at 1.0 generally cold meat and soup, tea at 5.0. Dinner or supper at 7.30, seldom get meat then, usually bread and butter, cheese, salad and plenty of onion. Can walk five or six miles without feeling tired; I am out of doors as much as possible." To this satisfactory account of himself he adds that his weight went up gradually from 9 stone four lbs. to 12 stone 6 lbs. and he concludes his letter by saying, "I have not weighed so much for 12 or 14 years but remembering that I am 71 years old I cant expect to keep this weight up although I dont feel my age."

I saw this patient again in the early part of June, 1904, twenty two months after the operation. He was in good health, maintained his weight and was passing through London to visit some grandchildren in Canada. The trip was successful for he writes to me again from Devonshire in October 1904 "I have just returned from a visit to the North West Territory where I had to rough it considerably. I have been travelling day and night since October 2nd and do not feel the least ill-effects – I hear, 1908, that he is still in good health.

The general symptoms of duodenal obstruction may be gathered from what has already been said. There is usually pain of the nature of dyspepsia felt an hour or two after taking food. The pain depends more upon the quantity of food taken than upon the quality. It is relieved by vomiting and the severity of the vomiting increases with the length of time the symptoms have lasted. It is usually copious and often painful. It is not a mere emptying of the stomach, for, when the patient has vomited a large quantity, he will in an hour vomit as much again, although he has taken nothing in the interval. The attacks of vomiting are often worse at night than in the daytime. This seems to be particularly the case with business men, perhaps because they make a light breakfast, have but little lunch and make their chief meal in the evening. The attacks of vomiting therefore, like the pain, bear a definite relation to the quantity, rather than to the quality of the food taken. The quantity of fluid vomited and the small amount of food digested and absorbed lead to very obstinate constipation. It is the relief of this symptom which is hailed with the greatest joy by a patient who has been cured by a gastro-jejunostomy and the regularity of the bowels is one of the best proofs to the surgeon that his anastomosis is working successfully many months after the operation. The same loss of absorptive power leads to diminution in weight, to a harsh and dry skin, to a brittleness of the nails and to loss of the subcutaneous fat; in other words, the patient shows many of the signs of chronic starvation.

A systematic physical examination of the abdomen should be made in every case where there is reason to think that the patient is suffering from duodenal obstruction. The patient should lie flat on his back on a couch, with the knees bent and the shoulders slightly raised by a pillow. A good light should be allowed to fall upon the abdomen and the surgeon should at first merely watch the abdominal movements without touching the patient. In thin people and in a case of marked duodenal obstruction the outline of the dilated stomach can often be seen with slow waves of peristalsis passing across the upper part of the abdominal wall from left to right. These waves in themselves are characteristic of some obstruction to the outflow of the gastric contents and the more healthy and active the person the more marked are the waves. The surgeon now places his hand flat upon the abdominal wall and his practised touch readily discovers the outlines of the enlarged stomach, even if there be no tumour or nodule perceptible in it. The position of the pylorus is often marked in these cases by a thickened nodule, which is easily mistaken for cancer, especially if, as in the case related above, the patient vomits a little blood from time to time. But the actual position of the pylorus varies greatly when the stomach is dilated and its exact position may not be detected at the first examination. The absence of a tumour does not preclude the diagnosis of duodenal constriction. Percussion is not of any great value in determining the size of the stomach, because a dilated stomach is often associated with a distended colon, and it is difficult to distinguish the note yielded by one from that of the other. Auscultation, too, is of no great service except to elicit the succussion splash. A dilated stomach can be easily distended by pumping in air, a proceeding which, though painless, is unpleasant to the patient, or by the cruder method of administering separately the constituents of a Seidlitz powder. With these guides, there is really no excuse for overlooking a dilated stomach, or for being doubtful as to the existence of such a condition.

The teeth and gums should always be examined, as a matter of routine, to eliminate the possibility of the dyspeptic symptoms and constipation being due to chronic lead poisoning. It is better not to give a definite diagnosis until the bowels have been satisfactorily emptied by means of an enema, repeated if necessary, and it is wise to examine the abdomen more than once, and at different times after meals.

A test meal should be given, and the presence or absence of free hydrochloric acid should be noted. The usual test meal consists of a thick slice of bread and butter with a breakfastcupful of weak tea sweetened, but without milk. The meal is given at breakfast time, and is withdrawn from the stomach an hour later by means of a stomach tube. The material withdrawn is filtered, and the residue is examined microscopically to see how far digestion has proceeded. The filtrate is tested with Günsberg's reagent for free hydrochloric acid. A few drops of the filtrate are mixed in a porcelain dish with an equal quantity of a solution consisting of phloroglucin 2 parts, vanillin 1 part, and absolute alcohol 30 parts. The mixture is evaporated to dryness at a gentle heat, and, if free hydrochloric acid is present, red crystals will form. As a broad rule, free hydrochloric acid is present in simple duodenal constriction, it is deficient or absent in cancer of the stomach.

Microscopically too the Oppler-Boas bacillus should be absent in cases of non-malignant constriction of the duodenum.

Palliative treatment in cases of duodenal constriction is chiefly directed to relieve the vomiting. This is done by rectal feeding and washing out the stomach, since the indications are clearly to keep the stomach empty, and prevent putrefactive changes. The stomach is washed out with a warm solution of bicarbonate of soda (20 grains to the pint). A soft tube is passed into the stomach and its contents are evacuated, half a pint of the solution is then poured into the tube and is allowed to run out again, and this is repeated several times. In the early stages of duodenal constriction, the stomach needs only be washed out every other day, and this is done most conveniently before breakfast; but in the later stages, when the vomiting is most distressing at night, the stomach should be washed out every evening just before the patient goes to bed, and about four hours after the last meal.

It is obvious that this treatment is only palliative, and it follows, from what has been said already, that patients, who suffer from painful vomiting, with loss of flesh and constipation, should always be examined carefully to find out whether there is any dilatation of the stomach. When the stomach is dilated, and diet, combined with simple remedies, fails to bring about a cure, there should be no hesitation in recommending an exploratory incision with a view to the performance of a posterior gastro-jejunostomy by direct suture.

The operation should not be postponed until the patient has exhausted himself, because early operation is attended with comparatively little risk, and has a twofold advantage. If the patient is found to be suffering from cancer of the stomach, much more radical measures can be pursued in the early stages of the disease, than if delay has allowed the growth to infiltrate all the surrounding tissues. But even if the constriction proves to be due to malignant disease, and removal is impossible, gastro-enterostomy serves excellently as a temporary expedient. It has, too, the advantage over colotomy for the relief of an analogous condition in the rectum, that it leaves no open wound. The patient, therefore, is able to go about his ordinary work, until the progress of the disease renders him incapable of further effort. But if, on the other hand, the patient is suffering from duodenal constriction, which is not due to cancer, the surgeon can promise him a speedy relief from all the disagreeable symptoms, and a prolongation of his active life for many years in comfort.

Contribution à l'étude de la splénectomie

Par M. CAILLAUD, Monaco.

La splénectomie ou extirpation de la rate est une opération bien réglée et assez simple quand elle se pratique sur une rate flottante, facilement mobilisable. On peut alors attirer l'organe au dehors et lier le pédicule sans difficultés.

Ces conditions particulièrement favorables ne se trouvent pas souvent réalisées; elles sont même assez rares. Dans la majorité des cas, la rate profondément située ne se laisse pas aisément déplacer. Deux causes peuvent ainsi la rendre fixe: la brièveté de certains ligaments et les adhérences.

Les ligaments qui fixent la rate en arrière et en haut: le pancréatico-splénique et le phréno-splénique sont souvent très courts.

Le premier n'aurait en moyenne que 2 centimètres, d'après Poirier, et il pourrait faire défaut dans un grand nombre de cas. Le second également très bref peut aussi manquer. Habituellement et du fait de ces ligaments, la rate ne pourra donc se porter que très peu en bas et en avant.

En outre, des adhérences se rencontrent assez fréquemment entre la face convexe et le diaphragme.

Ces adhérences, on n'est pas surpris de les rencontrer quand il existe ou qu'il a existé une lésion de la rate ou des parties voisines.

Elles peuvent alors être très solides. Mais on est beaucoup plus étonné d'en trouver encore même quand la rate est normale et chez des personnes dont les antécédents morbides ne comportaient rien qui pût attirer l'attention de ce côté.

Dans un assez grand nombre d'autopsies nous avons constaté de semblables adhérences sans qu'il fût possible d'en trouver l'explication dans l'histoire pathologique du sujet.

Il est vrai de dire qu'elles étaient en général assez peu résistantes mais suffisantes quelquefois pour déterminer des déchirures de la pulpe, si on les rompait, ce qui aurait amené une hémorragie sur le vivant.

Ainsi donc, que la difficulté vienne des ligaments ou des adhérences, quand la rate est immobilisée, son extirpation est souvent très malaisée en raison du peu de commodité que l'on a pour aborder son pédicule et le lier, aussi n'est-il pas rare de voir à la suite de cette opération des insuccès dûs à des hémorrhagies.

Nous croyons cependant que de tels accidents peuvent être évités, même dans ces mauvais cas, en modifiant la technique généralement adoptée. La technique que nous proposons ne consiste pas à exercer des tractions sur l'organe pour le dégager malgré tout, pas non plus à vouloir pincer le pédicule en bloc comme on le fait d'habitude.

Elle consiste à aller avant tout droit au danger; aux gros vaisseaux : artère et veine, sans toucher tout d'abord en quoi que ce soit à la rate. Si on pouvait pincer, lier en premier lieu les deux vaisseaux dans de bonnes conditions, toutes les autres manœuvres seraient ensuite exemptes de danger. L'artère et la veine splénique, après avoir longé le bord supérieur du pancréas, passent sur sa face antérieure dans leur partie terminale. Elles se trouvent comprises entre la face antérieure de l'extrémité externe du pancréas et le feuillet postérieur de l'arrière-cavité des épiploons, puis entre les deux feuillets du ligament pancréatico-splénique.

C'est là, dans ce ligament, tout près du hile qu'il faut aller prendre ces troncs principaux.

En les pinçant ainsi, avant qu'ils n'aient fourni leurs branches de distribution : (divisions pour la rate, vaisseaux courts et même gastro-épiploïque gauche), on est sûr d'avoir une bonne hémostase préventive. Comment découvrir et aborder ainsi ces vaisseaux ? En ouvrant l'arrière-cavité des épiploons nécessairement, puisqu'ils se trouvent dans la paroi postérieure de cette cavité.

Voici d'ailleurs la technique complète que nous proposons après l'avoir étudiée plusieurs fois sur le cadavre.

I — Incision de la paroi sur le bord externe du grand droit depuis les côtes jusqu'à l'ombilic ou un peu au-dessous, suivant les cas.

À cette incision on peut adjoindre, si besoin est, une autre transversale intéressant le muscle droit.

II — Introduction de la main. Recherche de la rate. Examen de sa mobilité. Si elle est mobile, essayer de l'amener au milieu de l'incision. Pour faciliter son accès, exercer une traction sur l'estomac. Si elle est adhérente, cas qui nous intéresse surtout, respecter pour le moment ses attaches et passer au 3ᵉ temps.

III — Ouvrir le grand épiploon au niveau de la queue du pancréas. Pénétrer par cette ouverture dans l'arrière-cavité des épiploons. Écarter largement les lèvres de l'ouverture épiploïque pour que l'on puisse reconnaître sur la paroi abdominale postérieure le pancréas. Cette découverte doit se faire par la vue et le toucher. La vue suffit quand on est en présence d'une personne maigre. La légère saillie que fait la glande, sa coloration et son aspect la mettent en évidence. S'il y a beaucoup de graisse autour du pancréas, il s'y trouve comme enfoui et on l'aperçoit plus difficilement. C'est au toucher à donner alors le surcroît de renseignements nécessaire. La main sent en effet facilement la consistance spéciale de l'organe.

L'ayant saisi au niveau du corps, elle peut le suivre tout du long, jusqu'à la queue. A cet endroit elle arrive bientôt à saisir le ligament pancréatico-splénique dans lequel sont contenus les vaisseaux.

Durant toute cette exploration la main a senti le long du bord supérieur du pancréas les battements de l'artère splénique. Elle les sent encore plus nettement dans le ligament puisque les vaisseaux y sont isolés. On peut donc là, après les avoir sentis, appliquer sur eux deux pinces et les couper entre ces pinces.

IV — Le pédicule vasculaire étant ainsi traité et tout danger de grande hémorragie étant écarté, on peut rompre délibérément toutes les adhérences qui retiennent la rate et l'attirer fortement vers la ligne médiane. On peut alors sectionner les ligaments sur tout le pourtour du hile en pinçant au fur et à mesure les quelques vaisseaux indépendants des troncs nourriciers: branche de l'artère diaphragmatique inférieure gauche qui peut venir par le ligament suspenseur; branche de la gastro-épiploïque gauche qui se distribue quelquefois à l'extrémité inférieure de l'organe. La rate est alors extirpée.

V — Il ne reste plus alors qu'à jeter une solide ligature sur le pédicule des deux gros troncs, ligature qu'il sera prudent de mettre double, d'autres sur les quelques vaisseaux secondaires; à bien vérifier l'hémostase dans toute la loge splénique et à refermer la paroi.

DISCUSSION

M. D'ARCY POWER thanked Dr. Caillaud for his interesting paper. Mr. Power said that he had removed the spleen in several cases. Once or twice for rupture; once for enlargement which he believed was syphilitic in origin and within the last few months for a large sarcoma of the spleen. In each operation he had followed the method recommended by Dr. Caillaud, for he had avoided traction upon the pedicle and he had placed double ligature upon the artery and veins as far apart as possible and have divided the vessels between the veins. The patient with ruptured spleens had died, but the other two cases recovered. One of these cases — lady — had returned to her occupation as a teacher of dancing and she had been without her spleen for eight years. Mr. Power asked Dr. Caillaud whether he had observed any changes in the blood of the patients from whose he had removed the spleen. Mr. Power had been unable to observe a permanent alteration, although he had made repeated examinations and blood counts.

M. GARRÈ. Auf die Frage des Herrn Collegen d'Arcy Power möchte ich bemerken, dass mir nach einigen Milzexstirpationen die sorgfältige Untersuchung des Blutes zunächst deutliche Veränderungen ergab, die sich aber nach wenigen Wochen ausglichen, so dass schon nach kurzer Zeit das Blut normale Verhältnisse ergab die sich über Jahre hinaus gleichmässig erhielten. Diese Beobachtungen sind noch von anderer Seite bestätigt.

M. CAILLAUD. Je ne puis donner de renseignements sur l'état du sang chez les splénectomisés, n'ayant pas eu l'occasion de pratiquer cet examen.

De la Rachistovaïnisation au Brésil

(Contribution à l'étude de la rachianalgésie chirurgicale)

Par M. ALVARO RAMOS, Rio de Janeiro.

Les contributions à l'étude d'une méthode d'anesthésie chirurgicale ne seront jamais de trop, surtout quand ces contributions arrivent de très loin témoignant la participation des peuples les plus éloignés dans les progrès toujours croissants de la chirurgie.

La rachianalgésie chirurgicale est encore à l'ordre du jour. Ses partisans ne sont pas encore assez nombreux, quoique le nombre de ses adversaires diminue.

Chez nous, la ponction lombaire, *"lumbal ponction,,* de Quincke, (1) était déjà bien connue après les travaux de Léonard Corning, de New-York; des Congrès de Kensberg, 1893; de Wiesbaden, 1893 et 1896; de Lubeck, 1895; des observations rapportées par Fürbringer, Freydem, Hubner, Senator, Goldscheider; après les travaux de Chipault, Marfan, Weill, Degenès, Sabres et Demon, en France; de Gaübissi, et Rocco Jemma, en Italie; et M. Pasteur, à Londres; nous avons assisté pour la première fois le professeur Miguel Couto en 1897 à faire la ponction dans un cas d'hémorrhagie sur la queue de cheval.

Les observations du professeur Couto ont inspiré la thèse de J. Maria Corrêa (2) et ont aussi été rapportées à l'Académie de médecine de Rio de Janeiro par Silva Rabello et à l'Association des internes des Hôpitaux, de Rio, par Henrique Duque Estrada.

Les injections sous-arachnoïdiennes lombaires de cocaïne ont été faites par le professeur Brant Leme dans son service à l'hôpital «Misericordia» d'après les études de Bier et pendant que Tuffier faisait sa communication à la Société de biologie de Paris, au mois de novembre 1899 et avant son article dans la «Sémaine Médicale», n° 21, mai 1900.

Encouragés par les résultats qui confirmaient la description de Tuffier, sa méthode a été peu à peu suivie par d'autres chirurgiens brésiliens, quoique la plus grande partie se conservât encore douteuse et hésitât sur sa valeur.

Parmi les premiers qui ont adopté la pratique de Tuffier nous sommes, Daniel d'Almeida et moi, à essayer sa technique depuis le commencement de 1900.

Plusieurs thèses parues à Rio depuis 1901 confirment le succès de la méthode à Rio de Janeiro, telles sont celles de Campos da Paz (3), Cruz Moreira (4), Octacilio Pessoa (5).

A S. Paulo, notre confrère Oliveira Fausto (6), qui venait d'assister lui même à la manière de faire de Tuffier à l'hôpital Lariboisière, à Beaujon et à Gramont, a été aussi le premier à pratiquer dans le service de Amarante Cruz; il a obtenu les meilleurs résultats avec la cocaïne de Carrion et ses impressions, ainsi que l'étude de la ponction lombaire et les injections intrarachidiennes au Brésil jusqu'à 1902, font partie de son aperçu sur la chirurgie nerveuse rapporté par lui dans *l'État actuel de la chirurgie nerveuse*, de A. Chipault (7).

A Bahia, Cerquinta Lima, Lydio de Mesquita, Pacheco Mendes et d'autres l'ont pratiquée et Pereira de Carvalho (8) a écrit sa thèse sur ce sujet.

Jusqu'à la fin de 1902, Daniel d'Almeida et moi nous avons pratiqué plus de 300 opérations avec ce mode d'anesthésie, avec quelques modifications enseignées par la pratique et par l'acquisition de nouveaux produits.

Afin de supprimer ou, au moins, d'atténuer les troubles et les accidents qu'on a signalés à la suite de l'emploi des solutions de cocaïne, nous l'avons substituée par l'eucaïne z et par l'eucaïne β, sans avantages.

Après les recherches de Ravaut et Aubourg (9) sur la rachicocaïnisation, nous avons aussi adopté les solutions les plus concentrées que possible.

Quoique un peu moins et sans gravité, en tout cas, les accidents étaient encore lamentables, et n'encourageaient pas à insister devant les malades sur les avantages de la méthode, qui était toujours combattue par les adversaires qui s'appuyaient sur les accidents toujours redoutables.

La communication de Karl Schwarz (10) nous a indiqué un autre dérivé de la cocaïne jouissant des mêmes propriétés analgésiques, mais ayant une toxicité moindre, la *tropacocaïne*.

Tuffier (11) a considéré comme fugace ou nulle l'action des divers médicaments qu'on a tenté de substituer à la cocaïne, il ne parle que très légèrement des résultats obtenus à l'aide des solutions de tropacocaïne.

Ayant toujours en vue la conclusion de Guinard (12) sur les recherches de Ravaut et Aubourg, *que l'eau pure est un très mauvais véhicule pour la cocaïne, puisqu'à elle seule elle est nocive,* nous avons essayé de concentrer le plus possible les solutions de tropacocaïne.

En profitant de l'extrême solubilité de la tropacocaïne, Daniel d'Almeida a imaginé son procédé particulier de préparer et stériliser la solution la rendant le plus concentrée que possible, de manière à ce que chaque goutte contienne un centigramme du sel.

La solution de Daniel d'Almeida, rigoureusement préparée, est bien dosée et très bien stérilisée par l'ébullition, elle nous a donné toujours de bons résultats.

Ainsi, la ponction faite, le liquide céphalo-rachidien recueilli dans la seringue même, nous n'avons qu'à verser la quantité de gouttes de la solution telle que le nombre de centigrammes de tropacocaïne que nous voulons injecter.

Cette manière de procéder nous a aussi autorisés, Daniel d'Almeida et moi, à faire plusieurs communications à l'Académie de médecine, de Rio de Janeiro, à la Société de médecine et chirurgie, de Rio (13), et aussi des publications dans les revues de médecine (14). Vieira Souto (15), F. Vaz, Brandão Filho et d'autres chirurgiens ont suivi la pratique de Daniel d'Almeida.

La tropacocaïne que nous avons employée pendant presque trois ans ne nous a jamais donné des accidents graves; d'une valeur analgésique moindre que la cocaïne, il faudrait employer une quantité plus grande et, tout de même, l'analgésie de certaines régions n'était pas tout à fait complète, comme nous dirons ensuite.

Nous n'avons jamais dépassé la dose de 7 centigrammes pour chaque injection; ordinairement, 2 à 4 centigrammes, c'est assez pour les opérations qui ne demandent pas trop de temps.

Avec ce mode d'anesthésie nous avons pratiqué toutes les opérations sur les membres inférieurs, le périnée, la vessie, le vagin, l'anus et le rectum, les bourses, le testicule, le col de l'utérus et la région de l'aine; il faut déclarer pourtant, comme nous avons déjà annoncé, que même avec 7 centigrammes de tropacocaïne l'analgésie n'était pas complète dans le curettage de l'utérus, au moment de sa dilatation; aussi pour l'évidement de l'aine, la traction sur le cordon pendant les opérations de la hernie étaient douloureuses dans presque tous les opérés.

La découverte de Fourneau est venue pour affermir le crédit de la rachianalgésie; c'est la *stovaïne* qui vient de dire le dernier mot sur cette méthode, au commencement si combattue par des adversaires autorisés, mais qui changeront d'idées certainement devant le nombre de faits tous en sa faveur.

M. Sonnenburg (16) était réfractaire jusqu'ici à l'anesthésie médullaire par injection sous-arachnoïdienne de cocaïne ou de ses dérivés, en raison des effets toxiques parfois mortels qu'on a signalés à la suite de l'emploi de ces substances, mais il s'est laissé tenter par le nouvel anesthésique qu'on a substitué dans ces derniers temps à la cocaïne et qui, tout en possédant des propriétés anesthésiques aussi énergiques, est infiniment moins toxique. M. Sonnenburg a eu recours, jusqu'au mois de février 1905, 57 fois, dans son service de l'hôpital Moabit, à l'analgésie médullaire par injection sous-arachnoïdienne de stovaïne.

Présentée au monde médical par Reclus (17) dans son rapport sur la communication faite à l'Académie de médecine, de Paris, par Billon, lu en séance du 5 juillet 1904, la stovaïne a été expérimentée par le père de la cocaïne dans son service pendant plus de huit mois, et il a fini par proclamer ses qualités analgésiques et sa moindre toxicité.

Comme l'ont très bien écrit Keudirdjy et Berthaux (18), «la stovaïne, venue sous un tel patronage, ne pouvait que tenter ceux qui étaient restés fidèles — en principe du moins — à la rachianesthésie».

Le 7 mai de cette même année, Chaput (19) communiquait à la Société de biologie ses premiers essais d'injections sous-arachnoïdiennes de stovaïne et il conclut:

L'action analgésique de la stovaïne locale à $\frac{1}{200}$ est identique à celle de la cocaïne. La stovaïne est moins toxique que la cocaïne. Elle a une action vaso-dilatatrice qui, en congestionnant le bulbe, supprime la syncope et permet aux malades d'être opérés assis et de se lever aussitôt après l'opération. Pure ou associée à la cocaïne, la stovaïne améliore considérablement l'anesthésie lombaire, car elle ne fait pas pâlir les malades et elle supprime les chances de syncope. La stovaïnisation lombaire permet d'entreprendre toutes les laparotomies, même les plus difficiles, et de les conduire à bien quand les malades ne sont pas très émotifs.

Dans son étude pharmacodynamique de la stovaïne, le professeur Pouchet (20) considère aussi la stovaïne comme un des analgésiques locaux possédant en outre, à faible dose, des propriétés antithermiques manifestes. Elle possède une action analogue à celle de la cocaïne, elle abolit les propriétés vitales des cellules avec lesquelles elle vient en contact et agit comme poison du système nerveux central.

La toxicité beaucoup plus faible de la cocaïne, son action tonique sur le cœur, son pouvoir analgésique considérable, ses propriétés antiseptiques, en font un médicament auquel on peut prédire un bel avenir au point de vue thérapeutique.

Les expériences du professeur Lapersonne viennent aussi confirmer les résultats obtenus par Billon.

Au mois d'octobre 1904, Daniel d'Almeida et moi nous avons fait nos premières injections avec la stovaïne, nous basant sur les résultats que nous venons de lire.

Nous avons employé la solution préparée à la manière de Daniel d'Almeida, c'est-à-dire, que chaque goutte de la solution contenait un centigramme de *stovaïne*.

Depuis 1900 que nous avons pratiqué plus de 500 injections sous-arachnoïdiennes pour la rachianalgésie, nous avons commencé par la cocaïne et aujourd'hui nous n'employons plus que la stovaïne.

Chez une malade opérée 4 fois d'une fistule vésico-vaginale nous avons pratiqué, dans le délai de 2 ans et demi, 4 injections, une avec la cocaïne, deux avec la tropacocaïne et la dernière avec la stovaïne; cette malade qui auparavant avait été opérée dans un autre service par le chloroforme n'a plus jamais voulu l'anesthésie générale. Avec la dernière injection (avec la stovaïne) elle n'a en rien souffert après l'opération.

La méthode avec la stovaïne commence à obtenir la confiance de plusieurs confrères qui l'avaient abandonnée à cause des accidents de la cocaïne. Plusieurs de nos éminents confrères nous ont déjà honoré de leur confiance en nous permettant de pratiquer la rachistovaïnisation chez plusieurs de leurs opérés et le résultat ne s'est jamais fait attendre.

A S. Paulo aussi, la rachistovaïnisation a été pratiquée avec succès; nous devons à notre distingué confrère Oliveira Fausto nos remerciements pour les informations qu'il a bien voulu nous donner.

Oliveira Fausto (21) a pratiqué avec la solution de stovaïne à $^{40}/_{100}$ en 16 cas et il a obtenu 12 résultats positifs; deux cas importants, qu'il faut noter, furent: une extirpation de veines variqueuses et une suture osseuse avec une analgésie très complète.

Les cas négatifs, selon l'opinion de Oliveira Fausto, sont dus à la petite dose de stovaïne et les autres à un défaut de technique dans la stérilisation de la solution.

Il a observé dans un cas une parésie de la vessie qui a duré 48 heures.

La rachistovaïnisation n'a pas trouvé d'opposition à S. Paulo, nous rapporte Oliveira Fausto; d'autres confrères l'ont pratiquée avec succès. Amarante Cruz l'a pratiquée à l'Hôpital militaire, surtout dans les opérations sur les organes génitaux et sur le rectum;

Luiz do Rego l'a employée ainsi que notre confrère Camargo, de Limeira; Alves Lima l'a pratiquée dans plusieurs de ses opérations, relevant celle d'un cas d'hypospadias, avec bon succès; Baeta Neves en a réussi dans des prostatectomies; Oliveira Fausto, Arnaldo de Carvalho, Luiz do Rego et d'autres l'ont pratiquée aussi dans leurs cliniques privées.

Technique. — Nous nous sommes servis de la solution titrée par Daniel d'Almeida. Cette solution est stérilisée par l'ébullition et recueillie dans de petits flacons à compte-gouttes très bien fermés et protégés par du coton et de la gaze stérilisée. Avant de nous en servir nous avons toujours la précaution de flamber le flacon, de laisser couler une ou deux gouttes dehors, et, tout de suite après, le flacon est enveloppé avec du coton et de la gaze stérilisée, de manière que le même flacon avec une solution préparée depuis plus de 6 mois ne perd jamais son pouvoir analgésique ni ne devient septique.

Nos instruments sont seulement: une seringue en verre, de Luer, et une aiguille en platine iridié de 8 à 10 centimètres de longueur avec un biseau court à la manière de Tuffier.

Jamais nous n'employons le mandrin, quand l'aiguille est obturée nous essayons une légère aspiration avec la seringue; si l'on ne réussit pas, nous préférons retirer l'aiguille pour la planter en un point différent, ayant toujours soin de vérifier sa perméabilité au moyen de la seringue avec eau stérilisée.

Pour la ponction nous préférons le troisième espace lombaire, mais souvent nous ponctionnons le deuxième ou le quatrième, toujours à droite de la ligne médiane quand le patient est assis et de l'autre côté s'il est en décubitus gauche.

Avant de donner l'inclination à l'aiguille, en dedans et en haut, au moment de la piqûre, pour pénétrer les masses musculaires, nous la plaçons verticalement sur la peau, qui offre toujours plus de résistance à l'aiguille à biseau court et qui peut glisser et faire perdre les points de repère, et jamais on ne réussirait.

Cette précaution, qui semble inutile, est très importante surtout pour ceux qui n'ont pas l'habitude de la ponction lombaire et qui veulent suivre la technique telle qu'elle est décrite.

Il faut qu'on sache qu'un des plus grands embarras pour la divulgation de la méthode de la rachianalgésie n'est plus que la difficulté qu'éprouvent ceux qui essayent la ponction pour la première fois, sans y réussir; une ponction blanche de la première fois donne presque toujours naissance à un ennemi de la méthode; alors, il faut tâcher de montrer clairement tous les petits détails de la technique pour la rendre plus facile et accessible à tous les praticiens.

La position du malade doit être: assis en travers de la table, les pieds appuyant sur un tabouret de manière à faire gros dos. Dans quelques cas nous sommes forcés de faire la ponction dans le décubitus latéral et, quoique avec un petit peu de difficulté, on réussira.

Nous avons toujours la précaution de suivre l'avis de Tuffier, et nous répétons les mots: « *Je vais vous piquer, vous ne sentirez que peu de chose, ne bougez pas* »; avec cet avertissement nous n'avons jamais été surpris par un mouvement brusque ni jamais nous n'avons eu besoin de faire l'anesthésie de la peau.

Les détails de la technique ont été très bien décrits par Tuffier et aussi par Keudelly et Leguen et dernièrement dans le livre de Keudelly (22).

Ayant traversé le ligament jaune, l'aiguille entre facilement, et le liquide céphalo-rachidien paraît et suinte au bout de l'aiguille; cette preuve est indispensable pour être sûr qu'on a pénétré dans le canal rachidien.

Quand le liquide ne filtre pas et nous croyons avoir pénétré, nous faisons une petite aspiration avec la seringue pour déboucher l'aiguille, jamais nous n'injectons quoi que ce soit, ni nous n'employons le mandrin; nous sommes tranquilles avec cette manière de procéder.

Si le liquide apparaît, nous le recevons dans la seringue sur laquelle nous versons le nombre de gouttes de la solution de stovaïne que nous voulons, selon l'importance de l'opération.

Le mélange du liquide céphalo-rachidien et de la solution de stovaïne devient opalescent et un peu savonneux. Ensuite, on remet le corps de pompe de la seringue, on fait sortir l'air de l'intérieur de la seringue et on l'adapte à l'aiguille qui est en place et on repousse lentement; on n'a pas avantage à faire l'injection rapidement.

Nous employons la dose de 5 à 10 centigrammes selon la durée probable de l'opération, jamais nous n'avons eu d'accidents, il nous semble qu'au-dessous de 4 centigrammes l'analgésie ne s'obtient pas chez tous les malades.

La dose de 10 centigrammes, notre maximum, peut être dépassée sans produire aucun accident grave; nous avons vu injecter 12 centigrammes, sans la moindre perturbation. Au delà de 10 centigrammes on n'obtient pas une extension plus grande de la région anesthésiée, mais les grandes doses maintiennent pour longtemps la durée de l'anesthésie, c'est la raison pourquoi nous préférons, pour les opérations de longue durée, la dose de 10 centigrammes, quoique nous puissions obtenir la même analgésie avec 6 ou 8 centigrammes, seulement pendant moins de temps, et, une fois que le malade recommence à acquérir la sensibilité, il empêchera d'aller à la fin; il serait dégoûtant de faire une nouvelle ponction pour finir l'opération.

Statistique. — Notre statistique comprend seulement la série de rachistovaïnisations que nous avons pratiquées jusqu'au mois de mars dernier, dans le service de Daniel d'Almeida, à la 24e infirmerie de l'hôpital «Misericordia» de Rio de Janeiro, et dans notre clinique privée, aussi bien que dans celles de nos amis Fernando Vaz et Augusto Brandão Filho; elle comprend 193 cas comme suit:

1 amputation du pied.
4 amputations de la jambe.
4 amputations de la cuisse.
2 désarticulations métatarso-phalangiennes.
1 désarticulation du genou.
1 désarticulation coxo-fémorale (cas du prof. Pereira Guimaraes).
1 ablation de l'ongle du gros orteil.
2 phlegmons de la jambe.
3 phlegmons de la cuisse.
1 arthrite suppurée du genou.
1 extirpation d'hygroma prérotulien.
1 suture du fémur.

6 curettages osseux.

2 élongations forcées des genoux.

1 raclage du genou.

2 élongations du sciatique.

1 extirpation de veines variqueuses de la jambe.

1 extirpation d'un anévrysme supposé fémoral.

1 abcès et fistule crurale.

2 évidements de l'aine (1 cas, Vieira Souto).

11 cures radicales de hernie inguinale.

3 cures radicales de hernie ombilicale.

1 appendicite suppurée (cas Olympio Pereira).

1 anus iliaque.

8 circoncisions.

2 uréthrotomies externes.

12 cures radicales d'hydrocèle vaginal.

3 hématocèles.

3 tailles de Dupuytren.

29 grattages uterus.

21 hystérectomies vaginales.

17 cautérisations et raclage du col de l'utérus par cancer inopérable.

4 hystéropexies abdom. et périnéorraphies.

6 fistules vésico-vaginales.

2 cautérisations d'ulcère rectal.

3 abcès et fistules de l'anus.

1 papillome de l'anus.

11 cures d'hémorrhoïdes (Whitehead).

3 rectococcypexies.

1 amputation partielle du rectum.

9 rectotomies linéaires.

2 ablations de tumeur des fesses.

2 kystes dermoïdes de la région sacrococcygienne.

198

Nous devons signaler que le seul accident que nous ayons observé c'est la parésie de la vessie pendant 24 à 48 heures après l'opération sur le rectum, sur l'utérus et sur l'aine, surtout quand le thermocautère de Paquelin a été appliqué; nous savons que cela n'arrive pas seulement avec la stovaïne, au contraire, c'est un phénomène habituel des opérations dans ces régions avec le Paquelin. En tout cas, on n'en trouve pas toujours et l'accident ne persiste pas.

De tout ce que nous avons observé et de ce que nous a enseigné une pratique de plus de 1.000 rachianalgésies, nous pouvons conclure que:

1° La stovaïne remplace avec avantage la cocaïne dans la méthode de la rachianalgésie.

2° La rachistovaïnisation est la méthode de choix pour les opérations sur les membres inférieurs : le périnée, la vessie, le vagin, l'anus et le rectum, les bourses, le testicule, le col de l'utérus et la région inguinocrurale.

BIBLIOGRAPHIE

(1) *Quincke*: Die Lumbalpunction des Hydrocephalus, Berliner Klinische Wochenschrift, 21 sept. 1891, n.° 38.

(2) *J. M. Corrêa*: Valor diagnostico e therapeutico da puncção lombar. These, Rio, 1897.

(3) *Campos da Paz*: These, Rio de Janeiro; 1901.

(4) *Cruz Moreira*: These, Rio de Janeiro; 1903.

(5) *Octavião Pessoa*: These, Rio de Janeiro; 1905.

(6) *Oliveira Fausto*: Revista Medica de S. Paulo, n.° 10, anno IV, 31 de maio de 1904.

(7) *Oliveira Fausto*: A. Chipault — L'état actuel de la chirurgie nerveuse. Tome troisième, pag. 800, Paris 1903.

(8) *O. Pereira de Carvalho*: Analgesia cirurgica por meio das injecções sub-arachnoideanas lombares de cocaina, Th. de Bahia, 1902.

(9) *Ravaut et Arbeury*: Le liquide céphalo-rachidien après la rachicocaïnisation, Gazette des Hopitaux, pag. 608, 1901.

(10) *Karl Schwarz*: Zur Frage der medullaren Narkose, Centralblatt für Chirurgie, n.° 9, 1901.

(11) *Tuffier*: La Rachicocaïnisation, Paris, C. Naud, 1901, pag. 23.

(12) *Guinard*: XIV Cong. franç. de chir., Paris, 22 oct., 1901, in Presse Médicale, 13 nov. 1901, pag. 277.

(13) *Daniel d'Almeida*: Analgesia pela tropacocaina, Sociedade de medicina e cirurgia, 29 de outubro de 1901, Brazil Medico, 1901, pag. 416.

(14) *Alvaro Ramos*: Analgesia cirurgica por via subarachnoideana pela tropacocaina, Brazil Medico, anno XVI, n.° 33, 1.° setembro 1902, pag. 325.

(15) *Vieira Souto*: Anesthesia cirurgica pela cocaina, Academia nacional de medicina, 9 de maio de 1901.

(16) *Sonnenburg*: Réunion libre des chirurgiens de Berlin, Presse Médicale, 12 avril 1905, pag. 229.

(17) *Reclus*: L'analgésie locale par la stovaïne, Presse Médicale, 9 juillet 1904, pag. 433.

(18) *L. Kendirdjy et R. Berthaux*: L'anesthésie chirurgicale par injection sous-arachnoïdienne de stovaïne, Presse Médicale, 15 octobre 1904, pag. 660.

(19) *Chaput*: Presse Médicale 14 mai 1904, pag. 311.

(20) *Pouchet*: Bulletin de l'Académie de médecine de Paris, 12 juillet 1904.

(21) *Oliveira Fausto*: Lettre du 5 janvier 1906.

(22) *Kendirdjy (Dr. Léon)*: L'anesthésie chirurgicale par la stovaïne, Paris, 1906.

Die Thymus-Stenose und der Thymus-Tod.

Par M. L. Rehn, Frankfurt a. Main.

Meine Herren!

Ich würde Ihre Zeit heute nicht in Anspruch nehmen, wenn die Störungen der Gesundheit von Seiten einer grossen Thymus ausgesuchte Seltenheiten wären, gewissermassen ein Curiosum. Das ist sicher nicht der Fall. Schon die eine Tatsache mag Ihnen zu denken geben, dass einzelne Autoren über eine Reihe von Fällen verfügen — ich selbst sah deren fünf. — Zweimal habe ich mit Erfolg operiert, dreimal erlebte ich einen völlig unerwarteten und deshalb um so erschütternden tötlichen Ausgang. Ich führe Sie freilich auf ein sehr strittiges Gebiet. Dunkel wie die Physiologie der Drüse ist ihre Pathologie. Nur bezüglich der rein mechanischen Wirkungen beginnt sich der Schleier zu lüften. Und gerade hierfür erbitte ich Ihre Aufmerksamkeit. Dann wird sich schon die alte Erfahrung geltend machen, dass ein anscheinend seltenes Krankheitsbild um so häufiger wird, je mehr der Blick des Arztes dafür geschärft ist. Und ich darf die sichere Hoffnung aussprechen, dass bei richtiger Deutung des Krankheitsbildes manch junges Menschenleben durch einen relativ einfachen Eingriff gerettet werden wird.

Sie wissen Alle, welche bedeutsame Rolle die Thymus schon einmal in der Geschichte der Medicin gespielt hat. Es würde sich gewiss verlohnen, historisch der Entwicklung der Lehre von den Schädigungen durch eine grosse Thymus nachzugehen. Das sei einem Anderen überlassen. Für uns genügt zu wissen, dass die Thymus im 17ten, 18ten und der ersten Hälfte des 19ten Jahrhunderts bestimmt als eine Ursache von Atmungsbehinderungen angesprochen wird. Es wurde i. J. 1821 sogar von Allan Burns auf Grund zweier Leichenversuchen ein Verfahren angegeben, die Drüse zu entfernen. Astley Cooper (Anhang 1) hinterliess eine vortreffliche anatomische Arbeit über die Thymus. Am Schlusse derselben schildert er eine bemerkenswerte Erkrankung, über die er sich in vivo nicht klar werden kann. Ein 19 jähriges Mädchen mit Kropf ging unter chron. zunehmender Atemnot kachektisch zu Grunde. Die Sektion deckte eine grosse Thymus auf — Cooper spricht von einem Thymus-Schwamm — es war aber offenbar nur eine grosse Thymus persistens. Diese Thymus und nicht etwa der Kropf hatte, wie Cooper ausdrücklich hervorhebt, die Luftröhre durch Umwachsen seitlich zusammengedrückt und dadurch zum

Tode geführt. Zum ersten Male meines Wissens ist damit das gleichzeitige Vorkommen von Kropf und Thymus persistens, zum ersten Male die deutliche Druckspur einer grossen Thymus an der Luftröhre beschrieben. Es ist auffallend, dass Cooper in seiner Epikrise, obwohl er Burns vorher bei der Beschreibung der Fascien erwähnt, nichts von der Möglichkeit einer Operation spricht.

Wie so oft in der Medicin die Bedeutung einer Tatsache überschätzt, eine richtige Beobachtung kritiklos zur Erklärung anderer dunkler Krankheitserscheinungen herangezogen wird, so geschah es auch bei der Thymus. Kopp (¹) setzte alle Fälle von Laryngospasmus auf Rechnung der Thymus und nun folgte die Arbeit Friedlebens (²), eine äusserst sorgfältige mühsame Studie, welche so gründlich mit allen bisherigen Anschauungen aufräumte, dass das Wahre an der Sache mit allen Hypothesen für Jahre hinaus begraben wurde. Noch heute beherrscht Friedleben's Lehre in ihrer reinen Negation die Köpfe der Aerzte. «Es giebt keinen Druck von Seiten der Thymus weder auf die Atmungsorgane, noch auf Gefässe oder Nerven». Vergeblich erklärte Virchow (³) auf Grund seiner Erfahrung, es gäbe doch eine solche Compression. Auch Cohnheim's (⁴) Stimme verhallte ungehört. Vergeblich traten immer wieder einzelne Aerzte auf, welche gestützt auf ihre Beobachtungen für die Existenz eines Thymustodes eintraten, so Clar (Anh. 2) und Abelin (Anh. 18).

Erst in den letzten Jahrzehnten kam ein allmählicher Umschwung. Somma (Anh. 3) beschrieb im Jahre 1884 zwei Thymus-Todesfälle, deren einer eine Compression der Luftröhre in Gestalt von Druckmarken erkennen liess. Das war ein sehr wichtiger Befund. Neben Anderen traten Hennig (Anh. 29), Pott (Anh. 27), Grawitz (Anh. 26), Beneke (Anh. 5) lebhaft für das Vorkommen eines Thymus-Todes ein. Das Interesse der Gerichtsärzte wurde wachgerufen.

Vor 10 Jahren hatte ich dann Gelegenheit am Lebenden den Nachweis zu führen, dass die Thymus schwere Atmungsstörungen hervorrufen kann (⁵). Bald darauf wurden von Fritz König (⁶),

---

(¹) Kopp. Denkwürdigkeiten in der ärztl. Praxis, 1830.
(²) Friedleben. Die Physiologie der Thymus. Frankfurt a/M, 1855.
(³) Virchow. Die krankh. Geschwülste, Berlin 1863. Band II.
(⁴) Cohnheim. Allgemeine Pathologie, 1880, Band II.
(⁵) E. Bircher. Ueber die Pathologie der Thymus. Berl. klinische Wochenschrift, 1896, n.° 40.

(⁶) König. Centralblatt f. Chirurgie, 1897, n.° 21.

dann von Purrucker (¹), in letzter Zeit von Ehrhardt (Anh. 15), durch operative Eingriffe an der Thymus schwere Erstickungssymptome beseitigt. Ich habe kürzlich einen weiteren Fall operiert. Unterdessen haben sich auch die Fälle rasch vermehrt, die Druckmarken an den Luftwegen erkennen liessen, so dass wohl der ungläubigste Arzt die Möglichkeit einer Compression der Luftwege von Seiten der Thymus einräumen muss. Wohlverstanden, es handelt sich hier nicht um den Druck maligner Neubildungen des Thymus-Gewebes, sondern um grosse, hyperplast. Brustdrüsen.

Bekanntlich hat von Recklinghausen gegenüber Nordmann (²) die Bedeutung der Thymus hinsichtlich dreier von letzterem beschriebenen Todesfälle geleugnet und den exitus als Herzschlag lymphat. Individuen bezeichnet. A. Paltauf (³) hat sich von Recklinghausen angeschlossen und alle sogenannten Thymus-Todesfälle auf Rechnung einer lymphat. chlorot. Constitution gesetzt. Er hat die Lehre vom status lymphat. resp. thymicus aufgestellt. Individuen dieser Art sind fett, haben oft eine enge Aorta und sind widerstandslos. Paltauf leugnet jeden Einfluss der Thymus auf den üblen Ausgang des Leidens und verlangte von seinen Gegnern den Nachweis, dass die Luftröhre wirklich beengt gewesen sei.

Dieser Standpunkt lässt sich heute nicht mehr festhalten, nachdem durch die Autopsie und beim Lebenden schwere Compression der Luftwege nachgewiesen ist. Es kann sich nur noch darum handeln, ob im gegebenen Fall eine gross Thymus für den Tod verantwortlich gemacht werden kann, wenn Druckspuren an den Luftwegen fehlen. Weigert pflegte darauf hinzuweisen, dass man den Druck einer Thymus nur durch eine besondere Art der Sectionstechnik erkennen könne. Die gewöhnliche Technik wäre dazu unbrauchbar. Das ist sicherlich sehr wahr und wird mehr und mehr anerkannt. Nach meiner Ansicht wird manchmal auch die zuverlässigste Art von Section ein negatives Resultat ergeben, weil sich die Teile nach dem Tode noch verschieben können und Druckmarken trotz eines Erstickungstodes nicht vorhanden zu sein brauchen.

Immerhin hat gewiss Paltauf insofern Recht, als eine Vergrösserung der Thymus nicht selten mit einer Hyperplasie des

---

(¹) Purrucker, Medic. Gesellschaft Magdeburg, 26. Mai 1899.
(²) Nordmann, Korrespondenzblatt der Schweizer Aerzte, 1889.
(³) Paltauf, Wiener klin. Wochenschr. 1889, 1890, Berl. klin. Wochenschr. 1896.

lymphat. Apparates vergesellschaftet ist, er hat vielleicht Recht,
wenn er meint, dass Erkrankungen dieser Art mit einer geringen
Widerstandskraft des Individuums einhergehen. Hedinger (¹) teilt
mit, dass er bei seinen Untersuchungen bezügl. eines Thymus-
Todesfalls mit status lymphat. Befunde erhoben habe, welche für
Uebergänge zur Pseudoleukaemie und Leukaemie sprechen.

Wir werden nun sehen, dass es unter den beschriebenen
Thymus-Todesfällen eine Anzahl giebt, welche der strengsten Kritik
bezügl. einer Tracheo-Broncho-Stenosis thymica Stand halten, dass
eine weitere Zahl nicht ohne Zwang anders erklärt werden kann,
endlich dass ein gewisser Rest verschiedene Deutungen zulässt
je nach dem Standpunkt, welchen man einnimmt.

Die anatomie der thymus

Es ist wohl als sicher anzunehmen, dass die Thymus im em-
bryonalen Leben eine grosse Rolle spielt. Nach Beard entstehen
in der Thymus die ersten Leukocyten. Die Drüse nimmt bis zum
zweiten Lebensjahr an Grösse zu. Später wächst sie noch in die
Länge, gewöhnlich auf Kosten der Dicke. Reste der Drüse sind
bis in das späteste Lebensalter nachzuweisen (Waldeyer [²], Dwornitschenko [³]). Es kommt aber gar nicht selten vor, dass nach dem
zweiten Lebensjahr die Drüse in aussergewöhnlicher Weise wächst.
Bekanntlich sind auch bei Erwachsenen abnorm grosse Thymus-
Drüsen gefunden worden, namentlich bei Leukaemie, bei Morbus
Basedow, oder einfachen Kröpfen.

Die Form der Drüse ist so verschieden, dass man kaum eine
Regel aufstellen kann. Im Allgemeinen kann man sagen, dass sie
aus einem rechten und linken Lappen besteht, welche wie ein Pol-
ster zwischen die Mediastinal-Blätter und die grossen Gefässe hin
eingeschoben sind und nach unten hin dem Herzbeutel anliegen. Die Drüse ist von einer festen Kapsel eingeschlossen, welche dünne Septa in das Parenchym schickt. Diese Kapsel bildet
einen weiten Sack, in welchem der Drüsensubstanz mehr oder
weniger Bewegungsfreiheit gelassen ist. Will man über den man.
sterni die Drüse selbst freilegen, so muss man das der Hinterfläche der m. m. sterno hyoid. anliegende Fascienblatt spalten.

(¹) Hedinger. Deutsches Archiv f. klin. Medicin, 13 Dez. 1905.
(²) Waldeyer. Die Rückbildung der Thymus. Sitzungsbericht der Kgl. Preuss. Akademie der
Wissensch., Berlin, 1890.
(³) Dwornitschenko. Vierteljahrschrift für gerichtliche Medicin, 3 f., Bd. 14.

Man gelangt dann in das Spatium praetracheale, in welches die beiden Lappen mit ihren oberen spitz zulaufenden Enden von der Thymuskapsel überzogen hineinragen. An der Kapsel kann man die Drüse ziemlich weit hervorziehen. Man erkennt bei der Praeparation, dass sich das vordere Blatt der Kapsel in aufwärts geschwungenem Bogen an beiden Seiten in die Gefässscheide der Arteria carotis und vena jugularis fortsetzt. Die hintere Kapselwand geht in die praetracheale Fascie über, derart, dass nach der Schilddrüse hin ein mehr und minder ausgedehnter Raum entsteht. Bei starker Exspiration kann sich die Drüsensubstanz in diesen Raum vorwölben und wird dann als weiche Geschwulst wahrgenommen.

Die Kapsel ist mit dem sternum lose verwachsen, dagegen fest mit dem Herzbeutel und den Gefässen. Eine Totalexstirpation der Drüse mitsammt der Kapsel erscheint unausführbar, wohl aber kann man eine Ausschälung der Drüsensubstanz vornehmen.

Die Gefässversorgung ist nicht überall die gleiche. Für gewöhnlich laufen von der Art. thyreoid. inf. zwei Gefässstämmchen nach dem oberen Pol, und seitlich in die Drüse je ein Ast von der Art. mam. int. Die Venen sind stärker entwickelt. Die oberen münden in die thyreoid. ma. resp. inferior, die unteren in die v. v. anonym. und mamm. int. seltener Azygos und Hemiazygos.

Die dem Brustbein zugekehrte Seite der Drüse ist gewöhnlich glatt. Wichtiger ist die vertebrale Seite. Sie schmiegt sich beim Wachstum offenbar den gegebenen Formen an und schafft sich Nischen innerhalb der Kapsel, wo sie den geringsten Widerstand findet.

Die Drüse deckt bekanntlich zungenförmig auslaufend den oberen Teil des Herzbeutels, weiter nach oben vena anonym. sin., die art. anonym, und schiebt sich in den keilförmigen Raum zwischen art. anonym. u. carot. dextr. einerseits, art. carot. sin. andererseits, so dass sie auf die Trachea zu liegen kommt. Im Grossen und Ganzen kann man sagen, dass die Gefässe ihren Platz gegenüber dem Wachstum einer Thymus-Drüse zu behaupten wissen. Sie werden nicht selten umwachsen, aber nicht ohne dass sie sich weite Rinnen in der Drüsensubstanz gebildet haben. Für die unter einem hohen Druck stehenden Arterien ist das nicht wunderbar, weit eher sollte man in gewissen Fällen Verlegung der v. anonym. sin. erwarten. Doch scheint es ein seltenes Ereignis zu sein. Ich denke mir, dass der anormale Verlauf der

v. anonym. sin. vor der Drüse sternalwärts (v. Mettenheimer [1])
durch eine allmähliche Druckatrophie der Drüse zu Stande kommt,
worauf sich unter der Vene die Drüse wieder zusammenlegt.

Einer Entwicklung der Drüse in den oben geschilderten Raum
nach der Trachea hin sind günstige Bedingungen geboten. Hier
kann sie sich der Dicke nach ausbreiten und zwar direct nach
der Vorderseite der Trachea hin, wie auf die Seitenfläche derselben.

Die Nervi phrenici laufen seitlich dicht an der Drüsenkapsel.

Der linke n. vagus sowie der linke n. recurrens kommen mit
der Drüse in nächste Nachbarschaft.

Die eigentlichen Drüsennerven stammen, wie sehr lange
schon bekannt ist, vom Sympathicus.

Lymphgefässe sind spärlich.

Es giebt nur wenige Menschen, welche die Thymus oder wenigstens einen Teil derselben am Lebenden beobachten konnten.
Ich möchte nicht verfehlen auf Röntgendurchleuchtung hinzuweisen. Es scheint mir wichtig zu betonen, dass die Thymus sich
mit der Atmung verschiebt. Bei der Inspiration steigt sie in den
Brustraum hinab, bei der Ausatmung steigt sie herauf. Je forcier-
ter die Atmung, um so stärker ist ihr Excursion. Hat man die
feste Thymus-Kapsel gespalten, so kann man an der Drüse selbst
diese Bewegungen in aller Schärfe wahrnehmen. Die Drüse
wird bei tiefem Einatmen gleichsam aspiriert und bei starker
Ausatmung, beim Schreien, beim Husten aus dem Brustraum
hervorgepresst. Das letzte Symptom kann geradezu pathognomo-
nisch sein, indem sich bei Kindern mit grosser Thymus nicht
selten im Jugulum eine deutliche kleine Geschwulst bildet, welche die Fascien des Halses mitsammt den m. m. sternohyoid.
hervorwölbt. Dieses Verhalten der Drüse erklärt uns, dass bei einer Vergrösserung derselben so oft nur die Einatmung gehemmt
ist. Die Drüse wirkt ventilartig. Je ruhiger das Einatmen, desto geringer ist die Beengung, je tiefer je gewaltsamer, desto schwerer.
Das lässt sich mit aller Sicherheit behaupten.

Für die Richtigkeit dieser Darstellung bürgt auch der operative Erfolg in meinem ersten Fall, indem durch Anziehen und Fest-
nähen der Drüse das Atmungshindernis dauernd gehoben wurde.

---

[1] v. Mettenheimer. Jahrbuch f. Kinderheilkunde. Band 56.

Es ist zweifellos, dass nicht alle Fälle so liegen. Wir brauchen uns bloss vorzustellen, und diese Vorstellung entspricht öfters der Wirklichkeit, dass Drüsenteile die Luftröhre seitlich umwachsen haben. Dann wird ein Druck auf das Luftrohr gegeben sein, welcher nicht durch einfaches Anziehen der Kapsel gehoben werden kann. Es kann auch vorkommen, dass eine sehr dicke Drüse einen dauernden Druck ausübt, nicht bei der Exspiration gelüftet wird, oder dass eine Drüse, wie ein Fall Beneke's zeigt, gewissermassen im Mediastinum festgeklemmt sitzt. Dann würde man auch ein Hinderniss bei der Ausatmung erwarten müssen. In acut verlaufenden Fällen der Ventilwirkung wird man vergeblich nach Druckmarken an den Luftwegen suchen. Auch in chronischen Fällen wird man sie öfters vermissen, da bei jeder Ausatmung die Luftröhre frei wird, der Druck sich rasch wieder ausgleicht. «Bleibende Druckmarken sind in der Regel nur bei dauerndem Druck zu erwarten.»

Wir erkennen, dass die Form der Drüse eine grosse Rolle spielt. Es ist bekannt, wie ausserordentlich verschieden diese Form ist. Eine lang gestreckte flache Drüse ist vielleicht ganz bedeutungslos für unsere Betrachtung, eine kurze dicke, keilförmig nach hinten ragende macht weit eher schwere Störungen. Das Gewicht der Drüse allein ist nicht ausschlaggebend. Der Chirurg wird mit Erstaunen lesen, dass Scheele [1] nach Experimenten das Gewicht festgestellt hat, welches im Stande ist, eine Luftröhre zusammenzudrücken, und auf Grund dieser Feststellung es ablehnt, dass je eine Thymus die Luftröhre beengen könne. Welchem Chirurg würde es wohl einfallen, einen substernalen Kropfknoten, welcher die Luftwege beengt, zu wiegen. Die Thymus wirkt nicht durch ihr Gewicht, sondern durch Pressung in einem engen Raum.

Naturgemäss entsteht nun die Frage, wie verhält sich die Luftröhre gegen diese Pressung, wie weit kann sie einem Druck answeichen, welchen Widerstand kann sie leisten. Ich denke, je näher der Bifurcation, je weniger Bewegungsfreiheit hat die Luftröhre. Je gespannter sie ist, wie bei einem starken Rückwärtsbeugen des Kopfes, um so mehr ist sie in ihrer Lage festgehalten. In Zukunft wird man mehr darauf achten müssen, ob das Luftrohr im Ganzen abgesehen von Druckmarken eine besondere Weichheit erkennen lässt.

Es schliesst sich die weitere Frage an, an welcher Stelle der

Luftröhre der Druck der Thymus angreift. Das ist offenbar ganz verschieden. Die wenigen Operationen haben eins ergeben, dass der Druck nicht in der Höhe des oberen Randes des man. sterni stattfand, sondern tiefer. Er kann aber bewiesenermassen auch einmal in der Höhe der man. sterni, der grössten Enge der Brustapertur einwirken. Barack (Anh. 4), Strassmann und Flügge (Anh. 12) haben mit gutem Grunde die Ansicht aufgestellt, dass gerade dort, wo die art. anonyma schräg über die Trachea hinwegläuft, die ominöse Druckstelle zu suchen sei. Herr Stabsarzt Drüner, commandiert zu meiner Abteilung, hält gestützt auf die embryologischen Forschungen diese Stelle für besonders geeignet zu einer Compression bei Neugeborenen. Im Uebrigen findet man an positiven Befunden d. h. an sichtbaren Verengerungen der Trachea bald seitliche Compression, bald Abplattung von vorn nach hinten, oder im schrägen Durchmesser, ja es giebt Befunde, welche vornehmlich eine Compression eines Hauptbronchus erkennen lassen. Das ist ja auch ganz natürlich. Es giebt kein Schema in dieser Beziehung. So wechselvoll die Form der Thymus ist, so verschieden ist die Druckstelle.

Flügge hat eine zweite Druckwirkung der Thymus festgestellt, nämlich die seitliche Verschiebung der mediastinalen Gebilde.

Eine mündliche Mitteilung des Herrn Dr. Demmer spricht dafür, dass eine Thymus neben der Luftröhre sogar den Oesophagus comprimieren kann.

Wenn wir uns bezüglich weiterer Schlüsse auf absolut gesichertem Boden bewegen wollen, dann dürfen wir vorläufig nur unsere Operationsfälle sowie die Sektionsergebnisse in Betracht ziehen, welche Druckspuren an den Luftwegen erkennen liessen. Denn hier sind alle Zweifel an einer Compression von Seiten der Thymus ausgeschlossen. Ich habe im Anhang 28 Sektionsbefunde und einen operativen Nachweis von Verengerung der Luftwege zusammengestellt. Was lehren uns diese Fälle ganz im allgemeinen? Eine grosse Thymus kann allmählich oder plötzlich die Atmung behindern. Hauptsächlich gefährdet sind Säuglinge. Aber auch das spätere Kindesalter ist vertreten.

Lassen sich aus dieser immerhin sehr beachtenswerten Anzahl von Fällen Analogie-Schlüsse ziehen? Ich denke diese Frage bejahen zu müssen. Sie bilden Paradigmata. Avellis (¹) sah den qualvollen Erstickungstod eines Kindes mit grosser Thymus.

____

(¹) Avellis. Arch. f. Laryng. und Rhinol., Band VIII. Münch. medic. Wochenschr., 1898.

Dieser Fall führte ihn zum Studium der einschlägigen Literatur. Er kam zu dem Schlusse, dass der sogenannte Stridor der Säuglinge auf Thymus-Hyperplasie beruhe. Diese Erkrankung gilt in den Kreisen der Kinderärzte und Laryngologen als eine meist harmlose, spontan heilende Atmungsstörung.

Pröbsting (¹) schliesst sich Avellis an und in letzter Zeit hat Hochsinger eine höchst bemerkenswerte Arbeit über diese Erkrankung geschrieben. Er beobachtete 20 derartiger Fälle und konnte durch das Röntgenbild die Vergrösserung der Thymus nachweisen. Es ist zu hoffen, dass in Zukunft das Röntgenbild bei der Diagnose der Krankheit wichtige Fingerzeige geben wird.

*

Meine Herren! In der Tat, wenn man das Bild des inspirat. Säuglingsstridor mit unseren operativen Erfahrungen vergleicht, so wird man überzeugt, dass es sich um ein und dasselbe Krankheitsbild handelt, dass die Thymus weit öfter Compressions-Erscheinungen der Luftwege hervorruft als wir bisher angenommen haben. Diese Atmungsstörungen gehen allerdings sehr oft vorüber, heilen spontan, aber harmlos sind sie wohl niemals. Sie bedürfen der genauesten Ueberwachung, und die Zeit erst wird entscheiden, wie man sich therapeutisch am Besten zu verhalten hat.

Wenn wir das Wesen der Stenosis thymica richtig erfassen wollen, so müssen wir die enorme Gefahr plötzlicher Zufälle, von Katarrhen der Luftwege in Betracht ziehen, die schweren Erkrankungen dieser Art im Auge behalten und vor allem beherzigen, dass der Stridor thymicus nicht allein dem Säuglingsalter angehört, sondern auch bei älteren Kindern beobachtet wird.

Das Krankheitsbild muss weiter gefasst werden! Nehmen wir einen zweiten Fall! Ein Kind lässt von Geburt an ein leichtes Einsinken des Jugulum erkennen. Beim Weinen wird das inspirat. Einsinken stärker, es steigert sich bis zum inspirat. Stridor und zur Cyanose. Wird das Kind beruhigt, so wird das Atmen wieder geräuschlos. Im Anfall d. h. bei Erregung würde jeder Arzt an Glottiskrampf denken. Selbst ein so erfahrener Arzt wie Moritz Schmidt stellte in dem zuerst von mir operierten Fall diese Diagnose. Andere Kinder haben beständig den inspirat. Stridor. Wieder andere lassen daneben auch Störungen der Exspiration erkennen. Bald ist die Stenose von der Geburt an zu

---

(¹) Pröbsting. Münch. medic. Wochenschr., 1902.

beobachten, bald tritt sie später auf. Bald verläuft sie unter chronischen Beschwerden, stört das Befinden auffallend wenig, bald setzt sie acut ein mit heftiger Dyspnoe, geht vorüber, um rasch völligem Wohlbefinden Platz zu machen, vielleicht dauernd, oder sie endigt im zweiten oder dritten acuten Anfall mit dem Tod. Natürlich kann auch der erste Anfall letal endigen. Avellis beschreibt einen solchen. Ein stets gesunder, überaus kräftiger Knabe von 4 Jahren, erkrankt eines Morgens nach dem Frühstück an plötzlicher Atemnot mit inspirat. Stridor. Avellis sah noch den Erstickungstod. In zwei Stunden war der Knabe gesund und tot. Die Section ergab als Atmungshindernis eine blutreiche, namentlich in ihrem Dicken-Durchmesser vergrösserte Thymus.

Soweit halte ich das klinische Bild der stenosis thymica für gesichert. Vollkommen gesichert ist auch das familiäre Vorkommen. Avellis stellt es fest. Moritz Schmidt (¹) sah drei Kinder einer Familie an chron. Säuglingsstridor sterben, ein viertes Kind litt auch an Stridor, blieb aber am Leben. Und nun bitte ich die Fälle in Betracht zu ziehen, welche von plötzlichen Thymus-Todesfällen in einer Familie bekannt geworden sind. So erzählt schon Felix Platen (²) von drei Kindern einer Familie, welche unter heftiger Dyspnoe zu Grunde gehen. Aehnliches berichteten Weber, Barack; in letzter Zeit Hedinger u. a. a. Wir sehen also, dass nicht nur ein familiäres Vorkommen des Säuglingsstridor, sondern auch der Thymus-Hyperplasie und des Thymus-Todes festgestellt ist.

*

Können wir nun auf Grund unserer Erkenntnis eine kurze kritische Betrachtung der vielen strittigen Thymus-Todesfälle wagen? Wir wollen versuchen, Anhaltspunkte für unser Urteil zu gewinnen. Ich habe im Anhang eine weitere Reihe dieser Fälle zusammengestellt. Es sind 26 an der Zahl. Sieben davon wurden tracheotomiert. Allen diesen Todesfällen gingen prodromale Stenose-Erscheinungen voraus. Keiner zeigte eine anatomisch nachweisbare Beengung der Luftwege. Der letzte Umstand kann sowohl von der Art der Section abhängig gewesen sein, als davon, dass in der Tat eine Beengung in der Leiche nicht mehr vorhanden war. Nichtsdestoweniger müssen wir diese Todesfälle als Thymus-Wirkung anerkennen, gleichgültig ob die Kinder erstickten oder

<hr>

(¹) Moritz Schmidt. Halskrankheiten.
(²) Cité d'après Baginsky (Arb. ...

einige wenige derselben am Herztod gestorben sind. Wir denken
dabei nicht an eine Compression des Herzens, sondern an die
Schädigung des Herzens durch chronische Atemnot. Vielleicht
werden wir später einmal von einem Thymus-Herz reden, wie
jetzt von einem Kropfherzen. Die Mehrzahl obiger Fälle ist wohl
erstickt. Für die unter Stridor Verstorbenen ist es sicher.

Wie steht es nun mit den plötzlichen Todesfällen ohne
Vorboten? Einen Teil derselben haben wir bereits erledigt. Es
sind die Fälle mit mit deutlichen Spuren der Verengerung an
den Luftwegen. Der plötzliche Tod war mehr oder weniger lange
vorbereitet. Ein anderer Teil starb unter unzweideutigen Er-
stickungs-Symptomen. Da sich kein anderes Hindernis fand, als
eine grosse Thymus, so ist die Sache klar. In einer Anzahl erfolgte der Tod unbeobachtet oder so rasch, dass man kaum eine sichere Entscheidung treffen kann. Hören wir Hedinger an! In einer
Familie starben fünf Kinder mit und ohne prodromale Anfälle eines blitzähnlichen Todes unter starker Cyanose d.h. unter ähnlichen Erscheinungen wie sie Pott so classisch bei seinen Thymus-
Todesfällen geschildert hat. Die Kinder standen im Alter von 3-6
Jahren. Die Section des letzten Kindes ergab neben Thymus-Hyperplasie den stat. lymphat. Ein sechstes überstand einen schweren
Anfall und blieb am Leben. Hedinger gibt an, dass die prodroma-
len bedrohlichen Anfälle sehr bald von völligem Wohlbefinden
gefolgt waren. Spricht das für chronische Herzerkrankung? Doch
sicherlich nicht! Höchstens für acute Herzcompression.

Behalten wir einstweilen nur die Fälle im Auge, wo es sich
um anscheinend ganz gesunde Kinder handelt. Hier kommt in Frage
acuter Herztod durch Compression der grossen Gefässstämme
oder totale Aufhebung der Luftzufuhr. Sei dem wie dem sei! Die
Ursache liegt offenbar darin, dass eine plötzliche Aenderung in
den Raumverhältnissen des Mediastinums eintritt. Das kann in zwei-
facher Weise stattfinden. Entweder ist die Thymus gewissen Schwankungen ihres Volumens unterworfen, oder der ihr angewiesene
Raum wird plötzlich enger. Letzteres wird natürlich sofort eintreten, wenn sich Hals und obere Brustwirbelsäule lordotisch aus-
biegen. Es ist bezeichnend, dass diese Haltung bei so vielen plötzlichen Thymus-Todesfällen erwähnt wird, und überaus wahrscheinlich, dass diese Haltung allein genügt, in einzelnen Fällen
übergrosser Thymus tödliche Wirkungen herbeizuführen. Im Uebrigen aber sollte man meinen, dass nur Säuglinge, oder Kinder mit
kraftlosen vorderen Halsmuskeln, oder Menschen in Narkose so

sterben können, gewiss aber kein Mensch, der im Stande ist, sofort den Kopf vorwärts zu beugen.

Wir sind geradezu gewungen, bei gewissen Thymus-Todesfällen acute Anschwellungen der Drüse anzuschuldigen. Denken Sie an den Fall Avellis! Dieses acute Auftreten der Stenose-Erscheinungen der Luftwege, das anfallsweise Wiederkehren bei freien Intervallen lässt nur die eine Deutung zu. Der Streit über dieses Thema ist alt. Erst weitere sehr genaue Untersuchungen können ihn entscheiden. So lange diese ausstehen, müssen wir uns behelfen. Bekannt ist, dass der Turgor der Drüse je nach ihrer sekretorischen Tätigkeit wechselt. Die kleinen Arterien der Drüse sprechen nicht gerade für die Wahrscheinlichkeit einer plötzlichen arteriellen Hyperaemie. Wohl aber kann man vom gehemmten Venen-Abfluss eine Stauungshyperaemie erwarten. Die plötzlichen Todesfälle bei Kropf resp. Morbus Basedow und Thymus persistens lassen wohl kaum eine andere Deutung zu, als dass durch Veränderung der Blutcirculation eine rasche Anschwellung der Drüse zu Stande kommen kann. Ich erlebte, dass ein junges Mädchen mit Morbus Basedow nach glatter Operation einige Stunden später suffokatorisch zu Grunde ging. Die Sektion (Weigert) deckte als einzig nachweisbaren Befund eine sehr grosse Thymus persistens auf. Ich weiss hier keine andere Erklärung als, dass der Unterbindung der art. thyreoid. inf. und der unteren Venen eine Blutüberfüllung der Thymus folgte, welche direct zum Erstickungstode führte. (Siehe Gluck [1] u. a., auch Dwornitschenko.) Wenn wir sehen, dass ein Kind mit stenosis thymica beim Weinen cyanotisch wird und sofort stärkere Atembeschwerden bekommt, so möchte man doch eine momentane Stauungshyperämie sowie ein Anschwellen der Thymus nicht von der Hand weisen. Es muss aber noch andere Ursachen geben, welche sich völlig unserer Kentnis entziehen. So bleibt die Frage offen, ob und wie oft acute Infections-Krankheiten zu einer raschen Anschwellung der Drüse führen? Für Diphtherie liegen einige Anhaltspunkte vor. Ich begnüge mich, festzustellen, dass es klinisch gut characterisierte Thymus-Stenosen giebt, welche uns zu der Annahme einer acuten Drüsenschwellung zwingen.

Ich habe bisher noch nichts über die Möglichkeit der Compression der grossen Gefässe und des Herzens gesprochen. Zeichen einer Behinderung des venösen Abflusses kann man öfters finden. Schwere Störungen sind jedenfalls selten. Ich habe im Anhang drei Fälle

---

[1] Gluck, Berl. klinische Wochenschrift, 1844.

angeführt, welche über solche Druckwirkungen berichten, der eine ist von Hans Cohn (34), der andere von Lange (35) beschrieben, der dritte stammt aus von Ranke's Klinik (36). Lange hält auf Grund seiner Erfahrung Herzstörung durch Thymusdruck für häufig. Ich halte es für sehr möglich, dass die Ansicht Lange's in der nächsten Zeit noch weitere Bestätigung finden wird.

Was etwaige Reflexwirkungen betrifft, welche durch Thymusdruck ausgelöst werden, so handelte es sich bisher nur um Vermutungen. Die Möglichkeit kann natürlich nicht bestritten werden. Eine Recurrenslähmung durch Thymusdruck ist noch nicht bekannt geworden.

Der Vollständigkeit halber will ich noch erwähnen, dass Svehla den Thymus-Tod als eine Hyperthymisation auffasst. Ich komme nun zu meinem zweiten Operationsfall.

Krankengeschichte

Der 4 Monate alte Knabe leidet seit der Geburt an Schweratmigkeit, die bei jeder Aufregung so hohe Grade annehme, dass das Kind blau im Gesicht werde und ganz weg, sei. Eltern und 5 Geschwister gesund.

Das Kind sieht gut genährt und kräftig aus. Lungenschall voll. Keine Rasselgeräusche zu hören. Herzdämpfung nicht verbreitert, Herztöne rein.

Der Hals ist kurz, das Kind hält den Kopf nach hinten gebeugt, hat in der Ruhe ein rosiges Aussehen, bei der Inspiration ist ein leises Geräusch zu hören. Das Jugulum sinkt etwas ein, die Stimme ist klar. Beim Schreien wird das Kind rasch cyanotisch, die Atmung wird mühsam und zwar ist nur die Inspiration gehemmt. Sie dauert lang und ist von einem lauten langgezogenen Geräusch begleitet, die untere Thoraxapertur wird eingezogen, die Halsvenen schwellen an, im Jugulum bildet sich eine tiefe Grube. Die Exspiration ist nicht behindert, sie erfolgt kurz und stossweise, das Jugulum wird dabei durch einen weichen bei der Inspiration hinter dem manubrium sterni wieder verschwindenden Tumor vorgebuckelt. Die Lordose der Hals und Brustwirbelsäule wird vermehrt. Atemnot und Cyanose nehmen zu mit der Dauer des Anfalls, bei längerem Schreien nimmt die Dyspnoe einen bedrohlichen Character an, der Gesichtsausdruck wird ängstlich, die Haut lässt sich bläulichweiss und bedeckt sich mit warmem Schweiss. Wird das Kind durch Aufnehmen oder Verabreichung der Flasche beruhigt, so lassen die Erscheinungen bald nach. Operation: Hautlängsschnitt vom Schildknorpel bis aufs Sternum, stumpfes Auseinanderdrängen der praetrachealen Muskulatur, Spaltung der tiefen Halsfascie. Jetzt wird die Thymuskapsel sichtbar, sie reicht bis gegen den Isthmus der Schilddrüse herauf. Bei der Exspiration wird sie durch die emporgeschleuderte Thymus ballonförmig ausgedehnt, bei der Inspiration zu einer tiefen Mulde eingezogen. Anziehen der Kapsel verringert den inspiratorischen Stridor, beseitigt ihn aber nicht vollständig, deswegen quere Incision der Kuppe der Thymuskapsel. Der Lappen der weissröttlichen Thymus, der bei der Exspiration hervorgeschleudert wird, wird mit Pincetten gefasst, das Thymusgewebe ist aber so weich, dass die gefassten Partikel bei der inspiratorischen Aspiration der Thymus abreissen. Durch öfteres Nachfassen während der Inspiration wird allmählich ein im ganzen wallnussgrosses Gewebestück ohne nennenswerte Blutung aus der Thymus stumpf entfernt. Die Thymus reicht weit auf den Herzbeutel herunter, man sieht deutlich die sie flankierenden grossen Gefässstämme, an der Trachea sind keine Veränderungen zu erkennen. Die Thymuskapsel wird mit drei Cagutfäden an die Fascie über dem manubr. sterni angenäht, und ein Iodoformgazstreifchen hinter den so in elevierter und anteponierter Stellung fixierten Thymusrest geschoben. Vereinigung der m.m. sterno-hyoidei mit 2 Cagutfäden. Hautknopfnaht.

Nach der mikroskopischen Untersuchung (Dr. Albrecht) handelt es sich um eine Hyperplasie der Thymus, in den grossen Hassal'schen Körperchen finden sich reichlich Leucocyten-Einschlüsse.

Der Erfolg der Operation war gleich am ersten Tage ein auffallender. Das Inspirationsgeräusch bei ruhigem Atmen ist weggefallen, selbst bei heftigen Erregungszuständen tritt keine Dyspnoe mehr auf, das Kind behält beim Schreien seine rosige Farbe, auch eine am Ende der ersten Woche einsetzende Bronchitis verlief ohne Atmungsstörungen zu verursachen. Das einzige Ueberbleibsel der Stenose ist ein kurzes inspiratorisches Atmungsgeräusch bei starkem Schreien.

Die Operation der Stenosis thymica

Es wird sich gleich bleiben, ob man eine Beengung der Luftwege oder einen Druck auf die grossen Gefässe und das Herz annimmt. Die Indication bleibt dieselbe. Der schädliche Druck von Seiten der Thymus muss gehoben werden. Dass diese Indication nicht durch eine Intubation oder einen Luftröhrenschnitt erfüllt werden kann, ist einleuchtend (Siegel, Anhang 17-23). Ich zähle, dass unter den mir bekannten Fällen achtmal der Luftröhrenschnitt ausgeführt wurde — einen neunten Fall (Bode) zähle ich nicht mit, weil am bereits verstorbenen Kind operiert wurde.

Es ist nicht verwunderlich, dass in den meisten Fällen von Tracheotomie ein Erfolg ausbleibt. Das Hindernis sitzt zu tief. Bieder (Anh. 20) konnte diese tiefe Stenose nach der Tracheotomie mittelst eines Katheters feststellen. In einigen Fällen brachte allerdings die Tracheotomie Erleichterung. Man kann sich vorstellen, dass die Tracheotomie-Wunde einen freieren Luftzutritt gestattet, dass die Aspiration der Stimmbänder fortfällt und somit deren inspiratorische Einkrempelung. Vielleicht übt auch die Kanüle hie und da einen directen günstigen Einfluss aus auf die Stenose durch Spannung der Wand der Luftröhre. Ein dauernder Erfolg ist durch den Luftröhrenschnitt niemals zu Stande gekommen. Alle Kinder starben (zwei von denselben nach Entfernung der Kanüle).

Es ist einleuchtend, dass die Thymus selbst durch die Operation in Angriff genommen werden muss.

Eine Narkose ist nicht ungefährlich und daher besser zu vermeiden.

Vermittelst eines Längsschnittes dringt man in den Zwischenraum zwischen dem m. m. sternohyoid. ext. muss eine vena communicans am oberen Ende des Sternum doppelt unterbunden werden. Nach Spaltung der tiefen Halsfascie gelangt man in den praetrachealen Raum, in welchem die vena thyreoidina und die kleinen Arterienäste der Thymus nach der Brust hin verlaufen. Man wird schon jetzt bei jeder Exspiration sich die Thymus-Drüse umhüllt von ihrer Bindegewebskapsel hervorwölben sehen. Der Wundspalt muss gut auseinander gehalten werden. Dann fasst man die Drüsenkapsel mit Pean'schen Klemmen und versucht, sie mit mässiger Kraftanwendung nach aussen zu ziehen. Folgt die Drüse dem Zug nicht, so dringt man mit dem Finger vorsichtig zwischen Sternum und Kapsel und trennt stumpf die lockere Verbindung der Kapsel mit der Hinterfläche des Brustbeins. Um in den Raum hinter die Kapsel zu gelangen, muss man vermittelst eines kleinen Querschnitts die Verbindung der Kapsel mit der praetrachealen Fascie trennen. Beim Eingehen in diesen Raum ist besondere Vorsicht geboten.

In dem ersten von mir operierten Fall liess sich durch Anziehen der Kapsel die Drüse über den Rand des sternum hervorziehen und das genügte, um die Atemnot zu beseitigen. Es hat sich erwiesen und das war von vornherein zu erwarten, dass ein derartiges Vorgehen nicht immer zum Ziele führt. König resezirte ein Stück der Drüse und fixiert den Rest nach aussen. Purrucker und Ehrhardt haben ein grosses Stück der Drüse entfernt, letzterer spricht von einer totalen Entfernung.

Ich möchte betonen, dass niemals eine extracapsuläre Ausschälung versucht werden soll. Sie ist unausführbar aus anatomischen Gründen. Wenn ein Anziehen der Drüse nicht genügt, so muss die Kapsel in ihrem oberen Zipfel gespalten und die Drüsen-Substanz enukleirt werden. Das wird sich in jedem Fall ausführen lassen. Man hat nur wenig von einer Blutung zu fürchten. In den Fällen Purrucker und Ehrhardt konnte auf diese Weise leicht ein grosser Teil der Drüse hervorgezogen und entfernt werden. Ich sage mit Absicht ein grosser Teil, wahrscheinlich der grösste Teil. Ob es sich in diesen Fällen um die gesammte Drüsensubstanz gehandelt hat, erscheint mir zweifelhaft. Auf jeden Fall aber genügte die Operation zur Hebung des Hindernisses und das ist der springende Punkt.

Nicht immer wird man so leicht die Drüsensubstanz hervorziehen können, wie mein zweiter Fall beweist. Das wird vorkommen, wenn die Drüse weich ist, bei einem Zug einreisst. Dann wird man stückweise evt. mit Hülfe eines stumpfen Löffels soviel wegnehmen müssen, als es zur Beseitigung der Stenose bedarf. Darauf ist die Drüsenkapsel auf der Aussenfläche des Sternum zu befestigen und nach Einführung eines kleinen Drainage-Rohrs in den Kapselraum die Wunde durch Naht zu verschliessen.

Ich glaube, es wird höchst selten vorkommen, dass man mit den geschilderten relativ einfachen Massnahmen nicht zum Ziele kommt. In diesen Ausnahmsfällen würde ich nicht anstehen, eine Resection des manubrium sterni zu empfehlen. Damit wird eine weit bessere Uebersicht des Operationsfeldes gegeben sein. Man bedarf zu dieser Operation nicht der Sauerbruch'schen Kammer, da eine Verletzung der Pleura-Höhle leicht vermieden werden kann.

Schluss-Sätze

1). Eine grosse, es ist nicht festgestellt ob in allen Fällen hyperplastische Thymus kann einen Druck auf die im mediastinalen Raum liegenden Gebilde ausüben.

2). Dieser Druck benachteiligt in den meisten Fällen und in erster Linie die Luftwege, seltener Herz und Gefässe.

3). Die Tracheo-Broncho-Stenosis thymica ist eine klinisch und autoptisch sicher gestellte Erkrankung, nicht zu verwechseln mit dem Glottis-Krampf. Sie ist häufiger als man bisher annahm.

4). Das Krankheitsbild zeigt je nach dem Grad der Stenose Verschiedenheiten. Es giebt Uebergänge vom leichten Einsinken des Jugulum, vom scheinbar unschuldigen Säuglingsstridor, zu gefahrdrohenden Dyspnoe-Anfällen, vom langsamen suffokatorisch. exitus zu blitzähnlichem Tode infolge totaler Compression der Luftwege.

5). Die Stenose kann sich allmählich oder plötzlich bemerkbar machen.

6). Sie kann spontan heilen, oder auch im ersten unerwarteten Auftreten zum Tode führen.

7). Es giebt ein familiäres Vorkommen der Erkrankung.

8). Selbst die scheinbar harmlosesten Formen, bei welchen das Befinden der Pat. kaum gestört ist, müssen prognostisch sehr vorsichtig beurteilt werden, weil nicht vorherzusehende Ereignisse rasch zu einer schlimmen Wendung führen können.

9). Die sofortige Indication zu einer Operation ist gegeben, wenn suffokatorische Anfälle eintreten. Die Zeit und die Erfahrung werden entscheiden, ob prophylaktisch zu operieren ist.

10). Eine Operation hat sich direct auf eine Hebung des Atmungshindernisses d. h. auf die Thymus zu richten. Wenn eine Ectopexie nicht genügt, so muss die Drüse nach Einschneiden der Kapsel mehr weniger ausgeschält werden. Eine extracapsuläre Ausschälung der Drüse ist nicht ausführbar.

11). Die bisherigen Thymus-Operationen waren nicht nur vom besten Resultat begleitet, sondern sie waren relativ einfache, ungefährliche, technisch leicht auszuführende Eingriffe.

12). Eine Narkose ist zu diesen Eingriffen weder wünschenswert noch erforderlich.

ANHANG

29 Fälle von durch Sektion oder Operation (Fall 15) nachgewiesener Compressionsstenose der Trachea

1) *Astley Cooper* (The Anatomy of the Thymus gland, London 1832): 19 jähriges Mädchen, mehrwöchentliche Atemnot, die beim Zurücklegen des Kopfes zunahm. Die mit weisser breiiger Substanz durchsetzte Thymus hatte die Trachea eingehüllt und in ihrem Quer-Durchmesser verengt.

2) *Clar* (Jahrbuch für Kinderkrankh. 1855) spricht in einer Epikrise zu seinem dritten Falle von der erst an der Leiche nachgewiesenen Compression der Trachea durch die grosse Thymus, aus dem Sektionsbericht lässt sich jedoch nicht entnehmen in welcher Weise die Trachea comprimiert war.

3) *Somma* (Archiv di patologia infant. 1884, cit. nach Flügge, 12): 4 Tage alt, grosse Zahl von Erstickungsanfällen, stark vergrösserte Thymus, Trachea über eine Länge von 3 Knorpeln abgeplattet und verengt in ihrem Lumen.

4) *Barack* (In Dissertation 1891, Berlin): 6 Monate altes Kind, keine Prodrome. Luftröhre erscheint deutlich abgeplattet, nach ihrer Eröffnung und bei hinten übergesunkenem Kopf berühren sich Vorder- und Hinterwand. Die grösste Verdickung entspricht der Stelle, wo die Art. anon. mit der linken vena anonym. über die Luftröhre hinwegzieht.

5) *Rehn* (Berl. klin. Wochenschr. 1894): 8 Tage alt, keine Prodrome. «Sehr grosse Thymus, die im oberen Teile ziemlich fest zwischen Manubrium sterni und Trachea eingebettet war, die Trachea ist daselbst deutlich abgeplattet und kann durch leichte Rückwärtsbeugung des Halses sofort vollständig geschlossen werden.

8 Monate alt, manchmal Röcheln, unter Erstickungserscheinungen gestorben. Von der Bifurkation an erscheinen die Bronchen bis in die feinsten Verzweigungen auffallend eng, vor ihrem Eintritt in die Lungen abgeplattet und gestat.

6) *Morfan* (Ref. Centralblatt für allg. Path. und path. Anat. 1895): Sehr aufverlaufender Fall von Erstickung bei einem 2 1/2 Monate alten Mädchen. Der Thymus wog 31 gr. Die Trachea war abgeplattet, die lymphatischen Organe zeigten keinerlei Hyperplasie.

7) *Lange* (Jahrbuch für Kinderkrankh. Bd. 48, 1895): Ca. 4 Monate alt, morgens ot aufgefunden, nachdem es in der Nacht unruhig gewesen. Die vergrösserte Thy

mus umgriff die Trachea fast vollständig und comprimierte dieselbe etwa 2 cm oberhalb der Bifurkation in einer Ausdehnung von ca. 1,5 cm von links hinten nach rechts vorne säbelscheidenförmig. Die membranösen Spatien der Luftröhre waren an der verengten Stelle deutlich verbreitert, die Knorpel jedoch nicht geschädigt.

8. *Farret* (Thèse de Paris, 1896, cit. nach Hedinger, Jahrb. für Kinderheilk., 1905): 8 Stunden alt, trotz künstlicher Atmung und guter Herztätigkeit Exitus. Thymus sehr blutreich, hatte die Trachea von hinten nach vorne leicht comprimiert.

9. *Weigert* (Cit. bei Siegel, Deutsche medic. Wochenschr. 1896) fand bei einer Sektion eine bedeutende Compression der Trachea durch hyperplastische Thymus und demonstrierte sie dem ärztlichen Verein.

10. *Clessin* (Münch. med. Wochenschr. 1896): 2 Monate, nie Atembeschwerden, morgens tot im Bett. «Nach Entfernung des Brustbeins fiel die grosse braunrote Thymus auf, welche etwa 2/3 des Herzens bedeckte und mit Petechien übersät war». Die Trachea war etwa 2 cm oberhalb der Bifurkation so von der Drüse zusammengedrückt, dass sich in den mittleren Partien nahezu vordere und hintere Trachealwand berührten, während zu beiden Seiten je ein kaum für eine Stricknadel durchgängiger Kanal bestehen blieb. Die Luftröhre war makroskopisch nicht verändert.

11. *Jessen* (Aerztl. Sachverständ. Zeitung, 1898): Acuter Erstickungstod bei einem 5½ Wochen alten Kinde. Thymus 20,5 gr. schwer, derb. Trachea völlig abgeplattet und in sagitaler Richtung comprimiert.

12. *Flügge* (Vierteljahrschr. für gerichtl. Medicin 3. f. 17. Bd., 1899): 2 Stunden alt. Asphyxie bei normaler Herztätigkeit, Wiederbelebungsversuche erfolglos. «Der Hauptbronchus und die Trachea sind vollkommen säbelscheidenförmig abgeplattet».

8 Monate alt, keine Prodrome beobachtet, «die Trachea ist im untersten Teil säbelscheidenförmig platt, mit scharfem Knick in den Knorpeln. Die Abplattung beginnt schon kurz unter dem Pharynx. Sehr stark wird sie erst an der Stelle, wo die art. anonym. über die Trachea hinwegzieht.

Neugeboren, scheintot, Herztätigkeit hört bald auf. Die Bronchi I. Ordnung sind etwas platt, die Trachea ist oberhalb der Bifurkation durch die vorüberziehende Art. anonym. stark eingebuchtet, ganz platt.

Totgeborenes Kind. Neben einer grossen Thymus mässige Compression der Trachea an der Kreuzungsstelle.

12 Stunden alt. Nach 4 stündigen Wiederbelebungsversuchen erfolgten sehr angestrengte spontane Inspirationen. Die Trachea zeigt an der Kreuzungsstelle eine tiefe Rinne und dementsprechende Abplattung ihres Lumens. Die Bronchien sind von der Bifurkation ab sehr platt, säbelscheidenförmig, eng.

2½ Stunden. Scheintot, keine spontane Atmung zu erzielen. Querschnitte durch das gehärtete Präparat lassen eine deutliche Compression der Trachea erkennen. An der Stelle der stärksten Compression ist die Trachea etwas nach rechts, der Oesophagus etwas nach links abgewichen. An der Verengungsstelle teilt sich gerade die Art. anonym. In der Höhe der Bifurkation ist die Abplattung noch deutlich, die Hauptbronchi dagegen scheinen kaum verändert.

3 Stunden, scheintot, genügende Atmung nicht zu erzielen. Bronchien von normaler Grösse, Trachea gleich oberhalb der Bifurkation hochgradig abgeplattet, entsprechend dem Verlauf der Art. anonym. Die Abplattung reicht nach oben hinauf bis ca. 2 cm unterhalb des Larynx.

13) *Tuilleus* (Rev. medic. de la Suisse rom. XXI, Schmidt's Jahrb. 273, 1902): Ein 2 Wochen alter gesunder Säugling wurde asphyktisch im Bett gefunden, starb nach mehrstündiger Dauer der Asphyxie. Thymus 38 gr schwer. Luftröhre am Uebergang vom Halsteil zum Brustteil abgeplattet. Die Abplattung glich sich auch nach Entfernung des Thymus nicht aus.

14) *Peukert* (Deutsche med. Wochenschr. 1902): 6 Monate alt. Unter Erstickungserscheinungen rasch gestorben. «In der Luftröhre sieht und fühlt man eine Verengerung in querer Richtung in der Gegend der oberen Brustapertur, sie ist fast säbelscheidenförmig zusammengedrückt».

15) *Ehrhardt* (Archiv für klin. Chirg. 1905): 2 jährig. Atembeschwerden und Heiserkeit, später dauernde Atemnot und inspiratorischer Stridor. Bei der Inspiration zeigte sich die Trachea in ihrem antero posterioren Durchmesser deutlich fühlbar abgeplattet.

16) *Hedinger* (Jahrbuch für Kinderheilkunde, 1906): Totgeborenes reifes Kind. An dem in Spiritus fixierten Präparat finden sich die Trachea und die Bronchien durch die sehr grosse Thymus so stark comprimiert, dass die vordere Wand die hintere fast berührt.

Etwa 20 Stunden alter Hemicephalus mit unregelmässiger krampfartiger Atmung. Thymus liegt in ungewöhnlicher Grösse vor, die Trachea erscheint oberhalb der Bifure. deutlich abgeplattet.

5 Fälle von Mors thymica. «In sämtlichen Fällen konnte man nach Fixierung der Hals- und Brustorgane in Formol eine meist exquisite Abplattung der Luftröhre an der Kreuzstelle mit der Art. anon. nachweisen. Die Abplattung fand sich auch dann, wenn die Masse der Thymus die als Normalmasse angegebenen Zahlen nicht oder nur wenig übertrafen.

26 Todesfälle nach vorausgegangenen Stenoserscheinungen ohne anatomisch nachweisbare Kompression der Trachea, davon tracheotomiert. Fälle17-53 incl.)

17) *Clar* (Jahrbuch für Kinderh. 1858, cit. bei Jacobi 1888): «Bei einem Knaben von 1 Jahr und 9 Monaten, welcher an Croup litt, erwies sich die Einführung der Tracheotomiekanüle als unmöglich wegen der gleichen Ursache (hypertrophischer Thymus).

18) *Abelin* (Journal für Kinderkr. 1870, B. 55, cit. bei Flügge): 7 Jahre alter Knabe erkrankte ganz plötzlich an Erstickungsangst, Cyanose. Nach Einlegen der Tracheotomiekanüle trat sofort Besserung ein. Wurde die Kanüle entfernt, so traten die alten Beschwerden wieder auf. Nach 4 Wochen wurde die Kanüle herausgenommen, das Kind starb 1 Stunde darauf ganz plötzlich. Bei der Sektion fand sich ausser einer übergrossen Thymus nichts Besonderes, vor allem keinerlei Anhaltspunkte einer überstandenen Rachitis.

19) *Kraus & Cahen* (Deutsche med. Wochenschr. 1890, Demonstration im Greifswalder ärztl. Verein): 2 jähriger Knabe mit den Erscheinungen hochgradiger Tracheastenose in der chirurg. Klinik bei hängendem Kopf tracheotomiert. «Mit dem Angenblicke wo wir anfingen, die Schilddrüse stumpf nach unten abzulösen, wurde die Atmung oberflächlich, der Puls setzte aus, das Gesicht färbte sich cyanotisch. Nach Eröffnung der Trachea stockte die Atmung völlig. Bei künstlicher Atmung gelang es nicht den geringsten Luftwechsel durch die inzwischen angeführte Trachealkanüle zu erzielen». Bei der Sektion zeigte sich eine erheblich vergrösserte Thymus, geringfügige Diphtherie beider Stimmbänder und Schwellung und Röthung der Trachea bis zur Bifurcation.

20) *Bader* (Berl. klin. Wochenschr. 1895); 10 Monate alter Knabe mit stenotischem Atmen, ohne diphtheritischen Belag, geringes Fieber, Dämpfung in der oberen Sternalgegend, starke Einziehungen. Erfolglose Intubation und Tracheotomie. Der Katheter stiess unterhalb der Wunde auf Wiederstand.

Sektion: die geschwollene Thymusdrüse ist zwischen Schilddrüse und 2 Paketen geschwollener Bronchialdrüsen eingekeilt.

21) *Demmer* (nach mündlicher Mitteilung). Ein Neugeborenes litt an Atemnot und einem Schluckhindernis. Im Heilig-Geist-Hospital zu Frankfurt a. Main wurde eine Tracheotomie ohne Erfolg vorgenommen. Die Sektion zeigte eine sehr grosse Thymus als Ursache.

22) *Noetzel* (Chir. Journal, städt. Krankenhaus, Frankfurt a. M. 1902/03, 1193); 10 jähriges Mädchen, pastös, mässig guter Ernährungszustand. Zeitweise Atembeschwerden, Rachen und Gaumenmandeln geschwollen. In Halbnarkose Tonsillotomie und Auskratzen des Nasenrachenraums mit Ringmesser. Das Kind hustete gut aus und war vollkommen wach, bis auf dem Wege vom Operationssaal ins Krankenzimmer plötzlich Cyanose und Asphyxie auftrat. Tracheotomie und 2 Stunden lang fortgesetzte künstliche Atmung erfolglos. Die Autopsie ergab eine abnorm grosse Thymus, die die Trachea verengerte.

23) *Marfan* (Rev. mens. des mal. de l'enfant, 23, Schmidt's Jahrb. Bds 286, 1905); 15 Monate, von Geburt an Atembeschwerden, die sich sowohl beim Ein- als Ausatmen bemerkbar machten. Bei Aufregungen traten mitunter förmlich asphyktische Anfälle auf. Intubation, Tracheotomie. Der Zustand bessert sich, doch blieb das strindulöse Atmen. Nach 3 Monaten erneute asphyktische Anfälle und im Laufe eines solchen Exitus. Sektion: bedeutende Thymushypertrophie und Milzlues.

24) *Abelin* (Jour. für Kinderkrankh. 1870, B. 55); 6 jähriges Mädchen, plötzlich acute Atembeschwerden. Sektion ergab sehr grosse Thymus.

25) *Sommer* (l. cit.); 3 Tage alter Knabe, hatte etwa 15 Erstickungsanfälle, starb in einem solchen.

26) *Grawitz* (Deutsche med. Wochenschr. 1888); 6 Monate alter Knabe bekam auf dem Arm seines Vaters plötzlich Atemnot, ballte die Faust, wurde blass, ungewöhnlich grosse Thymus.

27) *Patt* (Jahrb. für Kinderkr. 34. 1892) berichtet über 6 Autopsien von Kindern, welche plötzlichen Erstickungsanfällen erlagen, nachdem zuvor schon wiederholt dyspnoische Attaquen aufgetreten waren, und bei welchen vergrösserte Thymusdrüsen gefunden worden.

28) *Thiergarten* (I. Dissertation, Halle 1893). 9 Monate alt; längere Zeit kurzathmigkeit, 3 Anfälle von krächzendem Character. Im Letzten blieb das Kind weg.

29) *Henning* (Gerhardts Handb. für Kinderkr. 1893, Nachtrag III); 4 Jahre. Ab und zu Atembeschwerden, plötzlich tot im Bett gefunden. Entschieden vergrösserte Thymus.

30) *Kayser* (I. Dissertation, Giessen 1895); 4 Tage alt, Anfälle von Atemnot, Nachts unerwartet gestorben.

31) *Glöckler* (Cit. bei Siegel); 3 Fälle, in denen man als Todesursache für die jedesmal nach schon längerer chronischer Dyspnoe eingetretene Erstickung nichts anderes als eine vergrösserte Thymus fand.

32) *Kobé* (Bull. de la Société Anat. de Paris, 1897, Schmidt's Jahrb. 98); 2 ½ Monate altes, mit Harnkatarrh und Otitis purulenta im Krankenhaus behandeltes Kind sollte schon entlassen werden, als es Dyspnoe bekam und 3 Tage darauf starb. Sektion: Die vergrösserte Thymus umfasst mit zwei von ihrem oberen Rand entsprin-

genden Ausläufern die Trachea. H. nimmt an, dass die Erkrankung des Kindes eine vermehrte Leukocytenbildung hervorrief und dass hierdurch eine plötzliche Schwellung der ohnehin vergrösserten Thymus entstanden sei.

33) *Zander & Keyhl* (Jahrb. für Kinderkr. 1901) 5 1/2 Monate Atemnot, moribund eingeliefert. Intubiert. Exitus 4 Stunden nach Beginn der Atemnot. Kalbshühnereigrosse Thymus.

4 Monate alt, stirbt nachts plötzlich unter Erstickungserscheinungen. Sehr grosse Thymus.

6 Monat alt. Temperatur morgens 5 Uhr plötzlich 40, 3) Atmung beschleunigt, keuchend, angstvoller Ausdruck des Gesichtes, Bulbi nach oben verdreht 8 1/2 Uhr Exitus. Thymus vergrössert.

3 Todesfälle durch Druck der Thymus auf Blutgefässe

31) *Hans Kohn* (Deutsche med. Wochenschr. 1901): Demonstriert dem Berliner Verein für innere Medicin die Praeparate eines Falles von Thymustod.

7 Monate altes Kind wurde nach einer Erkältung 2 Tage vor dem Tod cyanotisch und dyspnoisch, keine Lungenaffection. Sektion: stark vergrössertes und hypertrophisches Herz, Erweiterung des aufsteigenden Astes des Aortenbogens. Die vergrösserte 40 gr schwere Thymus drückte wie eine Pelotte auf die Aorta in der Mitte des Bogens.

35) *Lange* (Verhandlungen der 19. Vers. der Gesellschaft für Kinderheilkunde, Karlsbad, 1902): 8 Monate altes Kind stirbt unter Erstickungserscheinungen nachdem es seit 8 Tagen unruhig gewesen und Abends zuvor starke Atemnot bekommen hatte. Die Thymus umgreift die grossen Gefässe und die Bifurcation der Trachea. Luftröhre nicht comprimiert, dagegen sind die grossen Gefässe mehr oder weniger flach gedrückt. Das Herz ist ausserordentlich stark vergrössert, hypertrophisch und dilatiert.

36) *Zander & Keyhl* (loc. cit.) 5 Monate alt, gut entwickelt, etwas pastös Kind wird Mittags apathisch, verweigert die Nahrung, es tritt plötzliche Pulsverlangsamung und erschwerte Atmung auf, keine Cyanose, keine Krämpfe. Sektion «Die linke vena jugularis int. ist auf der Höhe des Jugulum bei ihrem Eintritt in den Thorax thrombosiert auf 1/2 cm Länge. Die obere und untere Fortsetzung der Vena ist frei. Thymus stark vergrössert, besonders der Tiefendurchmesser.»

Chirurgie des Brustkorbes unter Ueberdruck

Par M. FRANZ KUHN, Kassel.

Wie Sie alle wissen, streitet in Fragen der Chirurgie der Brusthöhle das sog. Unterdruckverfahren gegen das Ueberdruckverfahren. Jedes der beiden Verfahren hat seine Freunde und Gegner.

Es kann keinem Zweifel unterliegen, dass das Unterdruckverfahren das physiologisch natürlichere ist. Als solches wurde es auch von physiologischen Autoritäten auf dem Congress in Lüttich anerkannt.

Um dies zu beweisen, bedürfte es kaum der eingehenden Begründung von Sauerbruch und Tiegel.

Sosehr jedoch es feststehen mag, dass das Unterdruckverfahren das physiologischere, ebenso wenig sicher ist andererseits, dass mit der Anwendung des Unterdruckes das Problem für die Praxis gelöst ist. Denn das Prinzip und die prinzipielle Lösung des Problems ist für die Praxis nicht allein massgebend; massgebend bleibt die praktische Durchführbarkeit und Anwendbarkeit einer Methode in der Praxis.

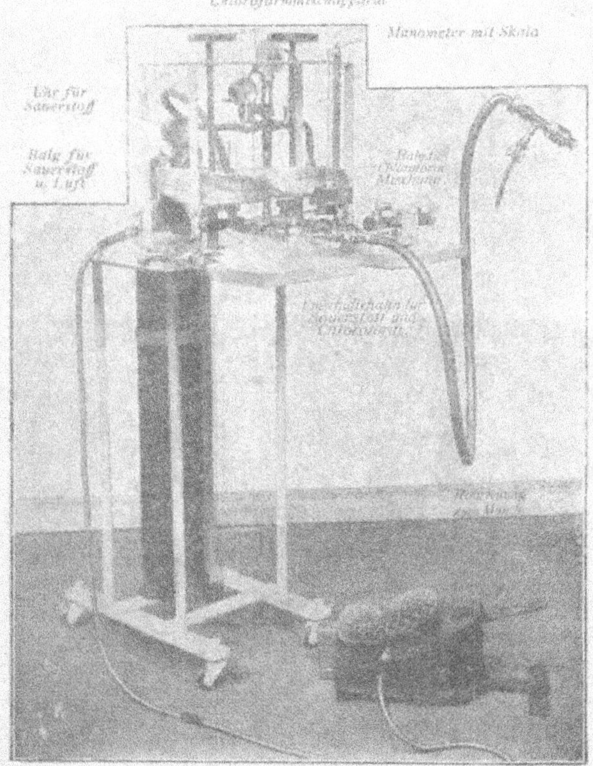

Fig. 4. Narkoseapparat für Überdrucknarkose Kuhn-Dräger.
II. Phase (Letztes Modell).

Es kann kein Zweifel sein, dass die Sauerbruch'sche Kammermethode enorme Anforderungen stellt, sowohl was die Anschaffung als Unterhaltung, als Bedienung der Apparate betrifft.

Von diesem Standpunkte ist sie im praktischen Leben schwer durchführbar; am wenigsten kann sie Allgemeingut breiter chirurgischer Kreise werden. Dazu kommen noch zahlreiche Vorwürfe für die Benützung der Kammer, die Lichtverhältnisse und Raumverhältnisse, die Asepsis und Ventilation, etc.

Es kann nicht wundern, dass man nach Substituten für diese teuren Unterdruckanlagen gesucht hat und wieder etwas zum älteren Ueberdruckverfahren zurückgekehrt ist. So hat man verschiedene *Kammern* gebaut mit Ueberdruckanwendung, hat *Masken* verwendet und *Intubationsröhren* eingeführt; und während noch der Streit tobt, ob Ueberdruck oder Unterdruck das für die Praxis bessere Verfahren, erhebt sich im Lager der Ueberdruckfreunde der Kampf um den besten Apparat, um die einfachste, billigste und beste Application des Ueberdruckes.

Es stehen sich da gegenüber:

1) Der *Brauer'sche Ueberdruckkasten*, in welchen der Kopf des Patienten kommt, während der Narkotiseur mittels luftdichter Aermel die Narkose besorgt.

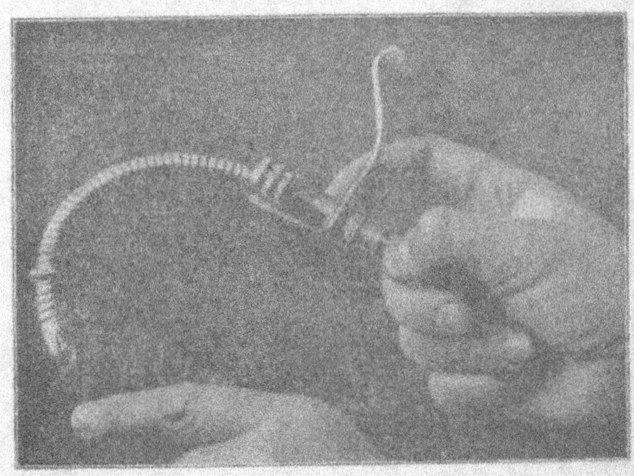

Fig. 2

2) *Engelken'sche Kasten*, in welchen der Kopf des Patienten zu liegen, und der Narkotiseur zu sitzen kommt. Ein besonderer Injektor saugt das verbrauchte Chloroform ab.

3) *Mein Ueberdruckapparat*, der mittels Blasebalgs und Chlo-

roformsauerstoff arbeitet, Luftbälge einschaltet, und die Druckluft und Narkoseluft mittels Maske oder Intubationsrohr appliciert.

Noch muss dahingestellt bleiben, welcher Apparat für die Praxis der bessere ist; allein die praktische Verwendung kann entscheiden.

Mir ist an dieser Stelle nur darum zu tun, mein Verfahren, wie es sich für die Praxis gestaltet, zu erläutern.

Der Apparat zerfällt in zwei Teile.

1) einen Teil, der die Druckluft und die Narkosegase liefert und aufbewahrt und an den Patienten leitet.

2) einen Teil, der die Gase luftdicht der Lunge des Patienten übermittelt; er besteht in einer Maske oder dem Tubus der peroralen Intubation.

Der druckliefernde Apparat hat folgendes Aussehen: Sein Oberteil ist abnehmbar, und transportabel construiert, und hat dann die Form eines Reisekoffers.

Die Druck applicierenden Apparate bestehen in folgendem:

Für Fälle, in denen die Lunge selbst affiziert, und Patient keine gesunden Luftwege hat, tritt eine Maske in Tätigkeit. Dieselbe besteht ganz aus weichem Stoff, mit einigen Gummiverstärkungen.

a) Der innere Teil, der dem Gesichte sich anschmiegt, ist ein Zwischending von Jagdkappe und Bartbinde; er lässt Augen, Nase und Mund frei.

b) Der äussere Theil ist ein mit Glasfenster versehener kleiner Ballon, welcher dem inneren Teil luftdicht angefügt ist. In ihn münden die Luft zuführenden und abführenden Ventile. Die Weichheit der Kappe gestattet über dem Gesichte eine Summe von Handgriffen.

2. Der Tubus ist der Tubus der peroralen Intubation und hat die bekannte Form.

Akute Perforationen des Magendarmkanals und der Gallenblase

Par M. Tilmann, Cologne.

Die Entwicklung der Bauchchirurgie hat die Erkenntnis der Erkrankungen der Bauchhöhle ausserordentlich gefördert. Wir wissen in welchen Fällen noch radikal zu helfen ist und wir wissen, dass durch Palliativoperationen das Leben auch bei anscheinend sehr schweren Erkrankungen noch verlängert werden kann. Der Fortschritt der Chirurgie hat einerseits darin bestanden, die Technik zu heben. Man gab Methoden an, bei vorgeschrittenen

Carcinomen auch die Lymphdrüsen noch zu entfernen, um einem
Recidiv vorzubeugen; man glaubte den ganzen Magen entfernen zu
können, man rechnete aus, wieviel Meter davon der Mensch entbeh-
ren könne. Und doch müssen wir uns heute sagen, dass es ein
undankbares Amt ist, zu weit vorgeschrittene Carcinome zu operieren, oder Palliativoperationen zu machen, deren Wesen der
Patient nicht versteht. Er glaubt, durch den überstandenen Eingriff geheilt zu werden, und ist schwer enttäuscht, wenn die un-
ausbleibliche Verschlimmerung nicht ausbleibt. Der Chirurg ist gewiss befriedigt, wenn er im einzelnen Fall ein gutes Resultat erzielt, aber die Befriedigung ist keine volle, es ist ja doch nur Flick-
werk. Wir kommen nur vorwärts durch Besserung der Diagnose. Wir müssen dahin kommen, dass wir die Erkrankungen der
Bauchhöhle zu einer Zeit operieren, wo eine radikale Hülfe, eine
Rettung noch möglich ist. Leider ist ja der deutsche Chirurg, der
am meisten in diesem Sinne gearbeitet hat, Mikulicz, selbst einem zu spät diagnosticierten Magencarcinom zum Opfer gefallen.
Daran sehen wir, wie weit der Weg noch ist, und wie manches
Hindernis noch beseitigt werden muss, ehe wir zu dem erstreb-
ten Ziele gelangen.

Dass eine anatomische Diagnose bei *chronischen* Erkrankungen
des Magendarmkanals schwer ist, soll nicht bestritten werden.
Wenn aber jeder Arzt bei jedem Kranken, den er behandelt, nicht
eher ruhig ist, bis er eine Diagnose hat, dann kämen wir schon
weiter. Bedeutend wichtiger und verhängnisvoller für den Kranken
ist das Warten mit der Diagnosenstellung bei den *akuten* Perforationen des Magendarmkanals und der Gallenblase. Durch die Ver-
vollkommnung der chirurgischen Technik sind wir fast soweit
gekommen, dass man die akuten Perforationen kaum noch fürchtet,
wenn sie früh in Behandlung kommen, und sondert man die grossen Veröffentlichungen, so sieht man deutlich dass Alles darauf
ankommt, die Fälle früh in Behandlung zu bekommen. Für die
akuten Perforationen eines Magengeschwürs hat man eine Frist
von 6 Stunden gesetzt, innerhalb derer eine Operation noch Erfolg
hat; bei den Perforationen des Processus vermiformis eine solche
von 48 bis 60 Stunden. Diese Fristen sollen aber nur besagen, dass
innerhalb der angegebenen Zeit bei einer Operation noch ein Erfolg
zu erwarten ist. Es kann kein Zweifel sein, dass das beste eine sofortige Operation ist. Bekommt man einen derartigen Fall in Behandlung, so sind schon Zweifel berechtigt, ob man den Kranken noch ins Hospital transportieren soll. Ich selbst operiere aku-

te Perforationen des Magen- und Darmkanals grundsätzlich in der Wohnung des Erkrankten, da ich mich in einzelnen Fällen der Erkenntnis nicht erschliessen kann, dass der Transport den Verlauf ungünstig beeinflusst habe, oder umgekehrt, dass ein günstiger Verlauf bei sehr schwerem abdominellen Befund dem Ausbleiben eines Transportes zu verdanken ist. Man wird gezwungen, die Laparotomie bei akuten Perforationen des Magendarmkanals als Nothoperation anzusehen, die ebenso wie die Tracheotomie und Unterbindung der Arteria meningea media von jedem Arzt ausgeführt werden muss. In Städten wird ja stets noch Zeit sein einen Chirurgen zuzuziehen, aber auf dem Lande, bei grossen Entfernungen von Städten, wird es oft schwer zu verantworten sein zu warten. Allerdings wird durch die Erfindung der Automobile auch diese Besorgnis erheblich eingeschränkt.

Die Aufgabe der Chirurgie ist also eine doppelte, einmal die Diagnose der Perforationen möglichst zu präcisieren und sichern und weiterhin die operative Behandlung so einfach zu gestalten, damit sie auch unter einfacheren Verhältnissen eines Privathauses und nicht nur in grossen aseptischen Operationssälen ausgeführt werden kann.

Die akuten Perforationen sind dadurch charakterisiert, dass sie plötzlich erfolgen, und zwar meist in die freie Bauchhöhle; hat sich die Perforation langsam entwickelt oder sich sogar schon vorbereitet, dann tritt der Durchbruch in Verwachsungen ein, und kann man dann schon hoffen, das der Process lokal verläuft und abgekapselt bleibt.

Die Ursache der Perforation liegt in der Entwicklung des Erkrankungsprocesses der die Grundlage bildet. Wenn der Ulcerationsprocess die Serosa erreicht hat, wenn die Gallenblase ihre höchstmögliche Spannung erreicht hat, dann bildet sich ein Loch, oder die Gallenblase platzt. Ich habe mich überzeugen können, dass in vielen Fällen ein Trauma, ein Stoss, ein Schlag der Grund der Perforation ist.

Bei den meisten Fällen trat sie im Schlaf, beim Absteigen von der elektrischen Bahn oder beim Gehen ein. «Ich muss wohl einen Fehltritt gemacht haben», heisst es dann gewöhnlich. Dass sich vor der Perforation keine Verwachsungen mit der Umgebung bilden, die einen Durchbruch in die freie Bauchhöle hindern, liegt wohl beim Magen darin, dass dieses Organ einen starken Wechsel seiner Lage und Füllung aufweist, beim Blinddarm darin, dass der Process sich zu schnell entwickelt.

Das Loch im Magen bei der Perforation eines Magengeschwürs ist gewöhnlich erbsengross und nicht etwa stecknadelspitzengross. Es scheint also als ob auch nach der Perforation noch eine Erweiterung des Loches statthat. Wichtig für die Behandlung ist die Tatsache, dass oft noch einige mm in der Umgebung der Oeffnung die Schleimhaut fehlt und dass der umgebende Schleimhautrand sich verwölbt und den Anschein erweckt, als ob nur ein kleiner Defect in der Schleimhaut wäre. Bei der Excision muss man beachten, dass man die Schleimhaut auch wirklich im Gesunden exstirpirt.

Der Durchbruch des Wurmfortsatzes bietet wohl das meiste Interesse.

Ein sehr interessanter Fall zeigt den Vorgang in einem besonderen Lichte.

Ein junger Mann von 17 Jahren erkrankte unter Erbrechen nach einer argen Magenüberladung an Schmerzen in der Blinddarmgegend. Unter Fieber nahm die Schmerzhaftigkeit zu, der Leib war namentlich in der Blinddarmgegend enorm schmerzhaft, aber eingezogen. Die Palpation war bei den stark gespannten Bauchdecken zweifelhaft. Ich nahm eine drohende Perforation an und schlug sofortige Operation vor. Ich fand den Wurmfortsatz wie ein erigirtes Penis, daumendick, stark injicirt und geröstet. Als ich nach seiner Herausnahme die Ligatur löste, spritzte sein Inhalt 50 cm. weit, stand also unter schwerem Druck. In einem zweiten Falle öffnete sich der ebenso straff gespannte Wurmfortsatz beim Anheben aus seiner Lage und spritzte seinen Inhalt im Bogen nach der Umgebung. Wenn man dann weiter bedenkt, wie schwer es oft ist, die stecknadelspitzgrosse Oeffnung zu finden aus der sich der Inhalt des Processus vermiformis entleert hat, dann muss man angeben, dass nicht nur Decubitalgeschwüre die Ursache der Perforation sind, sondern die pralle Füllung und Dehnung des Organs durch seinen Inhalt der nicht heraus kann. Das Hinderniss, das den Zugang zum Coecum verlegt, ist sonst der Kothstein, der wie ein Ventil den Kanal versperrt und oft in die Wand des Coecums und des Wurmfortsatzes eingepresst wird. Die mikroskopische Untersuchung aller von mir bei akuten Perforationen entfernten 49 Wurmfortsätze hat ergeben, dass in der Umgebung der Perforationsöffnung oft keine Entzündung und keine Ulceration als Ursache der Perforation angesprochen werden kann. Kommt es zur Gangrän des Wurmfortsatzes, so ist dieselbe auch meist circulär, d. h. von einer bestimmten Stelle circulär bis zum Ende reichend. Wäre die gangränöse Entzündung der Schleimhaut die Ursache dieses Processes, so wäre schwer verständlich, warum der Process so scharf linear abschneidet. Das ist wohl nur dadurch zu erklären, dass der Stein an der Stelle des Centrums der Gangrän gesessen hat, dass durch den Druck des peripher sich ansammelnden Secretes derselbe immer fester eingepresst wird, bis er schliesslich die Blutzufuhr zu dem Blinddarmende abschneidet. In zwei Fällen von Gangrän des Processus, die ich beobachtete, war der Kothstein noch in dem schwarz verfärbten Organ zu sehen, man konnte aber mit der Sonde den Rest des Anhangs passiren bis in das Coecum hinein, ein Beweis, dass ein sonstiger Grund der Versperrung der Passage nicht vorlag.

In allen Fällen von Perforationen des Magendarmkanals ist das erste Symptom der Schmerz. Alle Kranken geben einen heftigen reissenden Schmerz als erstes Symptom an, der besonders heftig bei Magengeschwüren ist. Es kann wohl kein Zufall sein, dass von meinen 8 Fällen von Magengeschwürsoperationen 7 die Angabe machten, dass sie vorher ein eigentümliches Gefühl von Völle und Aufgeblasensein in der Magengegend empfunden hätten, das ihnen die Luft benahm. Alle hatten das Bedürfnis, sich Luft zu machen, und es ist ein eigentümlicher, aber bedeutungsvoller Zufall, dass alle 7 zur Behebung dieser Beschwerden Ricinusöl genommen haben, 4 auf eigene Eingebung, 3 sogar auf ärztliche Anordnung. Bei keiner der sonst von mir beobachteten Perforationen ist mir eine ähnliche Angabe begegnet, sodass ich diesem Symptom jetzt eine gewisse Bedeutung zumesse. Die Erklärung derselben ist wohl eine einfache. Das Vorschreiten des Ulcerationsprocesses bis an die Serosa ruft reflektorisch eine Magenlähmung hervor, die zur Aufblähung und deren Konsequenzen führt. Bald nachher kam die Perforation. Ich will nicht glauben, dass das Ol. Ricini den Durchbruch bedingt oder beschleunigt habe, da derselbe doch von dem Vorgeschrittensein des anatomischen Processes abhängt.

Der heftige Schmerz ist wohl bedingt durch den Eintritt von Darminhalt in die Bauchhöle. Auch hier wieder sind die Verhältnisse am Magen am ungünstigsten, da hier grosse Mengen sauren Inhaltes sich in die freie Bauchhöhle ergiessen. Das Netz ist meist nach unten geschlagen und kann nicht schützen. Mit dem einmaligen Erguss ist es nicht geschehen, sondern andauernd fliessen neue Massen von frisch secernirtem Magensaft nach, sodass man den langdauernden Schmerz und den argen Collaps versteht, unter dem der Kranke leidet. Bretthart gespannte Bauchdecken und enorme Empfindlichkeit bei Betastung sind die äusseren Zeichen. Das begleitende Erbrechen fehlt bei Magengeschwürsperforationen nicht. Wenn man aber nichts per os giebt, dann kehrt es gewöhnlich nicht wieder. Jeder Tropfen Wasser ruft neues Erbrechen hervor.

Aehnlich ist das Bild bei der Perforation eines Typhusgeschwürs, nur mit dem Unterschied, dass man es mit einem schon schwerkranken Mann zu thun hat, dessen Zustand sich plötzlich verschlimmert, während die Magengeschwürsperforationen gewöhnlich bei sonst gesunden und kräftigen Menschen eintreten, die vorher an Magengeschwüren gelitten haben. Es kann zweifelhaft sein, ob der Darminhalt allein als die Ursache der enormen Schmerzen anzusehen ist, denn wir wissen, dass bei traumatischen Darmzerreissungen zunächst Stunden lang Schmerzanfälle fehlen können. In den Fällen von traumatischer Darmzerreissung, die ich gesehen habe, kamen 2 erst nach 36 bezw. 48 Stunden in Behandlung, die beide der begleitenden Peritonitis erlagen, einer indes schon nach 3 Stunden. Derselbe hatte bald nach dem Hufschlag erbrochen, zeigte bei der Untersuchung nur leichte Spannung der Recti und ein Symptom, das mir besonders wichtig erscheint, nämlich eine kostale Athmung. Ich habe noch keine Perforation des Magendarmkanals gesehen, bei der dieses so wichtige Symptom gefehlt hätte. Bei einfacher Appendicitis bei Ileus ist die Athmung oft kostoabdominal, bei Perforationen meist rein kostal. Das kommt von dem Reiz der ergossenen Flüssigkeit ins Peritoneum. Denn bei geplatzten Extrauteringraviditäten, wo sich nur Blut in die Bauchhöhle ergiesst, ist die Athmung ebenfalls kostoabdominal. Der Gallenerguss bei geplatzten Gallenblasen macht eine fibrinöse Peritonitis ohne grosse Schmerzen. Hier fehlt auch meist eine ausgesprochene Spannung der Bauchdecken, während das Erbrechen meist in sehr ausgesprochenem Maasse vorhanden ist. Auch hier handelt es sich um einmaligen Erguss einer gewissen Menge Flüssigkeit, die sich infolge Verschlusses des Ductus cysticus in der gedehnten Blase ansammelt, bis diese platzt. Auch bei der Appendicitis ergiesst sich der Inhalt des Appendix in die Bauchhöhle, dann hört der Erguss auf. Beim Magengeschwür dagegen und in geringerem Grad auch bei der Darmzerreissung ergiessen sich andauernd neue Massen in das Peritoneum, solange das Loch offen bleibt. Daraus ergiebt sich auch die Prognose, die beim Magengeschwür zweifellos am schlechtesten ist, während sie bei der Darmzerreissung etwas besser wird. Innerhalb der ersten 6 Stunden ist die Prognose bei allen Perforationen gut, und diese wichtige Thatsache, dass alle innerhalb der ersten 6 Stunden nach der Perforation operirten Kranken geheilt sind, zeigt, wo der Hebel anzusetzen ist, um diesen Kranken zu helfen. Von den 8 Magengeschwürsperforationen, die ich operirt habe, kam 1 sechs Stunden, 2 je 24 Stunden, die übrigen 48-72 Stunden nach der Perforation in die chirurgische Behandlung. Der erste wurde gesund, die beiden nach 24 Stunden operirten überstanden die Operation, einer starb nach 4 Wochen an Blutungen aus einem zweiten Magengeschwür, einer 3 Wochen nach der glücklich überstandenen und geheilten Bauchoperation, an Lungengangrän und Empyem, die übrigen 2-6 Tage nach der Operation, au Peritonitis. Bei den traumatischen Darmzerreissungen wurde auch der nach 3 Stunden operirte geheilt, die anderen starben. Bei den Perforationen des Processus vermiformis wurden alle geheilt, die innerhalb der ersten 62 Stunden nach der Perforation operirt wurden. Von 8, die bis 72 Stunden nachher operirt wurden, starben 2, 6 wurden geheilt; von den 7 noch später operirten starben 4 und drei wurden geheilt. Bei allen Gestorbenen lag allgemeine diffuse Peritonitis vor.

Die Behandlung der akuten Perforationen des Magendarmkanals und der Gallenblase hat zuerst die Aufgabe das Loch zu schliessen, und dann die Peritonealhöhle so zu behandeln, dass die schon bestehende Infection derselben keine weiteren schädlichen Folgen zeitigt, dass sie zurückgeht. Ersteres wird erreicht durch Exstirpation des Wurmfortsatzes, nach dem man bei akuten Perforationen stets suchen muss, weil sonst stets neuer Darminhalt in die Bauchhöhle sich ergiesst und sich fast stets eine Darmfistel entwickelt, die schwer zu schliessen ist. Bei Abscessen die lange schon bestanden haben, ist der Wurmfortsatz meist schon obliterirt, sodass man sich die oft schwierige Operation der Ausschälung dieses Organes sparen kann. Die Behandlung des Stumpfes ist einfach. Ist schon Eiter da, dann binde ich bloss ab; findet sich in der Bauchhöhle nur strict seröse Flüssigkeit, dann kann man es wagen, den Stumpf zu übernähen, die Bauchwand zu nähen und durch einen Tampon für Abfluss des Secretes zu sorgen. Bei Magengeschwürsperforationen liegt die Sache insofern anders, als es sich bei Excision des Ulcus um eine Magenresection handeln muss. Die Geschwürsfläche ist oft erheblich grösser als das Loch in der Serosa, die Schleimhaut ist stark hyperämisch und überdeckt die Ränder des Geschwürs. Demnach soll man die Excision des Ulcus als die Normaloperation bezeichnen. Liegt es am Pylorus, so habe ich in 2 Fällen trotzdem excidirt und, da der Pylorus zu eng wurde, gleich die Gastroenterostomie angeschlossen. Das scheint mir noch einfacher zu sein als die Pylorusresection, die ohnehin in dem so stark entzündeten Peritoneum etwas Missliches hat. Das erste Erfordernis ist, dass das Ulcus ganz herausgenommen wird. Die Perforationen von Typhusgeschwüren müssen mit Darmresection behandelt werden, wenn sie grösser sind als eine Erbse. Andernfalls genügt eine Excision in längsovalem Schnitt mit querer Naht. Die geplatzte Gallenblase näht man am besten in die Haut ein, da Operationen am Gallengangssystem im entzündeten Peritoneum zu unsicher in ihrem Erfolg sind.

Bei allen diesen Fällen von Perforationen steht nun noch eine Frage im Vordergrund, das ist die Frage der Spülung. Soll man die Bauchhöhle ausspülen oder nicht? Früher war ich ein Gegner der Bauchspülung, da es sehr schwierig war, Kochsalzlösung in der nöthigen Menge und vor Allem der erforderlichen gleichmässigen Temperatur zu beschaffen. Ich fand, dass zu hohe und zu niedrige Temperaturen, namentlich aber ein Wechsel der Wassertemperatur einen sehr starken Reiz für das Peritoneum darstellt, der als Choc in die Erscheinung tritt. Die mit Gas geheizten Apparate functionirten schlecht, wenigstens nicht so absolut sicher wie man verlangen muss. Nun construirte die Firma Lautenschläger in Berlin einen Kochsalzapparat mit elektrischem Betrieb, der im Operationssaal selbst, ohne die Luft irgendwie zu beeinträchtigen, leicht anzubringen ist. Derselbe sterilisirt zunächst die eingefüllte Kochsalzlösung durch Erhitzen auf 110°. Dann wird sie durch kaltes Wasser, das durch Kühlschläuche läuft, abgekühlt bis 45° C., dann durch Einschalten von 2 Ampère andauernd auf 45° C. gehalten und zwar Tag und Nacht, sodass die ganze Klinik andauernd sterile Kochsalzlösung von 45° zur Verfügung hat. Der Apparat funktionirt bis jetzt ausgezeichnet, und zu meiner vollsten Zufriedenheit. Seit ich im Besitz dieses Apparates bin, spüle ich jede Magengeschwürsperforation mit grossen Mengen Kochsalzlösung aus, und zwar brauche ich jedesmal bis zu 50 Liter. Bei frischen Perforationen des Appendix habe ich noch nie gespült, nur wenn es sich um eine diffuse Peritonitis handelte, habe ich auch gespült.

Der Erfolg der Spülung war trotz Allem kein vollständiger. Trocknete ich nach vollendeter Spülung die Bauchhöhle aus, so fand ich unter dem Zwerchfell, im Douglas und auch zwischen Därmen stets noch trübe Flüssigkeit mit Eiter oder Mageninhalt untermischt, sodass ich nie mit dem Resultat zufrieden war, auch wenn die Flüssigkeit zuletzt klar abgeflossen war. Aus diesem Grunde habe ich dann in einer weiteren Serie von Fällen nicht mehr gespült, sondern die ganze Bauchhöhle mit trockenen Töpfern ausgetupft, wozu natürlich ein grosser Schnitt erforderlich ist. Vergleiche ich die Resultate, dann kann ich einen wesentlichen Unterschied der Fälle nicht finden. Ich will nicht mit Zahlen operiren. Es mag auch ein Zufall sein, dass die mit Spülung operirten fast sämtlich starben, während die geheilten fast alle

nicht gespült waren. Alle drei Magengeschwüre, die mit Spülung
behandelt waren, haben die Operation mehrere Wochen überstanden, alle die nicht gespült sind, sind innerhalb einer Woche gestorben. Ich glaube das darauf zurückführen zu müssen, dass in
den meisten Fällen von akuten Perforationen die Peritonitis zunächst noch keine diffuse ist, sondern lokal bleibt. Beim Blinddarm
sind die zunächstliegenden Darmpartien, beim Magen der Raum
zwischen Leber und Zwerchfell, vor dem Netz, im Douglas und
zu beiden Seiten die Umgebung des Colon ascendens und descen-
dens betroffen. Das Netz selbst schützt aber den ganzen Dünndarm, wie eine grosse breite Schürze, lange vor dem Mageninhalt.
Spült man ein, dann vertheilt man den ergossenen Mageninhalt
über das ganze Peritoneum in verdünnter Form und macht so
eine Art von Aussaat über eine grosse Fläche. Dann kann ich
mich des Eindrucks nicht erwehren, dass das nach einer Perforation sich bildende Serum, das zunächst nur getrübt erscheint, die
schädlichen Keime der ergossenen Flüssigkeit gewissermaassen
einhüllt und unschädlich macht. Denn sonst kann man kaum
verstehen, wie nach einer Perforation des processus vermiformis,
wenn die Operation früh gemacht wird man, vorausgesetzt, dass
noch kein Eiter sich gebildet hat, nach sorgfältiger Austupfung
die Bauchwunde oft nähen kann, und prima Heilung eintritt. Eine
Spülung würde diese seröse Flüssigkeit verdünnen und dadurch
schaden.

Weiterhin kann ich mich des Eindrucks nicht erwehren, dass
die ausgedehnte Spülung der Bauchhöhle im Sinne eines Chocs
schwächend auf den Kranken einwirkt. Bei Thieren habe ich grosse
Massen dieser erwärmten Kochsalzlösung durch den Bauch laufen
lassen, ohne dass ich einen sichtbaren Schaden gesehen hätte. Aber
das beweist nichts, da es sich um Thiere handelt, und eine Perforation nicht vorlag.

Ich stehe also auf dem Standpunkt, dass man bei akuten frischen Perforationen des Magendarmkanals nicht spülen, sondern
nur trocken austupfen soll; besteht schon ein wirklich allgemeine
Peritonitis, so habe ich nicht viel gegen die Spülung einzuwenden;
ich kenne aber noch keinen Fall, der durch eine Spülung gerettet
wäre. Bei akuter Perforation des Processus vermiformis halte ich
eine Spülung für kontraindicirt.

Betreffs der weiteren Behandlung der Operirten will ich noch
erwähnen, dass ich es für sehr richtig halte, dass die Kranken 48
Tage nichts per os geniessen. Tritt Erbrechen ein, so mache ich

nene Magenspülung. Die Ernährung besteht nur in subkutanen, nicht intravenösen Kochsalzinfusionen, und zwar pro Tag etwa ein Liter. Sind die Kranken schwach, so bekommen sie die erste Injection schon auf dem Operationstisch.

Eine weitere Gefahr erwächst dem Kranken noch durch die Pneumonie, die sich so oft an Laparatomien anschliesst. Leider stehen uns keine Mittel zu Gebote, um dieser grossen Gefahr zu begegnen. Je mehr wir fortschreiten in der Erkenntnis der Ursachen dieser Erkrankung, umso trostloser ist die Prophylaxe. Wir kennen schon die Schluckpneumonie die durch grosse Sorgfalt bei der Narkose wohl zu vermeiden ist. Schwieriger ist es schon bei vor der Operation bestehendem Bronchial-Katarrh. Hier liegt der Grund der Operationspneumonie in der Unmöglichkeit des Kranken, den angesammelten Schleim durch Husten zu entfernen, da Husten zu schmerzhaft ist. So sammelt sich der Schleim in den Bronchien an, und ruft schliesslich eine Bronchopneumonie hervor. Gänzlich hülflos stehen wir der Embolie kleinster Lungengefässe durch Blutgerinsel oder durch Fett gegenüber. Erstere sind ja nur möglich im Gebiete des Plexus hämorrhoidalis und der Vena spermatica, da diese allein ihr Blut in die Vena cava ergiessen. Der Annahme von Pneumonien auf dem Lymphwege stehe ich etwas ungläubig gegenüber, da eine Infection der Lymphe des Zwerchfells auf die Bronchialdrüsen und von diesen aus erst auf die Lungen einwirken kann. Alle diese Erklärungen passen auch nicht auf 2 Fälle von Operationspneumonie die ich beobachtet habe. Ein völlig gesunder Arbeiter erhält einen Fusstritt gegen das Abdomen; 4 Stunden später mache ich eine Darmresection wegen Darmzerreissung. Die Narkose verläuft ohne Erbrechen. Sofort nach der Operation zeigt der Mann eine mühsame Athmung von 28 in der Minute, bei normalem Puls von 72. 4 Stunden später steigt die Temperatur auf 38,5°. Am zweiten Tage waren einzelne pneumonische Heerde in beiden Lungen nachzuweisen, nach 8 Tagen starb er an der doppelseitigen Pneumonie. Bei der Obduction war die Bauchhöhle normal, die Resection war glatt per primam geheilt. In beiden Lungen fanden sich zahllose Heerde, die vielfach konfluirten und am meisten der croupösen Pneumonie ähnelten. In einem zweiten Falle handelte es sich um eine Gastroenterostomie bei einem Manne wegen Pyloruscarcinom. Auch hier sofort nach der Operation eine Beschleunigung der vorher ruhigen Athmung bis 26, nach 8 Tagen Exitus an Pneumonie. Alle bisherigen Erklärungen versagen hier. Eine Embolie grösserer Aeste der

Arteria pulmonalis lag nicht vor. In beiden Fällen war am Darm
bezw. am Magen operirt worden, es waren also Chylusgefässe in
grosser Anzahl eröffnet, da ist es nun sehr wohl möglich, dass
in diese Chylusgänge Darminhalt eingetreten ist und nun durch den
ductus thoracicus dem Blute und dann den Lungen zugeführt
wird. Anatomisch ist dieser Weg sehr wohl möglich. Versuche die
ich bei Thieren machte haben kein positives Resultat ergeben,
was indes an und für sich noch nichts beweist.

Nimmt man diese Möglichkeit an, dann sind eine ganze Reihe
von Operationspneumonien erklärt, für die wir bisher eine Erklärung noch nicht hatten.

Le prolapsus du rectum; sa pathogénie et son traitement

Par M. N. NAPALKOW, Moscou.

Les infirmités, appelées ordinairement prolapsus du rectum, ne
représentent pas une forme de maladie déterminée, mais plusieurs
lésions de nature différente. De là, l'impossibilité d'une définition
précise, d'un côté, et la nécessité de classification des diverses formes, de l'autre. D'abord nous devons exclure de cette catégorie
les maladies appelées par les chirurgiens allemands prolapsus
coli-invaginat; elles n'ont aucun rapport avec les maladies du rectum, car cet intestin ne sert que comme canal, donnant passage
au côlon prolabé.

Toutes les autres formes du prolapsus, réunies sous le nom
commun de prolapsus du rectum, peuvent être ramenées à deux
groupes: le prolapsus de la muqueuse rectale et le prolapsus du
rectum in toto.

Le prolapsus de la muqueuse se limite, d'après l'opinion
commune, à la région de l'anus et, par conséquent, est identifié au
prolapsus de l'anus. Cette dernière dénomination manque tout à
fait de précision, car la formation la plus caractéristique de l'anus,
son appareil obturateur, n'est jamais soumis au prolapsus. En surplus, la muqueuse peut prolaber non seulement dans la région
de l'anus, mais à un niveau plus élevé; on a observé des cas de
prolapsus de la muqueuse d'une longueur de 5 à 8 cent. et même
de 12 cent. Le trait le plus caractéristique du prolapsus de la muqueuse qu'on peut constater dans tous les cas, c'est un état catarrhal du rectum. Cet état catarrhal ne se limite pas seulement à
la partie prolabée de la muqueuse, mais s'élève à une hauteur
assez considérable. En surplus, dans un certain nombre de cas

j'ai pu constater avec toute la précision que le catarrhe ne s'était pas produit comme suite du prolapsus, mais l'avait bien précédé. Enfin, à l'occasion d'opérations pratiquées sur des hémorrhoïdes, j'ai pu pronostiquer le développement du prolapsus d'avance, me basant sur l'observation d'un état catarrhal très prononcé de la muqueuse rectale; effectivement le prolapsus se développa à une échéance plus ou moins longue. Toutes ces observations me donnent des raisons pour insister sur ce que le prolapsus de la muqueuse rectale est une suite de son état catarrhal. Les données étiologiques correspondent entièrement à ces conclusions, car le prolapsus représente presque toujours une complication du catarrhe intestinal ou des hémorrhoïdes. Les enfants et les individus atteints d'hémorrhoïdes sont les plus exposés à cette lésion. Pourtant les adultes peuvent en être atteints même en l'absence d'hémorrhoïdes; nous citerons comme exemple le prolapsus après la dysenterie.

L'influence du catarrhe, favorable à l'évolution du prolapsus de la muqueuse, influe dans deux directions: prémièrement il se produit une tumeur de la muqueuse, secondement il se développe un œdème et un relâchement du tissu conjonctif sous-muqueux. La muqueuse devient spongieuse, épaisse, forme dans l'intérieur de l'intestin une quantité de grands replis, saigne souvent, se couvre d'ulcères et donne lieu quelquefois au développement de tumeurs polypeuses. La stase veineuse et l'œdème de tissu sous-muqueux causent souvent la néoformation exagérée de tissu conjonctif. Dans les cas d'un prolapsus prolongé, on observe aussi une affection de la tunique musculaire du rectum, les fibres musculaires sont remplacées par du tissu conjonctif. Il se produit encore plus tôt une dégénérescence des faisceaux de fibres musculaires lisses qui traversent le tissu cellulaire sous-muqueux en le parcourant de la tunique musculaire à la tunique muqueuse; de cette manière la solidité de la tunique muqueuse est affaiblie. Nous observons souvent aussi une atténuation de la sensibilité au toucher de la muqueuse anale. Cet affaiblissement semble être une suite des troubles de la circulation; on peut émettre en faveur de cette supposition l'observation que ce fait se retrouve très souvent dans les cas d'hémorrhoïdes rectales. Cet affaiblissement de la sensibilité, joint à l'influence du procès inflammatoire et à l'influence de la dilatation constante du sphincter anal par la muqueuse prolabée, produit l'atonie du sphincter; cette atonie favorise de son côté la formation du prolapsus. Voilà les conclusions principales, concernant la pathogénie du prolapsus de la muqueuse rectale, auxquelles je suis arrivé en me basant sur les observations que j'ai faites à la clinique du prof. Diakonow, à Moscou.

Quant au traitement du prolapsus de la muqueuse rectale, c'est la lésion catarrhale du rectum, qui doit avant tout être prise en considération. Dans les cas récents, surtout chez les enfants, le prolapsus peut être guéri par le traitement du catarrhe. Mais dans les cas invétérés on doit avoir recours non seulement au traitement du catarrhe, mais à une excision de la muqueuse, partielle ou circonférencielle, car les lésions anatomiques ont pris dans ce cas un caractère permanent. On doit bien remarquer que non seulement la partie prolabée de la muqueuse est soumise aux lésions, mais encore ses parties situées plus haut. C'est la raison pourquoi on observe souvent la récidive du prolapsus de la muqueuse après son excision. Pour contribuer à l'atrophie de la muqueuse, épaissie sous l'influence du procès inflammatoire, j'ai pratiqué dans plusieurs cas, après l'excision de la partie prolabée, la torsion du cylindre supérieur de la muqueuse à 180° et j'ai obtenu des résultats excellents. En tout cas, le traitement de la lésion catarrhale ne doit jamais être négligé.

Le prolapsus du rectum in toto a donné occasion à un nombre considérable d'hypothèses concernant sa pathogénie et à un plus grand nombre encore de procédés opératoires pour sa guérison. Néanmoins, les causes de son développement ne sont pas claires jusqu'à présent et les résultats de son traitement restent incertains. Une des causes principales de cette incertitude, c'est l'insuffisance des observations anatomiques à l'égard des modifications qui se produisent dans les relations topographiques entre le rectum prolabé et les tissus et les organes du plancher pelvien. J'ai tâché de suppléer à cette insuffisance en cherchant à provoquer un prolapsus artificiel sur le cadavre, et j'y ai réussi. J'introduisis une canule par l'ombilic dans la cavité de l'abdomen, ensuite je remplis les deux cavités pleurales de plâtre et j'entourai l'abdomen de bandes plâtrées. Pompant ensuite de l'air ou de l'eau dans la cavité abdominale et en élevant lentement la pression jusqu'à 1,5—2 atmosphères, j'obtins d'abord une saillie considérable du périnée et ensuite la chute du rectum. Sur les cadavres d'enfants j'obtins les mêmes résultats sans plâtrer les plèvres et l'abdomen, mais à condition d'élever la pression intraabdominale très lentement, si l'augmentation de la pression est trop rapide, les tissus se rompent et l'expérience ne réussit pas.

Ces expériences nous ont démontré que le prolapsus rectal commence par la paroi antérieure du rectum au niveau du pli transversal de Kohlransch. Cette partie de la paroi intestinale s'invagine dans la lumière du rectum, qui dans cet endroit forme ampoule; successivement sont entraînées les parois latérales du rectum, qui finalement sont suivies par la paroi postérieure. La partie du rectum qui la première est soumise au prolapsus correspond au niveau du fond de l'excavation vésico-rectale. Le sac péritonéal descend dans la courbe de la paroi intestinale antérieure, passe accompagné de cette dernière entre les bords médiaux des releveurs de l'anus et fait saillie par l'anus. Dans mes observations, le péritoine ne recouvrait jamais la partie postérieure du prolapsus; je dois remarquer ici, que je cessais mes expériences quand j'obtenais un prolapsus d'une langueur de 3 — 5 cent. Je renonçais à une saillie plus volumineuse craignant la rupture de l'intestin. Lorsque le prolapsus, chez les hommes vivants, se produit très lentement et atteint un volume considérable, par suite d'une dilatation progressive des tissus, l'abaissement du péritoine à la face postérieure de la partie prolabée est possible. Des viscères peuvent être entraînés dans le cul-de-sac péritonéal, comme par exemple l'ovaire, les anses intestinales. Autour de l'orifice anal, entre la partie prolabée de l'intestin et l'anus, se forme un sillon, dont la profondeur diminue à mesure que le prolapsus augmente. De cette manière j'obtins un prolapsus en forme de trois cylindres. Je dois faire observer pourtant que le cylindre extérieur n'est autre chose que la partie anale du rectum. Tant qu'elle reste en place, il n'y a aucune raison à la rapporter au prolapsus.

Lorsque les dimensions de la masse prolabée augmentent, elle peut être entraînée, mais alors elle formera une partie du second cylindre. Entraînée entièrement dans le prolapsus, le sillon à l'orifice anal disparaît et le prolapsus ne sera composé que de deux cylindres. C'est pourquoi on a plus de raison de parler de deux cylindres. Quant à l'état des muscles releveurs de l'anus, mes observations fournissent les données suivantes: si l'on introduit le doigt du côté du péritoine jusqu'au fond de l'excavation vésico-rectale, qui descend dans la masse prolabée, les bords des muscles font l'impression de bandes résistantes qui enserrent le doigt. Lors de la dissection, je constatai que la fente entre leurs bords à la face antérieure du rectum était de 1,5 à 3 cent. La surface concave supérieure des muscles releveurs de l'anus s'approche de la circonférence cutanée de l'anus, ce qui cause l'allongement considérable des fibres musculaires. Si le prolapsus est réduit, la tension des fibres musculaires est affaiblie et la face supérieure du diaphragme pelvien s'élève. Les fibres des muscles releveurs de l'anus, rencontrant la paroi du rectum, s'entrecroisent avec la couche musculaire de la paroi et longeant cet intestin jusqu'à la peau, forment une espèce de canal musculaire destiné au passage du rectum. Je lui propose la dénomination de canal périnéo-rectal. Son orifice abdominal est situé au niveau de la surface supérieure du diaphragme pelvien musculaire; son orifice cutané est formé par l'anus. Dans le cas du prolapsus du rectum ce canal est traversé par la paroi antérieure du rectum et par le sac péritonéal; le canal s'élargit, mais devient plus court, et son orifice abdominal s'approche de son orifice cutané. Quant aux lésions des muscles releveurs de l'anus chez les malades, j'ai eu l'occasion de les étudier durant l'opération même, ou bien au microscope sur des coupes faites de petits morceaux de tissu musculaire, excisés pendant l'intervention chirurgicale. Dans tous les cas, je trouvai les muscles atrophiés et pâles; l'examen microscopique montrait leur dégénérescence en tissu conjonctif. De même, les fibres musculaires lisses du tube intestinal sont aussi soumises à des lésions considérables, qui portent le caractère d'atrophie et de la dégénérescence en tissu conjonctif.

Il serait fastidieux d'énumérer tous les faits que j'ai eu l'occasion de constater durant mes recherches anatomiques et cliniques; je ne m'arrêterai pas non plus sur les principes de la théorie herniaire du prolapsus du rectum, bien exposée d'ailleurs par *Waldeyer* et *Laudloff*. Je pense avoir donné à cette théorie une nouvelle base, une base expérimentale. Les observations cliniques ne m'ont rien donné qui fût contraire à cette théorie, c'est pourquoi je l'adopte entièrement et je la pose comme base du traitement opératoire du prolapsus du rectum. Envisageant le prolapsus comme une hernie, je dois établir les propositions suivantes comme but auquel doit tendre l'intervention chirurgicale; il est indispensable de supprimer le sac herniaire et de fermer l'orifice abdominal du canal herniaire par du tissu musculaire. Quant à la résection de la partie prolabée du rectum, vu l'absence de lésions considérables, elle est inutile, car la paroi intestinale n'est entraînée dans le prolapsus que successivement sous l'influence de l'abaissement du sac péritonéal. En pratiquant l'ex-

cision du sac herniaire, il faut avoir en vue que pendant la réduction du prolapsus le péritoine se retire en haut, et qu'il se
trouve situé dans la masse du tissu adipeux de l'espace pelvi-rec-
tal supérieur. Pour la fermeture de l'orifice abdominal du canal,
il est indispensable d'obvier à la faiblesse des muscles releveurs
de l'anus et de la tunique musculaire du rectum. On peut rassembler les fibres musculaires de la paroi intestinale à sa face
antérieure comme un hernia par 2-3 sutures transversales qui ne
doivent pas pénétrer dans la lumière de l'intestin. De cette manière on obtiendra une paroi intestinale plus rigide et plus résistante à la pression du sac péritonéal.

Pour fortifier les muscles releveurs de l'anus il sera urgent
de rétrécir la fente entre leurs bords médiaux et de supprimer
l'allongement de leurs fibres détendues. On rétrécit la fente en
unissant les bords des muscles par suture sur la ligne médiane,
et on supprime l'allongement en pratiquant la plicature transversale des muscles releveurs. Voici la technique à mettre en pratique sur le malade; par une incision courbe prérectale du périnée on découvre la surface inférieure des muscles releveurs de
l'anus. Passant à travers la fente des releveurs de l'anus, on
partage avec précaution le tissu cellulaire au moyen des pinces
en y cherchant le cul-de-sac péritonéal. On le détache ensuite du
tissu cellulaire, on le dissèque, on en éloigne les viscères prola-
bés, on le lie très haut et on le résèque; ensuite on passe au renforcement des muscles de la paroi antérieure du rectum et du
diaphragme pelvien. On fait de droite à gauche 2-3 sutures à travers les bords des deux releveurs de l'anus et de la couche musculaire intestinale. Sans nouer ces sutures, on pratique un
plissement transversal de chacun des muscles releveurs de manière à les rendre plus courts et plus épais. Chaque pli est fixé
par une suture. Ce n'est qu'à ce moment qu'on tire les fils,
passés auparavant à travers la paroi intestinale et les bords
des releveurs. Tous les fils peuvent être conduits jusqu'à la peau
pour pouvoir les enlever dans quelque temps; dans ce but, on
croisera les bouts des fils des sutures correspondantes sous la
peau de manière à former le chiffre 8. Ces bouts peuvent être
employés pour la réunion de la plaie cutanée; de chaque côté de
la plaie on introduit une bande de gaze.

Dans la période post-opératoire, les malades doivent s'abstenir
pendant quelque temps de faire des efforts et l'évacuation des
matières fécales se fera dans une position horizontale. Dans quel-

ques cas de reposition du prolapsus, je n'ai pas réussi à trouver le péritoine en forme de sac herniaire; je me contentai alors d'un renforcement des muscles de la paroi intestinale et du diaphragme pelvien et j'obtins des succès. Ce procédé opératoire a été pratiqué dans neuf cas, et chaque fois avec succès. Deux sujets furent examinés plus de 18 mois après l'opération et furent trouvés guéris. Quelques malades ont été opérés depuis plus de 4 ans et nous avons toutes les raisons de supposer qu'en cas de rechute ils seraient revenus à la clinique.

Deux fois, j'ai rencontré dans le cours de mes opérations une complication qu'il faut avoir en vue: dans un cas, aussitôt après l'opération, sur la table même, par suite d'un effort du malade, il se produisit un prolapsus de la muqueuse; je fis de suite la torsion de la muqueuse à 180° et le malade guérit. Dans le second cas, le prolapsus de la muqueuse se développa chez une femme après sa sortie de la clinique. Modéré dans ses dimensions, il inquiétait peu la malade en comparaison du prolapsus précédent. Ayant en vue que le prolapsus du rectum est toujours compliqué par la lésion catarrhale et que cette lésion est la cause principale du prolapsus de la muqueuse, cette complication sera facile à comprendre.

J'ai tâché de baser le traitement du prolapsus du rectum sur l'étude des modifications des conditions topographo-anatomiques et je suis convaincu que le succès ne dépend pas de l'invention de nouvelles méthodes opératoires, mais de l'exploration de la topographie pathologique de la lésion.

Erfahrungen über einzeitige Resektion von Colon- und Cœcaltumoren

Aus dem öffentl. Kaiser Franz-Joseph-Hospital in Trebitsch

Par M. J. BAKES, Trebitsch.

Die chirurgische Therapie der Dickdarmtumoren ausschliesslich der Rectalgeschwülste bewegt sich, durch hervorragende Arbeiten Hohenegg's, Mikulicz's und Schloffer's gefördert, vorwiegend in den Grenzen des mehrzeitigen Verfahrens, welches mit Recht so allgemein sich eingebürgert hat, dass die einzeitige Resection nun wenig in Betracht kommt.

Dank den oberwähnten Arbeiten sowie den Erfahrungen über Ileus wissen wir, dass Kranke mit Stenosenerscheinungen keinem grösseren Eingriffe, insbesondere in tiefer Allgemeinnarkose gewachsen sind, und dass eine Operation hier auf das möglichste Minimum beschränkt werden müsse.

Wir wissen nun auch, dass bei jeder Darmresection trotz strengster Asepsis und bester Technik eine Aussaat von Keimen auf die anliegende Serosa erfolgt, mit welchen die resorptive Kraft d. Peritoneums fertig werden muss. Diese ist aber bei den zumeist sehr herabgekommenen Kranken erheblich gestört, sodass man ihnen auch in dieser Hinsicht nicht viel zumuten darf.

Deshalb besitzt das mehrzeitige Verfahren unschätzbare Vorteile, welche insbesondere in Fällen von acutem und chron. Ileus eclatant zu Tage treten.

Es gibt jedoch Fälle von Colontumoren, in denen man es unter Beobachtung gewisser technischer Maassnahmen wagen darf, das Neoplasma *einzeitig* zu entfernen, ohne die Gefahr für den Kranken zu erhöhen.

Dadurch wird dem Kranken ein langes Krankenlager und eine ganze Reihe von Nachoperationen, von denen insbesondere der Verschluss des Anus praeternaturalis nicht immer ungefährlich und technisch leicht ist, erspart.

Wir wollen daher an der Hand des operierten bescheidenen Materiales für die in den Hintergrund gestellte einzeitige radicale Resection von Coecal und Colontumoren eine Lanze brechen, um sie in geeigneten Fällen wieder zur Geltung zu bringen, ohne die glänzenden Erfolge der mehrzeitigen Methoden schmälern zu wollen.

Welche sind nun die geeigneten Fälle?

Es ist bekannt, dass nahezu jedesmal erst die Stenosenerscheinungen uns das Vorhandensein eines Darmtumors anzeigen. Diese Symptome der gestörten Darmpassage allein geben nach unserem Dafürhalten durchaus keine Contraindication gegen das einzeitige Verfahren ab, wenn der Allgemeinzustand und insbesondere das Herz der Kranken noch leistungsfähig befunden werden, und weiter bei der Laparotomie sich herausstellt dass die Mobilisierung des Neoplasmas auf keine technischen Schwierigkeiten stossen dürfte.

Bei der Beurteilung der zu operierenden Fälle kommt es also *auf die Dauer und den Grad der Stenose*, welche der Resorption giftiger Darmproducte proportional ist, und *auf die vorgefundenen jeweiligen localen Verhältnisse* an, ob ein- oder mehrzeitig operiert werden soll.

Ein wichtiges Postulat scheint uns dabei zu sein, dass der Eingriff unter *möglichster Schonung der Körperwärme des Kranken und ohne allgemeine tiefe Narcose* vorgenommen werde. Rigo-

roseste Asepsis und extraperitoneales Operieren nach Mobilisierung und Eventration des Neoplasmas sind ganz selbstverständ-
lich.

Wenn hingegen der Organismus des Kranken durch Toxinresor-
ption geschwächt erscheint (Herz!) überdiess die Mobilmachung
des Tumors Schwierigkeiten bereitet, oder es sich um eine Attaque
von Ileus handelt, dann werden wir am besten nach der Methode Schloffer's durch Anlegen eines Anus vor der Stenose (in Localanaesthesie!) dem Kranken Zeit lassen sich von seiner Auto-
Intoxication nach Möglichkeit zu erholen und dann eventuell radical
operieren.

Aus unserem Material ist ersichtlich, dass wir ziemlich vorgeschrittene Fälle sehr eingreifenden Operationen unterzogen haben, ohne dass der geringste Schaden den Kranken daraus er-
wachsen wäre, denn sämtliche sieben [*] einzeitig Resecierte sind
geheilt entlassen worden.

Diesen eben erwähnten Erfolg bei unseren einzeitigen Resectionen schreiben wir zwei Umständen zu:

1) *der Methode unserer combinierten Narkose;*

2) *einigen technischen Modificationen des Eingriffes selbst.*

Die combinierte Narkose ermöglicht es in erster Linie die
Eingriffe, abgesehen vom temporär applicierten Aetherrausch eigentlich ohne Narcose auszuführen; die Operation selbst wird mit
grösster Exactheit und Ruhe ohne Hast, ohne Furcht vor Narcose-
complicationen durchgeführt. Das bei Allgemeinnarkose so wichtige rascheste Beenden des Eingriffes fällt weg, da die Kranken
gut gegen Wärmeverluste geschützt die längere Operationsdauer
garnicht empfinden. Unsere sämtlichen grossen Magendarmopera-
tionen beanspruchen ungefähr drei Stunden zu ihrer Vollendung,
und die Patienten sind trotz der langen Operationsdauer *in so
guter somatischer Condition, wie es sonst nach keinem Eingriffe
in tiefer Allgemeinnarkose der Fall ist.*

Die Technik ist kurz folgende: der in dicke Flanellanzüge ge-
hüllte und auf einen Thermophortisch bequem gebettete Kranke
wird 20 Minuten vor Beginn der Operation durch subcutane Injection von 0,015-0,02 Morph. morphinisiert und vom Narcotiseur
über den Verlauf der vorzunehmenden Maassnahmen genau ins-

---

[*] Inzwischen wurden weitere vier Fälle ausgedehnten Resectionen wegen mal. Colonmo-
tren nach den hier beschriebenen Principien unterzogen, und gehe ... entlassen, sodass nun die Reihe
geheilt einzeit... er Colonresectionen ... beträgt.

truiert. Der Eingriff beginnt mit Infiltrationsanaesthesie, in welcher d. Abdomen eröffnet wird. Nun kommt der erste Aetherrausch, in dem das Peritoneum parietale gespalten, die Orientierung im Bauche vorgenommen und die des Eingriffes bedürftigen Organe eventriert werden. Zu diesem Rausche werden ca. 10—30 gr. Aether verbraucht.

Hierauf erfolgt die ganze eigentliche Operation schmerzlos bei vollem Bewusstsein der Kranken. Bei starken Verwachsungen verursacht der Zug an den Mesenterien, dem Peritoneum parietale, überhaupt der Zug an den fixen Puncten der Bauchhöhle dem Patienten ein Gefühl des Druckes und manchmal nicht unerhebliche Schmerzen, welche durch Wiederholung des Rausches oder durch Infiltrationsanaesthesie coupiert werden müssen. Die Toilette der Bauchwunde, sowie die Reposition der Organe geschieht unter reichlicher Spülung von warmer (40°C) physiologischer Salzlösung, worauf die Bauchdeckennaht mit Infiltrationsanaesthesie beendet wird.

Die Bauchspannung bekämpfen wir durch energisches Fordern von tiefem Ein- und Ausathmen. Das lästige Aufstellen der Beine beim Erwachen aus dem Rausche machen wir durch Anbinden der Kniegelenke mit breiter Compresse zur Platte des Operationstisches unmöglich.

Diese Narkosemethode basiert auf genauer Kenntniss der Schmerzhaftigkeit und Schmerzlosigkeit diverser Gewebe und Organe des menschlichen Körpers. Zu ihrem vollständigen Gelingen ist eine Operationstechnik von nöthen, welche der bei grossen Eingriffen in Localanaesthesie üblichen am nächsten steht.

Das Anfassen der Gewebe muss zart geschehen, jedweder brüsker Zug muss vermieden werden. Reichliches Benetzen des Operationsfeldes mit physiologischer Kochsalzlösung, sowie Verwendung feuchter Tupfer und Gummihandschuhe, welche durch in Kochsalzlösung angezogene Tricothandschuhe geschützt werden und ihre Schlüpfrigkeit verlieren, unterstützen das Gelingen dieser Methode.

Der zweite Umstand, dem wir das oberwähnte Resultat zuschreiben, sind einige *technische Modificationen.*

Vor Allem sind wir bestrebt, *möglichst viel vom Dickdarm mit dem Neoplasma,* ohne uns darum zu kümmern, ob die Darmenden aneinander gebracht werden können oder nicht, zu entfernen, was mehrfache Vorteile in sich birgt:

1. wird mit grösserer Sicherheit alles Krankhafte entfernt

und die Möglichkeit des Recidivs entsprechend in die Ferne
gerückt;

2. wird die angelegte Naht insoferne geschont als der Darminhalt breiig und noch ungeformt die Nahtstelle passiert; die nicht
selten vor der Stenose angehäuften Kotmassen werden mitentfernt;

3. kommen Darmteile mit physiologisch noch intacter Wand
zur Vereinigung; denn es ist bekannt, dass der vor der Stenose
befindliche Darm nicht nur hypertrophisch, sondern durch Ueber-
dehnung und andere Noxen pathologisch verändert ist, was selbst-
verständlich die Festigkeit seiner Naht beeinflussen kann.

Die Enden werden nach Doyen blind geschlossen, und die
Vereinigung durch laterale Apposition im Sinne der Peristaltik mit
Naht (3 schichtig) vereinigt. Wo dies infolge Wegfalles zu grosser
Darm-Abschnitte unmöglich wird, stehen wir nicht an durch *Mobi-
lisierung der fixen Flexuren* die Enden so zu nähern, dass keine
Spannung bei Vereinigung derselben besteht.

Die Mobilisierung der Flexuren wird durch bogenförmige Spal-
tung des Peritoneum parietale und stumpfes Abschieben des fixen
Darmteiles von seiner Unterlage — analog der Mobilmachung des
Duodenums — ausgeführt.

Bei Resection zu grosser Colonabschnitte wird die Passage
durch Ileocolostomie hergestellt.

Beim Anlegen der Anastomose legen wir das Hauptgewicht
auf das exacte Ausführen der Mucosanaht. Die fertige Anastomose
sichern wir noch durch ausgiebige Netzplastik.

Nach der Toilette des Operationsterrains und Reposition der
Organe wird der Eingriff in der Regel ohne Tamponade durch mehr-
schichtige Bauchdeckennaht, nachdem in die Bauchhöhle Kochsalzlösung eingegossen wurde, beendet.

Zu den technischen Behelfen behufs frühzeitiger Diagnosenstellung gehört die *Coloscopie*, wenn Kranke mit Tumoren unter der
Flexura lienalis in Betracht kommen. Es gelingt insbesondere in
Fällen mit unsicheren Stenosenbeschwerden durch Coloscopie das
manchmal sehr kleine Carcinom zu entdecken. So passierte uns
in einem Falle, dass die kleine Stenose der unteren Flexura sigm.
bei der Laparotomie der Palpation entgieng und erst durch später
vorgenommene Coloscopie gefunden wurde. Der Patient wurde fäls-
chlich als Appendicitis operiert. Bei dem bekannten heimtücki-
schen Charakter der Colontumoren sollte bei jedem leisesten Verdacht auf Tumor von der Coloscopie der ausgedehnteste Gebrauch
gemacht werden.

Eine erfreulicherweise seltene Eigenschaft der malignen Dickdarmgeschwülste sind die sogenannten *Doppeltumoren*. Einen einschlägigen Fall beschrieb Körte in seiner Arbeit über Dickdarmgeschwülste, einen Fall beobachtete ich als Assistent der Klinik weiland Albert in Wien; derselbe kam nach dem Eingriffe zur Obduction, wobei der bei der Operation zurückgelassene Secundärtumor am Dickdarme erst entdeckt wurde — und einen Fall hatte ich das Glück vor 2 Jahren mit Erfolg zu operieren — die Frau erfreut sich heute des besten Wohlseins.

Trotz der Seltenheit d. Vorkommnisse wäre es von Wichtigkeit bei malignen Colontumoren während der Orientierung im Bauche den ganzen Dickdarm bis in den Douglas gründlichst abzutasten.

Das zweite Carcinom ist in der Regel klein. In dem oben erwähnten glücklich operierten Falle wurde palpatorisch vor dem Eingriffe nur das faustgrosse Carcinom der Flex. sigmoid. diagnostiziert; während der Operation musste unseren Principien gemäss die flexura lienalis mobilisiert werden, wobei zu unserer Ueberraschung am Colon transv. sich ein ganz kleiner carcinomatöser Ring mit infiltrierten Drüsen im Netze entdecken liess und natürlich in toto sammt dem entsprechenden Stück des Querdarmes exstirpiert wurde. Die laterale Apposition der blind geschlossenen Enden gelang dann nach Mobilmachung der Flexura hepatica anstandslos.

Zu betonen wäre noch, dass Doppelresectionen bei diesen Doppeltumoren als zeitraubend und den Patienten gefährdend grundsätzlich zu vermeiden sind — es ist technisch leichter und für den Kranken schonender den ganzen erkrankten Darmabschnitt mit einem Schlage zu entfernen, zumal die vielseitig schon erprobte Tatsache feststeht, dass der Organismus den Verlust ganz grosser Darmabschnitte gut verträgt.

Das Material auf Grund dessen wir es wagen auf den einzeitigen Operationsweg zu verweisen beläuft sich auf 12 Fälle (*) welche binnen 3 jähriger Tätigkeit im Trebitscher Hospitale unter ca. 340 Laparotomien zur Ausführung gelangten.

Sieben Fälle (**) sind einzeitig radical reseciert worden mit sieben Heilungen, fünf Fälle sind palliativ operiert worden mit 3 Todesfällen, welches ungünstige Resultat nicht etwa den ange-

---

*) Nun 16 Fälle unter 412 Laparotomien. 31.X.1905.
**) Nun 11 Fälle sämtlich geheilt.

wandten mehrzeitigen Methoden, sondern eben der Schwere der Fälle selbst zuzuschreiben ist.

Von den sieben geheilten Fällen habe ich sechs theils selbst nach-untersucht, theils Bericht von praktischen Collegen erhalten. Bis dato sind alle sechs gesund und gehen ihren Lebensbeschäftigungen nach.

Der älteste Fall (I) ist jetzt drei Jahre drei Monate, Fall II 2 Jahre 8 Monate, Fall III 1 Jahr 11 Monate und Fall IV 1 Jahr 5 Monate nach dem Eingriffe, die übrigen sind jüngeren Datums.

Reseciert wurden:

3 Mal Coecum und Colon ascend. (Fälle III, V, VI).

1 Mal Coecum, Colon ascend., Flex. hepat. und Colon transversum (Fall I).

1 Mal Colon transv. und Flex. lien. (Fall II).

1 Mal Colon transv., Flex. lien. und Flex. sigmoid. (Fall IV).

1 Mal Magen und Colon transversum (Fall VII).

Nun folgen in Kürze die Krankengeschichten der einzeitig operierten Fälle:

FALL I. Ca. coeci, coli ascend. et flexurae hepaticae. — Resectio, Ileocolostomia. Sanatio.

Marie B. Gutsbesitzersfrau aus Oblistov (Mähren), Aufg. 16-IV, — geh. entl. 14-V-1903.

Die Familienanamnese der Patientin ist insoferne interessant als 2 von ihren Brüdern an ähnlichen Darmgeschwülsten unoperiert gestorben sind und ihre Schwester auch an Colontumor (Fall IV) ein Jahr später bei uns operiert wurde. Patient selbst ist sehr herabgekommen, bemerkt seit zwei (?) Jahren einen sich stets vergrössernden Tumor an der Ileocoecalgegend, welcher ihr insbesondere in der letzten Zeit grosse kolikartige Schmerzen verursacht. Im Stuhl Schleim und schwarze Massen.

Stat. praes. Vollkommen kachektische, gänzlich abgemagerte Frau mit einem kindskopfgrossen, höckrigen, harten auf der Unterlage kaum beweglichen Ileocoecaltumor.

23-4. Operation — Ileocolostomie. Heilung per I. (?). Entlassen 13-V-1903.

FALL II. Diagn.: Ca. coli transv. — Resectio, Colo-coloanastomosis. Sanatio.

Marie J. 63 jährige Private aus Trebitsch (Mähren). Anz. 11-XI, geheilt entl. 21-XII-1903. Anam. Anhaltende schmerzhafte Defaecationsbeschwerden zwingen Patient auf Anraten des Hausarztes zur Spitalsaufnahme.

Stat. praes. Bei der ihrem Alter entsprechend aussehenden Frau leichter Meteorismus. Zwischen Symphyse und Nabel taucht während starker Blähungen ein leicht beweglicher runder harter Tumor aus d. Tiefe, um nach Application von hoher Irrigation zugleich mit den Beschwerden spurlos zu verschwinden.

---

(1) Pat. hat sich persönlich in d. Anstalt 20-XI-1906 vorgestellt: sieht gut aus, hat guten Stuhl u. Appetit, fühlt sich völlig wohl. Objectiv alles normal.

Bei der Laparotomie zeigt sich, dass der apfelgrosse Tumor in der Mitte des abnorm langen Colon transv. sitzt und ins kleine Becken herabhängt. Resection.

Heilung per I.

Revision durch den Stadtarzt ergibt völliges Wohlbefinden.

FALL III. Diagn. Tumor coeci ihr. Resectio, Ileocolostomia. Franziska V. 33 jährige Tagelöhnerin aus Batschitz (Mähren), Aug. 18.VIII), geheilt entlassen 18.IX. 1904.

Anamnese: Pat. hereditär nicht belastet, hat vor ca. 4 Jahren Schmerzen in d. Ileocoecalgegend bekommen, zu denen allmälig Koliken hinzutraten. Seit Frühjahr 1904 deutlicher Ileocoecaltumor — höchst unregelmässiger Stuhl.

Stat. praes.: Entkräftetes mittelgrosses Weib mit normalen Lungen, kindskopfgrosser Coecaltumor, hart, druckempfindlich, von glatter Oberfläche, wenig beweglich, in der Lende ballotierend. Durch Cystoskopie und Harnbefund Nierentumor ausgeschlossen.

Resectium. Ileocoecotomie durch Implantation d. Ileum in die Taenie des Colon transv. Mikulicz-Tampon zur Niere wegen zu grossem Peritonealdefect. Heilung. Nach Mitteilung d. Collegen Dr. Belvar Patient völlig gesund.

FALL IV. Diagn. Ca. flex. sigmoid, et ca. coli transversi. Resectio, Colodoanastomosis. Franziska K., 50 jährige Bäuerin aus Christor (Mähren). Anfg 20. II, geheilt entl. 13.III.1905.

Anamnese: Diese Pat. ist die Schwester der Marie B (siehe Fall I) welche 1903 hier an Coecalcarc. operiert wurde, und deren 2 Brüder an ähnlichen Darmgeschwülsten unoperiert gestorben sein sollen. Patient selbst leidet an Stuhlunregelmässigkeiten und Kolikschmerzen.

Stat. praes.: Gutgenährte mittelkräftige Frau mit starkem Hängebauch. Im l. Hypogastrium ein beweglicher bis zum Rippenbogen reichender, bei Palpation schmerzhafter harter spindelförmiger Tumor.

Operation 23 II in combin. Narcose (Morph. 0.02 subcut.), vier(10 graduirte) Spritzen schwacher Schleichlösung, Aetherrausch 80 gr. Mobilisierung d. unteren Tumors und d. flex. henalis; dabei findet man einen zweiten Tumor am Colon transv. Daher Resection des ganzen Convolutes. Anastomose der mittels Quetschmethode verschlossenen Darmenden nach Mobilisierung der flex. hepatica. Operationsdauer 3 1/2 Stunden. Die Pat. hat den Eingriff sehr gut überstanden, spricht mit uns, lässt sich das Praeparat zeigen — kurz ist in ausgezeichneter somatischer Condition. Der Aetherrausch wurde in diesem Falle bei der Mobilisierung und Ligatur der Mesenterien protrahiert so dass ein Mehrverbrauch von ca. 40 gr. Aether resultierte. Per I. geheilt entlassen. Die letzten Nachrichten, Februar 1908, melden völliges Wohlbefinden.(1)

FALL V. Diagn. Ca. coeci et coli ascend. Resectio, Ileocolostomia. Adolf I. 31 jähriger Gastwirt aus Romanily (Mähren). Anfg. 5.IX. geheilt entlassen 13.X.1905.

Anamnese: Seit Winter 1904 appetitlos, im Frühjahr Rauschschmerzen um den Nabel. Auftreten einer harten Geschwulst in der Ileocoecalgegend.

Stat. praes.: Kachektisch aussehender Mann. Ileocoecaltumor kindskopfgross, hart, höckrig, wenig beweglich, auf Druck eminent schmerzhaft. Im Harn Indican.

Operation 11 IX in comb. Narkose Morph. 0.015, drei Spritzen Schleichlö-

---

(1) Pat. stellte sich zugleich mit d. Schwester (Fall I) am VII noch persönlich in der A... vor. Sie ist vollkommen gesund, hat eine feste Laparotomienarbe.

...sung) dreimalige Wiederholung des einmal protrahierten Aetherrausches (140 gr.) Operationsdauer 3 Stunden. Bei Mobilisierung des Tumors welche bis zur Flexura hepat. reicht musste ein grosses Teil des Perit. parietale mitexstirpiert werden (protrahierter Rausch).

Resection. Ileocolostomie der blind geschlossenen Enden. Deckung d. Peritonealdefectes gelang durch Heranziehen der benachbarten Partien. [*] Heilung per I.

FALL VI. Diagn. Tumor circ. Ileo. Resectio. Ileocolostomia. Josef T. 20 j. Comm. aus Pohrlitz (Mähren) Aufg. 5/IX. entlassen 27/I 1903. Wiederaufnahme wegen anderer the. Erkrankungen März 1905. — Anamnese. Mutter starb an Lungenphthise. Pat. leidet lange Zeit an Diarrhoe mit Kolikschmerzen um d. Nabel herum.

Stat. praes. Sehr herabgekommener junger Mann mit Ileocoecaltumor mit gelinden Stenosenerscheinungen. Diarrhoe. Operation 10/X in comb. Narkose, bei welcher viermal Aetherrausch zu je 50 gr. zur Verwendung kommen musste. Bei d. Exstirpation des den, zahlreiche Verwachsungen zusammenhangenden Tumors wird bei der Lösung im retroperitonealen Räume mit grosser Vorsicht der in Schwielen eingehefteten Ureter durchschnitten.

Nach Resection des Coecum und Colon ascend. Ileocolostomie. Allr. Acte der Darmoperation durch abnorme Brüchigkeit der Darmwände erschwert. Hierauf Naht des Ureters; Mikulicz Tampon zur Niere in den ungedeckten Peritonealdefect.

Pat. heilte sehr langsam da sich eine feine Ureterfistel etablierte, welche bei seiner Entlassung bestand.

FALL VII. Ca. ventriculi et coli transvers. Resectio ventriculi et coli transv. Entero-enteroanastom. Sanatio [?].

Eine Resection des Colon transversum wurde gelegentlich einer nahezu totalen Magenexstirpation wegen Ca. desselben, welches das Colon transv. durchwucherte, ausgeführt. Pat. überstand den grossen Eingriff es etablierte sich ohne nachweisbare Ursache an der Vereinigungsstelle d. Darmenden eine Fistel, welche 2 Jahre später andernorts geschlossen wurde, jedoch bald wieder an derselben Stelle sich erneuerte [†].

Contribution au traitement des corps étrangers de l'œsophage

Par M. SUAREZ DE MENDOZA, Paris [‡].

Fort nombreux sont les moyens dont dispose le chirurgien pour extraire les corps étrangers de l'œsophage. Cette grande diversité dans les méthodes et dans les instruments employés tient aux nombreuses particularités qui accompagnent chaque cas nouveau. L'on se trouve, en effet, souvent fort embarrassé devant

---

[*] Pat. stellte sich im Mai 1906 persönlich vor, sieht blühend aus und fühlt sich völlig wohl.

[†] Pat. starb an allgemeiner Bauchtuberculose 9/VIII 1906.

[‡] Die Publication d. Falles und Abbildg. d. Praeparates erfolgte im Langenbeck's Archiv für klin. Chirurgie, Bd. 76, Bft 4. Bakes: Zur operat. Therapie des coli. Magengeschwürs.

[§] Pat. erlag im April 1907 — also ca. 2 ½ Jahre nach dem grossen Eingriff weiteren Metastasen.

[‖] A la suite de la lecture du rapport de M. le dr. Richelot sur ce travail, l'Académie de médecine, dans sa séance du 17 mai 1910, vota que des remerciements seraient adressés à l'auteur M. le dr. Suarez de Mendoza, de Paris. Voir le Bulletin de l'Académie de Médecine, nᵒ 21, séance du 17 mai 1910.

une complication tout à fait imprévue; et c'est alors que l'esprit imaginatif de l'opérateur trouve libre carrière et qu'il crée des appareils spéciaux, suivant les circonstances.

Nous allons rapidement passer en revue tous les procédés qui furent mis en vigueur pour extraire par la bouche les corps étrangers arrêtés dans l'œsophage et nous exposerons ensuite, au cours des observations, la technique opératoire que nous avons adoptée dans les quatre cas qui font l'objet de cette communication.

Procédés anciens. — Comme nous l'apprend Hévin dans son remarquable mémoire présenté à l'Académie royale de chirurgie de Paris en 1743, les moyens les plus anciennement employés semblent être: la *propulsion* dans l'estomac, soit avec des substances alimentaires, figues, purées, morceaux de viandes, soit avec des poireaux, des navets, des tiges de laitue, etc., soit encore avec une bougie graissée d'huile et chauffée au préalable. On eut recours plus tard à des tiges métalliques qui se terminaient par un renflement conoïde ou à l'extrémité desquelles on fixait une éponge. Quel que soit l'instrument employé, la propulsion est un procédé dangereux, unanimement condamné et qui expose à des complications souvent graves.

Nous ne ferons que mentionner les autres moyens tout aussi inefficaces et qui sont totalement abandonnés ; la *tape dans le dos* avec la main qui, combinée avec la propulsion, aurait donné, paraît-il, des succès à Ambroise Paré; la *position déclive; l'ingestion de glace ; la saignée ; le massage du canal œsophagien à travers les parois du cou*, etc.

Quant à la *méthode des vomissements*, qui a joui pendant quelque temps d'une grande faveur, elle consistait à administrer le vomitif par la voie stomacale. Quand le corps étranger obstruait le calibre de l'œsophage au point de s'opposer même au passage des liquides, on avait recours aux injections sous-cutanées et intra-veineuses de substances vomitives. La méthode des injections intra-veineuses d'émétique fut surtout employée en Allemagne. Par la voie hypodermique on utilisa les propriétés émétisantes de l'apomorphine. Enfin, on provoqua encore les vomissements à l'aide de lavements d'infusion de tabac.

Cette méthode de vomissements est aujourd'hui à peu près abandonnée. Le professeur Duplay ne l'a recommandée qu'avec une très grande circonspection, et le professeur Terrier la condamne absolument.

Extraction par la voie buccale. — La méthode d'extraction par la voie buccale des corps étrangers de l'œsophage offrait des avantages si marqués sur la propulsion et les vomissements qu'elle ne tarda pas à avoir la préférence. Les nombreux instruments qu'on a imaginés témoignent à la fois de son importance et de ses difficultés ; leur variété est grande mais on peut les ranger un peu arbitrairement, peut-être, en trois catégories.

1° Nous faisons entrer dans la première catégorie tous les instruments chargés de *saisir le corps par sa partie supérieure et de le tirer au dehors*, c'est-à-dire tous les différents genres de pinces (pinces de Cloquet, de Collin, de Tiemann, etc.) ;

2° Dans la deuxième catégorie nous plaçons tous les *instruments destinés à saisir le corps étranger par sa partie inférieure et à le pousser de bas en haut*. Tels sont les crochets et leurs variétés dont les plus employés sont le *panier de Graefe* et le *crochet de Kirmisson*, ce dernier employé surtout pour l'extraction des pièces de monnaie. Grâce à ces instruments le nombre est grand des malheureux qui ont été débarrassés d'un danger menaçant. Mais si le succès de ces instruments est l'habitude, il ne faut pas croire qu'il soit la règle absolue ; et il est bon d'être prévenu des mécomptes qui arrivent quelquefois.

3° Enfin dans la troisième catégorie figurent les *instruments destinés à saisir ou pousser le corps étranger par sa partie inférieure et à le ramener également de bas en haut après avoir dilaté les parois œsophagiennes*. Tels sont : le parapluie de Fergusson, le parasol de Rivière, la pince avec dilatateur de Blondeau, les éponges que l'on faisait passer sèches au-dessous du corps étranger et qui dilataient l'œsophage par suite de l'augmentation de volume qu'elles prenaient après ingestion de grandes quantités de liquides. Rentrent aussi dans cette catégorie les procédés qui consistent à injecter des liquides dans l'œsophage et à employer des sondes élastiques (sondes uréthrales, sondes molles de Nélaton, etc.).

On eut recours également à des vessies ou à des ballons fixés à l'extrémité d'une sonde et que l'on introduisait vides dans l'œsophage. On leur faisait ordinairement franchir le corps étranger ; puis on les gonflait soit avec du liquide, soit avec de l'air, ils déterminaient ainsi de la dilatation de l'œsophage et, en les ramenant, ils entraînaient le corps étranger.

Au cours de nos recherches bibliographiques, nous avons trouvé quelques cas de dilatation de l'œsophage à l'aide de vessies en baudruche et un cas de dilatation avec le pessaire de Gariel (cas de Gautier). Mais nous n'avons pas trouvé de cas où la dilatation au-dessus du corps étranger ait été faite pour libérer celui-ci de la pression œsophagienne et le livrer ainsi au panier de Graefe.

En présence des succès que nous avons obtenus depuis 1888, avec l'appareil dilatateur de Collin-Verneuil, et du beau résultat que cet appareil nous a donné dans un cas difficile, en l'associant au ballon de Tarnier, nous avons cru intéressant de faire cette communication pour éveiller à nouveau l'attention sur ce procédé qui, depuis l'élogieuse communication de notre premier cas, faite par le professeur Verneuil à l'Académie de médecine [1], est tombé dans un oubli tout à fait immérité à notre avis; car il nous semble que l'opinion autorisée du grand chirurgien aurait dû porter davantage.

Notre procédé comporte donc l'emploi : 1° de l'appareil dilatateur Collin-Verneuil (longue bougie conductrice, olives creuses, sonde œsophagienne ouverte) ; 2° du panier de Graefe et, au besoin, du crochet de Kirmisson [2] et du ballon de Tarnier modifié par moi pour la circonstance.

Nous n'insisterons pas sur le *modus faciendi* qui se trouve décrit, comme nous l'avons dit plus haut, au cours de nos observations et qui peut se résumer ainsi :

1° Passage d'une fine et longue bougie en baleine, entre le corps étranger et l'œsophage.

2° Dilatation de l'œsophage contre le corps étranger, à l'aide de la sonde œsophagienne munie d'olives creuses de l'appareil Collin-Verneuil.

3° Au besoin, à travers de la sonde œsophagienne à ouverture axiale, introduction dans l'estomac de substances alimentaires ou de liquides médicamenteux, calmants, toniques ou reconfortants.

4° Introduction du panier Suarez de Mendoza (modification du panier de Graefe) sur la bougie conductrice, jusqu'au-dessous du corps étranger qui, en général, cède aux tractions.

5° Dans le cas contraire, introduction, guidée par la bougie, d'un ballon de Tarnier, modifié à cet effet; gonflement, à l'air ou à l'eau, du ballon; dilatation œsophagienne au-dessus du corps étranger.

---

[1] *Bulletin de l'Académie de médecine.* Séance du 4 septembre 1888.

[2] Bien que jusqu'à présent nous ayons su utiliser tel quel cet excellent instrument de M. Kirmisson, nous l'avons adapté aussi à notre procédé en le munissant d'un ordre [illegible] pour pouvoir l'introduire [?], le cas échéant, sur la bougie conductrice.

6° Extraction du corps étranger sans danger pour les parois œsophagiennes, protégées qu'elles sont par le ballon demi-gonflé qui précède le corps étranger dans son ascension.

OBSERVATIONS

Avant de relater nos observations nouvelles, nous croyons utile d'exhumer l'observation enterrée depuis 14 ans, en rapportant textuellement les paroles du maître:

«L'Académie a reçu, dans ces derniers temps, dit M. le professeur Verneuil, deux communications importantes sur les affections de l'œsophage: l'une due à M. le dr Nicaise, l'autre à M. le dr. Kirmisson, tous deux chirurgiens fort instruits et fort distingués de nos hôpitaux.

Dans le mémoire de M. Kirmisson, il a été question d'un instrument auquel j'ai collaboré avec l'un de nos plus habiles et plus ingénieux fabricants et qui porte pour cela le nom de sonde Collin-Verneuil. Cet instrument a servi bien des fois déjà à franchir et à dilater les rétrécissements de l'œsophage et à y porter des sondes à demeure, dont Krishaber, de regrettée mémoire, nous avait déjà montré les avantages. Il est assez connu des chirurgiens français pour qu'il soit nécessaire d'en faire ici l'histoire et d'en montrer les avantages, mais je crois bon d'exposer devant vous une de ses applications que, jusqu'à plus ample informé, je crois tout à fait nouvelle.

Elle a été faite, il y a quelques mois déjà, dans un cas grave de corps étranger dans l'œsophage, par un praticien de province, M. le dr. Suarez de Mendoza, qui exerce avec distinction la médecine et la chirurgie dans la ville d'Angers.

Le cas était grave, la cure difficile et dangereuse. Néanmoins, notre honorable confrère a conçu son procédé d'une façon si ingénieuse et manié les instruments avec tant d'habileté qu'il a obtenu une guérison complète, rapide et qu'aucun accident n'est venu troubler.

L'observation m'a paru si intéressante et elle plaide si fort en faveur de notre instrument que je crois utile de lui donner la publicité qu'elle mérite:

Corps étranger de l'œsophage, arrêté à 23 centimètres des arcades dentaires et enlevé au cinquième jour, à l'aide de la sonde œsophagienne Collin-Verneuil, par le docteur F. Suarez de Mendoza, d'Angers (1).

OBSERVATION I. — Jeudi soir, 9 février 1888, je fus appelé à la hâte pour voir Mᵐᵉ G...., fermière aux environs d'Angers. Cette femme, âgée de quarante huit ans, et d'une bonne santé habituelle, avait avalé, le lundi 6, à midi, un os de bœuf qui s'était arrêté dans l'œsophage. Elle nous raconta que son médecin habituel en la voyant le lendemain, à midi, et sans avoir fait aucune tentative d'extraction, l'engagea à ne prendre que du liquide et à ne pas se faire ouvrir la gorge, car, disait-il, l'opération était dangereuse.

---

(1) A cette époque, j'habitais la capitale de l'Anjou.

Le lendemain, l'état de la malade empirant et la déglutition même des liquides étant presque impossible, on fit demander un autre confrère, qui ordonna un vomitif, trouvant que, ne voyant pas l'os, il n'y avait pas autre chose à faire. Le vomitif fut pris non sans peine et, malgré de grands efforts de vomissement, le résultat fut nul. C'est alors que nous fûmes prévenus. Nous trouvâmes la malade dans un état de faiblesse considérable. Nous pratiquâmes le cathétérisme, et malgré une persistance d'une heure, on ne put franchir ni repousser l'obstacle ; la sonde était arrêtée à 23 centimètres des arcades dentaires. Le lendemain matin une nouvelle séance n'étant pas plus fructueuse ni avec les sondes œsophagiennes (28, 21, 15), ni avec le panier de Graefe, j'ai eu recours au dilatateur œsophagien Collin-Verneuil. Après quelques essais, j'ai pu enfin introduire la bougie et, sur elle, je fis passer les olives 1, 2, 3 ; mais il fut impossible de faire passer le panier de Graefe.

Vu l'état de faiblesse de la malade, qui, depuis quatre jours, n'avait rien pris, je suspendis la séance après avoir fait passer sur la bougie conductrice la sonde et fait prendre un demi-litre de lait, trois œufs, un verre de vin, et avoir constaté un changement dans l'os, qui permettait le passage de l'olive n° 4.

Le lendemain, à huit heures du matin, je commençai par essayer le passage d'une sonde 16. Après plusieurs tentatives infructueuses, je réintroduisis la bougie et sur elle je fis glisser les olives 3, 4 et 5. Ces olives passèrent facilement, vu leur forme conique ; mais, en les retirant, on se sentait un instant arrêté par l'os, qui finissait par livrer passage à l'olive sans se laisser entraîner par elle. L'olive retirée, nous pûmes faire passer le panier de Graefe, muni d'une échancrure ad hoc faite pour la circonstance (1) qui, après quelques tentatives, accrocha l'os lequel, malgré des tractions très fortes, demeura immobile, m'obligeant à suspendre la séance pendant quelques minutes pour reposer la malade, qui était exténuée.

Le panier introduit de nouveau, laissé sans conducteur cette fois, et de nouvelles tractions donnant toujours le même résultat, je fis glisser, laissant le panier en place, sur la bougie qui n'avait pas été enlevée, la petite olive de la série et, en arrivant sur l'os, je poussai fortement en bas, pendant que, de l'autre main, je tirai fortement en haut le panier.

Un léger craquement est perçu à travers la sonde métallique ; après, on sent la résistance vaincue, et le panier, la sonde et la bougie sont enlevés entraînant avec eux l'os entouré d'une couche de mucosité sanguinolente. Huit jours après, la malade est tout à fait remise, et, à partir de ce jour, elle reprend sa vie habituelle.

Il me paraît certain que, sans l'aide des instruments précités, l'extraction du corps étranger, dont la présence menaçait la vie de ma malade, aurait été de tout point impossible : 1° parce que le panier de Graefe ne pouvait être introduit ; 2° parce que, sans faire basculer la lamelle osseuse, il aurait été impossible de la mener au dehors sans produire de lacérations probables des tissus, et cela est d'autant plus certain qu'avant d'introduire pour la dernière fois l'olive, nous avons fait de très énergiques tractions.

Ce fait donc me paraît devoir appeler l'attention sur une nouvelle indication de l'ingénieux appareil instrumental de MM. Collin-Verneuil.

Je mets sous les yeux de mes collègues le corps étranger ; c'est un fragment osseux fort irrégulier, mais de forme plutôt lamellaire, épais de 7 à 8 millimètres

____

(1) Voir *Bulletins de l'Académie*.

long de 22 et large de 15, lisse sur une de ses faces recouverte de tissu compact, rugueux sur l'autre constituée par du tissu spongieux, ce qui indique qu'il provient d'un os plat. Sa périphérie, partout extrêmement tranchante, offre en outre quatre dents aiguës qui ont dû facilement pénétrer dans les parois œsophagiennes et y être fixées par le spasme de la tunique musculaire; d'où la résistance aux tractions et au déplacement.

On remarquera, dans l'observation de M. Suarez de Mendoza, les points suivants :

1° L'impossibilité de franchir l'obstacle avec les instruments ordinaires, même après une heure de patientes tentatives;

2° La facilité relative du passage de la bougie conductrice et des olives perforées;

3° La possibilité d'introduire, séance tenante, et malgré la présence du corps étranger, des aliments liquides en assez grande abondance pour soutenir la malade très affaiblie par quatre jours de diète forcée;

4° Le passage du panier de Graefe au-dessous du corps étranger, rendu facile grâce à la bougie conductrice;

5° Le dégagement ou propulsion de haut en bas du corps étranger avec l'olive placée au-dessus de lui et pressant sur lui;

6° La fixation solide de l'os entre l'olive sus-jacente et le panier sous-jacent permettant l'extraction simultanée de tous les instruments et du corps étranger.

Parmi les trois cas où, après avoir échoué par les méthodes ordinaires, nous avons eu recours avec plein succès à notre méthode, deux ont été presque la répétition de cette première observation si aimablement commentée par feu le professeur Verneuil. Dans le troisième, le corps étranger étant pointu et résistant une fois accroché aux tractions, nous dûmes introduire une nouvelle modification à notre façon de faire en ajoutant, pour ménager l'œsophage, l'action dilatatrice et protectrice du ballon de caoutchouc. Ce qui nous a permis de compléter notre méthode de la façon que nous venons de l'indiquer.

OBSERVATION II. — Le 12 septembre 1895, je fus demandé, à la hâte, à huit heures du soir, pour aller voir un enfant de 15 ans qui, disait-on, étouffait parce qu'un noyau de pêche lui était entré dans le « tuyau » du poumon. A mon arrivée, je trouve un enfant bien constitué, très intelligent, légèrement oppressé mais pas étouffant comme on l'avait dit.

L'enfant prétendait que, après avoir avalé trop vite, par peur d'être grondé, une pêche mal mâchée prise dans le verger paternel, il avait eu pendant quelque temps le « tuyau » de la respiration bouché, que plus tard le noyau était descendu et ne l'empêchait plus de respirer; mais en échange cela lui faisait grand mal dans le haut de la poitrine, comme ferait un morceau de pain sec avalé trop vite.

Bien que la gêne respiratoire n'eût rien d'inquiétant, j'ai procédé à l'examen laryngologique qui ne révéla rien d'anormal. J'essayai de faire boire l'enfant, mais l'eau fut rejetée et l'effort fait par l'enfant produisit de la souffrance; un morceau de pain bien mâché eut le même sort.

Une sonde œsophagienne, introduite alors, s'arrêta à dix centimètres de la gorge. J'essayai de pousser, ayant à plusieurs reprises obtenu des succès par la propulsion, mais l'obstacle ne bougea pas.

Après plusieurs tentatives de propulsion, j'eus recours au panier de Graefe, mais il me fut impossible de l'insinuer entre le corps étranger et l'œsophage; j'ai essayé alors de passer la bougie du dilatateur Collin-Verneuil, et j'eus la chance de l'introduire entre le noyau et la paroi œsophagienne; comme dans ma première observation, j'ai dilaté à l'aide de plusieurs olives et finalement j'ai passé le panier qui m'a permis de faire l'extraction sans grande difficulté. Quelques jours après, le malade était tout à fait revenu à l'état normal, ne gardant de cet accident qu'une sainte horreur des pêches et du pêcher.

OBSERVATION III. — Mme X..., âgée de soixante ans, habitant à la campagne, me fit demander le 20 mars 1897, parce que, pendant le repas, elle avait avalé un ratelier en caoutchouc muni d'agrafes en or. Son médecin habituel avait essayé d'abord de prendre avec de longues pinces le corps du délit et ne pouvant y réussir avait essayé de le pousser dans l'œsophage à l'aide d'une sonde urethrale munie d'un mandrin.

La gêne éprouvée par la malade ayant beaucoup augmenté depuis la veille, on me fit demander pour savoir s'il fallait intervenir chirurgicalement. Me rappelant un malade auprès duquel j'avais été appelé assez tard pour n'oser rien tenter et qui succomba quelques heures après ma visite à la suite des énergiques tentatives d'extraction faites par le médecin traitant, je décidai d'être plus prudent.

J'essayai d'abord inutilement de la propulsion, puis du panier de Graefe, qui ne passa pas; j'eus recours ensuite à la pince de Collin. Le corps étranger ne venant pas (peut-être par la crainte que j'avais de noire), j'employai alors le dilatateur Collin-Verneuil avec l'espoir de dégager l'œsophage des adhérences qu'il pouvait avoir prises avec les parties pointues du ratelier. La bougie passa facilement et à sa suite plusieurs olives franchirent le corps étranger. Mon panier œsophagien glissa aussi facilement sur la bougie et accrocha de bas en haut le corps étranger; des tractions répétées furent inutiles. Craignant de faire des déchirures, je laissai en place le panier et introduisant sur la bougie un ballon de Tarnier muni d'un anneau métallique, je le conduisis jusqu'au corps étranger. J'injectai alors de l'eau dans le ballon, l'œsophage se dilata doucement et, sans savoir exactement comment, je dégageais le corps étranger, qui fut ramené au dehors avec le panier, la bougie et le ballon Tarnier, dilaté par l'eau.

OBSERVATION IV. — Le 18 mars 1904, un de nos compatriotes, atteint de dysphagie consécutive à des accidents spécifiques, me fit demander en toute hâte dans l'après-midi, au commencement de ma consultation, en me priant d'apporter de quoi lui enlever un morceau d'os qu'il venait d'avaler et qui le gênait horriblement.

Je me rendis chez le malade qui, très impressionnable, exagérait d'une façon extrême les symptômes éprouvés (étouffements, gêne et douleurs provoquées par la déglutition).

Après l'avoir calmé moralement, je fis de larges pulvérisations de cocaïne dans l'arrière-gorge et, au bout de quelques minutes, la sonde œsophagienne put être introduite; elle s'arrêta à 24 centimètres des arcades dentaires; la propulsion étant très douloureuse, j'essayai le passage du panier de Graefe qui, très mal supporté, arriva cependant sur le corps étranger sans pouvoir le franchir malgré l'emploi de la cocaïne que j'avais portée, à l'aide de la sonde, au niveau du corps étranger.

Ne possédant plus le dilatateur Collin-Verneuil, je courus chez M. Collin, l'habile et aimable fabricant d'instruments de chirurgie, pour en demander un, ainsi qu'un panier de Graefe ayant la modification apportée par moi en 1888. Les dits instruments ne se trouvant pas prêts, et l'heure de la fermeture étant arrivée, il me fut aimablement promis de faire veiller un ouvrier afin de m'arranger un appareil pour le lendemain, à la première heure.

À huit heures le lendemain, j'étais en possession du dilatateur et d'un panier de Graefe muni de la cannelure nécessaire pour glisser facilement sur la tige conductrice.

À la vue de l'instrument, le malade, surexcité par la mauvaise nuit, refusa d'abord toute intervention, prétendant qu'il préférait la mort à la souffrance. Une injection de morphine, plusieurs pulvérisations de cocaïne, une forte dose de patience et de persuasion eurent à la fin raison de l'entêtement du malade. J'introduisis alors sans peine une longue baleine conductrice qui, après quelques tâtonnements, franchit l'obstacle; puis je fis passer trois olives sans difficulté, et finalement je pus introduire mon panier œsophagien qui ramena, non sans peine, un gros morceau d'os à bord rugueux, dont j'ai négligé de prendre les dimensions, ne pensant pas, au moment, publier l'observation.

Le malade, remis de cette intervention, eut au bout de dix jours une petite hématémèse qui fut arrêtée par l'emploi d'une potion à l'adrénaline et par l'usage de la glace pilée en petites cuillerées souvent répétées.

Cet incident n'empêcha pas le malade de partir deux mois après, complètement guéri de sa dysphagie.

Comme le malade était en puissance d'avariose tardivement traitée, je me suis souvent demandé s'il fallait attribuer la petite hématémèse à l'avariose, au traitement intensif, ou à la chute d'une petite escare produite par une légère mortification de la paroi œsophagienne.

CONCLUSIONS

Le résultat obtenu dans les quatre observations que nous venons de relater nous autorise, croyons-nous, à tirer les conclusions suivantes:

1° Lorsque le corps étranger de l'œsophage résiste ou a résisté à la propulsion, et que l'introduction du panier de Graefe n'a pas été possible, soit à cause du spasme œsophagien, soit à cause du volume excessif du corps étranger, la dilatation partielle de l'œsophage à l'aide du dilatateur Collin-Verneuil permet quelquefois d'introduire le panier de Graefe, et partant, de faire l'extraction du corps étranger;

2° Lorsque le corps étranger, accroché par le panier de Graefe ou par le crochet de Kirmisson, résistera aux tractions exécutées méthodiquement, et que l'on sera tenté d'abandonner la séance par crainte de déchirures possibles du conduit, la dilatation de l'œsophage par le ballon dilatateur de Tarnier, mis en place à l'aide de la bougie conductrice de l'appareil Collin-Verneuil, pourra permettre le dégagement et l'extraction du corps étranger sans blesser les parois œsophagiennes;

3° Cette méthode a, en outre, l'avantage d'assurer l'alimentation du malade, même dans les cas extrêmes, grâce à l'emploi de la sonde creuse, qu'on parvient toujours à glisser sur la bougie conductrice.

(Présentation d'instruments.)

SÉANCE DU 25 AVRIL

(Matin)

Présidence : M. MAYO ROBSON

Chirurgie artérielle et veineuse. Les modernes acquisitions

Par MM. d'ARCY POWER, Londres (v. page 1).
et PIERRE DELBET, Paris (v. page 393).

DISCUSSION

M. D'ARCY POWER read his report on recent advances in the surgery of the vascular system. He drew attention to the important work on shock and collapse which had been carried out by Prof. Crile in the United States of America. Mr Power said that he had obtained some satisfactory results in consequence of this work by the injection of adrenalin in cases of extreme shock.

The advances in the ligature of arteries were then passed under review and Dr Power expressed his preference for sterile silk over catgut and silkwormgut.

The treatment of aneurysm was then discussed and Dr Power explained an apparatus for wiring aneurysms with subsequent electrolysis which had been invented by Dr G. H. Colt, one of his house-surgeons.

The advances in connection with the surgery of the venous system was considered and Mr Power expressed his opinion that Trendelenburg's method of treating varicose veins was satisfactory in the majority of cases, though it was unsuitable where there were many very large and thin walled veins. He called attention to the advances in the treatment of varicocele and of hæmorrhoids, concluding his report with an account of the methods in use for nævi whether vascular or lymphatic.

Mr Power summed up his report in the following questions which he thought might form the subject of discussion in the section.

(1) Do the members present prefer silk, catgut or silkwormgut for the ordinary ligature of blood vessels? Mr Power trusted silk only.

(2) What results had been obtained by the surgeons present with the gelatin treatment of aneurysm? Mr Power's results had not given him satisfaction.

(3) In the opinion of those present, what cases of varicose veins gave the best results from Trendelenburg's operation? Mr Power thought in those cases where there were many small veins or where the varix was only of moderate severity.

(4) What is now the usual operation for varicocele? An incision over the external abdominal ring with ligature and subsequent excision of the spermatic veins or complete excision of the whole pampiniform plexus? Mr Power contented himself with the former method as he had found it impossible to remove the whole of a large varicocele as was advocated by many surgeons.

M. GARRÉ: Auf die Frage des Herrn D'Arcy Power möchte ich antworten:

1. Dass ich als *Ligaturmaterial* die *Seide* ausschliesslich anwende, und zwar dünnste Seide (N° 0) nicht im Dampf sterilisirt, sondern in Sublimat-Alcohol eingelegt. Die Resultate sind sehr gut.

2. Die *Gelatine-Behandlung* der Aneurysmen hat mir keine befriedigenden Erfolge gegeben.

3. Die *Trendelenburg'sche Operation* pflege ich nur dann anzuwenden, wenn das sogenannte Trendelenburg'sche Phaenomen deutlich vorhanden ist; sonst mache ich ausgedehnte Excisionen der Varicen.

4. Bei der *Varicocele* mache ich die Ligatur der Vena spermatica im Ing.-Canal nicht allein, sondern füge die Exstirpation des ganzen venösen Plexus an.

M. OLIVEIRA FELIÃO: Il emploie toujours la soie bouillie en solution phénique; catgut à l'iode (Clausius), lavé au sérum. Il n'a aussi aucun cas favorable des injections de gélatine dans les anévrysmes. Sur le traitement des varices il est d'accord avec Garrè; les chirurgiens portugais font l'excision de la saphène en bloc, ou par sections. Il vote aussi pour l'excision complète des veines du cordon dans le varicocèle.

Une nouvelle méthode d'anastomose vasculaire et ses applications à la replantation et à la transplantation des veines, des artères, des membres et des organes

Par MM. ALEXIS CARREL ET C. C. GUTHRIE, Chicago (v. page 238).

DISCUSSION

M. REYNALDO DOS SANTOS: Il a personnellement assisté à quelques-unes des intéressantes expériences de Carrel; il l'a vu transplanter un corps thyroïde d'un chien à un autre. Seulement les expériences de la transplantation de la cuisse d'un chien à un autre chien ont été faites après son passage en Amérique.

M. GARRÉ: Die mitgetheilten experimentellen Resultate sind glänzend und überraschend; indessen möchte ich doch davor warnen gar zu optimistische Hoffnung in Bezug auf die Anwendung solcher Methoden am Menschen zu hegen. Ich will hinsichtlich der Implantation von Organtheilen auf andere Individuen nur daran erinnern wie schwer schon Hautstückchen beim Menschen anheilen, wenn sie von andern Individuen genommen sind, selbst von Blutsverwandten des betr. Patienten. Sollte im Hinblick hierauf die Implantation ganzer Organe beim Menschen, besonders wenn es sich um empfindliche Gewebe handelt, die Möglichkeit einer reactionslosen Einschaltung eines solchen Organs nicht eine geringe sein? Ich möchte deshalb vor übertriebenen Hoffnungen, die sich an diese Experimente anschliessen, warnen, ohne damit den hohen Werth der Mittheilung irgendwie zu beeinträchtigen.

(Après-midi)

Du traitement opératoire des pleurésies purulentes

Par M. N. NAPALKOW, Moscou.

Il est fréquent d'observer que les pleurésies purulentes prennent une tournée chronique, même dans les cas opérés à temps et sans faute dans la technique opératoire. L'observation clinique a peu contribué jusqu'à présent à l'éclaircissement des conditions qui favorisent cette chronicité. Voici brièvement les données les plus importantes, obtenues dernièrement par la clinique. La marche chronique est observée souvent à partir de l'âge de quinze à quarante ans et encore plus souvent de vingt à trente ans. On la trouve quelquefois chez les enfants. Je connais un cas où une pleurésie d'origine traumatique a duré cent-quarante-trois jours chez un enfant de deux ans. Des résections répétées de la 6e, 7e et 8e côtes durent être pratiquées pour obtenir la guérison. La chronicité est comparativement plus rare chez les malades d'un âge avancé et surtout chez les vieillards. Elle se rencontre trois fois plus souvent chez les hommes que chez les femmes et le même rapport, quant au sexe, existe chez les enfants. Il n'y a nulle différence à cet égard entre les pleurésies du côté droit ou gauche. Il n'est pas possible non plus de lier la marche des pleurésies à une forme quelconque de leur origine. Les pleurésies qui compliquent les inflammations du poumon, les lésions traumatiques du thorax ou les maladies infectieuses, peuvent toutes prendre une marche chronique, dont les causes intimes restent inconnues. Seules les pleurésies d'origine tuberculeuse doivent être considérées comme particulièrement enclines à prendre un cours chronique. L'examen bactériologique des pleurésies chroniques découvre les formes les plus variées de microorganismes: des staphylocoques, streptocoques, pneumocoques, bacilles de la grippe, colibacilles, bacilles de la tuberculose et d'autres sous la forme de l'infection simple ou combinée. Il faut attacher une grande influence sur le cours des pleurésies purulentes au moment où a lieu l'intervention chirurgicale: plus l'opération sera faite tôt, plus il y aura de chance à la suppression de la suppuration. Néanmoins une suppuration prolongée peut s'observer quelquefois même après une intervention précoce.

L'incertitude des données cliniques à l'égard de la durée des pleurésies purulentes a forcé les chirurgiens à chercher une issue dans de nombreux procédés opératoires. On a discuté sur le meilleur procédé pour ouvrir la cavité pleurale, avec ou sans résection costale, à quelle hauteur, sur quelle ligne du thorax; sur les meilleurs procédés de drainage et d'irrigation de la plèvre. Des procédés ingénieux d'aspiration de l'exsudat furent inventés, mais, malgré tous ces efforts, l'observation nous montre qu'aucun des procédés opératoires et des traitements post-opératoires ne garantira la cessation de la suppuration.

On pourrait donc douter de l'exactitude du principe qui sert de base au traitement contemporain des pleurésies purulentes, et qui consiste à admettre qu'elles ne sont pas autre chose que des abcès de la cavité pleurale. Je pense pourtant que nous n'avons pas le droit d'en vouloir à cette déduction, car il faut convenir que dans notre mode opératoire, jusqu'à présent du moins, nous n'avons pas assez rigoureusement suivi le principe lui-même. Aujourd'hui encore la cavité pleurale, en cas de pleurésie purulente, n'est pas considérée comme la cavité d'un abcès ayant différentes positions et dimensions et confiné dans des parois où se déroule un processus morbide, mais comme une cavité anatomique, adaptée aux fonctions des viscères du thorax, ayant un contenu anormal — l'exsudat purulent, qu'on n'a qu'à éloigner pour que tout revienne à l'état normal. C'est là où est la faute. Dans aucun cas de suppuration nous ne nous contentons seulement d'évacuer le pus, toujours nous explorons avec soin toute la cavité purulente, tous les coins et recoins, nous en examinons les parois, et nous prenons toutes les mesures nécessaires pour que leur *affrontement* se fasse dans les meilleures conditions nécessaires pour le développement de leur adhérence. Nous excisons quelquefois même une partie des parois de l'abcès, si cela favorise la guérison, comme par exemple dans les cas d'abcès osseux.

Dans la plupart des cas de pleurésie, même après l'opération, l'état du poumon et de la plèvre reste inconnu. Il est évident qu'on omet deux moments de la plus grande importance; l'examen de la cavité et les mesures à prendre que cet examen pourrait indiquer. Il en résulte que, souvent après l'opération, la suppuration se prolonge quand même et qu'il se forme des fistules pleurales très opiniâtres à la guérison.

Depuis *Estländer* les suppurations pleurales chroniques sont opérées en pratiquant de larges ouvertures dans la plèvre et grâce à cela nous sommes en état, à l'heure actuelle, de nous rendre compte des conditions favorables à la guérison des pleurésies purulentes à marche chronique. Ces conditions, il faut les avoir en vue dans les opérations primitives, dans tous les cas.

Pour les suppurations pleurales, il n'y a pas d'autre possibilité de guérison, que par oblitération de la cavité. (Nous n'avons aucune donnée sur la possibilité d'une régénération de l'épithelium [endothélium] de la plèvre après une pleurésie suppurative). La rapidité de la guérison de la pleurésie dépend de la rapidité avec laquelle se développera l'adhérence des deux feuillets pleuraux, et pour cette adhérence leur attouchement complet est indispensable. Cet attouchement est obtenu grâce à la dilatation du poumon après l'évacuation de l'exsudat qui le comprimait. La dilatation du poumon jusqu'à l'attouchement complet des deux feuillets pleuraux forme la base de la guérison. Si le poumon se dilate complètement, il suffit d'une simple évacuation de l'exsudat et d'un drainage d'une courte durée. C'est la raison du succès des opérations aujourd'hui usuelles dans les cas de pleurésie aiguë—évacuation du pus avec drainage consécutif. Si le poumon ne se dilate pas suffisamment, la pleurésie prendra inévitablement une marche chronique, à moins qu'on aie recours à d'autres moyens pour provoquer l'attouchement des feuillets pleuraux. Par conséquent, dans chaque intervention, nécessitée par une pleurésie purulente, il est indispensable de se rendre compte jusqu'à quel degré le poumon a conservé le pouvoir de se dilater. Lorsque l'ouverture de la plèvre est assez large on peut se faire une idée de la mobilité du tissu pulmonaire par la vue et le toucher. C'est une erreur de croire qu'une fois la plèvre ouverte, le poumon se contracte à sa racine. Cela ne s'observe guère que sur le cadavre; chez l'homme vivant, le volume du poumon continue à changer sous l'influence des mouvements respiratoires de la cage thoracique et c'est d'après ces changements du volume pulmonaire qu'on pourra juger si le rapprochement des feuillets pleuraux sera possible ou non. On peut faire trois groupes des causes qui empêchent dans ces cas la dilatation complète du poumon: 1) L'infiltration inflammatoire diffuse du poumon, 2) les fistules bronchiales, 3) l'épaississement de la plèvre pulmonaire.

Dans les deux premiers cas, il faut toujours chercher à produire des mesures qui favorisent le rapprochement de la paroi thoracique vers la plèvre pulmonaire et non pas la plèvre pulmonaire de la paroi thoracique. Pour la guérison des fistules bron-

chiques on sera obligé ou de les exciser avec le tissu pulmonaire
sclérosé qui les entoure, ou, comme l'a fait le chirurgien russe
Abrajanoff, de les fermer avec les tissus mous de le paroi thoracique.

C'est l'épaississement de la plèvre que pourtant se rencontre
le plus souvent dans les pleurésies purulentes. Pour rendre dans
ce cas au poumon la possibilité de se dilater, *Delorme* a préconisé
la décortication du poumon. Jusqu'à présent on n'est pas encore
d'accord sur la valeur de ce procédé. C'est pourquoi j'exposerai
ici les résultats de mes recherches personnelles. La plèvre pulmonaire épaissie, formant autour du poumon une enveloppe compacte et immobile, n'a pas de limites nettes, qui la séparent du tissu
pulmonaire. Ce dernier, dans ses couches superficielles, est remplacé par du tissu conjonctif au milieu duquel on remarque par
endroits des alvéoles pulmonaires comprimées et déformées. Par
endroits, des bandes de tissu conjonctif pénètrent dans l'épaisseur
du tissu pulmonaire. Ces bandes de tissu conjonctif recèlent aussi
des restes d'alvéoles pulmonaires et des particules de charbon.

Il ne faut pas croire que la dégénération fibreuse du tissu
pulmonaire ne se produit que dans les pleurésies prolongées. J'ai
pu l'observer très développée dans un cas de suppuration de 7
semaines. Il en résulte que la décortication sera parfois une opération très difficile, impossible même, et qu'elle peut être suivie
de fistules bronchiques. C'est ce qu'a fait observer *Rehn*.

Constatant que le poumon perd son extensibilité sous l'influence des pleurésies purulentes, je ne veux pas, ce qui serait ba-
nal, insister sur la conclusion que tout cas de pleurésie purulente
doit être opéré le plus tôt possible. Je cherche à bien faire res-
sortir que dans toutes les opérations l'élasticité du poumon doit
être établie avec toute la précision possible et que, si la mobilité
du poumon est restreinte, il faudra augmenter la mobilité de la
paroi thoracique.

Il peut aussi exister des obstacles pour l'accolement des
feuillets pleuraux et pour l'oblitération de la cavité pleurale dans
la cavité pleurale elle même. Je range dans cette catégorie: les
adhérences partielles qui forment cloison et divisent la cavité purulente en plusieurs parties tout à fait isolées ou bien réunies entre elles par d'étroites communications; la disposition de la cavité purulente et la formation de caillots fibrineux très volumineux.

Les adhérences forment assez souvent une série de cloisons

dans la cavité. Comme pour tous les abcès, il est nécessaire de les inciser et d'ouvrir largement la cavité avec toutes ses poches. La disposition de la cavité purulente est d'une grande importance, car c'est un fait d'observation que l'accolement des feuillets pleuraux ne se produit pas avec la même facilité dans toutes leurs parties. Cela s'observe d'une manière particulièrement fréquente dans les parties postérieures de la cavité pleurale.

C'est pourquoi, lorsque la cavité purulente s'étend vers la colonne vertébrale et sous l'omoplate, une limitation même insignifiante de l'élasticité normale du poumon suffira pour que la suppuration se prolonge. C'est alors qu'il faut surtout chercher à rapprocher par un moyen opératoire le feuillet pariétal de la plèvre à celui du poumon.

On n'observe que rarement des caillots volumineux de fibrine dans les pleurésies purulentes. Il faut prendre soin de les extraire, car, suppurant ou s'organisant, toujours ils soutiendront la suppuration.

Outre l'expansion du poumon, le rapprochement des feuillets pleuraux se produit aussi par rétraction de la paroi thoracique. Celle-ci se produit dans tous les cas de pleurésie purulente chronique. Chez les hommes mûrs, j'ai observé une différence entre les deux moitiés de la poitrine, d'environ 6—8 cent., chez les adolescents une différence de 10 cent. Ces observations, je les ai faites dans des cas où pour l'évacuation du pus on n'avait réséqué qu'une petite partie d'une côte, ou lors même qu'il n'y avait pas du tout de fistule pleurale, et que la cavité de la plèvre communiquait avec l'air par des fistules bronchiques. Il faut avoir cela en vue lorsqu'on cherche à se rendre compte des causes de rétraction du thorax, après une résection costale large. La forme des côtes elle-même change dans le cours des pleurésies purulentes chroniques. Les côtes deviennent plus grosses et perdent leur forme plate. Un examen plus attentif nous montre que cette déformation dépend de l'élargissement des bords inférieurs des côtes. La lèvre intérieure du sulcus costal semble s'allonger en dedans, le sulcus lui-même s'élargit. La section transversale de la côte déformée montre une figure triangulaire. Les surfaces des côtes ne sont pas plates, les deux surfaces latérales deviennent bombées, l'inférieure concave; seulement dans les cas où la surface intérieure est très petite en comparaison avec l'extérieure, la surface inférieure a une forme plate.

La rétraction de la paroi thoracique doit suppléer à l'insuffisance d'expansion du poumon. Donc chaque fois que nous observons cette rétraction, nous devons provoquer l'accolement des feuillets pleuraux en faisant une large résection de la paroi thoracique. Voici le procédé à suivre: nous dénudons les côtes en faisant un lambeau en fer à cheval, et nous faisons la résection sous-périostale des côtes dans toute la hauteur et la largeur de la cavité purulente. Si la cavité s'étend en arrière jusqu'à la colonne vertébrale, nous ne réséquons pas les côtes, mais nous les cassons simplement avec la main. Les côtes se brisent à la hauteur des sommets des processus transversaux et il ne reste que de petits tronçons d'environ 3 cent. liés aux vertèbres. Nous n'excisons pas les parties molles du thorax, comme l'a préconisé *Schede*, parce que c'est non seulement inutile, mais même nuisible. Elles ne doivent pas être excisées parce qu'elles sont capables d'adhérer à la plèvre pulmonaire, pourvu qu'elles s'y accolent par toute leur superficie, ce qui doit être pris en considération lors de l'opération. Dans ce but, il vaut mieux réséquer les côtes sur une étendue dépassant les limites de la cavité purulente, inciser les parties molles de la paroi thoracique sur toute l'étendue de la cavité purulente et même quelquefois les tailler en lambeaux qui peuvent plus facilement combler la cavité et s'accoler à la plèvre pulmonaire. Il est nuisible de les exciser, car, étant conservées, elles corrigent jusqu'à un certain degré la déformation du thorax causée par la résection des côtes et donnent au poumon une protection assez forte. En plus le périoste, resté dans les parties molles, donne naissance à du tissu osseux et alors les larges dimensions de la résection primitive ne portent pour ainsi dire plus qu'un caractère provisoire. A l'aide des rayons de Röntgen, j'ai pu me persuader que la régénération du tissu osseux se produit déjà 55 jours après l'opération; à l'occasion d'une intervention complémentaire, j'ai pu observer dans un cas des lamelles osseuses nouvellement formées de plusieurs cent. de grandeur.

La déformation du thorax qu'on observe après des pleurésies purulentes prolongées, comme je l'ai déjà remarqué, ne dépend pas tant de la résection des côtes que de la cicatrisation de la plèvre pariétale. Plus la suppuration est de longue durée, plus la déformation est grande, et ce n'est pas en étant trop méticuleux sur la dimension des parties à réséquer que nous pourrons l'éviter, c'est en cherchant à supprimer le processus suppuratif aussi promptement que possible que nous y arriverons. Cela se manifeste d'une manière encore plus éclatante par rapport à la colonne vertébrale, dont les déviations sont presque nulles après les grandes

résections des parois thoraciques et très fortes après les pleurésies purulentes prolongées; dans ces cas, la force rétractile du
tissu cicatriciel agit sur les vertèbres par l'intermédiaire de longues côtes qui forment leviers.

Je crois donc pouvoir conclure que, pour la suppression des
pleurésies purulentes, l'évacuation du pus ne suffit pas; l'accolement des feuillets pleuraux est indispensable; l'accolement en est
obtenu par l'expansion du poumon, et, si elle est insuffisante, par
une large résection des côtes.

Jusqu'à présent j'ai parlé avec intention simplement des pleurésies purulentes, sans distinguer les pleurésies aiguës et chroniques. Au point de vue opératoire il n'y a pas de différence entre
les unes et les autres. L'accolement des feuillets pleuraux est toujours indispensable et c'est alors seulement que la guérison sera
garantie. Commençant l'opération par une incision large de la
plèvre avec résection d'une ou de deux côtes, il faudra toujours
examiner la cavité purulente, s'assurer de l'extension du poumon
et agir comme l'indiqueront les circonstances. Dans les cas de
pleurésies comparativement récentes, la résection large des côtes
peut être nécessaire autant que pour les cas chroniques, mais certainement moins souvent. Le mode d'opérer, usuel actuellement,
donne souvent comme résultat des fistules pleurales, non parce
que l'opération est faite trop tardivement, mais parce qu'une simple évacuation du pus, seule, est dans ces cas insuffisante. Une
opération bien conduite est toujours accompagnée d'un examen
détaillé et se règle sur cet examen. L'opération des pleurésies
purulentes est soumise à la même loi.

Encore quelques mots concernant les pleurésies tuberculeuses. Leur opération doit être faite d'après le même principe: explorer la cavité purulente, ses parois, et provoquer leur accolement complet. De cette manière nous n'obtiendrons peut-être pas
la guérison complète, mais en tout cas nous limiterons la suppuration et l'absorption du contenu de la cavité et par conséquent
nous placerons nos malades dans les conditions les plus favorables à leur nutrition et leur guérison.

Sans m'arrêter aux détails, j'ai cherché ici à tracer en grandes lignes les principes qui servent de base au mode opératoire
en vigueur dans la clinique du prof. *Diakonow* à Moscou, principes
à l'élaboration desquels j'ai contribué en raison de mes forces,
et que je me permets aujourd'hui de soumettre à votre bienveil-
lante attention.

DISCUSSION

M. AUGUSTO VASCONCELLOS: Les inconvénients de l'opération de Delorme (décortication du poumon) ne sont pas seulement ceux indiqués par M. Napalkow. Dans le cours de cette opération des hémoptysies, parfois très graves, ont été observées. L'orateur a même connaissance d'un cas où l'hémorrhagie a été foudroyante.

M. OLIVEIRA FEIJÃO: Nous pouvons avoir un guide pour l'étendue des côtes à réséquer dans l'examen du pus de la pleurésie, l'extensibilité du poumon étant plus grande et se perdant plus tard, s'il s'agit d'une pleurésie à pneumocoques que s'il s'agit d'une pleurésie due à des streptocoques par exemple. Quant au besoin de juxtaposition des deux plèvres, elle est nécessaire à la guérison de la pleurésie; la physique le dit, mais il suffit de juxtaposition sans qu'il faille que l'adhérence existe entre la plèvre pulmonaire et la plèvre costale. Un examen nécroscopique me l'a prouvé. Quant à l'accolement des deux plèvres, il est obtenu par l'extensibilité du poumon et par les déformations du squelette, et ces déformations peuvent aller jusqu'à l'élévation du bassin, l'abaissement de l'épaule, l'incurvation de la colonne vertébrale et la déformation des côtes, comme j'ai vu dans un cas de très ancienne pleurésie purulente.

M. BRANT P. LEME prend la parole pour observer que lui aussi, comme M. le prof. Feijão, croit que la nature du pus peut donner d'avance une indication pour l'espèce d'opération qu'on devra faire dans les pleurésies purulentes. En fait, par exemple, il n'y a aucune comparaison entre la pleurésie purulente à pneumocoques et les autres variétés à staphylocoques, streptocoques et plus encore, le bacille de Koch. Les premières guérissent, en règle, facilement avec des interventions relativement simples, quelquefois même avec simples pleurotomies, avec ou sans contre-ouverture à quelque point déclive qu'on puisse rencontrer, ce qui n'arrive pas aux autres variétés.

Il croit aussi, comme M. le prof. Vasconcellos, que l'opération de Delorme est bien plus périlleuse et difficile qu'on ne peut penser par quelques références faites, et que toujours elle sera une opération d'exception.

M. NAPALKOW: Je n'ai pas dit qu'une résection large des côtes soit nécessaire dans tous les cas. Quant à la bactériologie des pleurésies purulentes, les observations des chirurgiens russes montrent que les pleurésies d'origine pneumococcique sont capables de prendre une marche chronique, comme les pleurésies d'origine strepto staphylococcique, etc. Les auteurs français et allemands le disent aussi.

Quant à la possibilité de la guérison d'une pleurésie sans l'oblitération de la cavité pleurale, je dois remarquer que jusqu'à présent nous ne savons rien de la régénération de l'épithélium pleural.

Résultats de l'immunisation active contre le micrococcus Doyen dans les cas de néoplasmes malins

(Travail du laboratoire bactériologique du service de M. Krajewski à l'Hôpital de l'Enfant-Jésus à Varsovie)

Par M. LÉON DE KARWACKI, Varsovie

De tous les parasites trouvés ou cultivés des néoplasmes malins, tels que levures, bacilles acido-résistants, staphylocoques, streptocoques, spirochaetes, bacilles pseudo-diphthériques, une variété des staphylocoques découverte et étudiée par Mr. Doyen présente le type le plus constant.

Au cours de mes recherches sur la flore des néoplasmes, j'ai réussi à cultiver 7 espèces identiques à celle de M. Doyen.

Les études sur l'agglutination de ce microcoque ont prouvé que le sérum de plusieurs malades atteints de néoplasmes pouvait donner la réaction spécifique au titre de 1/40—1/150. Le sérum normal de l'homme ne donne jamais une réaction pareille.

Bien que je ne partageasse pas l'opinion de M. Doyen sur la spécificité de son microcoque, il me paraissait admissible que ce microcoque pouvait exercer une certaine influence sur l'évolution des maladies néoplasiques. J'ai donc résolu d'essayer si l'immunisation des malades contre ce parasite pouvait modifier de quelque façon l'évolution naturelle des tumeurs. L'immunisation passive, à l'aide du sérum spécifique, me paraissait susceptible de deux objections.

1° Jusqu'ici tous les sérums antistaphylococciques, parmi lesquels devrait être rangé le sérum antinéoplasique, possèdent les propriétés spécifiques dans un degré bien infime, aussi bien dans les recherches de laboratoire, que dans les observations de clinique.

2° L'application fréquente de sérum dans une maladie chronique aboutit presque toujours à toute une série de manifestations d'ordre pathologique, phénomènes post-sériques. Pour ces deux raisons j'ai choisi la méthode de l'immunisation active.

Une culture de quarante-huit heures de microcoque sur bouillon glycériné a été portée pendant une heure à 60° et mise à l'étuve pour quelques jours. Ensuite j'ajoutai un 1/2 % d'acide phénique et sous cette forme je l'employai chez les malades en injections sous-cutanées. Selon l'état du malade, la dose de l'injection était de 0,5 à 1 centimètre cube. J'injectais d'abord deux fois par semaine, ensuite une fois par semaine en doublant la dose. J'essayais ces injections sur moi-même et sur les sujets normaux. Or, ces injections sont indolores, et, à part une légère infiltration, ne provoquent aucun trouble. Il en est autrement chez les sujets atteints de néoplasmes: sur 20 cas, j'ai obtenu 15 fois l'élévation thermique dans des limites de 0,5° à 1,5°. Le plus souvent la température revenait à la normale au cours des premières 24 heures, pourtant, par trois fois, après plusieurs injections, l'état sub-fébrile durait des semaines, en s'élevant le jour de l'injection jusqu'à 39°.

Dans deux de ces cas, la réaction thermique élevée coïncidait avec la régression des tumeurs. Je n'ai pas observé cette réaction thermique dans des cas de cancer d'estomac et d'œsophage. A côté de la réaction thermique apparaissaient, chez quelques malades, des phénomènes du côté du cœur, se traduisant par l'insuffisance cardiaque. Après une seule injection chez un malade atteint d'une tumeur sous-maxillaire, la réaction cardiaque fut si forte qu'elle entraîna la mort du malade après 5 jours. J'ai observé les manifestations cardiaques six fois sur vingt malades traités de cette manière.

Quant à la réaction locale, elle s'est manifestée par une légère et peu stable infiltration sur la place même de l'injection et par un retentissement dans le foyer néoplasique. Je n'ai observé cette dernière réaction que 5 fois sur 20. Les contours de la tumeur devenaient plus nets, sa consistance devenait plus compacte. Ensuite, ou l'évolution de la tumeur suivait son cours habituel (2 fois), ou la tumeur devenait de plus en plus dure et diminuait assez vite (3 fois).

Je me permets de faire des observations plus détaillées sur ces trois cas où les injections ont provoqué la régression des tumeurs.

Le 1er cas concerne un malade avec une tumeur dans la région de deux vertèbres cervicales inférieures. Au moment où je commençais le traitement, la conductibilité de la moelle épinière était complètement abolie. Je lui ai fait, en somme, 10 injections; 5 à 1 centimètre cube, à l'intervalle de trois jours chacune, et 5 à 2 centimètres cubes à l'intervalle d'une semaine.

Après chaque injection la température s'élevait jusqu'à 39°. Il va sans dire que l'état fonctionnel du système nerveux restait in statu quo, mais les dimensions de la tumeur diminuaient progressivement. Le malade mourut subitement dans un accès de dyspnée.

Un autre cas concerne une malade opérée à cause du cancer du sein, qui avait une récidive dans les ganglions sous-axillaires. Quand je vis la malade pour la première fois, la tumeur sous-axillaire était de la grosseur d'un œuf de poule. Au toucher on sentait une tuméfaction dans la région pylorique et des bosselures sur la surface du foie qui était augmenté de volume. Après une série d'injections, la température devint sub-fébrile continue. La tumeur sous-axillaire devenait dure et diminuait visiblement. Après 6 semaines, elle n'était presque plus palpable, cependant le foie grossissait toujours, les bosselures s'accentuaient davantage; ensuite apparurent l'ascite et les signes de l'insuffisance cardiaque. Vers cette époque, je perdis la malade de vue et je n'ai plus eu de ses nouvelles.

La troisième malade, âgée de 48 ans, avait les deux seins pris par le processus néoplasique. Les tumeurs immobiles étaient de la grosseur de deux poings. La peau adhérait à leur surface. Au voisinage, le système lymphatique était pris également. Les ganglions du cou des deux côtés étaient sensiblement augmentés de volume, ainsi que les ganglions inguinaux. Malgré cette grande étendue du processus la malade ne présentait aucun signe de cachexie, se plaignant seulement de douleurs névralgiques du côté des seins. Le traitement durait 4 mois. Au commencement je lui faisais 2 injections par semaine, puis une fois par semaine en doublant la dose. À la suite de ce traitement toutes ces tumeurs disparurent. Les seins diminuèrent de volume, devinrent mous et les adhérences avec le thorax disparurent. Des cicatrices se produisirent sur les lieux de lymphangite néoplasique. Les ganglions du cou diminuèrent de volume également, quelques cicatrices se produisirent à la place de quelques-uns de ces ganglions. Mais en même temps apparurent les signes de l'insuffisance cardiaque qui me forcèrent de cesser le traitement. Vers cette époque-là entra en scène toute une série de foyers métastasiques. De novembre 1905 au mois de février dernier, j'ai compté chez ma malade plus de cent nodules néoplasiques. Ces métastases se localisaient toujours dans le tissu sous-cutané, atteignaient le volume d'une noisette et disparaissaient au bout de deux ou trois mois, laissant à leur place une cicatrice. Les nodules occupaient la peau du ventre, du thorax, des épaules, du dos et des fesses. Sur le visage, ces nodules occupaient les paupières, le foyer dans la paupière supérieure gauche poussait dans la cavité oculaire, ce qui empêchait la malade de fermer l'œil gauche. La peau des extrémités supérieures et inférieures était indemne de cette éruption. Vers le mois de janvier de cette année, apparurent les douleurs abdominales s'accompagnant de l'état sub-fébrile. Il en résulta l'ascite. Comme au palper on ne sentait rien, j'identifiai le processus péritonéal avec celui des nodules cutanés, ce qui fut ensuite confirmé par l'examen cytologique. Après la centrifugation, j'ai trouvé, dans le dépôt, des cellules néoplasiques bien caractérisées. Malgré les métastases et les ponctions répétées, la malade ne présentait aucun signe de cachexie. L'état des organes respiratoires, du cœur et des organes digestifs était tout à fait satisfaisant. La malade reste encore actuellement sous mon observation.

Passant aux autres cas, je dois dire que presque tous les malades étaient dans un état de cachexie bien avancée et pour cette raison hors d'état de bénéficier d'un traitement quel qu'il fût. Je leur faisais, à leur demande, mes injections, quoique à priori on ne pouvait plus rien espérer. Deux cas pourtant, dont le premier concerne un cancer du sein en cuirasse, et le second un cancer de la langue, ne peuvent pas expliquer le résultat négatif du traitement. L'état général était bon, à part la tumeur primitive, il n'y avait pas de métastase dans les organes et malgré les injections répétées il n'y avait ni réaction thermique, ni arrêt du processus néoplasique.

Sous forme de conclusion, je dois dire que les résultats du traitement n'apportent pas une preuve bien évidente en faveur de la spécificité du microcoque. L'influence de l'immunisation dans un certain groupe de malades ne se manifestait par aucun signe objectif; dans un autre groupe, les injections provoquaient l'élévation thermique sans modifier aucunement l'évolution de la tumeur. Ce n'est que dans un nombre très restreint de cas que les injections provoquèrent une réaction générale et une réaction locale sous forme de régression de la tumeur. Sous ce rapport nous ne trouvons aucune analogie avec l'action des poisons spécifiques tels que la tuberculine ou la maléine. Nous trouvons une certaine analogie si nous nous adressons à l'action d'autres poisons bactériens tels que protéines streptococciques, protéines de bacilles de pus bleu ou celles de bacillus prodigiosus. De certaines tumeurs, sous l'influence de l'érysipèle évoluant sur la tumeur même ou à la suite des injections de microcoques ou de cancroïne, peuvent subir la régression et disparaître. Il ne s'agit pas ici évidemment d'une action spécifique. La nutrition des cellules néoplasiques peut subir une modification sous l'influence des poisons bactériens ou cellulaires, en même temps les cellules conjonctivales peuvent prendre le dessus sur les cellules néoplasiques et provoquer la dégénérescence de ces dernières. Comme fait curieux, je n'ai à noter aucune amélioration, même passagère, dans les cas de sarcomes. Le caractère abortif des métastases dans mon 3e cas prouve que dans la régression des tumeurs la moindre vitalité des cellules néoplasiques joue un certain rôle à côté des modifications vasculaires et conjonctivales.

La seule difficulté, et elle n'est pas la moindre, qui nous empêche de bien profiter de ce vaccin en thérapeutique, c'est que nous ne savons jamais d'avance sur quelle tumeur épithéliale il peut agir. Il en est de même pour les rayons de Roentgen, pour le radium et les autres méthodes employées dans les épithéliomas cutanés.

Avant que nous ne possédions une telle classification thérapeutique des néoplasmes, le résultat favorable du traitement sera plutôt une exception, soit en suivant la méthode d'immunisation passive, soit en suivant la vaccination active.

Das Wesen und die Behandlung der Neuralgie

Par M. BARDENHEUER, Cologne.

Auf dem diesjährigen Chirurgencongresse hatte ich Gelegenheit, 2 Fälle von geheilter Neuralgie des Trigeminus, welches ich mittels der Herausmeisselung des Nerven aus dem zugehörigen Kanale und Einbettung desselben in Weichteile, behandelt habe vorzustellen. Gestatten Sie mir mit einigen Worten der

Operation hier zu gedenken. Da ich aber ferner an einem andern Orte des längeren über das gleiche Thema gesprochen habe, so fasse ich mich hier kurz und verweise auf den Aufsatz, welcher in der *Zeitschrift für ärztliche Fortbildung* von Prof. Dr. Kuttner erschienen ist.

Auf der Naturforscherversammlung in Hamburg habe ich über 6 Fälle von hartnäckiger Ischias berichtet, in welchen ich vor 6-8 Jahren zur Behandlung einer äusserst heftigen Ischias die gleiche Operation, nämlich die partielle Resection der Synchondrosis sacro-iliaca ausgeführt habe um die Nervenwurzeln freizulegen. Die Patienten sind heute noch gesund. Diese Operation hat nur dann Berechtigung wenn die Nervendehnung im Stiche gelassen hat, da obige Operation eine eingreifende zu nennen ist.

In welcher Weise die Operation ausgeführt wird, habe ich in den Berichten der Hamburger Naturforscherversammlung niedergelegt.

Ich reiche hiermit einige Moulage herum, an welchen der Gang der Operation bei der Ischias leicht zu studieren ist.

Ich habe ausserdem 5 Fälle von Neuralgie des Trigeminus mittels ähnlicher Operation behandelt und reiche gleichfalls die Moulagen zur Demonstration der Operationsverfahrens herum. Ich lege bei der Operation den Accent darauf, dass eine Wand des Kanales, wodurch der Nerv verläuft (z. B. der N. infraorbit.), ohne Eröffnung der Highmore resp. der Mundhöhle z. B. des N. inframaxillaris entfernt und der Nerv selbst möglichst sanft aus dem Kanale hervorgehoben, in einiger Entfernung von der Knochenwandfläche gelagert wird. Damit keine Verwachsung zwischen dem translocierten Nerven und dem sich neubildenden Knochen, in dem aufgemeisselten Kanale entstehe, lagere ich einen subcutanen Muskel-Periostlappen, welcher aus der unmittelbarsten Nähe entnommen wird, unter den Nerven.

In welcher Weise die Operation ausgeführt wird, leuchtet aus den herumgereichten Moulagen hervor. Alle Fälle sind heute, nach 6 Monaten bis 2 Jahren frei von Schmerz.

Die Operation muss in Zukunft noch durch eine längere Beobachtungszeit den Beweis der dauernden Heilung liefern, indessen ist es doch heute schon ein gutes Resultat zu nennen, so dass die Operation mit der Neurectomie concurrieren kann.

Ich erkläre die Entstehung des Leidens durch die im Knochenkanale entstehende Hyperaemie, wie ich sie jedesmal bei den Operationen nachgewiesen habe und die eventuell folgende Verwachsung mit den Kanalwänden und secundäre Perineuritis. Durch die Entfernung der Knochenwände und Trennung des Nerven vom Knochen soll die Einengung des Nerven, welche die Hyperaemie verursacht und unterhält, sowie die Entstehung der Verwachsung des Nerven mit dem neu entstehenden Kallus und der Perineuritis verhütet werden.

Diese Theorie erhebt keinen Anspruch auf volle Berechtigung und fällt ev., was ich aber bisher nicht anzunehmen keine Ursache habe, mit der sich nachher herausstellenden Unzulänglichkeit der Operation; über letzteres muss die Zukunft durch eine grössere Zahl von wirksamen Operationen Aufschluss gehen.

Als stützende Beweismittel führe ich jedoch an:

1) den macroscopischen und vielen Aerzten demonstrirten Nachweis der venösen Hyperaemie, der Schwellung des Gefässbündelsch.

2) den augenblicklichen und bisher relativ langen Heileffect. — 2 Jahre.

3) den Umstand, dass an dem Nerven selbst nichts geschehen ist, welches die Leitung des Nerven unterbrechen konnte und dass trotzdem Heilung eintrat.

DISCUSSION

M. GARRÈ: Ist bei den Trigeminusneuralgien vorher ein operativer Eingriff anderer Art gemacht worden? Nein, dann würde ich doch in ähnlichen Fällen erst die Neurexairese empfehlen, ein Eingriff der meist zur Ausheilung führt und ein Eingriff der doch wesentlich weniger eingreifend ist und auch gewiss in cosmetischer Hinsicht vorzuziehen ist. Wir haben doch eben gehört, dass einmal eine Fractur des Unterkiefers und Knochennekrose eine recht unangenehme Complication zur Folge gehabt hat. Bei einem Recidiv nach der einfachen Neurexairese käme diser von R. empfohlen Eingriffe noch früh genug.

Contribution à l'étude du traitement des anévrysmes artério-veineux de l'aine par l'extirpation totale

Par M. BRANT PAES LEME, Rio-de-Janeiro.

Il s'agissait, dans le cas auquel je veux faire une petite allusion, d'un grand anévrysme artério-veineux de l'aine droite (racine des vaisseaux fémoraux), sans aucune difficulté pour le diagnostic, cela se comprend. Aussi ce n'est pas sur ce point, ni sur l'histoire du malade proprement, banale dans l'affaire, que je désire attirer l'attention, mais seulement sur les très grandes difficultés que j'ai eues pour mener heureusement à fin mon intervention, et aussi sur

l'heureux résultat qu'elle a eu, c'est-à-dire la cure du cas qui fut
obtenue. En fait, après avoir reconnu, sur le champ opératoire
même, qu'il ne pouvait aller autrement qu'avec la quadruple ligature pour l'extirpation totale, je l'ai faite, mais ayant contre moi
de très fortes hémorrhagies, qui m'ont donné des instants bien
embarrassants. Ce n'est pas du tout, il me semble, une situation
facile que celle de l'extirpation totale d'un anévrysme artério-veineux de l'aine; et c'est sur cela que je crois devoir attirer l'attention
des praticiens, en reconnaissant d'ailleurs la haute valeur de la
méthode.

Contribution à l'histoire des kystes du mésentère

Par M. BRANT PAES LEME, Rio de Janeiro.

Quoiqu'ils ne soient pas absolument rares, les kystes du
mésentère ne sont pas si nombreux qu'il ne puisse plus y avoir
intérêt à connaître des cas nouveaux. Dans celui auquel l'auteur
se réfère, il croit rencontrer l'intérêt: a) dans le volume de la
tumeur, énorme, remplissant tout le ventre, on peut le dire, comprimant tous les viscères, sans occasionner pourtant une très grande
souffrance, exception faite des derniers temps; b) dans sa condition multiloculaire au plus haut degré, innombrables poches kys-
tiques, depuis les plus petites, conglomérées, aux plus grandes
remplissant les loges profondes, loges rénales, de la cavité abdominale; c) dans le procédé opératoire employé, l'extirpation totale par
fragmentation de la volumineuse masse et avec un parfait succès,
quoique l'opération fût difficile, laborieuse, à cause des adhérences
des parois de plusieurs poches avec les viscères environnants, particulièrement les intestins, et aussi en conséquence de la présence
de quelques gros vaisseaux qui existaient dans les parois de quelques poches, en particulier au niveau du point du bourgeonnement primitif du kyste, au niveau de l'angle iléo-colique, selon ce
qu'on a pu vérifier après. Le malade, homme fort, quoique déchu
et maigre, n'apportait dans son histoire aucune référence digne
de mention; tout était au contraire obscur et confus; il a vu son
ventre croître petit à petit, sans souffrances, sans aucune perturbation de sa santé générale, excepté aux derniers temps, où il se
sentait étouffer. Du commencement de sa vie, pendant son enfance,
il ne donnait aucune information louable, peut-être a-t-il eu toujours un gros ventre, plus qu'il n'est commun. A l'examen, le diagnostic fait a été d'un «kyste multiloculaire» sans doute, sans

autre affirmation; pourtant, sur le point de départ, peut-être du
mésentère, on a bien pensé; mais kyste séreux, kyste hydatique?
on ne pouvait le dire. Aucune ponction n'a été faite et l'opération fut résolue. Laparotomie médiane, évidement de quelques
poches superficielles, pour ouvrir un chemin, manœuvre malaisée
à cause du petit volume de quelques-unes, surtout celles qui se
présentaient premièrement. Aussitôt qu'il fut possible de pénétrer plus profondément, le morcellement des masses des poches
évidées a permis de désenclaver les plus profondes et de reconnaître le point de départ du kyste au niveau de l'angle iléo-colique.
L'appendice adhérait à ce point, il fut réséqué; le reste du kyste
retiré; l'hémorrhagie qu'on a eu principalement alors, combattue;
l'hémostase absolue du ventre obtenue; le mésentère reconstitué
par une suture au point d'où le kyste avait été détaché, on pourrait presque dire son pédicule; et le ventre fermé. Cicatrisation
per primam. La nature séreuse du liquide des poches, et tout,
portait à placer le cas dans le groupe de ceux si bien étudiés par Arzagneur dans sa thèse d'agrégation de Paris, 1886,
et aussi dans la 6e catégorie de ceux étudiés par Terrier et
Lecène (*Rev. de Chirurgie*, n° 2, 1904); c'était un kyste juxta-in-
testinal, au bord mésentérique de l'angle iléo-colique, kyste dédou-
blant le mésentère. L'examen histologique a démontré la constitution typique des parois des poches qui étaient plus ou moins
épaisses, avec une enveloppe conjonctive, irrégulièrement vascu-
larisée, sans aucun vaisseau de grand calibre, exception faite
du point d'implantation, selon la mention qui en a déjà été faite.
L'intérieur des poches était constitué par une couche endothéliale,
analogue à celle des séreuses.

Seitliche Naht der Arterie bei Anenrysmaexstirpationen

Par M. C. GARRÈ, Breslau.

Seitdem *Murphy* (¹) im Jahre 1897 durch seine klassischen Versuche nachgewiesen hat, dass Arteriennähte und selbst eine Resection aus der Continuität der Arterie auszuführen ist ohne dass
das Gefäss thrombosiert, und nunmehr auch in einer ganzen Reihe
von Fällen am Menschen der Nachweis geliefert ist, dass die Arteriennaht mit Glück ausgeführt werden kann, lag es nahe den
Versuch zu machen Aneurysmensäcke zu exstirpieren und die Communicationsöffnung am Arterienlumen durch Naht zu schliessen.
Murphy selber hat diese Consequenz aus seinen Versuchen gezo-

gen und zum ersten Mal im Oktober 1896 bei einer Schussverletzung, welche Arterie und Vena femoralis gleichzeitig traf, die
Vene vernäht und die Arterie reseciert.

Es handelte sich um einen 22 jährigen Patienten, der am 19. September mit
einer Schussverletzung eingeliefert wurde. Der Schuss lag im Scarpa'schen Dreieck,
woselbst über der Arterie ein lautes, schwirrendes Geräusch gehört wurde. Ein
aneurysmatischer Tumor war nicht nachweisbar. Bei der Operation am 7. Oktober
fand sich die Arterie von der Kugel doppelt durchschlagen und die Vena femoralis
gleichfalls verletzt. Zu beiden Seiten der Arterie lagen Blutklumpen in kleinen
Höhlen; also eine kleine aneurysmatische Tasche. Die schlitzförmige Oeffnung in
der Vene konnte durch Naht geschlossen werden, von der Arteria femoralis hingegen musste ein Stück in der Länge von 3/8 Zoll = 9mm herausgeschnitten werden, worauf die beiden Enden durch die Invaginations-Methode vereinigt wurden.
Die Nähte wurden nur durch die Media gelegt. Es trat eine reactionslose Heilung
ein und der Puls an den Fussarterien war vorhanden.

Eine ähnliche Verletzung der Arteria poplitea gab *Koerte* (?) die
Veranlassung im Jahre 1901 die Arterie, sowie die Vene welche
mit derselben in Verbindung stand, voneinander zu trennen und
jedes der beiden Gefässe durch die Naht zu schliessen.

Es handelte sich um einen 13 jährigen Jungen, der am 8. Januar 1901 einen
Messerstich in die rechte Kniekehle erhielt. Die blutende Wunde wurde genäht und
es trat Heilung ein. 6 Tage später wurde auf Grund des arteriellen Schwirrens ein
Aneurysma arteriovenosum angenommen. Nachdem Druckverband, Bier'schen u. s.
w. erfolglos angewandt worden war, machte *Koerte* am 10. II. die Operation. Er
fand Arteria und Vena poplitea auf 8 mm. mit einander verwachsen, ohne dass
ein eigentlicher aneurysmatischer Sack vorhanden war. Das Loch in der Arterie
und in der Vene wurde mit Carbolzwirn genäht. Es trat Heilung ein.

In den beiden angeführten Fällen von offener Verbindung
zwischen Arterie und Vene hatte sich noch kein eigentlicher aneurysmatischer Sack gebildet. In beiden Fällen war die Zeit, welche
nach der Verletzung verstrichen war (18 Tage, resp. 32 Tage) zu
kurz für die Ausbildung eines wirklichen Aneurysma arteriovenosum. Nur in dem *Murphy*'schen Fall war eine Art Sack, mit Blut-
coagula gefüllt, vorhanden. Es war ein Aneurysma arteriovenc-
sum spurium, während bei *Körte* sich eine Verwachsung mit offener Communication der beiden Gefässe fand.

Ueber den ersten Fall eines wirklich sackförmigen Aneurysma,
der durch die Exstirpation des Sackes mit folgender seitlicher
Naht der Arterie geheilt wurde, kann ich nun in folgendem berichten. Er ist von mir im Jahre 1904 operiert worden.

Krankengeschichte

Der 26 jährige Instmann Friedrich Hülszau (J. nr. 210) stammt aus gesunder Familie und will früher niemals krank gewesen sein. Vor 10 Jahren verletzte er sich mit einem Taschenmesser an der Innenseite des rechten Oberschenkels, wo er sich eine tiefe Stichverletzung zuzog. Die Wunde heilte er sich selbst in etwa 3 Wochen zu. Unmittelbar nach der Verletzung will er an der Innenseite des Oberschenkels ein auffallendes starkes Sausen gefühlt haben, und es soll an der Stelle eine dicke Ader aufgetreten sein. Beides ist bis jetzt, also 10 Jahre lang, unverändert bestehen geblieben.

Im Sommer vorigen Jahres brach am rechten Unterschenkel eine Stelle auf und vergrösserte sich, da Patient weiter arbeitete, rasch. Er ging dann in's Krankenhaus (Goldap), wo er zunächst drei Wochen lang mit Chlorwasserumschlägen behandelt wurde; danach wurde das Unterschenkelgeschwür durch Thiersch'sche Transplantationen vom anderen Oberschenkel gedeckt. Patient lag dann noch 10 Wochen im Krankenhause, bis sie angeheilt waren. Unmittelbar nach seiner Entlassung, als er wieder zu arbeiten anfing, sollen die Hautstücke brandig geworden und abgefallen sein. Patient wurde abermals 3 Wochen lang ohne wesentlichen Erfolg behandelt. Als er zu arbeiten anfing, brach das Geschwür wieder auf.

Status vom 24.V.01. Mittelgrosser, kräftig gebauter Patient in gutem Ernährungszustand. Keine Oedeme, kein Exanthem. Fettpolster mässig entwickelt; Brust und Bauchorgane ohne nachweisbare innere Erkrankungen. Keine Drüsenschwellungen.

Etwa in der Mitte des rechten Oberschenkels vorne eine Zweipfennigstückgrosse glatte weisse, etwas vertiefte Narbe. Etwas nach oben und medianwärts davon breitet sich eine etwa handtellergrosse, flach aufsitzende Geschwulst aus, von weicher Consistenz, die sehr deutlich *pulsatorische Bewegungen* zeigt. Legt man die Hand auf, so fühlt man ein ausserordentlich starkes Schwirren und Sausen, welches sich auch über die Grenzen der Geschwulst ausbreitet und oben in der Inguinalgegend über der Femoralis ebensowohl wie in der Kniekehle fühlbar ist. Auskultatorisch hört man ebenfalls sehr starkes Sausen. Von der genannten Geschwulst ausgehend ziehen nach medianwärts herum zur Kniekehle starke Phlebektasien, die deutlich *Venenpuls* zeigen und über denen man ebenfalls starkes Sausen vernimmt. Puls in der dorsalis pedis erhalten und synchron und gleich stark wie links. Von der Mitte des rechten Unterschenkels nach der Knöchelgegend zu ist die Haut besonders auf der Innenseite stark gerötet und schillernd. Zahlreiche verheilte zum Teil mit Borken belegte bis pfenniggrosse Geschwürstellen. Etwa in der Mitte der geröteten Stelle eine grössere hammerförmige offene geschwürige Stelle, schmutzig belegt, darüber eine wallnussgrosse gleiche mit ziemlich scharfen Rändern. In der Mitte des linken Oberschenkels einige dunkelbraun pigmentierte Stellen.

28.V. Die Ulcerationen am rechten Unterschenkel haben sich unter Wasserstoffsuperoxydbehandlung bedeutend gereinigt.

4.VI. Operation. Blutleere mit Esmarch'schem Schlauch. In Aethernarkose. 12 cm langer Schnitt am vorderen Sartoriusrand entlang über die höchste Höhe der Geschwulst. Nach Spaltung der Fascie wird der Sartorius stumpf nach hinten gezogen und durch die Musculatur weiter bis auf die Sackwand vorgedrungen. Diese letztere wird allmälig freipräpariert, wobei eine *ganze Reihe von starken Collateralvenen* ligiert werden muss. Unter vieler Mühe gelingt das Ausschälen des

Sackes, der längliche Eiform hat. Der ganze obere Pol lässt sich etwas leichter auslösen bis fast zum untern Pol, wo stärkere Verwachsungen das Herauspräparieren erschweren. Hier am unteren Pol gelingt es dann endlich, die zuführenden Gefässe, Arterie und Vene, zu isolieren. Nun wird der Sack eröffnet, eine grosse Menge Coagula und flüssiges Blut stürzen hervor. Dabei war das Bein im Hüftgelenk gebogt worden, der Schlauch lockerte sich dabei offenbar etwas und es tritt venöse Stauung ein, die ziemlich störend ist und fortwährend Blutungen aus der Peripherie zur Folge hat. Die Verhältnisse sind nun folgende: Die Vene tritt an der medialen Seite am unteren Pol direct in den Sack ein und verlässt ihn nach ca. 1 1/2 cm. weiter oben wieder. Die Arterie liegt vor und etwas medialwärts von der Vene, läuft dicht an der Sackwand vorbei, tritt nicht direct in dieselbe hinein, sondern entsendet einen ca. 2 mm. langen Fortsatz in das Aneurysma hinein. Die Vene wird nun beiderseits von ihrem Eintritt in den Sack unterbunden, der periphere Stumpf noch mit 2 Nähten übernäht. Der arterielle Fortsatz wird dicht am Aneurysma durchtrennt. Der hierdurch entstandene Schlitz in der Arterienwand von ca. 1 cm. Länge wird verschlossen, indem zunächst die in den früheren Fortsatz hineinragende Intima etwas übereinandergeklappt und fortlaufend mit Seide genäht wird. Darüber wird die Adventitia durch 4 feine Knopfnähte vereinigt und über die Naht noch die Scheide herumgelegt und mit drei weiteren Knopfnähten darüber vernäht. Nach Ausräumung der Wundhöhle von Coagulis wird ein Jodoformgazestreif eingeführt und etwa in der Mitte der Wunde herausgeleitet, der Rest durch Naht geschlossen. Verband. Nach Abnahme der Blutleere stellt sich die Circulation langsam wieder her, der Fuss fühlt sich warm an. *Puls in der Poplitea wird konstatiert*, in der dorsalis pedis und tib. post. nicht zu fühlen.

Die Wunde verheilte bis auf die tamponierte Stelle reactionslos und der Puls war an der Arteria Poplitea zu fühlen, und blieb auch erhalten so lange der Patient in unserer Beobachtung blieb, d. h. 6 Wochen. Auffallend war, dass der vor der Operation vorhandene Puls in der Art. tib. post. und dorsalis pedis nachher nicht mehr zu fühlen war. Man hätte dies vielleicht auf eine durch die Naht bedingte Stenose der Arteria femoralis zurückführen dürfen, wenn nicht gleichzeitig auch der Puls an der *linken* Art. tib. post. unfühlbar geworden wäre.

Die tamponierte Stelle blieb lange Zeit offen und eiterte ein wenig; es wurde schliesslich durch die Auskratzung ein Seidenfaden von den vielen Ligaturen eine oder wahrscheinlich von der Adventitia entfernt.

Es unterliegt keinem Zweifel, dass diese Methode der Aneurysmabehandlung nicht nur als radical, sondern auch als ideal bezeichnet werden muss, denn wir beseitigen nicht allein den Aneurysmatumor, sondern im Gegensatz zu den anderen bekannten Methoden wird die Continuität der Arterie erhalten. Ich brauche wohl nicht besonders darauf hinzuweisen, welche Störungen die üblichen Unterbindungen des Arterienstammes bei der bisherigen Aneurysmabehandlung zur Folge hat, vornehmlich dann, wenn es sich um Aneurysma im Gebiet der Femoralis, Axillaris, Subclavia und Carotis handelt.

Ueber die Bedeutung der Arteriorrhaphie bei der Aneurysmabehandlung berichtet *Matas* (3) in einer ausführlichen theore-

tischen Abhandlung. Er folgt dabei einer Anregung die *Murphy* in
der oben genannten klassischen Arbeit giebt. Er geht des näheren
auf die verschiedenen Formen der Aneurysmen ein, mit bestimmten Vorschlägen über die jeweilige empfehlenswerte Art des
operativen Vorgehens. Er selbst hat aber trotz seiner eigenen und
hochinteressanten Erfahrungen in diesem Capitel keinen entsprechenden Fall operiert. Seine Vorschläge erstrecken sich auch auf
diejenigen Fälle bei denen aus irgend einem Grunde der Aneurysmasack nicht exstirpiert werden kann. Hier empfiehlt er nach
Eröffnung des Sackes die Zunähung der in den Sack einmündenden
Colateralen, sowie die Naht der Hauptarterie. Der von Coagula
gereinigte Sack soll nach *Matas* nun zusammengefaltet und durch
Nähte gerafft in sich selbst verkleben. Der Vorschlag ist gewiss
beachtenswert. Indessen muss ich bezweifeln, ob eine solche
Verklebung wirklich leicht zu Stande kommt und ob es überhaupt
möglich ist die starren Wände des Sackes soweit einzufalten, dass
sie in enge gegenseitige Berührung kommen. Lässt sich diese
Vorbedingung nicht erfüllen, so kann auf eine Heilung nicht
gerechnet werden.

Bei dem Aneurysma fusiforme, wo die Arterie sich schlitz-
förmig in den Sack öffnet, da will *Matas* die Arterie über einen
Drainrohr vernähen und darüber den gefalteten Sack schliessen.
Auch hier habe ich meine Bedenken und glaube diese stützen zu
können durch eine eigene Erfahrung.

Bei einem Kranken mit einem Aneurysma popliteum, der im
Jahre 1904 zu mir kam, wollte ich den Versuch der Arteriennaht
ebenfalls machen. Es war ein Aneurysma fusiforme mit breiter
schlitzförmiger Oeffnung in der Arterie. Die Präparation des
Sackes war sehr schwierig, da bestimmte und sichere Grenzen
nicht zu finden waren. Die beiden Lappen die ich aussparte um
sie über dem Arterienlumen durch die Naht zu schliessen, waren
so morsch und brüchig, die Arterie selbst atheromatös degeneriert,
so dass kein Nahtstich darin hielt. Ich war deshalb gezwungen
von der Arteriennaht abzusehen und nach althergebrachter Weise
die Unterbindung der Poplitea zu machen. Gerade dieses Beispiel
zeigt, wie sehr wir von den speziellen Verhältnissen abhängig
sind und dass wir nicht ohne Weiteres theoretisch die Aneurys-
menbehandlung construiren können. In dem angeführten Fall
hätte man noch an die Resection der Arterie und Vereinigung
durch circuläre Naht denken können, das war aber bei der Arterie
poplitea mit ihrer fettig degenerierten Wand und das durch das

Aneurysma infiltrierte umgebende Gewebe unmöglich auszuführen.

Mit wenigen Worten möchte ich noch auf die Technik der Arteriennaht zu sprechen kommen.

Es sind bisher mehr als 40 mal Arterien bei Menschen genäht worden, darunter sind 5 circuläre Nähte nach Resection des Gefässes, wovon der erste von *Murphy* ausgeführte und oben citierte Fall das glänzendste, bisher nicht wieder erreichte Resultat ergab.

Bei der Operation der Aneurysmen wird die Arterienresection voraussichtlich nur in Ausnahmefällen ausführbar sein. Denn abgesehen davon dass längere Arterienstücke, wie das beim Aneurysma fusiforme wünschenswert wäre, nicht zu exstirpieren sind, weil wegen der Spannung die nachträgliche Vereinigung unmöglich würde, vereitelt die in der Umgebung der aneurysmatischen Arterie fast ausnahmslos vorhandene Narben- und Schwartenbildung und die derbe Infiltration des Gewebes das Gelingen einer solch subtilen Naht.

Ist gar noch die betr. Arterienwand atheromatös, wie das bei meinen zwei Patienten der Fall war, so verbietet sich von vornherein die circuläre Naht.

Wesentlich grössere Aussicht auf ein Gelingen hat die *partielle* Naht des Arterienrohres und es ist zu hoffen, dass bei sorgfältiger Praeparation eines Aneurysmasackes sich öfter herausstellen wird, dass diese Methode ausreicht um die Circulation in der Arterie zu erhalten. Je subtiler man den Aneurysmasack herauslöst und besonders die Arterienwand davon abpräpariert, um so eher wird man sich von der Möglichkeit der partiellen Verschlussnaht überzeugen. Das zeigte sich auch bei meinem Fall sehr deutlich bei dem in Folge von Verwachsungen und schwerer Abgrenzbarkeit der Gewebe gegen einander es mir lange Zeit unmöglich schien ohne Unterbindung der Arteria femoralis auszukommen, bis bei weiterer Präparation immer deutlicher die Einmündungsstelle der Gefässe in den Sack sich differenziren liessen. So einfach wie es nach der Abbildung erscheint lagen ursprünglich die Verhältnisse nicht; die Abbildung ist schematisch gehalten und nach dem Spirituspräparat gezeichnet.

Nach den bisherigen Erfahrungen scheinen die unmittelbaren Erfolge der partiellen Arteriennaht recht günstige zu sein. Fast ausnahmslos erwies sich die Naht als sufficient und meist verblieb auch das Arterienrohr durchgängig.

Die Sorge wegen secundärer Thrombose der Arterien in Folge der Nähte liess *Murphy* u. A. die Durchlegung der Suturen lediglich durch die äusseren Schichten des Gefässes, mit Ausschluss der Intima empfehlen. Bei grösseren Gefässen (wie Carotis, und Femoralis) ist dies ebensogut wie z. B. am Ductus choledochus ausführbar; an kleineren Arterien versagt aber die Methode.

Die seitliche Naht einer Carotis nach *Murphy* ist mir im Jahre 1898 gelungen. Als ich bald darauf eine verletzte Arteria orbitalis zu nähen hatte, fasste ich mit dem Seidenfaden die ganze Wanddicke; eine Thrombose trat nicht ein.

Auf diese wichtige Erfahrung hin habe ich meine Assistenzärzte *Dr. Dörfler* und *Dr. Jacobsthal* zu einer experimentellen Untersuchung über die durchgreifende Naht der Arterien mit Seide veranlasst. Durch eine grössere Zahl von geschickt ausgeführte Tierexperimenten bewies *Dörfler* (4), dass eine aseptische ins Gefässlumen gelegte Seidennaht, wenn sie mit einiger Sorgfalt angelegt ist, keine Thrombosen erzeugt. Es handelt sich im Wesentlichen darum die Intima bei dem Eingriff möglichst wenig zu schädigen.

Aus den sorgfältigen histologischen Untersuchungen von *Jacobsthal* (5) geht hervor, dass die im Wundspalt sich bildenden feinkörnigen oder fädigen Gerinnsel kaum gegen das Lumen vorspringen; diese überziehen auch den Seidenfaden. Schon nach wenigen Tagen haben die proliferirenden Endothelien Gerinnsel und Fäden überkleidet. Damit ist der implantirte Fremdkörper unschädlich gemacht, gewissermassen ausgeschaltet.

Wo die Absperrung des Blutes während der Nahtanlegung nicht mit der *Esmarch*'schen Binde zu machen ist (wie an der Arteria femoralis, axillaris, carotis) werden mit Vorteil proximal und distal von der Nahtstelle, resp. der Communicationsöffnung mit dem Aneurysmasack Fadenschlingen um das Gefäss umgelegt. Durch einfachen Zug wird das Gefäss abgeknickt und damit verschlossen. Diese Methode ist schonender wie die Abklemmung mit Zangen (Pinces) auch wenn die Branchen derselben durch Gummiüberzüge geschützt sind. Auch durch die temporäre Ligatur ist eine Schädigung der Intima zu fürchten, wenn man nicht wie *Lejars* dies in praktischer Weise gemacht hat, die Arterienwand durch ein umgelegtes (längsgespaltenes) Gummidrain schützt.

LITERATUR

1. *Murphy*. Medical Record, 1897, 16 Jan.
2. *Körte*. Verhandlungen der Deutsch. Gesellschaft für Chirurgie, 1904, S. 14.
3. *Matas*. Annals of Surgery, 1904, feb.
4. *Dörfler*. Beiträge z. klin. Chir., 25. Bd. 1899.
5. *Jacobsthal*. Ibid. 27. Bd., 1900.

SÉANCE DU 24 AVRIL

(Matin)

Présidence : MM. OLIVEIRA FEIJÃO et BARDENHEUER

Fracture de la voûte crânienne : ablation de 3 grands fragments ; fracture comminutive et compliquée de l'humérus droit. Guérison

Par M. LATIS, Alexandrie.

Salomone Mizan — 51 ans — originaire de Corfou (Grèce). Son casier hospitalier est suffisamment chargé : hospitalisé il y a 4 ans pour une pleurésie bilatérale, on le trouve de nouveau interné du 10-I-911 au 23-I-911 pour un anthrax de la lèvre supérieure et du 5-II-911 au 10-III-911 pour un abcès pararénal à gauche. En plus Mizan, quand il était enfant, a eu une vaste brûlure qui lui a laissé des stigmates profonds, entr'autres une cicatrice allant du thorax à la moitié presque du bras droit et limitant en conséquence les mouvements.

Le 10 décembre 1905, ce pauvre homme se trouve dans une bagarre fameuse dans les annales d'Alexandrie ; il est blessé très gravement à la tête et au bras droit et on le transporte presque inanimé à l'Hôpital Israélite. On m'appelle d'urgence, j'accours de suite et je constate une fracture de l'humérus droit en correspondance à peu près de la moitié de l'os, comminutive et compliquée d'une large blessure de parties molles. A la tête, il y a une autre blessure, en correspondance à peu près de la circonvolution pararolandique antérieure. Les parties molles sont largement ouvertes sur une longueur d'au moins 7 centimètres, l'os pariétal droit est fracturé en plusieurs points de façon à donner un enfoncement de la voûte crânienne.

Deux gros fragments, l'un de mm. 70 × 22, l'autre de mm. 40 × 23 se sont implantés antérieurement et postérieurement avec une marge entre la dure-mère et la lamelle inférieure du crâne et l'autre dirigé en bas vers le centre de l'enfoncement de façon qu'il y a là comme un coin qui comprime très fort la substance cérébrale.

Un troisième fragment de mm. 20 × 19 s'implante dans le tissu cérébral se dirigeant perpendiculairement vers la base du crâne. Il y a une lacération des méninges et division de l'artère méningée moyenne, qui ne donne pas de sang, parce qu'elle est serrée entre deux fragments osseux.

Avec bien de difficultés, j'enlève les 3 fragments mentionnés et un très petit et je tamponne à la gaze iodoformée. Appareil amovo-inamovible au bras droit.

Les convulsions toniques et cloniques de la tête, des lèvres et du cou disparurent aussitôt (sic) l'opération ; il persista seulement une paralysie de la moitié gauche des lèvres qui disparut à son tour quelques jours après.

Ce qui me donna le plus de fil à retordre fut la fracture de l'humérus droit à cause de la cicatrice à la suite d'une brûlure très ancienne qui maintenait le fragment supérieur en adduction. Et c'est pour cela et peut être pour d'autres causes qu'il est resté une pseudo-arthrose du bras droit ; avec une petite intervention on pourra le libérer de cette difformité gênante.

J'ai eu en tout cas le plaisir de présenter Mizan parfaitement guéri de sa blessure au crâne à la séance de la Société médicale d'Alexandrie, le 2 février 1906.

J'ai revu Mizan avant mon départ pour Lisbonne, le 1er avril 1906; ses fonctions intellectuelles étaient évidemment plus éveillées qu'avant la fracture du crâne. La pseudo-arthrose du bras droit était presque tout à fait consolidée.

Sarcome de la voûte crânienne, ayant envahi le cerveau. Ablation d'une rondelle osseuse de cm. 10 × 12. Mort.

Par M. LATIS, Alexandrie.

Un autre cas de chirurgie crânienne n'a pas eu un résultat aussi heureux, mais il s'agissait d'une tumeur de mauvaise nature qui, ayant son point de départ dans la voûte, avait envahi le cerveau, déterminant des phénomènes très graves de compression.

C'était une femme de 33 ans, que j'avais opérée, il y a 5 ans, de résection d'une grande portion de la voûte crânienne: il s'agissait d'un sarcome à cellules fusiformes. Quatre ans après l'opération, reproduction de la tumeur en place et apparition de phénomènes cérébraux. Cette dame, à 3 mois de grossesse, refusa l'intervention proposée, la grossesse continua, il y eut accouchement normal, mais les symptômes cérébraux s'aggravèrent et il s'y ajouta aussi des phénomènes basaux. La pauvre femme souffrait tellement qu'elle accepta finalement l'intervention, que je pratiquai le 24-11-05, bien qu'ayant très peu d'espoir dans la réussite, parce que la tumeur ayant dû envahir trop de substance cérébrale, je fus obligé d'enlever de la voûte une très grande rondelle osseuse (cm. 12 × 10). Hémorrhagie très forte pendant l'opération, à cause de l'énorme dilatation des vaisseaux méningiens. La femme mourut pendant l'opération, peut-être aussi à cause du chloroforme.

A l'autopsie on put constater que presque tout le cerveau était envahi par la tumeur.

A propos de l'appendicite

Par M. LATIS, Alexandrie.

Étudier à nouveau tout ce qui se rattache à l'appendicite serait un travail trop long; je me bornerai seulement à provoquer votre opinion sur une question de traitement qui a passionné le monde chirurgical.

Quand on opère à chaud, doit-on chercher à enlever, coûte que coûte, l'appendice?

En me basant sur les cas que j'ai eu l'occasion d'opérer et ceux opérés par mes confrères d'Egypte, je me suis formé la conviction qu'il faut ouvrir largement l'abcès appendiculaire, mais respecter soigneusement les limites. Si même dans les limites parmi les adhérences on trouve l'appendice, certainement qu'il faut l'enlever; mais détruire le travail de défense naturel pour la recherche d'un appendice qui très probablement a déjà disparu dans l'abcès, c'est s'exposer à des dangers très forts et certains, puisque on va semer des matériaux septiques dans la grande cavité péritonéale, et on ne peut la drainer si facilement.

En 1903, j'ai eu l'occasion d'opérer 5 cas d'appendicite à chaud; dans un seul cas, opéré quelques heures après l'éclosion des accidents, j'ai réséqué l'appendice, qui présentait deux plaques gangrénées et qui adhérait dans toute sa longueur (14 cm.) au cæcum et au côlon ascendant.

Il en est résulté 5 guérisons; j'ai eu des informations sur les patients jusqu'à il y a quelques jours: aucun inconvénient.

En 1904, quatre opérations à chaud: 4 guérisons.

En 1905, quatre opérations à chaud: 3 guérisons, 1 mort. Dans le cas mortel il s'agit d'une opération tardive, un jeune russe de 27 ans qui abusait de l'alcool; l'autopsie confirma l'anamnèse: foie à noix muscade typique. On constata en plus que la cavité abcessuelle était bien ouverte: aucune trace d'appendice. On transporta le malade à l'hôpital plusieurs jours après la formation de l'abcès, quand il y avait déjà intoxication; mais, si son foie avait été dans un meilleur état, très probablement il aurait pu lutter avantageusement contre l'infection.

En tout cas, c'est le seul mortel que j'ai eu à enregistrer. Il est vrai qu'il s'agit d'une statistique très peu nombreuse, mais c'est un fait toujours impressionnant de n'avoir qu'un mort sur 13 cas opérés à chaud.

Je pense que cela dépend de la méthode suivie.

En plus de respecter la barrière naturelle formée tout autour de l'abcès, j'ai toujours eu soin d'éviter d'ouvrir des voies d'intoxication. C'est presque la règle que l'épiploon, une fois le ventre ouvert, se présente plus ou moins enflammé sur une étendue plus ou moins grande. Eh bien! Je ne le réséque jamais, je ne fais que le replier en dehors sur la blessure et le maintenir avec une gaze iodoformée de façon que bien vite il contracte des adhérences avec les parties sous-jacentes et constitue une barrière très valide au passage des secrets de la cavité abcessuelle dans la partie saine. Au premier pansement les adhérences sont très fortes, l'épiploon s'infiltre et s'épaissit pour perdre bientôt ses caractères, et après quelques jours il est résorbé.

Deux lésions rares du duodénum

Par M. REYNALDO DOS SANTOS, Lisbonne.

Dans le premier cas il s'agissait d'un homme qui avait été pris entre le marche-pied d'un wagon et une colonne de fer, celle-ci lui frappant l'épigastre.

Ayant déjà publié ailleurs des détails de cette observation (Bull. Soc. das sc. med. de Lisboa, sessão de 30 dez. 1905) je me borne, pour le moment, à rappeler qu'il a été opéré par le prof. Salazar de Souza, après avoir présenté, entre autres symptômes, des hématémèses répétées.

Laparotomie médiane. On trouve une *nécrose disséminée du tissu adipeux abdominal* et une rupture transversale du corps du pancréas. Rien à l'estomac. Tamponnement de la rupture et drainage. Les hématémèses ont persisté jusqu'à la mort qui eut lieu 20 heures après l'opération, 3 jours après le traumatisme. À l'autopsie on trouve, outre les lésions constatées pendant l'opération, *une contusion de la muqueuse de la première portion du duodénum*, face postérieure, à côté d'un estomac tout à fait sain. Elle siège à 3 centimètres environ du pylore, allongée dans l'axe longitudinal de l'intestin, de forme elliptique, 3 cent. de longueur et 1 cent. de largeur.

Le fond est presque noir, les bords légèrement irréguliers.

C'est, je crois, une lésion qui a été rarement constatée. Je ne connais que le cas de Pillet, cité par Jeannel, où, après contusion du duodénum sans perforation, s'est produit une péritonite suivie de mort.

Dans un cas de Kröulein, il y a eu déchirement de la muqueuse de la papille de Vater, qui a originé plus tard une sténose du cholédoque.

Il est bien probable que la contusion du duodénum soit une lésion plus fréquente que les comptes-rendus d'autopsies et d'opérations nous le font croire, et que plusieurs ulcères et sténoses se soient développés consécutivement à une contusion primitive non diagnostiquée; cependant les faits positifs comme celui que je viens de vous résumer doivent nous faire penser toujours à la possibilité d'une contusion du duodénum en face d'hématémèses à la suite d'une forte contusion de l'épigastre.

Le deuxième cas, dont je veux vous entretenir est celui d'une femme de 26 ans, ménagère, extrêmement émaciée et pâle, qui m'a été adressée le 17 mars 1906 avec le diagnostic d'ulcère de l'estomac.

Ant. héréd. Mère morte de pneumonie; le père encore vivant, hémiplégie, il y a 3 ans. La malade est mariée et elle a un fils de 2 ans et demi, parfaitement sain.

Ant. pers. Elle souffre de l'estomac depuis l'âge de dix ans, ayant eu des vomissements et des douleurs de temps en temps, presque toujours après les repas, parfois tout de suite après, d'autres fois 1 ou 2 heures plus tard; ils étaient aigres et accompagnés de pyrosis. Très souvent les douleurs cessaient lorsqu'elle mangeait. Malgré cela, elle était forte et pouvait travailler.

Cependant, les deux dernières années, les douleurs, les nausées et les vomissements aigres sont devenus plus fréquents et souvent il lui arrivait de vomir, la nuit, la nourriture prise vers l'après-midi.

Il y a un an et demi (août 1904), après une exploration prolongée d'un médecin qui lui palpait le ventre, elle a eu la première hématémèse. Elle a vomi du sang noir exhalant une mauvaise odeur. Dès lors de fréquentes hématémèses alternées avec des vomissements de nourriture, toujours aigres, qui lui emoussaient les dents.

La stase gastrique était telle qu'il lui arrivait de vomir des matières ingérées quelques jours avant. Les douleurs ainsi que les vomissements sont plus fréquents la nuit que le jour et celles-là si fortes que la malade s'évanouit. Elles siègent à l'épigastre, lui répondant dans le dos (douleur en clou), s'irradiant vers les épaules et les hypochondres, accompagnées de cuisson et sueurs.

Contrairement à ce qui lui arrivait étant enfant, les douleurs augmentent quand elle mange. Elle a une constipation obstinée qui ne cède qu'à des lavements et encore pas toujours. Parfois les selles sont noires comme du cirage. L'appétit s'est toujours conservé. Dernièrement l'intolérance gastrique est absolue même pour l'eau, et les vomissements constants avec la sensation de brûlure à la gorge et à l'épigastre suivis de sécheresse sont venus souvent mêlés de sang noir.

Obs. actuelle. 17-III-1906. — C'est une femme de grande taille, extrêmement maigre et pâle, pesant 36,200! Les bras et les jambes presque dégarnis de muscles et de graisse. La bouche édentée, surtout à l'arcade supérieure où il manque les couronnes de toutes les incisives et canines; il ne reste que les racines devenues noires, aux bords irréguliers.

La langue légèrement pâteuse et humide.

L'estomac n'est pas douloureux à la palpation et on ne sent aucune tumeur.

Par la percussion on ne parvient pas à le délimiter, pas de clapotement.

Les poumons et le cœur sont normaux, quoique la respiration et les sons cardiaques fussent affaiblis. 100 pulsations par minute. Vu l'état de grande faiblesse de la malade je m'abstins de plus d'explorations, les éléments obtenus étant considérés comme assez suggestifs d'une *sténose pylorique ou duodénale* avec ulcération.

Analyse du sang — 19-III-906
Hémoglobine — 45 % (Gowers)
Hématies — 4.230.000 (Zeiss)
Leucocytes — 7.200 { P. n. 76 %
{ Lymph. 19 %
{ Gd. mon. 4 %

Le 20-III-1906, sous éthérisation, j'ai fait la laparotomie médiane sus-ombilicale, incision de 10 cent. Lorsque le ventre a été ouvert, on a tout de suite vu le pancréas à travers l'épiploon gastro-hépatique, de lobulation très accentuée et dur à la palpation.

La petite courbure de l'estomac descendait à un chemin de l'ombilic jusqu'à l'appendice xiphoïdien. Une fois que la ptose gastrique et un épaississement du pylore ont été reconnus, on exécute immédiatement une gastro-entérostomie trans-mésocolique postérieure avec sutures (von Hacker).

Suture de la paroi abdominale en 3 plans.

L'anesthésie s'est passée sans incidents.

104 pulsations après l'opération, le pouls faible mais régulier.

La malade n'a eu que deux vomissements après l'opération, lesquels provenaient certainement de l'éther. Elle s'est réveillée sans signes de schok, mais on lui donne une injection de sérum artificiel 150 gr.); caféine et lavements salés. 92 pulsations l'après-midi. — Température 36°

Le 21, elle s'assied dans son lit. Sérum, caféine, lavements salés, et huile camphrée.

Elle boit quelques cuillerées de lait bouilli avec de l'eau de chaux. Température 36,5. Pouls 108. Elle a eu une selle.

Les suites ont été régulières pendant les premiers jours. La malade a toléré très bien sans vomissements une alimentation intensivement progressive (lait, farines, œufs, thé, bouillons peptonisés, etc.) et a eu des selles régulières et moulées.

Malheureusement, une pneumonie double des deux bases évoluant rapidement a enlevé la malade au neuvième jour.

Autopsie — à 9 heures du matin 29-III-904, 18 heures environ après la mort.

Femme extrêmement amaigrie et pâle.

Plaie opératoire à l'épigastre, ligne médiane, de la longueur de 10 cent. environ, réunion par première intention.

Incision du menton au pubis. L'autopsie de la cavité thoracique a démontré que les 2 lobes inférieurs des poumons étaient hépatisés. Le cœur normal.

Dans l'abdomen l'incision a passé à gauche de la plaie opératoire, laquelle montrait du côté abdominal une réunion parfaite aussi par première intention.

Occupant une grande partie de l'abdomen, surtout à gauche, on voyait l'estomac allongé de haut en bas et de gauche à droite descendant à plus de 10 cent. au-dessous du nombril. En le suivant du côté du pylore on voyait que celui-ci était très descendu et à un tel degré que le pancréas était presque entièrement à découvert au-dessus de la petite courbure; parfaitement visible à travers l'épiploon gastro-hépatique. De cette façon le duodénum était complètement modifié dans sa situation et ses rapports.

Au lieu de descendre formant une anse autour de la tête du pancréas, sa première portion montait directement à prendre contact avec cet organe et y restait adhérent dans une extension de quelques centimètres, correspondant à l'ampoule de Vater et voisinage de façon à recevoir le p. de Wirsung et le cholédoque, finalement il abandonnait de nouveau le pancréas pour descendre appliqué par le péritoine à la paroi abdominale postérieure jusqu'à l'insertion du mésocôlon d'où il se continuait avec le jéjunum. Celui-ci, après avoir formé une anse, montait et s'anastomosait avec la paroi postérieure de l'estomac près de la grande courbure et à la partie la plus déclive de celle-ci. Ensuite il suivait normalement.

Estomac — Par la palpation, on sent les parois très épaisses surtout dans la région pylorique. Extérieurement, pas d'indices d'ulcère.

En ouvrant l'organe suivant la petite courbure, on remarque qu'il est presque vide, ne contenant que du mucus et montrant ainsi que l'anastomose avait parfaitement fonctionné. Les parois présentent une épaisseur de 3 à 4 mm, dont 2 mm. appartiennent à la tunique musculaire. Au niveau du pylore l'épaississement de celle-ci atteint de 7 à 8 mm. environ et elle est couverte par une muqueuse également épaissie et lisse.

C'était le sphincter pylorique très développé qui par la palpation faisait croire à la tumeur que l'on avait déjà cru deviner pendant l'opération.

Le pylore, qui avant l'incision de la petite courbure s'était montré absolument perméable, se présentait maintenant complètement ouvert de 6 cent. environ de circonférence.

La muqueuse montrait beaucoup de plis et deux ulcérations au milieu de la paroi postérieure, une du diamètre d'un millimètre environ, et l'autre allongée avec la partie centrale noire représentant certainement l'origine des fréquentes hématémèses dans le passé de la malade.

À la partie la plus déclive de la paroi postérieure, au-dessus de la grande courbure, à 10 cent. environ du pylore, on voyait une ouverture circulaire de 3 cent. de diamètre, aux bords réguliers, communiquant avec le jéjunum et permettant facilement le cathétérisme avec un doigt. Quelques uns des points de suture qui entouraient cette ouverture étaient déjà en voie d'élimination.

Duodénum. — Par l'ouverture pylorique on essaye de cathétériser le duodénum, avant de l'ouvrir, mais à 5 cent. environ son calibre diminue tellement que c'est à peine si l'on peut faire passer les branches fermées d'une pince à dissection. En l'examinant on voit qu'à cet endroit un prolongement de la tête du pancréas, distinctement lobulé et dur comme le reste de l'organe, enveloppe le duodénum dans les ¾ de sa circonférence, de façon à l'étrangler, et ne laissant libre qu'une partie de la face antérieure. Sur les branches entrouvertes de la pince à dissection et le long de cette face on dresse la paroi duodénale mince à cet endroit et l'on continue cette ouverture jusqu'au jéjunum. La sténose duodénale produite par l'annexe pancréatique sclérosé devient alors évidente.

Pendant que la circonférence du pylore atteint 6 cent. environ, la première portion du duodénum ne mesure que 3 cent. et ne dépasse pas 15 mm. au niveau de l'anneau; ensuite le calibre s'élargit rapidement et à la hauteur de l'ampoule de Vater 5 cent. plus loin, il mesure 5 cent. de circonférence. La muqueuse duodénale est lisse et unie comme le pylore sans indice d'ulcère ni de cicatrice.

Le pancréas, de couleur jaunâtre, à une lobulation très prononcée, est dur à la palpation et à l'incision depuis la tête jusqu'à la queue. Il mesure à peu près 15 cent. de longueur. La veine splénique coule dans un sillon le long de sa face postérieure à un centimètre au-dessous du bord supérieur. L'artère splénique passe au-dessus de ce bord sans relation directe avec lui. De la partie droite inférieure de la tête se détache un prolongement glandulaire de 1 cent. environ d'épaisseur et qui entoure le duodénum dans la région et extension déjà indiquées.

De la partie moyenne du corps on a excisé un coin de tissu glandulaire pour l'analyse histologique.

Le long du bord inférieur du pancréas et de la petite courbure de l'estomac il existe des ganglions. Le foie, de grandeur sensiblement normale, est congestié. La vésicule biliaire est de grandeur et consistance normales sans calculs et avec un peu de bile jaunâtre. Les grands ductus sont perméables jusqu'au duodénum.

Rate normale. Reins pâles et avec des zones plus claires de dégénérescence.

Le jéjunum contenait du mucus coloré de bile.

Le cæcum, distendu avec l'appendice, long et normal; le côlon transverse et descendant est atrophié et de calibre réduit.

Organes génitaux normaux.

On n'a pas fait l'autopsie de la cavité crânienne.

L'analyse histologique du morceau de pancréas a montré qu'il était atteint d'une pancréatite chronique interstitielle.

Les cas de pancréas annulaire sont encore assez rares (6) pour justifier cette communication, et ceux où l'on est intervenu sont encore moins fréquents (je ne connais que le cas de Vidal [d'Arras], communiqué au dernier Congrès français de chirurgie), d'autant plus que c'est la première fois que l'on a recueilli l'histoire du malade, de son vivant.

Comme dans tous les autres cas de sténoses sus-papillaires du duodénum, les symptômes ressemblaient tout à fait à ceux d'une sténose du pylore et le diagnostic différentiel était impossible.

Ce cas diffère encore de celui de Vidal en ce que dans ce dernier il s'agissait d'un enfant de trois jours, porteur d'une malformation congénitale, tandis que chez la malade que j'ai opérée, quoique l'anneau (incomplet) fût sans doute congénital (les troubles digestifs dataient depuis son enfance), ce ne fut que plus tard, lorsque la pancréatite s'est développée, que la sténose s'est accentuée à ce point qu'elle ne laissait plus passer un porte-plume.

Le développement progressif est encore témoigné par l'hypertrophie des parois de l'estomac, traduisant une longue lutte contre l'obstacle duodénal.

DISCUSSION

M. MAYO ROBSON. — The section is greatly indebted to M. Reynaldo dos Santos for describing two such interesting and unique cases. The bruised duodenum shows admirably the origin of traumatic peptic ulcer which may occur both in the stomach and duodenum. I collected a series of traumatic peptic ulcers in my work on the Surgery of the stomach, but in no case was the process so well demonstrated as in the specimen here shewn, the bruising being the first stage and dissolution by hyperchlorhydria the second stage of ulceration.

The second specimen in which stricture of the duodenum was due to the pancreas encircling the bowel is I believe unique and it is quite clear that gastro-enterostomy was the only possible operation to afford a chance of relief; it is also of interest to know that the pancreas is the seat of interstitial pancreatitis which condition could tend to increase the obstruction which doubtless in early life was not so extreme, otherwise the patient could not have lived to be 26 years of age. Other specimens of stricture of the duodenum by deformed pancreas have been reported, but I believe this is the first case operated on.

Ueber die cauterisation der Haemorrhoiden

Par M. KOLEFFAROFF, Sofia,

Die Hauptmethoden operativer Natur, welche gegen Haemorrhoiden in Anwendung gebracht werden, sind: 1) Die Cauterisation

mittelst Thermocauter, 2) die Ligatur und 3) die Excision. Es
gibt noch einige Operations- und Behandlungsmethoden, welche an
zweiter Stelle in Betracht kommen, welche von einigen Chirurgen
empfohlen und prakticirt werden, und werden wir einige von denselben unten anführen. Doch konnte bisher nicht eine einzige
Operationsmethode sich in der Behandlung der Haemorrhoiden eine
dominirende Stellung sichern. Die Ursachen für das Fehlen einer
von allen Chirurgen allgemein acceptirten Operationsmethode liegen in dem Umstande, dass alle diese Methoden bei ihren Vorzü-
gen auch ihre Schattenseiten besitzen. Die Haemorrhoiden sind
eine genug ausgebreitete Krankheit und stellen eine wichtige Aufgabe für den Chirurgen bezüglich ihrer Behandlung. Bei der Aus-
wahl einer Operationsmethode muss man eine solche vorziehen, welche die wenigsten und die geringsten Complicationen gibt, welche für
den Kranken keine Gefahr und zwar in erster Linie für das Leben
desselben und in zweiter Linie für das Endresultat der Operation
bietet. Falls die Haemorrhoiden, sowie manche andere Tumoren,
auf einer zugänglicheren Körperpartie sich befänden, so würden
sie bei ihrer Extirpation keine besondere Schwierigkeiten darbie-
ten. Doch mit Rücksicht auf ihre specielle Localisation, sowie
die Schwierigkeit einer genauen Desinfection, bieten die Haemorrhoiden grosse Schwierigkeiten, sowohl für die Operation selbst,
als auch für die Nachbehandlung. Diese Schwierigkeiten werden
noch gesteigert durch die Function des Darmcanals, welcher mit
seinem Inhalte eine ständige Gefahr für die Infection der Wunde
darstellt und seiner Thätigkeit wegen der Wunde keine längere
Ruhepause gewährt.

Die Hauptgefahren, welche dem Chirurgen bei der Operation
vor den Augen schweben, sind besonders zwei: die Haemorrhagie
und die Infection. Die Infection kommt öfters bei den blutigen Behandlungsmethoden — die Exstirpation der Haemorrhoidalknoten,
dagegen die Haemorrhagie bei der Cauterisation mit dem Paquelin vor. Es gibt keine Chirurgen, die nicht kleinere oder grössere Blutungen bei dem Ausbrennen der Haemorrhoiden erlebt
hätten, hie und da sind auch Todesfälle infolge der Blutungen no-
tirt worden. Für die eventuelle Gefahr einer Infection spricht
schon das Operationsterrain an und für sich selbst.

In meiner 12 jährigen Praxis habe ich Gelegenheit gehabt,
sowohl eigene, als auch von anderen Fachcollegen Fälle zu beobachten, welche schlechte Folgen, entweder kurz nach Ausführung der Operation oder in ihrem Endresultate zeigen. Hier

spreche ich namentlich bezüglich des Ausbrennens der Haemorrhoiden mit dem Thermocauter. Speciell in lebhafter Erinnerung
ist mir ein Fall, bei dem sich die Haemorrhagie erst am achten
Tage nach der Operation zeigte, was für mich eine unangenehme
Ueberraschung war, umsomehr als für diese unerwünschte Complication, welche erst durch die Anheftung der Rectalschleimhaut
an die Analhaut beseitigt wurde, ausschliesslich der Thermocauter
beschuldigt werden konnte. Ueber die schlechten Endresultate
dieser Operation werde ich mich weiter unten äussern. Chirurgen, welche Gelegenheit hatten, die Schattenseiten der blossen
Cauterisation der Haemorrhoiden zu beobachten, können von
dieser Methode nicht befriedigt sein und sind daher gezwungen,
eine andere bessere Methode zu suchen, welche die obengenannten
Gefahren beseitigt. Diese Erwägungen haben mich veranlasst,
eine combinirte Operationsmethode in Anwendung zu bringen,
welche eine Gewähr gegen die Haemorrhagie bieten soll. Vor
der Beschreibung dieser combinirten Methode, die ich bei den
letzten 10 an Haemorrhoiden erkrankten Patienten angewendet
habe, möchte ich vorerst einen allgemeinen Ueberblick der bis
jetzt üblichen Operationsmethoden bei den Haemorrhoiden mit
besonderer Berücksichtigung der Mängel bei denselben, geben.

1. *Cauterisation der Haemorrhoiden.* Diese Methode reicht bis in die ältesten
Zeiten des Altertums zurück und besitzt noch viele Anhänger. Die Gefahren, welche sie im Gefolge hat, sind: die Haemorrhagie und die Strictur. Für die erstere —
die Haemorrhagie — ist ausschliesslich der Thermocauter zu beschuldigen, für die
Strictur, ausser dem Thermocauter auch der Operateur.

Die Blutung manifestiert sich manchmal unmittelbar im Anschlusse an die
Cauterisation, anderemale erst nach Verlauf von 5—8 Tagen, das ist um die Zeit,
wo die Brandschorfe abzufallen beginnen. Die mit dem Paquelin behandelten
äusseren Haemorrhoidalknoten bieten nicht eine derartige Gefahr von seiten der
Blutung dar, weil einerseits sich in denselben keine Arterien befinden, wie es
manchmal bei den inneren Knoten zu sein pflegt, ferner weil das nach aussen tre-
tende Blut sofort bemerkt wird, wogegen bei Blutung nach Cauterisation der inneren
Knoten eine Verblutung des Operirten unmerklich erfolgen kann.

Das in das Rectum eingeführte und mit Gaze umhüllte Drainrohr kann nur auf
das Operationsgebiet der operirten äusseren und intermediär gelegenen Haemorrhoiden eine Compression ausüben. Dagegen kann dieses Rohr bei den operirten
inneren, oberhalb der inneren Sphinkteren gelegenen Knoten, keine Compression
ausüben. Von einer Haemorrhagie unmittelbar nach der erfolgten Ausbrennung
kann ich folgenden Fall aus meiner Spitalspraxis anführen. Im Jahre 1898 operirte ich im hiesigen Militär-Hospital einen Officier, bei welchem ich drei innere
Haemorrhoidalknoten ausbrannte. Nachdem ich die Langenbeck'sche Zange von
dem letzten ausgebrannten Knoten entfernt hatte, habe ich ein Drainrohr, mit
Jodoformgaze eingehüllt, vorbereitet. Dieses Drainrohr führte ich vorsichtig

in das Rectum hinein. Mein Erstaunen war sehr gross, als ich beobachtete, dass aus dem Drainrohr ein starker arterieller Blutstrom hervorquoll. Sofort nahm ich das Drainrohr heraus, führte ein Speculum hinein, reinigte das Blutcoagulum, welches in einem Zeitraume von kaum 2 Minuten bis zu einem halben Liter sich angesammelt hatte, und entdeckte darauf in einem der ausgebrannten inneren Knoten einen spritzenden Arterienstamm. Nach Anlegung einer Seidenligatur hörte die Haemorrhagie auf. Wenn ich nicht die Gewohnheit gehabt hätte, was manche Chirurgen unterlassen, ein Drainrohr in das Rectum einzuführen, welches eigentlich dazu dient, um den Gazen freien Lauf zu geben, so stünde der Patient vor der unvermeidlichen Gefahr einer inneren Verblutung.

Ein Beispiel von einer Haemorrhagie, welche sich acht Tage nach erfolgter Ausbrennung der Haemorrhoiden mit dem Thermocauter eingestellt hat, ist folgendes. Im Jahre 1901 operirte ich den Kaufmann N. B. im hiesigen internationalen Clémentinen-Spital, welcher an inneren und äusseren Haemorrhoiden litt. Bis zum achten Tage ging es dem Patienten sehr gut, während welcher Zeit er das Drainrohr im Rectum hatte. Am 8-ten Tage entfernte ich das erste grosse Drainrohr, um es durch ein kleineres zu ersetzen. Das Einführen eines kleineren Drainrohres hat bei mir den Zweck, eine eventuelle nachträgliche Haemorrhagie zu controliren. Gegen abend desselben Tages bemerkte man, dass der Verbandstoff mit Blut durchtränkt war. Der Patient wurde auf den Operationstisch gebracht, man führte sofort das Speculum ein, dabei fand man, dass die Ampulle voll mit coagulirtem Blut war. Nachdem das angesammelte Blut entfernt worden war, sah man, dass aus allen ausgebrannten Flächen von neuem das Blut sickerte. Haemorrhagie en nappe, ohne dabei ein grösseres Gefäss zu entdecken. Wir haben das Rectum mit hydrophiler Gaze, mit Tanin bestreut, ausgefüllt. Am folgenden Tage bemerkte man wieder, dass die eingeführte Gaze mit Blut durchtränkt war. Daher wird dieselbe entfernt und mit neuer ersetzt. Am Abend desselben Tages, bei der Krankenvisite, bemerkte man, dass die Blutung noch nicht aufgehört hatte. Der Patient war blass, sein Puls schwach und schnell. In Anbetracht einer nachträglichen Haemorrhagie, welche diesmal für den Patienten ein tödtliches Ende nehmen könnte, schritt man zum Annähen des oberen Randes der ausgebrannten Mucosa an die Analhaut. Dadurch konnte man die Blutung gänzlich zum Stillen bringen. Bei diesem Falle konnte man recht deutlich constatiren, welche Unbequemlichkeit die Ampulle des Rectums darstellt, dass dort gar keine Tamponade hilft; man mag noch soviel Gaze hineinführen, sobald dieselbe einmal mit Blut sich durchtränkt, hebert sich der Tampon, schlüpft nach oben, und das Blut hat gar kein Hinderniss, weiter zu fliessen.

Das Operiren der Haemorrhoiden mit dem Thermocauter gilt als eine der leichtesten Operationen, welche alle Chirurgen und zwei manche praktische Aerzte täglich ausführen. Es unterliegt aber keinem Zweifel, dass die soeben erwähnte Complication manchen Operirten das Leben gekostet hat, obwohl in der Literatur solche Unglücksfälle wenig erwähnt sind. Wenn die Lage eines erfahrenen Chirurgen in solchem Falle eine unangenehme ist, um wieviel mehr muss sich dieselbe zu einer schwierigen gestalten für den soeben aus der Universität hervorgekommenen Arzt, der aus dem Lehrbuche der Chirurgie gelernt hat, dass die Cauterisation der Haemorrhoiden eine der sichersten und gefahrlosesten Operationen sei? Ich bin der Meinung, dass in einigen Lehrbüchern der Chirurgie die Gefahr, welche mit dem Ausbrennen der Haemorrhoiden verbunden ist, nicht mit dem erforderlichen Nachdrucke hervorgehoben wird. Ich glaube, dass eine solche

Operation, welche dem Patienten eventuell das Leben kosten kann, von allen Gesichtspunkten beleuchtet werden sollte.

Bis jetzt habe ich gesprochen von der Hauptcomplication der Haemorrhagie, als Folge des Ausbrennens der Haemorrhoiden. Nun wollen wir eine zweite Complication erwähnen, welche wieder eine Folge des Ausbrennens ist, und die sich erst zeigt, nachdem die Wunden bereits vernarbt sind. Diese sowohl für den Patienten als auch für den Operateur sehr unangenehme Complication ist die Strictur, welche hauptsächlich auf die schlechte Technik des Operateurs zurückzuführen ist. Eine Operation, wie das Ausbrennen der Haemorrhoiden mit dem Paquelin, mit 2 Complicationen, der Haemorrhagie an erster und der Strictur an zweiter Stelle, kann doch keineswegs als eine sichere und gefahrlose hingestellt werden.

II. Die zweite Hauptmethode der Haemorrhoidaloperationen ist die *Ligatur*. Diese Methode, von A. Cooper eingeführt, wird am meisten von den englischen Aerzten angewendet. Dittel ersetzte die Seide durch ein elastisches Rohr, welches den Vorzug hat, sich mit dem allmählig sich verkleinernden ligirten Theile zusammenzuziehen, was die Seide, einmal gebunden, nicht thun kann. Diese Methode hat gleichfalls viele Anhänger. Ich habe diese Methode selbst häufig angewendet und war mit dem Resultat zufrieden. Aber auch diese Methode entbehrt nicht mancher Nachtheile. Manche Chirurgen, welche diese Methode angewendet haben, erlebten Fälle von Pyämie, weil die Ligatur die Basis des Haemorrhoidalknotens nicht fest genug geschnürt hatte. Zu diesem Zwecke pflegen manche Operateure die Ligatur in zwei Portionen zu machen, indem sie einen doppelten Faden durch die Basis durchziehen. Eine andere Unannehmlichkeit, welche dieser Methode anhaftet, besteht darin, dass das Binden der äusseren Haemorrhoidalknoten mit grossen Schmerzen verbunden ist. Die elastische Ligatur, welche jedenfalls vor der seidenen vorzuziehen ist, hat noch diesen Nachtheil, dass mit derselben die kleinen Knoten nicht gebunden werden können. Lane und Gowland verloren von ihren 851 mit der Ligatur behandelten Kranken 3 an Tetanus, Allingham mit derselben Methode verlor von seinen 3213 Patienten 6 gleichfalls an Tetanus. Baumgärtner findet, dass diese Methode zuviel gesundes Gewebe vom Rectum wegnimmt, welches für die Function desselben notwendig ist.

III. Die dritte Hauptmethode der Haemorrhoidaloperationen ist die Excision und die Exstirpation. Das sind Methoden, welche dazu dienen, auf rein chirurgischem Wege die Haemorrhoiden zu entfernen, indem man dabei das Ziel verfolgt, nach ausgeführter Operation eine prima intentio der Wunde zu erzielen. Die radicalste Operation dieser Art ist die von Whitehead. Diese Methode, mit einigen abweichenden Modificationen von vielen Chirurgen angewendet, gilt als die radicalste, bei welcher jedes Recidiv ausgeschlossen ist. Die schlechten Seiten dieser Methode sind: man entfernt mit derselben die ganze gesunde Mucosa, welche sich zwischen den einzelnen Haemorrhoidalknoten befindet. Daraus folgt die Gefahr für eine eventuelle Strictur. Diese Operationsmethode ist sehr blutig, von langer Dauer und infolge ihrer schwierigen Technik nicht von jedem Arzte ausführbar. Ausserdem kann man gute Resultate nur dann erzielen, wenn die Aseptik vollkommen erhalten wird, und wenn man eine vollständige Vereinigung der Wundränder erhält, was aus leicht einleuchtenden Gründen nicht immer möglich ist. Wenn nicht eine prima intentio der Wundränder erfolgt, können sich nachträglich Stricturen bilden.

Zu dieser rein chirurgischen Methode gehört auch die von Braatz, welche nur etwas weniger radical ist, als die von Whitehead. — Es existiren noch ähnliche Methoden, wie die von Braatz, die wir anzuführen für überflüssig halten.

Von den anderen zahlreichen empfohlenen Methoden zur Behandlung der Haemorrhoiden, welche eigentlich nach den oben erwähnten die zweite Stelle einnehmen, sind folgende auszuführen:

IV. Die Methode nach Chassaignac mit dem von ihm erfundenen Ecraseur, mit dessen Hilfe man die Haemorrhoidalknoten zerquetscht ohne Anwendung von Ligatur oder Naht. Aehnlich Chassaignac operirten auch andere Chirurgen, indem sie zu diesem Zwecke das ursprüngliche Instrument modificirt haben.

V. South combinirt das Zerquetschen mit dem Ausbrennen, indem er den Rest des durch den Ecraseur zerquetschten Haemorrhoidalknotens ausbrennt.

VI. Garrod empfahl die Massage der Haemorrhoidalknoten.

VII. Die Methode der Ligatation, angewendet hauptsächlich von den französischen Chirurgen.

VIII. Landowski empfahl heisse Irrigationen per Rectum, wodurch die Knoten sich verkleinern und zusammenziehen.

IX. Schreiber bestreut die Knoten mit Pulver von Antipyrin. Dana empfiehlt das Chrysarobin als Salbe und als Suppositorien. Armstrong empfiehlt, ähnlich Dana, die Carbolsäure; Rauch, Suppositorien von Naphtalan; Mosen, starke Lösung von Adrenalin.

Einen mehr chirurgischen Charakter haben folgende Methoden:

X. Lisfranc empfiehlt die Scarification der Haemorrhoidalknoten.

XI. Andrews, die Electrolyse der Knoten.

XII. Einige amerikanische Chirurgen haben das Injiciren von Flüssigkeiten ins Innere der Knoten empfohlen. Kelsey hat die Carbolsäure als Injectionsmittel angewendet. Janzenko empfiehlt eine Combination von Ligatur und Einspritzen von Karbolsäure. Schwalbe gebraucht eine 3% Alcohollösung, welche er zwischen die äussere Haut und die Rectalschleimhaut injicirt. Richardson injicirt in jeden Knoten je 30 Tropfen Natrium salicylicum und eine Lösung von Alcohol mit Opium. Beck injicirt ins Gewebe, welches sich um jeden Knoten befindet, einige Tropfen von Jodoformaether. Lofton injicirt in den Knoten heisse physiologische Kochsalz-Lösung. Everett, Ergotin.

Von allen den soeben angeführten Methoden mit der Injection von Flüssigkeiten, konnte sich nur die mit Carbollösung Anhänger verschaffen.

Bis jetzt haben wir all die Haupt- und Nebenmethoden angeführt, welche bei der Behandlung von Haemorrhoiden angewendet wurden. Wie die einen, so haben auch die anderen ihre Nachtheile und einige von ihnen sind überhaupt unzureichend.

Bei dem aufmerksamen Analysiren der einzelnen Methoden gibt es nur drei, welche miteinander concurriren, und unter denen der Chirurg bei der Behandlung der Haemorrhoiden auszuwählen hat. Diese Methoden sind: das Ausbrennen mit dem Paquelin, die Ligatur und die Exstirpation. Wir haben oben gesehen, dass diese drei Methoden ihre Schattenseiten haben, und dass sie in sich Gefahren bergen, welche der Chirurg nicht aus den Augen verlieren darf, und seine Pflicht ist es, Mittel zu finden, um solche zu verhüten.

Die empfehlenswerteste, weil die meisten Vorzüge besitzende Methode, wäre das Ausbrennen der Haemorrhoiden mit dem Paquelin, wenn sie nicht die Gefahr einer eventuellen Haemorrhagie nach sich zöge. Beim Operiren mit dem Thermocauter braucht einerseits die Desinfection nicht so radical zu geschehen, was doch eigentlich an diesem Orte schwer ausführbar ist, anderseits wird die Operationsdauer und dadurch die Narcose auf ein Minimum reducirt, Umstände welche eine grosse Bedeutung haben, hauptsächlich beim Operiren in der Privatpraxis und für angehende Chirurgen.

In der letzten Zeit habe ich bei 10 Patienten mit Haemorrhoiden die Cauterisation derselben angewendet, *indem ich mich dabei vor einer eventuellen Haemorrhagie versicherte und zwar dadurch, dass ich 1-2 Seidennähte auf die ausgebrannte Fläche anlegte.* Nach der Entfernung der Langenbeck'schen Zange legt man 1, höchstens 3 Nähte auf die ausgebrannte Haemorrhoidalbasis. Die Nähte umfassen jenen Theil des Gewebes, welcher zwischen den Branchen der Zange eingeklemmt war, und nicht bloss die Rectalschleimhaut. Auf diese Weise wird die Naht fester und deren Herausfallen nicht so leicht. Als Nähmaterial kann Seide oder Catgut dienen.

Das Anlegen von einigen Nähten auf die ausgebrannte Haemorrhoidalbasis hat besonderen Wert bei den inneren Haemorrhoiden. Bevor wir diese Nähte angewendet haben, speciell bei den inneren Haemorrhoidalknoten, haben wir immer mit einer gewissen Angst den operirten Patienten verlassen, und konnten wir auch vom ersten bis zum 10. Tage nach der Operation uns der Angst einer eventuellen Haemorrhagie nicht erwehren. Man könnte uns entgegnen, dass diese Angst eine überflüssige, wenn nicht eine übertriebene für jeden einzelnen Fall sei, indem die Haemorrhagie doch eine seltene Erscheinung sei. Auf grund unserer und der von anderen Chirurgen gesammelten Erfahrungen aber, dass die Haemorrhagie nachfolgen kann und manchem Patienten das Leben gekostet hat, ziehen wir es vor, auf diese Art uns vor einer in allerdings seltenen Fällen gefährlichen Ueberraschung zu versichern.

Dabei möchten wir noch auf folgende Frage antworten. Stören die Nähte nicht etwa die leichte Ablösung der Schorfe? Die 1 bis höchstens 3 angelegten Nähte stören keineswegs die Ablösung der Schorfe, so wie wir bei unseren auf diese Art operirten Patienten constatirt haben. Die praktischen Vorzüge nun, welche das Anlegen einiger Nähte auf der ausgebrachten Haemorrhoidalbasis bieten, sind folgende:

1) Die Versicherung vor einer unmittelbar nach der Operation oder nachträglich gegen den achten Tag erfolgende Haemorrhagie.

2) Die angelegten Nähte verhindern das Auseinandergehen der Wundränder.

3) Die Verkürzung der Behandlung, indem wir dann nur einen dünnen Streifen haben, der, einmal von seinem Schorfe befreit, sich schnell vernarbt.

DISCUSSION

M. NAPALKOFF. Die Haemorrhoiden stellen eine diffuse Erkrankung der Venen und der Mucosa des Mastdarmes dar. Eine radikale Operation kann man nur ausführen nur von der Seite der Submucosa. Nur eine Resection des unteren Abschnittes der Mucosa kann eine radikale Operation sein. In der Mehrzahl der Fälle muss man eine circuläre Resection ausführen. Die circuläre Resection ist eine leichte, gefahrlose Operation. Die Recidiven kann man beobachten selbst nach dieser Operation; das ist eine Folge der diffusen Natur der Krankheit.

M. VASCONCELLOS préfère aussi l'excision et il insiste sur la nécessité de faire l'excision de tout l'anneau muqueux.

M. SCHLOFFER hat an der Wölfler'schen Klinik in Prag sowie hernach an der Innsbrucker Klinik fast ausschliesslich die Cauterisation ausgeführt und war nur ein einziges Mal gezwungen, secundär durch Unterbindung eine arterielle Blutung zu stillen. Um den Eintritt einer Blutung nach der Operation zu vermeiden, empfiehlt sich, die verschorften Stümpfe vorsichtig zurückschlüpfen zu lassen und keinerlei Instrumente, auch keine Gazestreifen und kein Drain in den After einzuführen. Der Strictur beugt man sicher vor, wenn man nur keine circuläre Verschorfung vornimmt.

M. KÜMMELL. Zur Vermeidung von Blutungen legt Kümmell, nachdem er die Knoten mit der Langenbeck'schen Flügelzange comprimirt und abgebrannt hat, eine fortlaufende Catgutnaht an. Auf diese Weise wird jede Blutung vermieden und vielfach tritt trotz des Schorfes eine primäre Heilung ein.

M. PAWLOWSKY: J'ai reçu des résultats très satisfaisants dans le traitement des hémorrhoïdes avec l'injection dans les hémorrhoïdes de la solution d'acide phénique constituée comme suit: Acide carbol. conc. 1, cocaïn. murrat. 0,1, glycérine 6,0, alcool 4,0. Les résultats dans les cas assez graves, observés pendant longtemps, étaient très satisfaisants. Un grand danger existe quelquefois ici dans la narcose générale. J'ai fait, dans quelques cas, l'opération de la cautérisation des hémorrhoïdes, par Paquelin, avec l'anesthésie locale et surtout avec l'injection de cocaïne en solution 0,1 %. L'opération marche très bien avec l'anesthésie locale par solution de cocaïne.

M. KOJOTNIKAROFF: 1) Il n'y a aucun doute que l'opération radicale des hémorrhoïdes est l'extirpation de la muqueuse, mais j'ai dit dans ma communication que cette dernière opération est très sanglante, de longue durée, et, si l'opération n'est pas suivie d'une prima reunio, l'effet est mauvais.

2) Quant à l'injection d'une solution quelconque dans les tumeurs hémorrhoïdales, j'ai aussi dit que ce sont des méthodes insuffisantes qui ne peuvent pas faire

concurrence aux 3 méthodes principales qui sont employées contre les hémorrhoïdes, comme la cautérisation, la ligature et l'excirpation.

3) L'opération des hémorrhoïdes avec anesthésie locale serait bien agréable pour le chirurgien, mais ce sont les malades dont les 3/4 ne se laissent pas opérer avec l'anesthésie locale et veulent être bien endormis.

Zufällige Zurücklassung eines sub operatione benutzten Fremdkörpers in der Bauchhöhle

Par M.M. Korotnanoff et Navon, Sophia.

Die Fälle von Zurücklassung eines sub Operatione benützten Fremdkörpers in der Bauchhöhle ist in der medizinischen Literatur wohl nichts Neues, obwohl sie zum Glücke nicht etwas alltägliches sind. Neugebauer hat anlässlich eines gerichtlich-medizinischen Gutachtens in der *Monatsschrift für Geburtshülfe und Gynaecologie* 108 solcher Fälle publicirt und seit damals ist die Literatur um noch einige solcher Fälle bereichert worden. Die in der Bauchhöhle vergessenen Fremdkörper sind meistens solche gewesen, deren sich der Operateur bei der Operation selbst bediente, als: Schwämme, Compressen, Tupfer, Drainröhren, Arterienpincetten, Nadeln, etc. In dem von uns beobachteten Falle handelte es sich um das Zurückbleiben einer Gazecompresse bei einer Keliotomia vaginalis, welche von einem bekannten Gynaecologen im Auslande vorgenommen worden war.

Anamnese. Patientin 42 J. alt, seit 23 Jahren verheiratet, hat in den ersten Jahren ihrer Ehe 2 normale Geburten gehabt. War nie ernstlich krank, zur Fettsucht geneigt (sehr adipeusm), weshalb sie zu wiederholten Malen Marienbader Cur durchgemacht hat, zu harnsaurer Diathese, in den letzten 2 Jahren an Angina pectoris zeitweilig leidend. Dieselbe unterzog sich am 5. Januar 1905 in einem ausländischen Privatsanatorium wegen Fibromyomata uteri einer vaginalen Hysterectomie. Diese soll einen normalen fieberlosen Verlauf gehabt haben, doch war Patientin seit der Operation zur Constipation geneigt, weshalb sie fast täglich Purgen nehmen musste. Zwei, drei Tage vor der am 22. März 1905 eingetretenen Erkrankung hatte sie täglich spontanen flüssigen Stuhl. Am 21. März nahm sie, da sie sich schwer im Leibe fühlte, ein Glas Bitterwasser, worauf zwei flüssige Stühle erfolgten. Tage darauf empfand sie kolikartige Bauchschmerzen, weshalb sie nochmals eine gleich grosse Dose Bitterwasser einnahm. Die bis dahin leichten Schmerzen steigerten sich derart, dass der Hausarzt (Dr. Navon) gerufen wurde. Da nichts objectives nachgewiesen werden konnte, verschrieb derselbe eine leichte Morphiumlösung und verordnete die Application von warmen Compressen auf den Bauch. Als die Schmerzen nachliessen, wurde ein Clysma verabreicht, auf welches aber abermals ein flüssiger Stuhl folgte. Einige Stunden darauf steigerten sich die Schmerzen wieder derart, dass eine Morphiumsinjection gemacht werden musste, deren Wirkung nur einige Stunden dauerte. Am 23. März wurden die Morphiumsinje-

einen nochmals wiederholt werden. Intern vergleichtes Ol. ricini und mehrere
einfache Clysmata mit Seifenwasser und Glycerinzusatz blieben erfolglos. Die
Flüssigkeit floss jedesmal nach einigen Minuten bis einer halben Stunde klar zurück. Dadurch stutzig gemacht, zog der Hausarzt den Chirurgen Dr. Kojecharoff
und den Gynäkologen Dr. Stavischeff bei, welche den Verdacht des Hausarztes auf
Ileus bestätigten. In der That entwickelte sich im Verlaufe desselben und der
nächsten Tage das vollständige Bild des Ileus, indem zu dem Bisherigen noch
wiederholtes Erbrechen, Meteorismus und Singultus auftraten. T = 36° bis 37°,8,
P = 75 bis 100. Therapie: Morphiuminjectionen, Eisbeutel auf dem Bauch, Kapillen,
absolute Diät, Intern: Tinct. opii. Es wurden beigezogen noch der Chirurg Dr. Petroff und der Hofarzt Dr. Grauder. Trotz des angenommenen Ileus erfolgte am
25. März spontan und auf hohe Irrigationen spärlicher Stuhl bestehend aus blassen
zusammengepressten Stücken mit Sand Beimischung und Abgang von Gasen in
geringer Menge. Als sich trotzdem der Zustand der Patientin verschlimmerte,
wurden die Angehörigen derselben auf die Nothwendigkeit einer Operation aufmerksam gemacht. Doch bestanden letztere darauf, dass bevor Zuflucht zum Messer
genommen würde, noch ein letzter Versuch unternommen werden sollte, Stuhlgang
hervorzurufen. Da der Ileus unvollständig zu sein schien, wurden noch 2 hohe
Irrigationen gemacht. Nach der ersten gingen abermals geringe Kotmassen von
derselben Beschaffenheit und Winde ab. Nach der zweiten kam ein 60 cm. langer, 40 cm. breiter lege artis zusammengefalteter Gazetampon per anum zum Vor-
schein. Patientin fühlte sich darauf sehr erleichtert. Auf weitere Irrigationen
erfolgte geringer Abgang von Fäkalien und Gaze. Die Schmerzen liessen bedeutend nach. Der Meteorismus und die anderen beunruhigenden Erscheinungen
schwanden in den nächsten Tagen, und Patientin erholte sich bald vollständig.

Als Sitz des Tampons wurde der obere Abschnitt des Colon ascendens angenommen, da bei der Anwendung der hohen Irrigationen das injicirte Wasser zu-
rückfloss, solange der eingeführte Darmkatheter weniger als 60 cm. tief eingeführt
wurde. Beim Versuch, denselben weiter vorzuschieben, fühlte die Hand eine Resistenz, nach deren Passiren das Wasser anstandslos hineinfloss und zurückgehal-
ten wurde. Nach Abgang des Tampons kein Zurückfliessen des Wassers auch bei
weniger tiefer Einführung des Catheters, keine Resistenz beim weiteren Vorschie-
ben desselben über die angegebene Stelle hinauf. Die diesbezügliche Annahme
wurde durch die nachträgliche Angabe der Patientin bestätigt, dass dieselbe 3
Wochen nach der Operation an der bezeichneten Stelle einen Tumor bemerkte, der
nach wiederholter Massage verschwunden sei. Nachträglich theilte der von diesem
Vorfalle verständigte Operateur mit, dass ihm thatsächlich nach Vollendung der
Hysterectomie ein Gazetupfer gefehlt, den er trotz sorgfältigsten Abtastens des Operationsfeldes nicht habe finden können, weshalb er sich entschlossen habe, ihn
dort zu belassen, umsomehr, als die Patientin die Narcose sehr schlecht vertrug, so
dass von einer anzuschliessenden Laparotomie Umgang genommen werden
musste.

Patientin fühlte sich den ganzen Sommer hindurch vollkommen wohl. Sie
machte im August wegen ihrer Neigung zur Fettsucht eine 4-wöchentliche Cur in
Marienbad und kehrte bedeutend gebessert nach Hause zurück. Am 12. October
1905 erkrankte dieselbe wieder plötzlich unter Ileuserscheinungen, welche diesmal
einen so stürmischen Verlauf nahmen, dass am 15. Oktober dieselbe behufs Laparotomie in ein Sanatorium transportirt werden musste. Da sie aber die Narcose sehr
schlecht vertrug, musste sich der Operateur (Dr. Michadovski) darauf beschränken,

auf der linken Bauchseite einen anus praeter naturalis anzulegen. Die drohenden Ileuserscheinungen verschwanden. Der Indicatio vitalis war Genüge geleistet. Trotz sorgfältigster Pflege entwickelte sich auf der linken Bauchseite ein starkes Exzem, welches der Patientin unsägliche Qualen bereitete.

Sechs Wochen nach der Operation hatte sich das allgemeine Befinden der Patientin soweit gebessert, dass sie nach Wien transportirt werden konnte, wo sie nach weiteren 2 Wochen von Hofrath Prof. v. Eiselsberg behufs Beseitigung des Anus praeter naturalis und der Ursache des Ileus laparotomirt wurde. Es wurden zwei dünne, kurze aber feste Stränge constatirt, welche den Dünndarm an 2 verschiedenen Stellen constringirten. Dieselben wurden durchschnitten und ligirt. Die vom Tupfer perforirte Darmstelle konnte nicht eruirt werden. Der Anus praeter naturalis wurde lege artis beseitigt, die Bauchhöhle vollständig verschlossen und ein Gazestück als Drainage an der Stelle des anus praeter naturalis eingeführt. Nach einigen Tagen war die tadellose Darmfunction wiederhergestellt. Patientin erholte sich sehr langsam nach diesem schweren Eingriff. Der Wundverlauf war ein normaler, doch kam Patientin am 18. Februar 1906 mit einer Bauchdeckenfistel nach Hause zurück. Dieselbe wurde nach den Angaben des Operateurs mit Wasserstoffhyperoxyd, Balsamum Peruvianum und Touchirung mit Jod und Lapis behandelt.

Am 3. März 1906 erkrankte Patientin plötzlich unter einem Schüttelfrost und Schmerzen in der Magengegend. Sofort wurde der Verband abgenommen, doch zeigte es sich, dass die Fistel wie gewöhnlich secernirte. Trotzdem wurde am nächsten Tage ein Chirurg (Dr. Petroff) beigezogen, der keinen Zusammenhang zwischen Fistel und jetziger Erkrankung der Patientin constatiren konnte. Am 5. März wurde die Fistel erweitert, wobei 4 ausgeeiterte Nähte entfernt wurden. Die Fistel mündete in eine ausgeweitete Nische aus, in welcher etwas retinirter Eiter mit Fäcalgeruch sich befand. Eine Communication mit der Bauchhöhle und deren Organen wurde trotz wiederhölter sorgfältiger Untersuchung nicht constatirt.

Der weitere kurz geschilderte Verlauf war nun folgender: Auf den ersten Schüttelfrost folgten in den nächsten Tagen mehrere solche, an manchem Tage 2—3 täglich, wobei unter Schweissausbruch die Temperatur bald wieder zur Norm fiel oder durch mehrere Tage hindurch ohne Unterbrechung zwischen 38°—40,5 schwankte. Es entwickelte sich eine Pyelonephritis, welche am 8-ten Krankheitstage gänzlich schwand, um einer Polyurie (Patientin secernirte bis zum 15-ten Krankheitstage 6—8 Liter Urin per Tag) Platz zu machen. Gleichzeitig klagte Patientin über heftige Schmerzen in der Lebergegend, wobei dieses Organ bedeutend schwoll, und ein schwerer Icterus auftrat (im Harne Gallenfarbstoff, acholische Stühle), so dass die Annahme von Entstehung multipler Leberabscesse bei jedem Schüttelfroste berechtigt erscheint. Gegen Ende der zweiten Krankheitswoche traten Schmerzen in der Herzgegend auf, wobei die Herztöne durch Geräusche ersetzt wurden (Endocarditis), Anfangs der dritten Woche eine allgemeine Peritonitis, Ende der dritten Woche beiderseitige Pneumonie. Der Exitus erfolgte spontot discrimina rerum am 24. März 1906 in einem Anfalle von Angina pectoris. Das klinische Bild der Pyaemie wurde durch zweimalige bakteriologische Blutuntersuchung bestätigt (vorgenommen von dem Bakteriologen Dr. Doctoroff), indem Bakterium coli, Staphylococcen und Streptococcen in grosser Anzahl nachgewiesen wurden. Im Verlaufe der 3. Wochen lang andauernden Krankheit wurden wiederholte Probepunctionen an verschiedenen Stellen der Lebergegend und des Abdomens mit negativem Resultat gemacht. Auch die Bauchwunde wurde noch zweimal erweitert. Das zweite Mal entleerte sich aus einer 8 cm. von der

Fistel entfernten subcutan gelegenen Stelle reichlicher localriechender Eiter, und es wurden noch 5 ausgeeiterte Seidenfäden entfernt. Die sonstige Therapie bestand hauptsächlich in subcutanen Injectionen von Streptococcenserum und physiologischer Kochsalzlösung. Als mitbehandelnder Arzt war schon in den ersten Krankheitstage Herr Dr. Graetzer beigezogen, später als Consiliarius Dr. Renvoll.

Was die Aetiologie dieser letzten Erkrankung anbelangt, so wäre wohl das nächstliegende anzunehmen, dass trotzdem keine Communication der Fistel mit der Peritonealhöhle constatirt werden könnte, doch durch die blosse Nachbarschaft mit dem Darme von diesem aus in die Fistel Infectionskeime aufgenommen wurden und in die Blutbahn eindrangen. Doch ist es wahrscheinlicher, dass die Fistel als Infectionsquelle gar nicht in Betracht kommt, vielmehr die seinerzeit durch den Tampon perforirte Darmstelle dieselbe abgegeben hat. Als Stütze für die letztere Annahme, mag der Fall 99 aus der Neugebauer'schen Statistik dienen: Rydygier (Pamietnik II Ziazdu Chirurg. Polskich 1898) verlor bei einer vaginalen Uterusexstirpation einen Tupfer in der Bauchhöhle, konnte ihn trotz energischen Suchens nicht wiederfinden und beschloss, spontane Ausstossung abzuwarten. Nach 7 Wochen fiel der Gazetupfer bei einer Spülung aus der Scheide heraus. Die Kranke starb dennoch später an Pyaemie am 16-4-1887.

Leider konnte in unserem Falle eine Obduction aus äusseren Gründen nicht vorgenommen werden.

In der von uns durchsuchten Literatur fanden wir wohl 30 von Neugebauer gesammelte Fälle von sub operatione in der Bauchhöhle zurückgebliebenen Tampons verzeichnet, doch keiner weist eine solche Aehnlichkeit mit dem von uns beschriebenen auf, insoferne nämlich, als keiner so reich an Peripetien ist, die schliesslich doch zu einem letalen Ausgang führten. Der Neugebauer'schen Statistik entnehmen wir, dass von den von ihm gesammelten 101 Fällen von sub operatione in der Bauchhöhle zurückgebliebenen Fremdkörpern 41 letal endigten und 59 genasen. Das Schicksal der zurückgelassenen Gazetupfer, Mullservietten oder Tupfern war folgendes:

In 7 Fällen wurde der Tupfer sub necropsia gefunden;

10 mal wurd der Tupfer per anum spontan entleert;

4 mal wurde ein Gazetupfer resp. eine Gazeserviette spontan entleert aus einem Bauchdeckenabscess;

4 mal kam es in der Folge zu einem erneuten Bauchschnitte;

1 mal trat am 21. Tage nach einer Symphyseotomie ein Ga-

zetupfer spontan heraus aus dem praevesicalen Raume. Genesung;

1 mal ein Gazetupfer zurückgelassen nach vaginaler Uterusexstirpation; nach acht Wochen tastete der Operateur den Tupfer hinter der Blase, liess ihn jedoch in situ in der Hoffnung, er werde früher oder später spontan herauseitern;

1 mal fiel der Tampon nach 7 Wochen aus der Scheide, aber Tod an Pyaemie (siehe oben);

2 mal wurde der Tupfer in der Bauchhöhle belassen in der Hoffnung, er werde spontan herauseitern.

Der unter Nᵒ 37 von Neugebauer citirte Falle ähnelt einigermassen dem von uns beschriebenen.

Eine Patientin konnte sich nicht recht erholen von einer gynaekologischen Koeliotomie und klagte namentlich über hartnäckige Verstopfung und Ileusattaquen.

Ein Jahr später trat aus der Mastdarmöffnung ein Zipfel eines Gazetampons hervor, und wurde jetzt eine grosse Gazecompresse extrahiert.

In der Folge musste noch in extremis wegen erneutem Ileus operirt werden. Man fand dabei unter den stark mit einander verwachsenen Dünndarmschlingen eine Stelle auf der Darmserosa, wo eine grosse strahlige Narbe vorhanden war. Es dürfte die Gazecompresse an dieser Stelle in den Darm gelangt sein. — Kader. La Semaine médicale, 1898, Nᵒ 17, pag. 132 (?)

Um zu resümiren, zeichnet sich unser Fall durch folgende Besonderheiten aus:

I. Dass der Tampon vom Operateur unmittelbar nach der Operation vermisst, aber nicht entfernt wurde, weil er nicht gefunden werden konnte;

II. Dass derselbe unter drohenden Ileuserscheinungen 11 Wochen nach der Operation per anum abging;

III. Dass 6 ½ Monate nach dem Abgange des Tampons neuerlich drohende Ileuserscheinungen auftraten, welche die Anlegung eines anus praeter naturalis erforderlich machten;

IV. Dass zur radicalen Beseitigung der Ursache des Ileus zwei Monate nach Anlegung des anus praeter naturalis eine Laparotomie vorgenommen werden musste, wobei eine Fistel zurückblieb;

V. Dass die dem Tode wiederholt entrissene Patientin schliesslich doch nicht ihrem Schicksale entging, indem sie der Pyaemie erlag.

DISCUSSION

M. J. BAKES: Das Zurücklassen von Gazetupfern in der Bauchhöhle ist eine wichtige Frage, welche noch nicht zur Zufriedenheit gelöst ist. Mir passierte trotz exacter Auszählung der Tupfer vor der Operation, dass ein Tupfer gelegentlich einer Sectio caesarea im Douglas zurückblieb. Derselbe wurde aus einem subcutis gebildeten Abscess durch die Laparotomiewunde herausgezogen und Patient heilte glücklicherweise vollständig aus.

Damit derartige höchst unangenehme Zufälle in Zukunft nicht vorkommen, haben wir bei der Ausstattung der Tupfer (welche von der Sterilizationsschwester mit dem abzustahlenden Assistenten vor der Sterilization, vor der Operation durch die Instrumentenschwester gezählt werden) eine dreifache Controlle eingeführt und alle Tupfersorten nach dem Vorschlage Mikulicz's mit langen Leinenbänden mit Glasperlen versorgt, dieselben hängen aus der Wunde heraus und verhindern das Zurücklassen der Tupfer.

Sur une maladie du tissu cellulaire sous-cutané

M. OLIVEIRA-FEIJÃO, Lisbonne.

La maladie dont je vais faire la description n'a été observée que deux fois par moi, pendant trente-sept ans de pratique dans les hôpitaux et en ville. Les malades, un homme et une femme, menaient une vie tranquille et aisée; il n'y avait nulle prédisposition chez la femme; on soupçonnait dans l'homme une syphilis qui n'était nullement avérée.

Dans les deux cas, la maladie s'est présentée tellement uniforme, elle eut un début et une allure tellement semblables que je crois pouvoir en faire une description que je ne sache avoir été publiée nulle part.

Les deux malades ont été observés aussi par mes collègues, MM. les professeurs José Gentil, Francisco Gentil, Carlos Tavares et encore par MM. Paes de Vasconcellos, Damas Mora et autres.

Dans l'homme, la maladie siégeait à la jambe droite et chez la femme dans la partie inférieure et interne de la cuisse droite.

Au début, il se présente une tumeur très dure, indolente, roulant sous la peau, à laquelle elle n'a pas d'adhérence, ni aux tissus profonds, et dont le siège est le tissu graisseux sous-cutané. Au bout d'un ou deux mois, la tumeur atteint le volume d'une petite noix et alors la peau commence à devenir rouge, violacée et proémine sur la peau voisine. La tumeur perd sa dureté et devient molle, la peau, continuant à s'amincir, s'ulcère et une perte de substance cutanée s'établit, régulièrement circulaire. En pressant sur la tumeur il en sort une matière d'un blanc jaunâtre, d'un aspect caséeux, et une caverne sphérique est formée.

Jusqu'ici on dirait qu'il s'agit d'une gomme syphilitique, mais l'ulcération et la maladie prennent ensuite une forme et une allure qui les séparent des productions dues à la syphilis.

Alors commencent les douleurs, qui accompagneront l'ulcère. Elles sont lancinantes, soudaines, intermittentes, spontanées, souvent atroces; au toucher on éveille aussi une douleur, mais pas si forte que les douleurs spontanées. Après l'ablation de l'ulcère les douleurs disparaissent.

Dès que l'ulcération caverneuse est formée on en trouve le fond couvert de matière jaunâtre et il en coule un pus fluide, mal lié, fétide. Les bords sont amincis, décollés, et le stylet montre que dans la profondeur l'ulcération dépasse beaucoup la perte de substance de la peau.

Le processus ulcératif marchant plus vite dans la profondeur qu'à la surface, çà et là apparaissent dans la peau des taches violacées qui s'ulcèrent, gagnent en étendue et vont rejoindre l'ulcération primitive, qui est agrandie ainsi par la destruction ulcéreuse de la peau.

Au bout de quelque temps un large ulcère est formé, en six mois il atteint un diamètre de douze à quinze centimètres.

Au commencement il peut être unique et il se présente plus ou moins rond, les bords décollés, la peau environnante est légèrement rougeâtre dans une étendue d'un demi centimètre et les tissus qui avoisinent l'ulcère sont très durs. Le fond est formé par des granulations bourgeonnantes, le plus souvent d'un rouge foncé, exubérantes par places, mais en d'autres points il n'y a pas de bourgeonnement et le fond se montre jaunâtre, couvert d'une couche formée par un mélange de pus et de cellules mortes.

La profondeur de l'ulcère peut être très grande et aller jusqu'à trois ou quatre centimètres, selon l'épaisseur de la couche du tissu adipeux. Mais à côté on trouve des points aussi où le fond de l'ulcère s'élève à la hauteur de la peau et peut même la dépasser. Des plaques de tissu blanchâtre de cicatrice épidermique peuvent se montrer, ou sur les bords de l'ulcère, ou au milieu de celui-ci.

Ainsi les bords sont taillés à pic, là où le processus ulcératif domine; ou se continuent avec l'ulcère dans un même plan, là où le bourgeonnement est vif. Un pus très fétide coule de l'ulcère.

Dans ces circonstances la maladie se présente sous un aspect qui ressemble fort à celui des ulcérations épithéliales, ce qui résulte des faits suivants: En même temps que l'ulcère ronge les tissus, un bourgeonnement très actif se produit sur quelques points, pouvant même devenir exubérant et combler très rapidement une partie de l'ulcère et se couvrir de tissu épidermique cicatriciel. La rapidité avec laquelle le bourgeonnement se fait est très remarquable, mais bientôt sur un point il devient faible, perd sa couleur rouge, devient pâle et l'on voit apparaître au milieu de ce bourgeonnement si vif un foyer de ramollissement, d'où sort une matière d'un blanc jaunâtre tout à fait pareille à celle décrite dans le noyau primitif; rapidement aussi l'ulcération partant de ce foyer détruit les bourgeons charnus et la cicatrice qui semblait être prête à se former. Ce rapide bourgeonnement de l'ulcère se fait sans l'influence d'aucun pansement, mais il est très remarquable comme conséquence du traitement topique; la destruction emportant toujours sur la réparation qui n'est qu'apparente, il en résulte que l'ulcère ne cesse pas de grandir.

Ce n'est pas seulement par une destruction de proche en proche que l'ulcère augmente en étendue. Plus ou moins loin de lui un noyau dur se présente et suit, beaucoup plus rapidement que la tumeur primitive, la même marche.

Il se forme une nouvelle ulcération qui en grandissant peut aller se joindre à l'ulcère antérieur; et dans la suite bien des tumeurs peuvent prendre naissance et former autant d'autres ulcères. J'en ai vu plus de quarante dans la jambe de mon premier malade.

Le plus souvent et même presque toujours, dans la profondeur, on trouve un fin trajet qui unit un ulcère à l'autre: fistule de communication. Dans la profondeur les aponévroses constituent, jusqu'à un certain point, une barrière à l'ulcération; mais cette barrière est enfin vaincue et c'est par les ouvertures par où traversent les vaisseaux et les nerfs que l'ulcération gagne les tissus sous-aponévrotiques. Il faut cependant dire que cet envahissement est rare.

Les ganglions lymphatiques ne sont pas atteints, ni même engorgés, ils conservent leur volume normal. Point de développement veineux. L'ulcère n'est pas saignant. Rien à remarquer dans l'examen des urines, rien dans les viscères thoraciques et abdominaux.

La durée de la maladie peut être très longue: mon premier malade a souffert pendant plus de huit ans, il est mort au bout de dix ans de souffrance et ce ne fut qu'à la fin que l'état général sembla être atteint. L'appétit s'est maintenu et la fièvre ne se présenta que quelques jours avant la mort.

Dans ce malade, l'extirpation étant impossible, à cause de l'étendue des lésions qui occupaient toute la jambe, et l'amputation ayant été refusée, j'ai eu recours au raclage, à la cautérisation au thermo-cautère, à l'acide lactique et aux antiseptiques. Un traitement anti-syphilitique employé auparavant n'avait donné aucun résultat.

Après bien des échecs et après avoir pendant deux ans fait des raclages répétés, cautérisations, etc., pris le plus grand soin à débrider les fistules, dès que j'en soupçonnais l'existence et à attaquer chaque foyer nouveau, dès qu'il se formait, je parvins à obtenir une cicatrisation complète.

Je fis à la malade l'ablation complète de l'ulcère et des tissus durcis qui l'environnaient et qui criaient sous le bistouri. La cicatrisation de la plaie est presque complète.

Avant, j'avais appliqué sans résultat un traitement anti-syphilitique. Sur l'ulcère l'eau oxygénée, sous l'action de laquelle le bourgeonnement fut très rapide, comme de même après l'ablation au thermo-cautère d'un des bords décollé dans presque la moitié de la circonférence de la lésion.

Bientôt après des foyers de nécrobiose apparurent au milieu du bourgeonnement actif, mais, averti par ce qui m'était arrivé avec mon premier malade, je me décidai à l'extirpation qui fut acceptée. J'appliquai ensuite, pendant quatre jours, un pansement à l'eau oxygénée pure, dans l'intention de détruire l'agent producteur de la maladie, quoique j'eusse fait une opération aseptique.

Donc, au point de vue de la cicatrisation, le pronostic de la maladie est sérieux, car elle est difficile à obtenir, et je considère l'extirpation de l'ulcère, faite dans les tissus sains, comme le moyen le plus sûr et rapide pour arriver à la guérison.

Le pronostic, cependant, peut devenir grave au point de vue de la vie du malade, si la lésion locale est ancienne. Peu de temps après la cicatrisation de l'ulcère, mon premier malade présenta des amnésies fréquentes qu'il n'avait pas auparavant. Les fonctions psychiques devinrent mauvaises, il lui fallait faire des efforts pour connaître les personnes qui l'entouraient. Il méconnaissait même sa chambre, il était hébété. Puis une fièvre de 39 degrés s'alluma, l'haleine prit une mauvaise odeur, sans toux ni dyspnée, sans que l'examen des poumons montrât aucune lésion, ensuite les abcès se formèrent sur les fesses et dans le dos; il tomba dans un état de stupeur et quelques jours après il mourut. La mort suivit de moins de deux mois la cicatrisation des ulcères.

On peut dire que la mort fut la conséquence d'une infection

secondaire, d'une pyohémie. Il n'en est cependant pas moins digne de remarque que la cicatrisation eût pu se faire sous l'influence de cette infection secondaire et que celle-ci ne se montrât qu'après la guérison des lésions locales. A mon avis la mort fût la conséquence d'une infection, mais celle-ci était aussi la cause de la maladie et les ulcères en étaient des localisations.

Pendant cette dernière période de la maladie l'appétit se maintint toujours. Le malade ne se plaignait de rien, pas même de maux de tête, et je ne pus rien découvrir par l'examen des organes thoraciques et abdominaux, digne d'être mentionné.

Malheureusement je n'ai pu faire d'autopsie, ni aucun examen des ulcères, ni du pus qui en suintait. Mais, comme à tous les points de vue les lésions locales étaient tout à fait pareilles dans ma seconde maladie, à laquelle j'ai fait l'extirpation de l'ulcère, j'ai prié mes collègues le professeur Pinto de Magalhães et le dr. Marck Athias de faire l'étude histologique de la pièce. Je laisse ici l'expression de mes remercîments à mes collègues, et je présente le résultat de leurs travaux.

L'épithelium cutané ne présente aucune altération appréciable. Sous lui, le corps papillaire du derme est en partie irrégulier; les faisceaux du tissu fibreux semblent épaissis, et l'on voit des rangées de petites cellules rondes, formant des amas qui vont jusqu'à l'intérieur des papilles.

Quelques vaisseaux sectionnés montrent une remarquable épaisseur de leurs tuniques et la lumière en est comblée par une prolifération cellulaire, qui doit provenir de l'endothélium.

Dans les points où l'ulcération détruisit l'épiderme on voit de grands amas de petites cellules rondes et de grands nodules déjà caséifiés.

Dans le tissu cellulaire sous-cutané on trouve des altérations plus étendues. Le tissu adipeux est altéré; et on y trouve surtout un épaississement des trabécules intercellulaires avec prolifération locale de petites cellules rondes; en quelques points, parmi les cellules adipeuses, cette prolifération est remarquable; en d'autres points les cellules graisseuses semblent manquer et à leur place il y a des lacunes; autour on voit une prolifération cellulaire de petits éléments et trois ou quatre cellules géantes.

Les faisceaux du collagène acidophile du tissu cellulaire sous-cutané ont, presque tous, souffert la dégénérescence hyaline; ils se présentent épaissis, gros, et au lieu de la structure fasciculée normale, ils ont un aspect homogène et brillant.

Les altérations vasculaires sont ici beaucoup plus considérables, aussi bien le processus d'endo-périartérite, que les oblitérations vasculaires.

Les infiltrations des petites cellules rondes, qui ont lieu surtout autour des vaisseaux, sont aussi plus nombreuses, mais on voit encore beaucoup de nodules parmi les faisceaux altérés du tissu conjonctif.

On rencontre aussi de nombreux nodules de petites cellules, dont le centre présente la nécrose de caséification et quelques cellules géantes.

Des injections faites dans les cobayes furent négatives au point de vue de la tuberculose.

Je suis d'avis que la maladie dont je viens de faire la description doit être due à un microbe et il est possible que ce soit une maladie parasitaire. La présence des cellules géantes fait penser à la tuberculose ou à la syphilis, mais d'une part l'injection dans les cobayes et l'absence de tout symptôme de tuberculose et de l'autre l'absence de symptômes et de lésions syphilitiques antérieures me font rejeter la nature syphilitique ou tuberculeuse de la maladie.

DISCUSSION

M. GARRÉ: Einen nicht gleichen, wohl aber analogen Fall, den ich vor Jahren beobachtet habe, der mir auch viel Kopfzerbrechen gemacht hat bezgl. der Diagnose, hat sich nach Monaten als *Malleus chron.* (morve) herausgestellt. Die histologische und die bacteriologische Untersuchung gibt beim chron. Rotz meist keine beweisenden Resultate. Das einzige ist die Einspritzung von den pathologischen Massen auf Meerschweinchen, was die Diagnose klären kann.

M. PEDRO S. DE MAGALHÃES: Je demanderai la permission à M. le prof. Feijão de le prier de nous informer si les inoculations dont il vient de nous parler ont été faites avec des matériaux provenant de ses malades, si elles ont été faites à des cobayes mâles et si des localisations se sont révélées dans les testicules, cas dans lequel le diagnostic de morve s'imposerait, aussi bien que la localisation aux mamelles. Strauss nous a même enseigné de profiter de la localisation spécifique de la morve après l'inoculation aux cobayes pour décider le diagnostic dans les cas douteux.

M. PAWLOWSKY. Il y a beaucoup de cas semblables aux cas publiés par M. le président avec étiologie variable.

J'ai observé un cas de morve chronique, dans lequel se sont formés les lymphangites chroniques, avec ulcération lente et production de petits foyer de pus le long des vaisseaux lymphatiques enflammés. Le malade a maigri peu à peu, l'élévation de la température a été jusqu'à 38,1-38,2. La maladie a été très longue, elle a duré quelques mois. Dans le pus on a trouvé les bacilles de la morve, et l'injection de Strauss a été aussi positive.

Il y a aussi des cas semblables, dans lesquels on ne trouve rien que les staphylocoques blancs, avec virulence affaiblie. Ce sont surtout les cas décrits par MM. Kocher et Tavel, et par d'autres, comme phlegmons en bois, chroniques.

Dans d'autres cas semblables, avec ulcération chronique et suppuration, il s'agit de cas de tuberculose et, surtout, de syphilis. L'ulcère de Pende et Mourgah, l'ulcère Madura et surtout l'ulcère des tropiques donnent quelquefois un tableau semblable à celui cité tout à l'heure par M. Feijão. Dans les cas de l'ulcère de Pende on a trouvé chez nous, en Russie, les staphylocoques blancs et, en dernier temps, des protozoaires. Eh bien, nous pouvons construire à présent beaucoup de diagnostics, mais toutes nos conclusions sur les cas publiés restent comme hypothèses. Pour obtenir les résultats définitifs dans le diagnostic des cas publiés, il faut faire aussi l'injection diagnostique de tuberculine. À présent nous pouvons seulement dire que les cas publiés par M. Feijão sont très intéressants et surtout il s'agit ici d'une maladie rare, d'un granulome chronique avec ulcération et suppuration.

M. FABRE (St. Denis de Pile): A la suite de la communication de M. Feijão, M. le prof. Garré a déclaré que la lésion pourrait être de la morve chronique, d'après les observations analogues qu'il avait pu faire d'une maladie semblable, mais que les inoculations faites aux cobayes ayant été mal opérées n'avaient rien donné, ainsi d'ailleurs que l'examen microscopique.

Les lésions de la morve chronique sont bien différentes de celles de la maladie qui nous intéresse, et viennent d'être très bien décrites par M. Pawlowsky.

Mais en admettant que ces lésions soient celles de la morve chronique ou de la tuberculose, comme le suppose M. Pawlowsky, ces deux maladies auraient bien pu exister sans que l'examen microscopique pût déceler aucun des bacilles générateurs de l'une d'elles. Car nous savons parfaitement que les lésions chroniques de la morve et de la tuberculose sont virulentes alors que l'examen microscopique reste négatif.

C'est donc aux inoculations révélatrices, et à elles presque exclusivement, qu'il faut s'adresser pour porter le diagnostic dans les cas suspects de morve ou de tuberculose — inoculations intra péritonéales faites aux cobayes qui, dans la tuberculose, donnent rapidement la maladie classique — et dans les cas de morve sur le cobaye mâle (procédé Strauss) amène la mort en 24 heures avec orchite double, caractéristique, procédé que vient de signaler M. Pedro S. de Magalhães.

Pour la tuberculose, en France, nous craignons les injections de tuberculine de Koch, qui ont bien souvent, pour ne pas dire toujours, amené la mort, lorsque le malade était tuberculeux.

Donc, dans les cas douteux de tuberculose ou de morve, à mon avis c'est aux inoculations révélatrices surtout qu'il faut accorder confiance.

M. KÜMMELL hat eine ähnliche Beobachtung gemacht, bei welcher nach langem Suchen erst nach Monaten Actinomycose festgestellt wurde. Man nahm Lues oder Tuberculose an; das charakteristische Bild der Actinomycose fehlte ebenfalls. Der Nachweis der Strahlenpilze stellte eine sichere Diagnose.

M. FEIJÃO: La maladie que j'ai vue ne ressemble point à une lymphangite chronique, j'en ai bien eu dans ma clinique, et j'ai dit que l'état général du malade ne fut atteint que quelques jours avant la mort; pendant des années le malade marchait, il n'a jamais maigri et ce ne fut que pendant que je lui ai prêté mes soins qu'il s'alita. L'examen des cobayes fut fait par mes collègues, dont la compétence est parfaite; il n'y avait chez eux nulle lésion tuberculeuse, rien dans les testicules, ce qui ne me fait pas penser à la morve chronique. Les injections furent faites dans le péritoine.

Aussi ces malades n'avaient aucun rapport avec des chevaux.

Il est vrai que la circonférence des ulcères est dure et leur tissu crie sous le bistouri, comme je l'ai dit, mais ça ne suffit pas pour porter le diagnostic d'actinomycosis, il ne s'y montra jamais ces anfractuosités que l'on voit au fond des ulcères d'actinomycosis, ni les grains de riz, et la marche de l'actinomycosis est égale à celle de la maladie que je viens de décrire.

Je dis donc: Pour moi, c'est une maladie microbienne, probablement parasitaire, mais je ne connais pas le microbe ou le parasite de la maladie, et j'ai présenté mes observations au Congrès en priant MM. les congressistes de vouloir bien me dire s'ils connaissaient quelques cas pareils. Je ne donne pas de nom à la maladie, puisque je ne connais pas l'agent qui en est la cause.

Contribution à l'étude des tumeurs de l'orbite. Un cas de fibro-enchondrome de la paroi externe absorbant le globe oculaire

Par M. Brant Paes Leme, Rio de Janeiro.

Il semble à l'auteur qu'ils ne sont pas communs les cas dans ces conditions, même au contraire ils sont très rares. Dans celui-ci, parfaitement documenté puisque cette communication va accompagnée par la photographie du malade et par des coupes microscopiques de la tumeur, est à noter l'énorme développement de la trame de la tumeur, suffoquant presque complètement le globe oculaire, très difficile d'être reconnu à la surface de la tumeur, et même dans les coupes, réduit à de très insignifiantes dimensions, presque totalement absorbé par la masse néoplasique. À la partie inférieure de la tumeur, au niveau de la paupière inférieure, on rencontrait, comme greffé sur lui, un *molluscum pendulum*.

Ce fut même principalement le poids de ce *molluscum*, selon le malade, qui l'a conduit à se laisser opérer, parce que la tumeur, proprement, ne le faisait pas souffrir à présent; dans le commencement, il y avait environ 20 ans, oui, le malade avait souffert les plus atroces douleurs, mais après, petit à petit, elles disparurent.

La tumeur était ulcérée depuis 2 ans, et même dans ces conditions elle n'était pas douloureuse. L'auteur a fait l'extirpation totale de la tumeur, c'est-à-dire l'évidement de l'orbite, et le malade a très bien guéri.

Sur la relativement moindre fréquence à Rio de Janeiro de quelques états morbides communs ailleurs, soit l'appendicite, les kystes hydatiques, les abcès du foie, etc.

Par M. Brant Paes Leme, Rio de Janeiro

Le point spécial sur lequel, à propos des états morbides susmentionnés, l'auteur veut attirer l'attention est, comme il a été dit dans le titre de la communication, leur fréquence relativement moindre à Rio de Janeiro comparée à ce qui arrive ailleurs, soit par exemple à propos de l'appendicite, en comparaison avec ce qui arrive en Europe et dans l'Amérique du Nord; à propos du kyste hydatique en comparaison avec ce qui arrive en Europe même et aussi dans la République Argentine, etc.; à propos des abcès du foie, en comparaison avec ce qui arrive dans les pays de climat chaud,

parmi lesquels on classe le Brésil, que volontiers et injustement on
considère d'habitude à l'étranger comme un héros de toutes les situa-
tions morbides. En considérant les états morbides mentionnés, si
différents les uns des autres, l'appendicite, les kystes hydatiques,
les abcès du foie, et tous en vérité très rares, mais très rares
même à Rio de Janeiro, tellement qu'on pourrait même douter
de leur fréquence ailleurs si ce n'étaient les statistiques publiées
et le nom des chirurgiens qui les rapportent, l'auteur croit trouver
d'une manière générale la cause commune du fait dans la pureté
de l'eau de boisson ordinaire, potable et pure, le plus qu'on peut
désirer, l'eau appelée et dite «eau Carioca», qui n'est pas conta-
minée et est la boisson préférée de tout le monde.

Ensuite, l'auteur croit aussi à l'influence du moindre abus des
boissons alcooliques, des liqueurs très spiritueuses, absinthe,
whisky, etc., etc., comme aussi au fait de la non-existence à Rio
de Janeiro, au moins dans les conditions graves et communes ailleurs, de la protéique «infection grippale».

Relativement aux abcès du foie en particulier, il faut noter
en plus la circonstance que Rio de Janeiro n'est pas la contrée
marécageuse qu'on s'imagine quelquefois, et que même l'impalu-
disme et la dysenterie, les causes ordinaires des abcès appelés
classiquement «abcès des pays chauds», y sont aussi rares.

L'auteur parle d'après ses observations cliniques en pratique
civile et hospitalière, et aussi d'après les résultats de ses études
au laboratoire d'anatomie à sa charge, où tous les cadavres sont,
depuis longtemps, soigneusement autopsiés en vue de l'investigation de ces questions, où ne peuvent pas passer des lésions mé-
connues et où ne peuvent pas exister non plus des erreurs de
diagnostic.

DISCUSSION

M. F. S. MAGALHÃES : Messieurs, n'ayant eu la certitude de me présenter à
ce Congrès qu'au dernier moment, peu de temps avant mon départ de Rio, je n'ai
pu emporter avec moi des données positives pour vous présenter quelques communications préparées d'avance. Mais le thème qui vient d'être présenté par l'orateur
précédent est si important que je me sens tenté de vous dire quelques mots sur
le sujet.

Celui-ci est en effet d'une importance très grande, et cette importance se
rapporte non seulement au point de vue de la géographie médicale, comme aussi
à des problèmes de pathogénie et d'étiologie. Ces problèmes, presque tous, sont
très difficiles à résoudre.

La rareté de beaucoup de maladies à Rio de Janeiro, maladies fréquentes
ailleurs, demande pour être expliquée que des matériaux abondants et positifs,

qui nous manquent encore, permettent de donner la solution scientifique aux problèmes qui s'y rattachent.

La rareté très notable de l'appendicite, explicable selon quelques auteurs qui se sont occupés de la question, par rapport à d'autres contrées, ne saurait trouver une explication ni dans l'alimentation, ni en d'autres conditions faciles à être connues. Étrangers et Brésiliens, vivant au pays dans des conditions à peu près les mêmes qu'en Europe, montrent une même rareté de fréquence (le morbidité pour l'appendicite.

Pour ce qui concerne la maladie kystique, pour les hydatides je ne connais que des cas très peu nombreux, et ceux-là même la plupart indubitablement étrangers au pays. Cette rareté contraste d'une manière frappante avec ce qui arrive dans la République Argentine où des chirurgiens ont pu rassembler des statistiques fort riches. Je sais que dans la République Orientale, les hydatides sont encore assez fréquentes, malgré que les faits soient bien plus rares dans quelques départements qu'en d'autres, elle y est très irrégulièrement distribuée.

Mais à Rio Grande do Sul, état brésilien le plus méridional, les cas de kystes hydatiques sont déjà observés encore plus rarement, et de préférence à la campagne.

A Rio Grande, à Montevideo, dans la République Argentine, la maladie paraît pouvoir s'expliquer par la vie commune menée par les individus qui s'occupent du bétail, avec les chiens qu'ils emploient pour les aider dans leur travail professionnel.

Je vous parlerai encore de l'actinomycose, également fort rare au Brésil; un seul fait a été enregistré jusqu'à présent. Ayant eu l'honneur d'étudier, en collaboration avec mon regretté ami Bulhões, dont la perte prématurée pour la science et pour la chirurgie brésiliennes ne pourra être comblée de sitôt, je pourrais bien vous le raconter si le temps ne me manquait pas.

Le cas a été considéré longtemps comme une tuberculose locale de la paroi thoracique, accompagnée de névralgie d'une grande intensité des nerfs intercostaux. L'examen a révélé les granules actinomycosiques. La maladie a duré de longs mois, et après la mort du patient la nécropsie a fait constater une généralisation fort étendue de l'infection à tous les viscères. Le cerveau, le cœur, les poumons, le foie présentaient de nombreux noyaux d'actinomycose. Le malade provenait du Ceará où il s'occupait de chevaux, et à son dire la maladie aurait eu une origine externe, le malade ayant fait une chute sur la partie la première affectée, un des côtés du thorax.

La localisation de la tuberculose dans les vertèbres, le mal de Pott, avec ses suites, les difformités de la colonne vertébrale ne sont pas si fréquentes que dans quelques pays européens; nos bossus sont bien peu nombreux en comparaison avec le nombre qu'on rencontre de tels individus à Vienne et dans bien d'autres villes d'Europe.

Il y aurait bien d'autres faits qui mériteraient d'être relevés à propos du thème en discussion. La supposée gravité et rapidité d'évolution de la syphilis dans les pays chauds est bien un fait très contestable. La plupart des fois ce sont des malades qui, étant restés sans soins médicaux pendant longtemps, ne se présentent au médecin que lorsque leur affection est bien avancée.

Je ne puis abuser plus longtemps de votre bonté et je dois terminer ici ce que j'avais à vous dire.

M. R. L. Kolle. A propos de la fréquence de certaines maladies dans l'Amétique du Sud et surtout au Brésil, je voudrais ajouter quelques observations à propos de la République Argentine, où j'avais fait mon éducation et ma pratique médico-chirurgicale.

L'appendicite devient en Argentine tous les jours plus fréquente, comme le démontrent les cas nombreux opérés dans les hôpitaux et en ville. Il arrive en Argentine comme en Europe pour la grossesse extra-utérine, dont les cas se multiplient à mesure que le diagnostic se précise.

L'actinomycose est assez fréquente en Argentine, méconnue encore il y a 5 ans. Déjà le dr. Cranwell a réuni dans une monographie récente plus de 30 cas. Au Brésil, on en a eu peut-être moins d'expérience.

Le kyste hydatique est très fréquent en Argentine et plus fréquent qu'au Brésil, car c'est un pays d'élevage de bétail et les chiens propagateurs de la maladie sont encore très fréquents, car l'hygiène prophylactique de tuer l'excès des chiens, etc., etc., n'est pas encore assez acceptée par le public. Dans la plupart des régions du Brésil le bétail n'est pas nombreux, donc manque de matériel pour la maladie parasitaire. Le chien devient ici moins important.

M. LEMOS: Sur les observations qui viennent d'être faites, j'ai seulement à dire deux mots relativement à la dernière. Du fait, à ce qui a été dit, il est d'avance répondu dans ma communication. Il ne peut s'agir d'erreur de diagnostic parce que je parle avec l'observation clinique et avec de très nombreuses autopsies dans le laboratoire d'anatomie de la Faculté, où tous les cadavres sont soigneusement examinés. On comprend facilement que sur les tables d'anatomie les appendicites, les kystes hydatiques, etc., méconnus par erreur de diagnostic, ne pourraient rester cachés.

À propos de trois cas personnels de suture du cœur

Par M. FRANCISCO GENTIL, Lisbonne.

J'ai eu l'occasion d'intervenir dans trois cas de blessure du cœur, un desquels me semble doublement intéressant par le siège excessivement rare de la lésion du myocarde et parce que la guérison s'est maintenue, il y a aujourd'hui presque trois ans, permettant à mon opéré de continuer sa profession de camionneur, profession qui parfois oblige à des efforts très grands. Il y a un léger degré de symphyse cardio-péricardique, ce qui n'empêche pas le bon fonctionnement du cœur.

Mon premier opéré, chez lequel j'ai suivi le procédé de Ninni, en faisant un lambeau thoracique quadrangulaire et à base interne, était un homme âgé de 51 ans, qui avait été blessé dix heures avant l'intervention. La blessure intéressait le ventricule gauche et avait quinze millimètres de longueur. Le blessé, profondément affaibli, présentait de l'hémopneumothorax gauche quand je l'ai opéré. Malgré l'intervention et le traitement je n'ai réussi qu'à lui conserver la vie pendant dix-sept heures. A l'autopsie j'ai constaté que la blessure du myocarde, à la paroi interne du ventricule, avait un centimètre de longueur et que le pilier antérieur avait été coupé net aux insertions pariétales. La suture était parfaite.

Chez mon second opéré, la blessure du myocarde était à l'oreillette droite. Les blessures des oreillettes sont très rares, et il est encore plus rare que l'intervention soit suivie de *guérison*, ainsi qu'il est arrivé pour mon malade. Il s'agissait d'un homme de vingt-huit ans, extraordinairement robuste, qui avait été blessé cinq heures avant. La blessure de l'oreillette avait un centimètre de longueur et l'hémopéricarde était abondant. La plèvre était légèrement entamée et on ne voyait pas de pneumothorax.

Le troisième opéré, au contraire, était excessivement faible. Homme de vingt ans, ayant subi une infection syphilitique il y avait 18 mois; il présentait des manifestations cutanées secondaires et souffrait aussi de tuberculose pulmonaire. Chez celui-ci, il s'agissait d'une blessure du ventricule droit avec hémopéricarde intense, pneumothorax gauche total et abondant hémothorax. J'ai opéré selon la technique de Fontan et le blessé a vécu 5 jours, puis il est mort d'une péricardite et des lésions pulmonaires tuberculeuses.

Les trois observations que je viens de résumer ont été décrites avec tout le développement possible dans un livre sur la chirurgie du cœur que j'ai publié en février 1905 (*Feridas do coração. Cardiorraphia*). D'après elles et les expériences auxquelles j'ai procédé, j'arrive à la conclusion suivante, au sujet de la technique de la cardiorraphie. Parmi les procédés de thoracotomie, applicables aux cas de blessure du cœur, je donne la préférence à celui de Wehr, d'après lequel on relève le sternum, dans sa portion comprise entre les 2e et 5e espaces intercostaux, en faisant charnière avec ce lambeau aux articulations chondro-costales droites. C'est une méthode qui permet d'atteindre le cœur de la façon la plus ample et directe et la cardiorraphie peut être faite avec le minimum de manipulations du myocarde; elle épargne les vaisseaux mammaires et l'ouverture de la plèvre. Elle permet aussi de soigner les blessures de la face postérieure du cœur et des lésions des autres organes du médiastin. Elle a, cependant, l'inconvénient de ne pas laisser facilement soigner le poumon et la plèvre. Dans mon travail publié en 1905, j'ai proposé de faire, dans ce cas, une incision dans le 5e espace intercostal gauche atteignant la ligne axillaire antérieure.

L'examen des espaces intercostaux et les expériences faites sur des cadavres montrèrent la grande ouverture que l'on peut obtenir en séparant la 5e d'avec la 6e côte, surtout si l'on a préalablement coupé le 5e cartilage gauche. C'est mon procédé de thoracotomie exploratrice dans les cas de blessure du thorax.

Spangaro, de Padoue, a tout dernièrement publié, dans le journal *La clinica chirurgica* du 31 mars 1906, un nouveau procédé de thoracotomie pour l'intervention dans les blessures du cœur, qui se résume à une incision du 5e espace tout à fait pareille à celle que j'ai proposée l'année dernière dans le traitement des complications pulmonaires et pour l'exploration.

Ce procédé, tel que Spangaro le propose et avant la thoracotomie de Wehr, a de réels avantages dans les cas de pneumothorax, car il est exceptionnellement simple et permet de traiter très aisément les blessures cardiaques les plus fréquentes, celles du ventricule gauche. Au cas où il n'y a pas de lésions pleuro-pulmonaires, je préfère le procédé de Wehr. Il est, cependant, si rare que le pneumothorax ne se produise pas, que la technique que j'ai proposée avant Spangaro a toutes les chances de se généraliser. Elle est facile, rapide et constitue un moyen de confirmer le diagnostic. On pourra lui associer, au besoin, un des procédés, n'importe lequel, de Lastasia, Ninni, ou Fontan, comme le propose Spangaro, ou celui de Wehr que je trouve préférable.

Un autre point important de la technique se trouve être celui du drainage du péricarde que l'on est presque toujours obligé de faire et qui, à mon sens, ainsi que je l'ai écrit en 1905, doit être fait indépendamment de la blessure opératoire en vue de la cardiorrhaphie. Je pense que l'on doit plutôt suivre la technique de Larrey et faire le drainage par péricardiotomie épigastrique. Je passe sous silence d'autres points de technique que j'ai étudiés dans tous leurs détails dans mon livre sur les sutures du cœur; je ne voudrais non plus trop allonger ma communication.

DISCUSSION

M. NAPALKOW. Le procédé de Wehr est le meilleur des procédés de résection temporaire du thorax pour la suture cardiaque. Mais il faut prendre en lambeau la 3e côte pour ouvrir les parties supérieures du cœur. Le diagnostic des lésions du cœur n'étant pas précis, c'est indispensable. En bas, il ne faut pas aller jusqu'au processus xiphoïdien pour conserver les adhérences du diaphragme et éviter ainsi l'ouverture de la cavité abdominale.

M. GENTIL. J'insiste pourtant sur ce point que l'incision du 5e espace, avec mobilisation du 5e cartilage costal moyennant sa coupe, ménage une large ouverture permettant de traiter la plupart des cas de blessures du myocarde. Comme, en général, le pneumothorax gauche se produit, cette incision n'a point d'inconvénients; bien au contraire, elle a l'avantage d'être simple et de permettre en outre la reconstitution facile de la paroi costale. On peut donc y avoir recours aux cas de diagnostic douteux dans un but d'exploration.

S'il n'existe pas de pneumothorax ou si, une fois produit, le traitement des lésions cardiaques devient impossible par la seule incision du 5e espace, alors je préfère la méthode de Wehr, car avec celle de Fontan le décollement de la plèvre est morose et difficile; en général, celle-ci se déchire, ce qui n'arrive pas pour la technique de Wehr, telle que je l'ai décrite dans mon travail en 1905.

(Après-midi)

Les anastomoses gastro-intestinales et intestino-intestinales

Par MM. Henri Hartmann, Paris (v. pag. 200),
Augusto de Vasconcellos, Lisbonne (v. page 227)
et H. Schloffer, Innsbruck (v. page 249)

DISCUSSION

M. Tillmann: Vortragender glaubt, dass man die Gastroenterostomie anterior ohne Enteroanastomose nicht verwerfen solle. Er empfiehlt eine Methode die darin besteht, dass er die zuführende Schlinge in grosser Länge an den Magen näht, wodurch der Circulus vitiosus vermieden wird, da bei jeder Magencontraction der Magen sich zusammenzieht und damit diese zuführende Schlinge mit hebt.

M. Kolbé: Il est bien établi aujourd'hui que le procédé Roux-Woelffer de G. E. est le meilleur et qu'il est le représentant de l'application de l'anatomie et de la physiologie la plus rapprochée de l'état normal.

Mais Roux même est éclectique; il fait toutes sortes de G. E. d'après l'indication spéciale du cas. Si le temps semble trop long pour le procédé de Roux, on peut, ce que Roux faisait quelquefois, faire la jéjuno-jéjunostomie avec un petit bouton, dont une moitié est glissée immédiatement dans l'anse ascendante après la section de l'intestin et avant la suture gastro-intestinale latéro-terminale. Au Paquelin on ouvre l'anse descendante et le bouton apparaît pour l'anastomose rapidement. Le circulus vitiosus est plus facile dans G. E. ant., mais aussi dans la G. E. postér. La bile aussi est un inconvénient dans l'estomac. Donc, G. E en Y est la meilleure quand elle est possible. Le rétrécissement est évité par la section oblique de la bouche intestinale, mais il y a dans le cancer, il peut y avoir une sténose du nouveau pylore et dans ma monographie (Kolbé. *Le Cancer de l'estomac et son traitement chirurgical*, 1901) je cite des cas avec trois opérations successives.

Le bouton Murphy est abandonné aujourd'hui tout à fait par Roux et Kocher.

M. Bakes: Die Technik der Gastroenterostomie ist derart ausgebildet, dass die Frage als erledigt betrachtet werden kann. Die hintere Gastroenterostomie mit kürzester Schlinge ist die Methode der Wahl, bei vorderer Gastroenterostomie ist die Suspension nach Kappeler, besser aber die Braun'sche Enteroanastomose anzuschliessen; kurz, der Circulus vitiosus ist lediglich auf technische Fehler zurückzuführen. Der springende Punkt der Technik scheint mir aber das zu sein, dass wir gelernt haben die allgemeine Narkose bei der Gastroenterostomie auszuschliessen, sodass die Kranken den Eingriff ohne Alteration ihrer Kräfte, ohne Erbrechen, etc. überstehen.

M. Doyen. — Je pratique exclusivement l'anastomose latérale par le procédé des sutures.

Le procédé des sutures est très supérieur à l'emploi des boutons anastomotiques pour deux motifs principaux:

1° La gastro-entérostomie par le procédé des sutures peut être faite avec une asepsie rigoureuse, tandis que l'introduction des pièces gastrique et intestinale des boutons anastomotiques, quels qu'ils soient, nécessite des manœuvres au cours desquelles le contenu de l'estomac ou du jéjunum risque de contaminer le champ opératoire.

2° Le procédé des sutures donne seul une coaptation exacte et sûre des parois gastro-intestinales et cette proposition est tellement vraie que les partisans des boutons anastomotiques considèrent comme indispensable d'assurer par des sutures la coaptation des séreuses gastrique et intestinale.

L'opération, par la méthode des sutures, ne dure que dix à quinze minutes de plus que l'application d'un bouton anastomotique.

Il y a donc un avantage indiscutable, puisque la sécurité est plus grande, à employer le procédé des sutures. Je fais trois plans séro-séreux postérieurs dont le dernier pénètre jusqu'à la muqueuse. Il s'agit alors de placer les pinces à mors élastiques que j'ai fait construire par M. Collin en 1894, et qui serront à former le calibre de l'estomac et de l'intestin. Deux pinces sont appliquées du côté de l'estomac, deux autres du côté de l'intestin. Ces pinces doivent être légèrement recourbées, de manière à pouvoir être appliquées sans gêner le champ opératoire.

L'estomac et l'intestin sont incisés parallèlement à 3 millimètres du troisième plan de suture, sur une longueur de 30 millimètres, et les lèvres antérieures de ces deux orifices sont réunies par un surjet séro-séreux profond. Ce surjet est effectué avec le même fil que le troisième plan postérieur, dont le chef terminal après la confection de la suture annulaire, est noué au chef initial. Les quatre pinces élastiques sont enlevées et l'on effectue les deux derniers plans antérieurs, dont les chefs initial et terminal sont noués aux chefs terminal et initial des deux plans postérieurs correspondants.

Je préfère trois plans de suture à deux, le plan circulaire qui borde l'orifice étant obligatoirement infecté.

L'orifice fonctionne bien lorsqu'on a su l'établir en un point déclive et où il n'existe pas de tiraillements.

La technique générale de l'opération étant déterminée, quel est le lieu d'élection des anastomoses gastro-intestinales ?

1° Gastro-duodénostomie avec section du pylore

Si la région pylorique de l'estomac et la première portion du duodénum sont très mobiles et qu'il s'agisse d'une contracture spasmodique ancienne du pylore ou d'une petite cicatrice pylorique, je pratique l'anastomose gastro-duodénale, avec section transversale du pylore, confection de deux plans séro-séreux postérieurs, verticaux, sous-pyloriques, application des pinces élastiques. Section verticale de l'estomac et du duodénum et section transversale du pylore ; plan muco-muqueux postérieur, qui se continuera en avant par un plan séro-séreux profond ; ablation des pinces et confection de deux surjets séro-séreux superficiels.

Cette opération est la meilleure quand elle est praticable, car elle rétablit le fonctionnement normal de l'estomac.

2° Gastro-entérostomie postérieure trans-méso-colique

Quand le pylore est très altéré ou bien adhérent, il faut pratiquer l'orifice gastrique, près de la grande courbure, au voisinage de la ligne médiane. Si la face postérieure de l'estomac et le méso-côlon transverse sont sains, le procédé de choix est l'anastomose trans-méso-colique. Le méso-côlon est perforé au centre de la grande arcade vasculaire et les bords de la perforation sont fixés à la face postérieure de l'estomac, sur une circonférence de six à huit centimètres de diamètre. L'anastomose gastro-jéjunale est pratiquée obliquement sur l'estomac et le jéjunum, tout près du ligament de Treitz, par la méthode des trois plans de suture.

3° *Gastro-entérostomie antérieure*

La gastro-entérostomie antérieure n'est indiquée que dans les cas où la gastro-entérostomie postérieure est impraticable. Il faut alors commencer par enfermer le grand épiploon, comme je l'ai recommandé depuis 1892, dans l'arrière-cavité de Winslow, par une perforation de l'épiploon gastro-colique, et fixer le côlon transverse à la grande courbure de l'estomac. On fait alors la gastro-entérostomie antérieure en prenant soin de laisser en avant de l'orifice une anse jéjunale assez longue pour la fixer à la face antérieure de l'estomac, à peu près verticalement, au-dessus du nouveau pylore. Cet artifice est indispensable pour éviter le reflux du contenu de l'estomac vers le duodénum.

On voit que je repousse absolument l'implantation termino-latérale, qui est plus longue à exécuter que l'anastomose latérale et expose davantage à l'infection du champ opératoire, puisque le calibre de l'intestin demeure ouvert beaucoup plus longtemps et dans des conditions beaucoup plus défavorables dans la première que dans la seconde.

4° *Pylorectomie avec gastro-entérostomie*

Il résulte de ce qui précède que je pratique exclusivement, lorsqu'il y a lieu de réséquer le pylore, la fermeture en cul-de-sac du duodénum et de l'estomac par mon procédé de ligature en masse après écrasement et de double suture en cordon de bourse.

Il faut prendre soin de faire cette suture, du côté de l'estomac, avec un fil de soie assez fort et pénétrant profondément dans la musculeuse. On pratique ensuite une gastro-jéjunostomie latérale. L'opération complète peut être terminée en cinquante à soixante minutes.

M. VASCONCELLOS fait remarquer que les orateurs précédents n'ont presque fait que défendre les conclusions de son rapport. Sur la gastro-entérostomie il s'en tient au von Hacker, parce qu'il le considère aussi efficace que le procédé en Y et beaucoup plus facile.

SÉANCE DU 25 DE AVRIL

Présidence: M. OLIVEIRA FEIJÃO

Chondromes multiples des mains

Par M. CIFUENTES DIAZ, Madrid.

Le cas sur lequel est basée la communication que j'ai l'honneur de présenter au Congrès se rapporte à un garçon de onze ans, fils de parents bien constitués et dont l'histoire n'indique que trois accès d'éclampsie aux premiers mois de sa vie.

Quand il n'avait que quatre mois apparurent les tumeurs dans la main gauche en commençant par la première phalange du doigt du milieu et continuèrent à se montrer successivement dans d'autres endroits de la même main aussi bien qu'à la main droite. Au moment de sa présentation, elles constituaient des élévations de la grandeur d'une lentille et quelques-unes plus petites encore, dures et indolentes; d'autres se montrèrent, par un grossissement partiel de la phalange, également indolentes, dures et sans empêcher les mouvements des doigts.

De cette manière, évoluant avec une grande lenteur, ce malade parvint, dans le cours des années, à présenter toutes les tumeurs que l'on pourra voir dans les figures ci-jointes, sans lui causer d'autres troubles que ceux du poids et du volume, spécialement dans la main gauche.

Il y a dix-huit mois, il a reçu un coup de pied à la main gauche, qui a produit une contusion dans la partie la plus remarquable de la tumeur située sur la

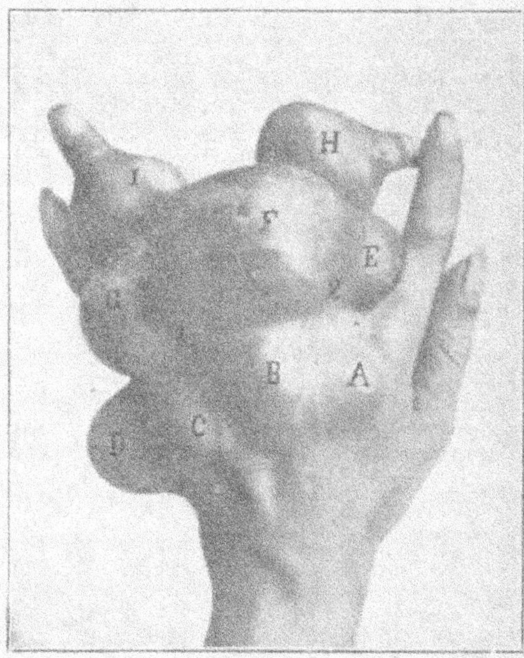

Fig. 1

première phalange du doigt moyen; depuis lors l'accroissement des tumeurs de cette main et surtout de la phalange indiquée a été plus rapide jusqu'à acquérir la grandeur qu'elle présentait au mois de mars, date où le garçon est entré à l'Hôpital de la Princesse.

La distribution des tumeurs est la suivante:

Main gauche: Un chondrome dans chacun des métacarpiens deuxième, troisième, quatrième et cinquième, faisant proéminence dans la partie dorsale, occupant la moitié inférieure de l'os (fig. 1 — A, B, C, D); les plus grands sont ceux qui sont situés dans le troisième métacarpien, lesquels sont aussi remarquables dans leur partie palmaire.

Doigt du milieu: Deux tumeurs dans la première phalange dont l'une occupe la portion dorsale, étant la plus grande de toutes; l'autre plus petite occupe sa portion externe et palmaire (fig. 1 — E, F). Une, de la grosseur d'une noix, située dans la seconde phalange. La troisième phalange se trouve libre.

Doigt annulaire: Dans la première et deuxième phalange, un chondrome dans chacune d'elles, de la dimension de l'antérieur, en faisant proéminence tout autour d'elles (fig. 1 — G, I). La troisième, libre aussi.

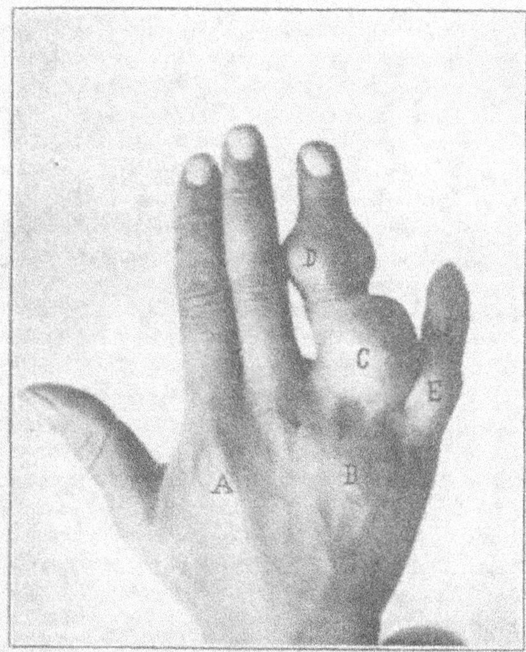

Fig. 2

Petit doigt: Une tumeur située dans la première phalange, de la grosseur d'une noisette, plus grosse dans sa face palmaire; une autre dans la seconde, d'accroissement nouveau, se remarquant bien le grossissement uniforme du corps de la phalange.

Les doigts pouce et index manquent de tumeurs.

Main droite: Une tumeur dans le second métacarpien occupant sa moitié inférieure, remarquable par sa face dorsale et grosse comme une noisette (fig. 2 — A); une autre située dans la quatrième, ayant les mêmes caractères (fig. 2 — B). Les doigts pouce, index et du milieu manquent de tumeurs. Doigt annulaire: Une dans la première phalange et une autre dans la seconde, la première plus grosse, du

volume d'une noix, et toutes deux avec accroissement vers la région dorsale et les
parties latérales. Dans le petit doigt, il y a deux autres tumeurs qui se rapportent
aux deux premières phalanges, plus petites et avec proéminence dorsale ; les troisièmes phalanges de ces doigts ne sont pas atteintes de tumeurs.

Du précédent rapport et par l'examen des photographies qui
l'accompagnent on peut voir que toutes ces tumeurs ont leur place
dans les métacarpiens et première et deuxième phalanges, parties
prédisposées au développement de chondromes, dont, d'après Virchow, l'échelle de fréquence va de la périphérie vers le centre,
de telle sorte que les phalanges des mains sont les parties les plus
facilement atteintes ; dans celles-ci, d'après Polaillon, elles se montrent plus souvent que dans les métacarpiens. Il se peut que les
chondromes n'affectent pas les troisièmes phalanges, comme dans
ce cas, fait déjà remarqué par d'autres auteurs : les lieux de préférence ce sont les deux premières phalanges. Mon maître, le dr.
Ribera, cite un cas de chondromes des mains dont tous les doigts
présentaient des tumeurs [1].

C'est dans la main que s'observent d'abord les cas de chondromes multiples, rarement aux doigts seuls ; au contraire, d'après
Weber, sur 103 cas de chondromes de la main, dans 77 la lésion était
multiple, et sur 92 cas de Polaillon, 57 étaient multiples et 35 de
tumeurs uniques. La présence de chondromes multiples dans les
deux mains est plus rare encore et il existe peu de cas publiés,
parmi eux quelques-uns cités par Polaillon [2] d'après Poulet et
Bousquet. Dans le cas présenté, le pouce et l'index des deux mains
ne sont pas affectés, circonstance digne de remarque, car les auteurs estiment le pouce avec une certaine immunité de même que
l'auriculaire. Dans notre cas, celui-ci est affecté dans les deux mains.

Les auteurs sont d'accord qu'il existe un rapport entre le développement de ces chondromes et le processus d'ossification ; voilà
pourquoi ils apparaissent quelquefois dans les premières années
de la vie, quand en vertu de l'activité cellulaire dans la période
de la constitution de l'os les îlots cartilagineux, qui restèrent comme
oubliés dans le sein du tissu osseux par une ossification que Virchow appelle irrégulière, entrent aussi en activité, prolifèrent, et
cette prolifération hétérotopique est le premier pas vers le processus chondromateux.

---

[1] Ribera, Éléments de pathologie chirurgicale général. Madrid, 1890.
[2] Poulet et Bousquet. Traité de pathologie externe.

Les articulations métacarpo-phalangiennes et phalangiennes en sont libres. Les chondromes ne se produisent jamais dans les cartilages préexistants, mais dans des terrains non cartilagineux; ils sont ainsi une production hétérologue; tandis que, si le cartilage donne lieu à une hyperplasie, celle-ci sera homologue et formera les appelés ecchondroses.

Nous admettons l'origine des chondromes dans la prolifération d'îlots de cartilage qui persistent dans le sein du tissu osseux dès la date du processus d'ossification (Virchow) ou bien dans la prolifération de cellules embryonnaires persistant dans les tissus jusqu'à l'âge adulte (Cohnheim). Par là s'établit le caractère hétérotopique de ces tumeurs.

Pour cette raison, les tumeurs n'affectant que les os, les mouvements articulaires sont possibles. Si dans quelques articulations ils sont diminués ou annulés cela est dû au volume et poids des tumeurs qui mécaniquement empêchent les mouvements, ce qui arrive à la main gauche de notre cas, dans laquelle les mouvements des trois derniers doigts sont presque annulés par le développement que les tumeurs les plus centrales ont acquis; outre cet accroissement de volume, il y a empêchement au bon fonctionnement des tendons fléchisseurs et extenseurs. Mais malgré cette immobilité l'indemnité des articulations peut se confirmer en provoquant des mouvements passifs, qui, quoique limités, sont appréciables et ne manifestent aucun signe de lésion articulaire.

Toutes les tumeurs sont plus ou moins sphériques, dures, élastiques, de plus grande consistance quand elles sont plus petites, fixées et immobiles sur l'os où elles s'implantent; celles de plus grand volume (main gauche) présentent une consistance plus molle et légèrement fluctuante, notamment dans celle qui reçut le traumatisme; celle-ci présente des caractères de fluctuation et est plus molle que les autres, quoique la fluctuation se remarque aussi dans d'autres de la même main. Le traumatisme que cette main souffrit a été une stimulation pour l'accroissement plus rapide de la tumeur.

Elles ne produisent pas de douleurs spontanées, pas même à la pression.

La peau est normale sur la plupart; sur celles de plus grand volume elle est distendue, de couleur rougeâtre foncée, avec quelques ramifications veineuses dilatées et glissant sur elles-mêmes.

La face dorsale de la tumeur qui souffrit le traumatisme déjà mentionné présente deux ulcérations d'un centimètre de diamètre, couvertes de croûtes. Celle qui est plus proche du bord cubital de la main exsude un liquide épais sanguinolent et présente un trajet fistuleux reconnaissable avec le stylet qui pénètre vers le centre de la tumeur; il appartient donc aux *ulcères chondromateux fistulaires*. Nous pouvons expliquer l'existence de ces ulcérations par l'action traumatique; la plaie contuse n'a pu se cicatriser à cause de la distension de la peau, toujours augmentée par la croissance de la tumeur; c'est une des manières d'ulcération des tumeurs qui s'ulcèrent ou bien parce que la peau est envahie par la néoplasie (tumeurs malignes), ou bien par un effet purement mécanique. La tumeur qui est adossée au doigt index de la main gauche présente un autre ulcère dans la surface de contact avec ce doigt, qui est dû aussi à l'effet mécanique de la compression et distension de la peau par le développement du néoplasme. Une des ulcérations plus haut mentionnées produisit, il y a deux mois, une abondante hémorrhage occasionnée par le détachement de la croûte qui la couvrait et la rupture d'une veine sous-cutanée, qui a pu être arrêtée par la compression.

Dans ces chondromes, peuvent se produire aussi ce que Gluge appelle des ulcères enchondromateux fistuleux, comme celui que nous avons mentionné, et dont Virchow explique la pathogénie de cette manière: Quand ces chondromes se ramollissent pour souffrir une dégénération granulo-adipeuse ou myxomateuse, le vrai ramollissement se produit dans la substance intercellulaire qui se transforme d'abord en un liquide épais, plus ténu après, contenant de la mucine; il arrive souvent qu'à ce liquide se joint le sang venant de la rupture des artères de la paroi, lui donnant par sa transformation en pigment une coloration rougeâtre ou jaunâtre. Eh bien, ces collections liquides peuvent s'ouvrir à l'extérieur donnant lieu à une ulcération fistulaire, ou bien elles sont ouvertes par le progrès de l'ulcération mécanique ou même par le histouri.

De l'observation comparée des deux-mains on peut remarquer que les portions terminales des doigts 3e, 4e et 5e de la main gauche n'ont pas la grandeur qu'elles devraient avoir d'après l'âge du malade et sont plus petites que les portions analogues de la main droite. C'est un degré d'atrophie par manque de fonction, explicable par la présence des tumeurs pendant le temps du développement de l'enfant, empêchant les parties saines d'acquérir leurs dimensions normales à cause de l'absence de mouvements.

En cherchant l'indication opératoire que le cas demande, on pense à l'ablation de ces tumeurs par l'amputation, puisque la résection est seulement possible dans les chondromes uniques. L'intervention s'imposait notamment à la main gauche à cause du développement qu'elles tumeurs y avaient acquis et de l'impossibilité des mouvements qu'elles produisaient.

En vue du lent accroissement de ces tumeurs, le traitement a commencé par la main gauche, la seule qui jusqu'ici soit tout à fait inutilisée.

L'opération a été une désarticulation des quatre derniers métacarpiens par le procédé elliptique à lambeau palmaire; c'était le traitement d'élection vu que les métacarpiens étaient affectés et qu'il fallait une opération radicale; ainsi que le disait Virchow, nous ne devons plus penser que l'enchondrome soit une tumeur tout à fait bénigne; il y a des cas de généralisation de chondromes mixtes (chondro-myxomes, chondro-sarcomes), etc., etc.

L'examen attentif des doigts amputés permit de faire l'étude anatomo-pathologique des tumeurs. Toutes présentent une configuration plus ou moins sphérique, sont implantées dans la diaphyse, occupant les régions palmaire et dorsale des métacarpiens. Dans le cinquième métacarpien la tumeur fait proéminence vers le bord cubital, ce qui doit être, vu qu'il n'y a pas un autre métacarpien pour en empêcher l'accroissement des tumeurs en dehors.

Les tumeurs présentent une couleur blanc-rosé avec de petites taches rougeâtres, dans quelques endroits elles offrent un aspect lobulé.

Est curieuse la modification soufferte par les diaphyses des os, surtout sur les os où la tumeur n'occupe pas toute la circonférence et se rapportant à la forme et à la direction de la diaphyse; le troisième et le quatrième métacarpien sont ceux qui offrent plus d'intérêt à cet égard. La conformation prismatique triangulaire du corps a disparu et il n'en reste d'autre vestige que le bord antérieur du quatrième métacarpien; elle est à présent cylindrique. En outre, le 4e métacarpien présente une courbure exagérée, concave en avant, fort remarquable parce que la tumeur est sur la face dorsale. Le troisième métacarpien présente deux proéminences, l'une dorsale et l'autre palmaire, entre lesquelles se trouve une zone formée par les bords latéraux de l'os non affectés, quoique grossis par l'accroissement externe du chondrome. En outre le corps de l'os se présente comme s'il avait souffert une torsion, l'extrémité antérieure en rotation externe. Tous les métacarpiens présentent des incurvations latérales comme si l'accroissement des tumeurs les eût repoussées les uns contres les autres. La deuxième et troisième phalanges du doigt moyen sont fortement inclinées vers le doigt index, formant avec celui-ci un angle droit.

La section des tumeurs est nette, régulière; elles ne résistent pas à la coupe, sauf pour celles qui sont revêtues d'une coque osseuse, en général très mince. Ce sont les tumeurs que Müller appela *chondrome avec coque osseuse* (1): la couche osseuse dépend de la grosseur de la tumeur, car, quand le développement du néoplasme commence par l'intérieur de l'os, le périoste forme extérieurement de nouvelles couches osseuses continuellement amincies par l'accroissement de la tumeur jusqu'à la totale disparition. Pour la plupart des tumeurs l'enveloppe est fibreuse, une véritable capsule formée par le périoste distendu; sa couleur est blanche, avec des reflets opalins, jaunâtres et roses dans d'autres endroits. Ça et là on voit de petites taches rouge-vineuses étoilées, de consistance osseuse, formées par des îlots de tissu osseux, d'autant plus rapprochées que le volume de la tumeur est plus petit. Dans quelques unes la coloration est à zones plus obscures; là aussi abondent les îlots osseux, et de petites lacunes jaunâtres constituées par du tissu adipeux.

Ces néoplasmes ne sont pas formés par une masse unique, car en leur section on peut voir surtout avec l'aide d'une loupe qu'ils sont formés de lobes séparés par un fin et délicat réseau. Cette lobulation des chondromes est due, d'après Virchow, à ce que ces tumeurs ne proviennent pas d'un seul foyer augmentant excentriquement, mais que leur accroissement dépend de nouveaux foyers toujours en formation. Dans le réseau interlobaire on voit les îlots osseux.

La consistance est d'autant plus molle que la tumeur est plus grande et entre la consistance dure et élastique, que présentent les plus petites, à la molle qu'offrent les plus développées, il y a plusieurs degrés.

On peut arriver à une telle mollesse que la tumeur se laisse écraser entre les doigts; c'est la consistance qui domine dans les tumeurs de notre malade.

Il est bien difficile de déterminer quel a été le point de départ de ces chondromes, l'os ou le périoste; c'est cette origine qui justifia leur division en médul-

---

(1) Joh. Müller. Ueber den feineren Bau der Geschwülste.

laires et périostiques (Cooper), centraux et périphériques (Vogel). D'après Virchow,
les chondromes des os de la main viennent rarement du périoste. Dans notre cas,
où quelques-unes des tumeurs font relief sur une seule face de l'os et ont res-
pecté une grande partie du tissu osseux de la diaphyse, l'origine est probablement
le périoste.

Les tumeurs que nous étudions n'envahissent pas le cartilage de conjonction
et les épiphyses; pour cette cause les articulations sont indemnes, leur fonction
est seulement diminuée ou annulée à cause de l'obstacle mécanique opposé par les
chondromes. Les tendons sont écartés de leur direction et situation, notamment
les extenseurs; tant que la tumeur est petite, le tendon suit sa direction normale
en passant par le point le plus élevé de la tumeur, mais lorsqu'elle s'accroît il
est dévié latéralement. Les muscles interosseux se trouvent tant soit peu atrophiés et en général tout l'avant bras gauche est plus mince que le droit, atrophié
par défaut de fonctionnement.

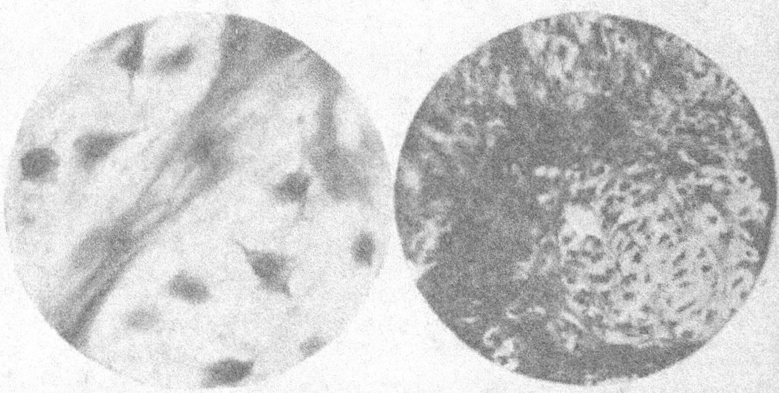

Fig. 3

L'examen microscopique des néoplasmes, fait au Laboratoire de l'École de
Médecine par mon collègue le dr. Tejta y Muñoz, démontre que leur structure est
celle du chondrome myxomateux. Auprès des éléments de cartilage hyalin très
abondant, on voit des cellules ramifiées rappelant la structure du cartilage des
céphalopodes. Le tissu myxomateux entre en partie dans la composition de la tumeur et en quelques points on voit aussi des îlots de tissu osseux. L'existence de
trabécules et îlots osseux dans les tumeurs permettrait de les qualifier de chondromes ossifiants dans lesquels le tissu osseux formé aux dépens du cartilage a une
existence transitoire et peut se transformer en tissu adipeux. Cette ossification
dépend du tissu cartilagineux, puisque dans les préparations microscopiques on
voit que les cellules de cartilage hyalin sont dans quelques endroits ordonnées en
séries comme il arrive au commencement de l'ossification normale. Les néoplasmes
dans leur commencement furent seulement des chondromes, après quoi ils éprou-
vèrent une transformation myxomateuse, laquelle prête à ces tumeurs un cara-

ctère de malignité évident; en effet les chondro-myxomes peuvent se généraliser produisant des noyaux métastatiques dans les poumons, plèvre, foie, etc., etc., ainsi que le démontrent les cas publiés par Volkmann, Weber et Müller, où la mort survint par généralisation.

Ce caractère myxomateux des chondromes doit constituer une indication remarquable pour la prompte intervention et leur ablation complète.

CONCLUSIONS

1° Bien que les chondromes se présentent avec quelque fréquence dans les os de la main, cette fréquence n'est pas la même au point de vue de leur extension sur tous les os de la main; les cas de ce genre sont peu nombreux. Leur apparition dans les deux mains est très rare.

2° La forme de ces tumeurs est toujours plus ou moins arrondie, plus ou moins modifiée par leur adossement réciproque, conséquence de leur continu, quoique lent, accroissement. Cette déformation est surtout observée sur la face dorsale et palmaire des métacarpiens, et tout autour des phalanges. La diaphyse de l'os est déformée.

3° Le développement de ces tumeurs laisse d'ordinaire libre le pouce et les troisièmes phalanges de tous les doigts; le siège de prédilection ce sont les métacarpiens et les premières phalanges.

4° Elles n'envahissent pas les épiphyses et le cartilage de conjonction, mais en altèrent la forme et la direction; cette altération est plus remarquable sur les faces articulaires, d'où il résulte non seulement la difficulté des mouvements, mais aussi une déviation en angle des os qui forment l'articulation, laquelle en constitue le sommet.

5° L'accroissement de ces chondromes peut s'activer quand ils éprouvent un traumatisme; ce traumatisme, si la tumeur est grande et si la peau qui la couvre se trouve fort distendue, joue un rôle important dans la pathogénie de l'ulcération.

6° Il est bien difficile de déterminer si l'origine de ces tumeurs a eu lieu dans le périoste ou dans le tissu osseux. Cette difficulté est évidente quand la tumeur a envahi toute l'épaisseur de la diaphyse, car dans le commencement de leur développement il est possible d'apprécier si la tumeur est d'origine centrale ou périphérique, sans oublier que dans ce dernier cas elle peut avoir son origine dans le périoste ou dans la couche la plus corticale de l'os.

7° Les troubles que les tumeurs produisent dans la main sont d'ordre purement mécanique; le fonctionnement de la main est empêché non seulement à cause du poids des néoplasmes, mais aussi parce que les mouvements articulaires sont limités et quelques tendons sont déviés.

8° La dégénération myxomateuse que les tumeurs peuvent souffrir leur donne un caractère de malignité qui aggrave le pronostic, car l'association du chondrome et du myxome produit facilement sa généralisation. Dans les cas de cette nature, l'ablation complète des tumeurs par amputation ou désarticulation s'impose; la resection doit être réservée pour les petits chondromes pas très nombreux. Nous tâcherons de la faire sur la main droite du malade.

Diagnostic opportun du cancer du sein; ses rapports avec l'intervention chirurgicale

Par M. DANIEL DE MATTOS, Coïmbre.

Par diagnostic opportun du carcinome du sein, j'entends le diagnostic précoce; cette désignation me paraît utile pour signifier combien le diagnostic fait à temps influe sur le succès opératoire et intéresse la survie des malades, car l'opportunité de l'intervention chirurgicale permet des résultats auxquels on n'est pas encore arrivé par d'autres moyens.

Il en est du carcinome du sein de même que de la tuberculose pulmonaire. Dans celle-ci le diagnostic opportun, indispensable à l'établissement d'un régime hygiénico-diététique — qui garantisse avec probabilité la guérison dans un temps relativement court — est quelquefois plein d'hésitations et de difficultés; tandis que ce diagnostic est facile, par suite de la netteté des symptômes et de leur synergie physiologique, pendant la période où la maladie est arrivée à produire l'ulcération pulmonaire.

Au début, dans le cancer du sein et même quelques mois après, le diagnostic est également difficile, délicat et hésitant; il est au contraire très facile quand, par sa marche rapide, son adhérence à la peau, les fréquentes douleurs lancinantes, l'engorgement ganglionnaire et lymphatique et plus tard l'ulcération, tous les doutes disparaissent, et cela quand l'exacte opportunité de l'intervention est perdue.

Et de même que dans la tuberculose où la guérison est le résultat fréquent de la thérapeutique hygiénico-diététique, guérison qui même si elle n'est pas définitive dans quelques cas est au moins économique dans beaucoup; de même aussi dans le cancer la thérapeutique chirurgicale opportune amène la guérison ou la prolongation de la vie pendant quelques années.

Si nous comparons la marche des deux maladies et leur évolution anatomo-pathologique, nous devons conclure que dans le cancer le diagnostic précoce est encore plus urgent, car généralement sa marche est plus rapide que celle de la tuberculose.

Sur quels éléments doit-on baser le diagnostic précoce du cancer du sein ?

1° — De même que dans la tuberculose il y a des âges de prédilection, de même pour le cancer il y a un âge où il se manifeste avec une plus grande fréquence; *l'âge des malades à tumeur mammaire* devient donc un élément important pour le diagnostic. En général la femme, qui a un cancer du sein, est plus près de la ménopause que de la puberté, ou alors elle se trouve pendant ou après la ménopause.

2° — *Absence de limitation de la tumeur*, qui se joint et adhère à la glande. Cette fusion de la tumeur avec la glande n'est toutefois pas mise en relief dans quelques publications autorisées; au contraire, elles indiquent même comme caractère la limite précise de la tumeur, et on dit qu'il existe une zone, un peu indécise, qui constitue un contour moins net que celui d'un fibrome, mais que la forme circulaire et la grande régularité de cette zone lui conservent le caractère d'un contour assez accusé.

Cependant, en observant des tumeurs récentes, de quelques mois à peine, en soulevant le sein avec une des mains et en explorant le contour de la tumeur avec l'index de l'autre main, on observe que dans quelques régions du contour la fusion est indécise; mais dans la plus grande partie du contour la fusion entre la tumeur et la glande est intime car le doigt sent nettement des prolongements qui vont de la tumeur à la glande.

3° — *La forme irrégulière* de la tumeur qui, quoique commençant par une nodosité qui occupe de préférence la partie externe et inférieure ou externe et supérieure du sein, est en peu de temps mélangée à d'autres nodosités.

4° — Il en résulte, dans son ensemble, une *superficie bosselée* qui s'accentue de plus en plus à mesure que la tumeur se développe.

5° — La palpation de la tumeur, faite suivant la technique considérée la meilleure, fait reconnaître une *consistance dure*, rigide, dans quelques segments, dans la variété la plus fréquente des cancers.

6° — Contrairement à ce qui arrive avec les tumeurs bénignes, à marche lente, le cancer a une *évolution progressive et rapide*,

si bien que quelques malades rapportent qu'un ou deux mois
après avoir reconnu leur tumeur, elles s'aperçoivent qu'elle a un
volume triple, ce qui est confirmé par de successifs examens cliniques.

7° — A mesure que le cancer se développe, la peau, avant
même d'être soulevée par la tumeur, présente certains caractères
spéciaux — en plus d'autres d'une observation plus facile et plus
courante — que je me permets d'indiquer comme étant d'une importance particulière. Je veux parler de l'examen de la peau super-adjacente à la tumeur, qui, *examinée à la loupe*, révèle de bonne heure des régions, où l'on observe un ton plus clair de la peau,
auquel correspondent des élévations épidermiques qui dessinent
des *lymphangectasies* des vases lymphatiques superficiels, quelquefois allongées, d'autres fois en ampoule.

Ce signe, qui sans un examen minutieux peut passer inaper-
çu, et qui précède l'adhérence de la tumeur à la peau, se rattache sûrement aux perturbations diverses, infectieuses, mécaniques
et dégénératives des lymphatiques profonds.

Il me semble que dans le tableau des symptômes d'une certaine phase de l'évolution du cancer du sein on passe des caractères qui s'obtiennent par la palpation des tumeurs à l'adhérence de la peau, sans donner aux altérations de la couche adipeuse
qui sépare la glande et la peau toute la valeur qu'elles méritent.

Or la couche prémammaire du tissu cellulaire adipeux sous-
cutané, qui manque seulement au niveau de l'auréole et du mamelon, où la peau se trouve directement en contact avec le tissu
glandulaire, est subdivisée en locules par des traînées fibreuses
qui vont de la surface de la glande à la partie profonde de la
peau. D'où il résulte que le processus de la carcinose chemine à
travers les lymphatiques de ces traînées jusqu'aux lymphatiques
profonds de la peau. Et de l'altération des traînées fibreuses et
de la propagation précoce de l'infection jusqu'aux lymphatiques
profonds de la peau il résultera les *lymphangectasies* des lymphatiques superficiels que la loupe permet de surprendre à leur début. Ce tissu cellulaire adipeux, avec le resserrement dû à la prolifération et à l'induration dans les traînées fibreuses inter-mam-
maires, tendra à immobiliser la peau avant qu'il ne s'établisse
une véritable adhérence.

Si nous comparons la *mobilité de la peau* qui correspond à
la partie la plus saillante de la tumeur avec la mobilité de la peau
sur la glande dans la région symétrique du côté opposé, on ob-

serve la *diminution de cette mobilité*. Ces deux signes sont moindres et on peut dire que seule une sensibilité tactile spéciale les
appréciera; mais il est certain qu'ils existent, qu'ils sont précoces

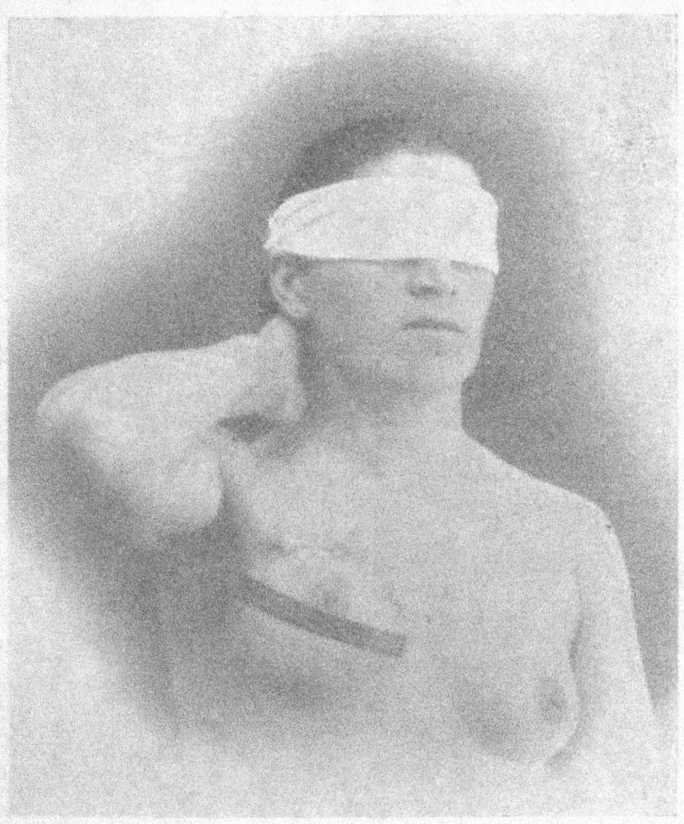

et que le diagnostic précoce d'une maladie quelconque est la réunion des signes moindres qui donnent la plus grande valeur de
probabilité à ce diagnostic.

8° — C'est consécutivement à ces altérations et à mesure
qu'elles avancent qu'on note *l'adhérence à la peau* par degrés divers; le premier se révèle par de petites dépressions entremêlées

de saillances papillaires, qui donnent à la peau l'apparence de
l'épicarpe d'orange plus ou moins fin; la peau quand on plie, en
la prenant entre les doigts, plus tard on observe un plus grand
degré d'adhérence ombilicale et la peau est retenue par des
brides.

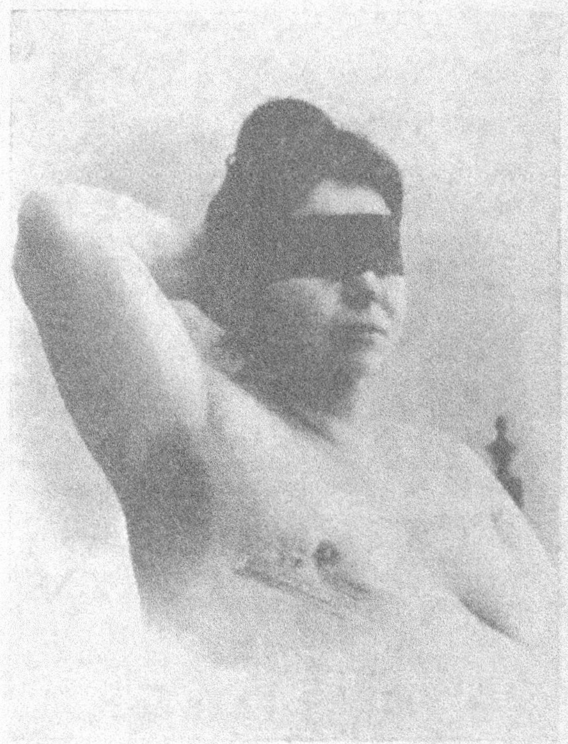

Fig. 1

Liée de très près à l'adhérence de la peau et par un mécanisme semblable, que des conditions anatomiques expliquent et
surtout l'absence de couches de graisse super-adjacente et la ri-
chesse lymphatique du plexus sous-aréolaire et mamillaire de
Sappey, dans lequel viennent également s'épanouir la plupart des
troncs issus de la glande mammaire elle-même, on observe la dé-

pression de l'aréole et la rétraction véritable du mamelon, signe
de grande valeur et qui, bien observé, est considéré par beaucoup
comme symptôme *presque certain* du cancer du sein.

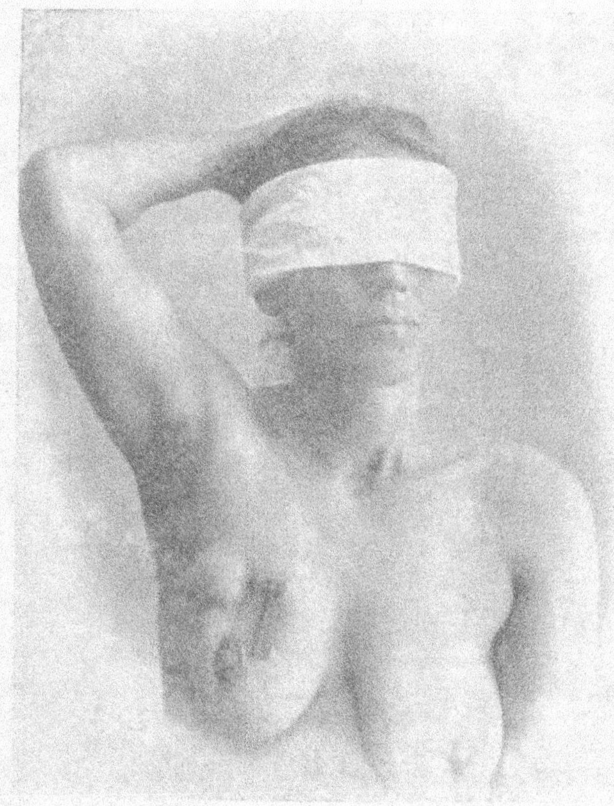

Fig. 3

A mesure que l'adhérence de la tumeur à la peau se développe, il y a une profonde adhérence, dans la région sous-mam-
maire, avec l'aponévrose du grand pectoral et avec le muscle lui-
même et, de là, la diminution de la mobilité du sein jusqu'à son
immobilité définitive.

Dans l'évolution du cancer de la glande mammaire, aussi bien que dans d'autres maladies de cette même glande, l'exploration de *tout le sein* a une importance spéciale et pour cela on doit toujours observer le volume, la forme et la consistance du prolongement axillaire de la glande et ensuite l'état des lymphatiques et des ganglions.

La carcinose du sein et de la peau de la région mammaire se répercute d'une telle manière sur tout le réseau lymphatique que l'exploration de toute l'aisselle doit être toujours faite soigneusement, car l'engorgement des cordons lymphatiques et celui des ganglions de l'aisselle ainsi que les ganglions infra et supraclaviculaires ont une signification diagnostique de grande valeur et sont des indicateurs du pronostic.

Si nous divisons l'évolution du cancer en trois périodes: — période initiale, — période de l'infection localisée aux tissus voisins — et période de l'infection généralisée — nous devons considérer la maladie à sa première période quand il existe seulement des symptômes indiqués jusqu'à ce qu'apparaissent des symptômes d'adhérence superficielle à la peau et de l'adhérence profonde; elle est à la seconde période quand ces adhérences sont nettes et accentuées et augmentent de jour en jour et qu'elles sont accompagnées d'engorgements lymphatiques et ganglionnaires de quelques uns des groupes de ganglions; et enfin nous devons la considérer dans sa troisième période quand l'infection a atteint des groupes plus élevés de ganglions et quand ceux-ci et d'autres symptômes, par leur extension et diffusion, passent par une phase pré-cachéctique à la cachexie qui correspond à la florescence de la période de l'infection généralisée.

Dans cette note, nous n'avons pas l'intention de faire l'énumération des symptômes de la cachexie cancéreuse et parce qu'on affirme encore quelquefois que la cachexie cancéreuse est le seul signe général certain du cancer. Je crois qu'en présence d'une tumeur mammaire, l'observation clinique minutieuse, la diagnose directe basée sur tous les symptômes observés et accompagnée dans sa marche par la diagnose différentielle soigneusement faite, doivent converger vers l'affirmation que le diagnostic du cancer de la glande mammaire peut être fait avec une telle probabilité que, en tenant compte de toutes les données, on arrive à la certitude, et on peut ainsi, au moins au début de la seconde période, faire un diagnostic opportun pour réaliser une intervention chirurgicale, que les statistiques modernes démontrent, dans tous les

pays, comme donnant les meilleurs résultats, aussi bien pour la
guérison définitive que pour la période de survie. Et si une technique chirurgicale plus large et plus complète a contribué à
cette amélioration de manière à éliminer tous les tissus considérés suspects dans des cas d'intense infection des lymphatiques et

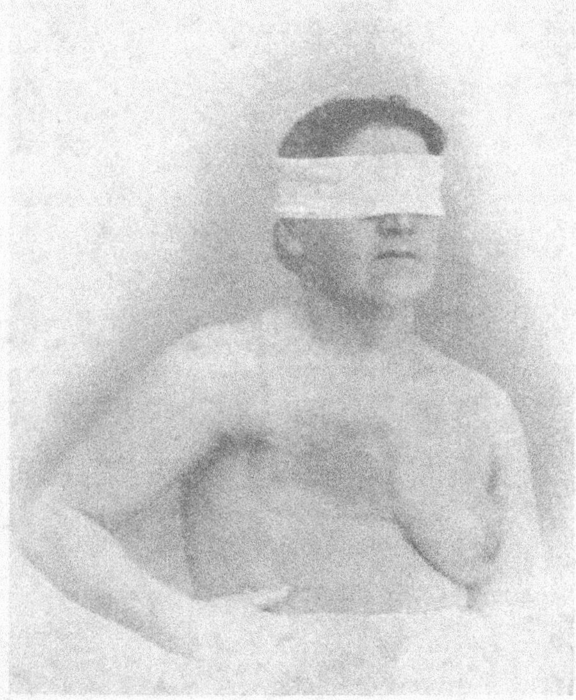

Fig. 4.

des ganglions, il est incontestable que le pourcentage des succès
augmenterait s'il y avait un diagnostic et une intervention précoces.

    Il est certain qu'aujourd'hui, dans toutes les cliniques d'en-
seignement ou dans tous les cours de clinique chirurgicale, on enseigne que pour une tumeur maligne de la glande mammaire
l'unique intervention rationnelle n'est pas l'extirpation de la tu-

meur et d'une partie de la glande, mais seulement l'amputation intégrale du sein, avec la peau qui le recouvre (ou même qui va plus loin que lui), des tissus, comprenant la peau, la paroi intéressée du thorax, où serpentent les vases et collecteurs lymphatiques qui viennent de la région mammaire et des divers groupes des ganglions de l'aisselle avec les tissus qui les enveloppent, et dans le même ordre où généralement ils sont envahis, de l'aponévrose du grand pectoral et des parties des muscles qui par eux et par leur tissu conjonctif proche sont devenus suspects.

On prend aujourd'hui un soin spécial, quand on fait l'évidement de l'aisselle, pour éliminer aussi complètement que possible les lymphatiques et les ganglions (suivant les cas et par leur ordre), le collecteur cutané des parois latérales du thorax, les groupes ganglionnaires infra-externe et super-interne, le ganglion du groupe central, les ganglions de la chaîne scapulaire, ceux de la chaîne humérale et les ganglions sous-claviculaires.

Cela veut dire qu'on réalise de larges éliminations inutiles dans quelques cas avancés, mais utilisables dans beaucoup. Cependant, en dehors des cliniques indiquées, il n'est pas rare que l'on exécute des opérations partielles qui ne touchent pas les ganglions de l'aisselle et qui laissent quelquefois une bonne partie du sein.

Quand le diagnostic est très hésitant, il vaut mieux réserver un bistouri pour faire une profonde incision dans la tumeur et, si on reconnaît à simple vue une erreur de diagnostic, faire rapidement une suture de la peau et procéder à une intervention chirurgicale plus large.

Choisissant parmi quelques cas les plus récents et les plus typiques, je citerai trois cas d'intervention vicieuse:

Mᵐᵉ N., de 34 ans, nullipare, a reconnu sa tumeur, encore très petite, dans la région supérieure de la mamelle droite, au début de 1904; elle augmenta rapidement en quelques semaines. L'été de la même année, elle souffrit quelques cautérisations d'un charlatan, et fut opérée dans son village en mars 1905. Le 7 mai, la cicatrisation était complète, mais aussitôt elle commença à sentir de l'induration dans la glande et en juin elle présentait en plus de la tumeur un engorgement ganglionnaire très grand de l'aisselle (fig. 1). Dans ce cas, il y a eu une récidive manifeste par continuation, elle fut opérée une deuxième fois en juillet 1905; on élimina la peau largement, on sectionna la plus grande partie du grand et du petit pectoral, en laissant du côté intérieur trois côtes à découvert, et du côté de l'aisselle, où on avait fait un large évidement (jusqu'au fascicule vasculo-nerveux) de tous les ganglions avec les tissus enveloppants.

La fig. 4 donne à peu près l'idée du traumatisme opératoire. L'aisselle était cicatrisée au bout de deux semaines, mais le reste de la surface prit des mois pour arriver à sa complète cicatrisation. Le résultat définitif n'est pas certain, car les opérations sur les tumeurs récidivées ne réussissent pas si bien.

Mme I. S., de 43 ans, mariée; a eu trois enfants, elle n'a pas eu d'accidents de lactation. Elle a reconnu sa tumeur en août 1903, en remarquant que le mamelon droit était déprimé et en trouvant dans la région aréolaire une nodosité dure qu'elle comparait à une noisette et qui était mobile.

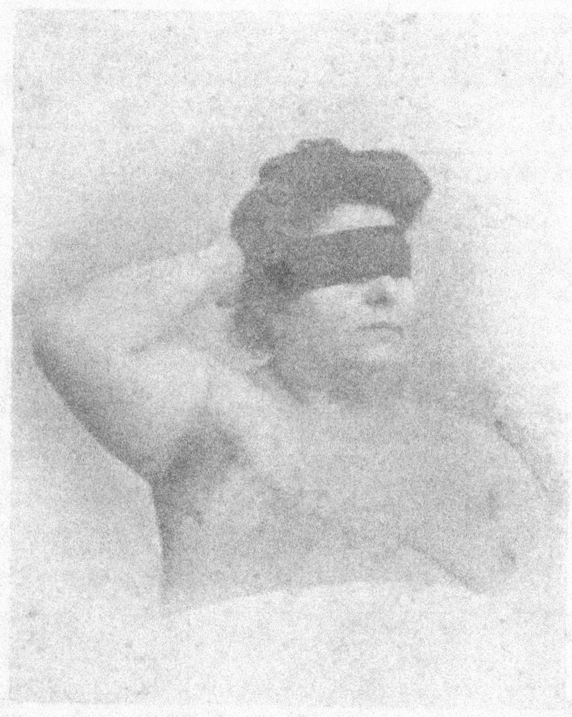

Fig. 7

En octobre, elle n'était plus mobile et avait un volume égal à celui d'un œuf de poule; elle adhérait aux tissus voisins et la malade avait des douleurs lancinantes. Elle fut opérée la première fois en Afrique (Loanda) en novembre 1903. La cicatrisation fut rapide; mais dans une des régions de la cicatrice, où la peau avait gardé une légère fente, les bords de cette fente durcirent et, dix mois après, c'est-à-dire 14 mois après la première opération, elle remarqua dans cette région une saillance qui lui rappelait un petit mamelon. Et la comparaison de la malade était exacte, car à première vue il semble que le mamelon était resté après la première opération. Autour de cette région le reste de la glande commença à durcir. En décembre 1905, avant d'être opérée, elle sent des douleurs lancinantes; il y a des indurations mal limitées dans la glande, et de légères infiltrations des ganglions axillaires.

Il s'agit d'une récidive par continuation, mais à évolution lente, ce qui contraste avec le premier cas. Serait-ce là l'effet de l'usage fréquent des sels de quinine qu'elle prit en Afrique, pour combattre les fièvres infectieuses? Elle fut opérée largement et profondément, la réunion presque immédiate étant possible à cause de la grande mobilité de la peau (fig. 5).

Mme J. C., de 43 ans, veuve, a eu 4 enfants; pas accidents de lactation. Elle dit qu'elle a été opérée en 1895 d'une tumeur, qui n'était pas récente. Aussitôt après l'opération elle sentit dans la partie intérieure de la cicatrice une masse additionnelle et elle en sentit une autre plus volumineuse du côté extérieur de la cicatrice (fig. 3).

Cette dernière augmenta lentement et il y a trois ans qu'elle est accompagnée d'adénopathie axillaire. L'adénopathie est générale dans l'aisselle, puisque à plus grande partie des ganglions sont réduits à une seule masse.

Les ganglions sus-claviculaires sont déjà suspects.

Elle accuse des douleurs thoraciques vives, à droite et à gauche et dans la direction des apophyses épineuses depuis la 4e vertèbre dorsale jusqu'au bas de la 6e. Elle souffre de très vives douleurs des membres inférieurs, douleurs qui ne sont pas soulagées par une thérapeutique variée.

Cette malade est en pleine cachexie cancéreuse; elle a probablement une carcinose pleurale et sûrement une carcinose vertébrale avec compression lente de la moelle; elle est dans la période des pseudo-névralgies. Dès qu'elle sut qu'elle n'était pas opérable, elle quitta l'hôpital et mourut un mois après, dans la période de paralysie flasque. D'après les renseignements recueillis, c'est un exemplaire très net de la paraplégie douloureuse des cancéreux de Charcot; c'est aussi un cas intéressant au point de vue de la longue durée de la maladie.

Ce serait probablement un cas de cure, si elle avait été opérée la première fois en éliminant non seulement la tumeur mais aussi tous les tissus voisins.

Ces trois cas sont typiques d'interventions partielles pour des tumeurs manifestement cancéreuses; en plus de ces cas, qui sont récents, j'en ai observé un grand nombre d'autres avec le même résultat.

Les conséquences de telles interventions sont des récidives immédiates, les tumeurs prenant, en général, une marche beaucoup plus rapide.

Chacun de ces trois cas, soit par leur histoire sommaire, soit par les dimensions des incisions effectuées, indicatives de tumeurs relativement volumineuses, aurait dû être tenu pour suspect de tumeur maligne. Et il aurait été préférable d'attendre quelques semaines, un mois ou plus, pour observer minutieusement les caractères et la marche de ces tumeurs, que de les opérer plus tôt, en les supposant bénignes et laissant ainsi des tissus déjà infiltrés.

Cette brève communication a la seule valeur d'être suggestive, par la représentation des cas typiques *de ce qu'on ne doit pas faire*; elle a également comme but de recommander une intervention thérapeutique rationnelle, basée sur un diagnostic opportun.

Ce diagnostic opportun est possible, car je l'ai démontré dans bon nombre de cas, après un examen répété, et, dans tous, l'examen histologique l'a confirmé.

Tout dernièrement encore, après avoir déjà ébauché cette note, j'ai observé avec mes collègues les prof. Angelo da Fonseca et Elysio de Moura deux cas de tumeurs mammaires récentes, pour lesquels sans divergence nous établîmes le diagnostic de cancer, qui fut confirmé. Pour le premier, opéré par le prof. Elysio de Moura, il s'agissait d'une malade J. J. de 44 ans; la tumeur fut reconnue par elle il y a 3 mois; elle a augmenté beaucoup pendant ces dernières semaines; malgré tout, elle est petite (volume d'une châtaigne); elle siège dans la partie supérieure du sein, près de l'auréole; elle se rattache nettement à la glande mammaire sans limitation; la peau qui la recouvre révèle, à la loupe, de légères dilatations lymphatiques, pas de douleur; les ganglions du 1er groupe sont légèrement augmentés.

Dans le second cas, opéré par le prof. Angelo da Fonseca, la malade, M. J., de 38 ans, a reconnu sa tumeur il y a un mois seulement; elle a augmenté depuis; elle a la forme d'une calotte sphérique de 6 centimètres environ de largeur; elle n'est pas très dure; son siège est près d'un ancien foyer de mastite (qui date de neuf ans), qui a suppuré et dont il reste une cicatrice sur le côté externe de la tumeur.

La peau correspondant à la tumeur en son point le plus culminant montre à la loupe des dilatations lymphatiques allongées; le pannicule adipeux est réduit et attaché à la tumeur; celle-ci est retenue au sein très nettement sur la plupart de son contour; elle est sans douleur; le prolongement axillaire de la glande mammaire est volumineux, et les ganglions qui suivent sont très peu tuméfiés si on les compare à ceux du côté opposé.

Ce sont là deux cas de diagnostic précoce qui, étant donnés l'âge des malades, l'absence de limitation, l'accroissement très accentué en un très court délai, les caractères de la peau sur lesquels j'ai insisté, le commencement de retentissement ganglionnaire et aussi la diagnose différentielle, ne permettent pas d'affirmer une mastite ou une tumeur bénigne.

CONCLUSIONS

1º — Le diagnostic précoce du cancer du sein est possible, peu après son début, à un degré de probabilité qui touche à la certitude.

2º — Ce diagnostic une fois fait, l'intervention thérapeutique, quelque petite que soit la tumeur, doit être large et profonde.

3º — L'extirpation de la tumeur, quelque petite qu'elle soit, en laissant une partie de la glande, doit être absolument rejetée comme inutile et nuisible.

Nouvelle méthode de suture des plaies intestinales

Par M. Cordero Lopez, Huelva.

Les difficultés aussi nombreuses que graves éprouvées par moi en pratiquant la suture de Gely m'ont amené à réfléchir sérieusement là-dessus et à me mettre à la recherche d'un procédé de suture, qui, sans dédaigner les avantages attachés à l'ancien système, fût débarrassé des désavantages considérables qu'il renferme.

Dans ce but j'ai étudié avec le zèle qu'exige un sujet d'une telle importance, et je suis parvenu moyennant l'effet de mes efforts à l'idée d'une méthode mixte dont deux qualités saillantes justifient, il me semble, de la désigner sous la dénomination de «Suture entrecoupée à point double».

Avec le nouveau moyen fourni par cette méthode, il est déjà possible de réaliser un parfait adossement des séreuses et une cicatrisation rapide, conditions qui d'elles-mêmes suffisent pour donner à la suture que je propose la supériorité désirable sur les autres systèmes actuellement connus.

Je vais donc prouver mon assertion et pour cela il me faut commencer par l'exposition des causes qui me poussèrent vers une poursuite scrupuleuse, aussi bien que vers la façon de pratiquer la suture dont il s'agit, en finissant par quelques considérations qui, en synthèse et comparativement, fassent voir les avantages de mon procédé sur tous les autres adoptés encore.

D'abord il convient de rendre compte des antécédents. En remplissant ma fonction comme médecin directeur d'un des établissements voués à l'assistance publique et dont l'objet spécial est le secours immédiat, de blessés surtout, il va sans dire que j'ai eu bien l'occasion de traiter plusieurs cas de plaies intestinales, et ce fut toujours la suture de Gely que j'ai suivie; mais en voici le résultat: J'ai tracé le premier point sans le moindre obstacle, mais, quand il était question de tracer le second, des inconvénients se présentaient à un si haut degré que je ne pouvais presque plus poursuivre, ce qui me contraignait d'effectuer l'opération tantôt au moyen de la suture entrecoupée simple, tantôt en faisant usage de la suture du pelletier. Or, je devais tâcher de découvrir l'origine d'où revenait l'insuccès de la suture Gely, et il me fallut reconnaître que le mal naissait d'une structure compliquée et de la continuité des points.

Si l'on trouvait un système où les deux difficultés pussent s'évanouir ou, ce qui revient au même, un système où l'on atteignît de la simplicité pour la structure et de l'isolement des points, la solution du problème serait une réalité flatteuse, indiscutable. L'un et l'autre résultats, sans faire mention d'autres avantages, constituent à l'avis du soussigné une suite aussi certaine que logique de la suture entrecoupée à point double. En voici l'emploi :

Un aide de chirurgien se place à main gauche de l'individu lésé, ayant soin de retenir l'anse intestinale en se servant du tenaculum ou d'un cordonnet, qu'on applique en guise de croc à l'un des angles de la blessure. L'opérateur doit se placer au côté droit, et pourvu d'un instrument de dissection à sa main gauche, tient à la droite une aiguille semi-courbe ou tout à fait courbe d'Agedorn, enfilée d'une soie sans rondeur et parfaitement cirée.

Grâce à la pince, l'une des lèvres de la plaie reste assujettie, tandis qu'au dehors, à une distance de quatre millimètres de l'un des bouts, on introduit l'aiguille depuis la séreuse jusqu'à la muqueuse inclusivement, avec le parcours d'un trajet de quatre millimètres parallèlement à la solution de continuité. Une fois cette partie opératoire terminée, la lèvre opposée se fixe, et l'aiguille est introduite de nouveau vis-à-vis de la deuxième ouverture du point antérieur, à la même distance de quatre millimètres du bord respectif, le parcours étant d'un trajet d'égale étendue dans un sens parallèle à la blessure, mais en direction contraire au premier point, aboutissant à se trouver tout en face de la ponction initiale. Quant au second point, il faut introduire l'aiguille à la distance de trois ou quatre millimètres du premier et à quatre millimètres de la plaie, avec un parcours tout égal au précédent. C'est de la même manière qu'il convient d'agir pour le reste. La seule chose à observer maintenant, c'est de bien serrer les points et de nouer dûment les bouts : cette partie de l'opération a lieu en tirant vers soi légèrement les fils de chaque point, et en même temps, au moyen d'une pince, les lèvres de la plaie sont déprimées afin d'obtenir l'adossement des séreuses. Cela fait, on noue les points l'un après l'autre avec celui de chirurgien et encore un simple, d'où le point double, pour acquérir plus de fermeté.

Après ce qui vient d'être exposé, rien de plus facile que d'envisager combien il est avantageux d'employer le nouveau système dont il s'agit. Point de doute après quelques considérations bien rapides. En effet, sur la méthode Gely, qui est aujourd'hui la plus recommandée, la mienne offre les côtés favorables qui suivent: premièrement les outils descendent jusqu'à la moitié, car une seule aiguille avec un seul fil suffit pour exécuter l'opération; d'ailleurs le nombre des points subit la même proportion, d'où il suit que les causes d'inflammation diminuent pareillement.

En outre, la nutrition vasculaire des bords ne se trouble point par suite d'une tension excessive; malgré les contractions intestinales les points ne peuvent pas s'affaiblir. Il faut se rappe-

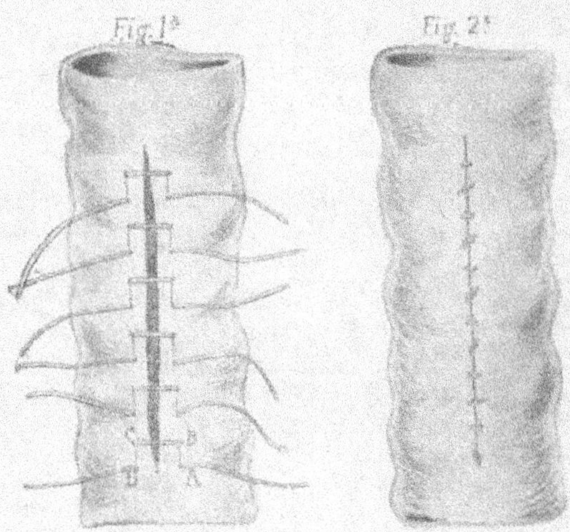

Fig. 1 — Suture sero-musculeuse. Tracé du premier point. L'aiguille, introduite dans A jusqu'à la muqueuse inclusivement, sort par B, afin de rentrer par C et trouver l'issue par D.
Fig. 2 — Suture nouée.

ler ces deux inconvénients du procédé Gely, lesquels disparaissent à présent. D'ailleurs aucun cas de laxité ne pourra occasionner le moindre risque.

A l'égard du système Lembert, fort vanté aussi pour les plaies transversales, il y a des objections à faire, et le fondement de ces objections donne la préférence à mon procédé. D'abord la hauteur, selon notre méthode, du repli membraneux est de quatre millimètres, précisément la même que celle des valvules conniventes, au lieu que suivant Lembert la hauteur atteint huit millimètres ou encore davantage, d'où la difficulté pour le cours des matières intestinales. Contrairement à ceci, dans mon système les points se manifestent fermes, tout sûrs, par cela même qu'ils comprennent toutes les membranes dans quatre millimètres et même moins de ce nombre; les fils, loin d'être réabsorbés, tombent dans la cavité intestinale au moment où la cicatrisation s'est accomplie.

Pour les sutures de Blatin et Cushing, continues à l'instar de celles de Gely, elles offrent presque autant d'inconvénients analogues, et celles de Jovert, Czerny et Halstead, quoique entrecoupées, partagent les défauts de Lembert.

En résumé, il résulte que la méthode «Suture entrecoupée à point double», tout en possédant la partie favorable des autres sutures, n'en a pas le côté défavorable. Il s'ensuit que cette dernière suture est à préférer dans les plaies, de quelque espèce qu'elles soient, longitudinales, transversales, complètes ou incomplètes.

DISCUSSION

M. KOLAR: La nouvelle méthode que M. Cordero Lopez propose n'a aucun avantage sur les autres méthodes, elle a encore les inconvénients de la période des tâtonnements des sutures intestinales. Il faut donc rester fidèles aux procédés bien admis, et surtout ne jamais laisser de soigner la suture séro-séreuse, qui dans le procédé proposé est très négligée.

Un cas de pygomèlle. — Intervention chirurgicale

Par M. AUGUSTO DE VASCONCELLOS, Lisbonne.

Un cas de goître; thyroïdectomie. Résultats immédiats

Par M. DANIEL DE MATTOS, Coïmbre.

Je présente ce cas en communication au Congrès, non seulement parce qu'il représente une contribution, encore que petite, pour la statistique de la thyroïdectomie dans ses résultats, mais aussi

a) parce que ce cas fait partie d'une série de goîtres de la même famille, qui va s'éteindre, et dans laquelle je crois qu'il y a eu un cas fatal de myxœdème, et

b) parce que je profite de l'occasion pour appeler l'attention sur l'utilité scientifique et humanitaire de dresser entre nous la carte des goîtreux.

Quelle que soit la pathogénie, encore très obscure, du goître, il y a de nombreux foyers anciens et il en apparaît quelques-uns de nouveaux; il est donc de tout intérêt d'examiner d'abord leur distribution géographique.

Les eaux ont-elles l'influence capitale dans l'étiologie du goitre comme beaucoup l'affirment?

Si elles l'ont, est-ce par leur composition chimique, ou bien parce qu'elles véhiculent des parasites?

À part la carte de répartition géographique, l'étude comparative des eaux fournies aux populations et la connaissance de toutes les autres conditions de la vie, on peut acquérir des éléments pour éclairer la pathogénie des maladies, ou au moins prendre des mesures de vigilance hygiénique qui réduisent le nombre des cas et guérissent ceux qui sont attaqués depuis peu.

La jeune fille N. A. a l'âge réel de 19 ans, ce qui est loin de concorder avec son âge apparent. Son visage presque enfantin, ses traits peu accentués, sa stature exiguë (1m,38), elle ne pèse que 30k,5, son petit développement général, lui donnent l'apparence d'une enfant de 12 à 13 ans. Elle n'a pas encore ses règles.

Elle habite le village de Pilez, canton de Goes, dans le district de Coïmbre.

Elle ne sait pas de quelle maladie mourut son père. Sa mère paraît être en bonne santé.

Une sœur plus âgée mourut il y a 6 ans, «Elle était, au dire de N. A., de petite stature, faible, très maladive, elle souffrait beaucoup des mains et des pieds qui se tuméfiaient, toujours plus en hiver qu'en été; les doigts des mains, assez difformes, étaient à demi-glacés sans qu'elle pût les mouvoir»

Elle a encore deux sœurs: l'une de 22 ans souffre d'une tumeur au ventre qui laisse toujours couler du pus; l'autre a aussi un goitre, mais il est bilatéral

Elle a un frère, plus jeune qu'elle, qui a un goitre unilatéral à droite, comme le sien, mais plus petit.

En général, quand le goitre est grand comme chez la malade N. A., il rappelle la forme générale de la glande normale, mais sa texture anatomo-pathologique n'est pas conforme; la tumeur avec ses bosselures irrégulières échappe à une description exacte.

Cependant, je reproduis ici La description du goitre de N. A., faite par mon cher Almeida Ribeiro, et qui se rapproche de ce qu'était réellement le goitre chez cette malade,

Symptômes objectifs. — À simple inspection on voit le cou très sensiblement augmenté de volume, augmentation qui, très accentuée à droite et aussi très apparente dans la partie antérieure, se trouve déjà beaucoup moins prononcée à gauche; à droite, au point de rencontre de deux lignes, respectivement horizontale et verticale, la première passant un peu au-dessous de l'os hyoïde, la deuxième un peu devant l'angle du maxillaire inférieur, surplombe à l'ensemble de la tuméfaction une élévation plus ou moins sphérique; de cette élévation, qui constitue un des foyers de l'augmentation, s'éloignent successivement et progressivement l'un de l'autre les bords limités de la tuméfaction; l'un, supérieur interne, rectiligne, descend tant soit peu obliquement vers le bas et vers le devant jusqu'à la partie antérieure du cou, puis à gauche de la ligne médiane pour se diriger alors, en un court trajet, obliquement vers le haut et par derrière, l'autre bord, inférieur externe, convexe se dirige un tant soit peu obliquement vers le devant et vers le bas, jusqu'à un peu au-dessus et hors de la région sternale, pour s'y doubler en un angle peu accentué et cheminer alors horizontalement, formant un bordelet saillant au-dessus du sternum, et monter alors dans la région gauche du cou, de manière à aller, en se perdant dans la tuméfaction moins accentuée de ce côté, s'unir d'une façon vague et en une courbe avec le premier bord considéré.

L'ensemble affecte la forme grossière d'un très gros rein, dont l'axe serait disposé obliquement de haut en bas, de dehors en dedans et de derrière en avant, et dont le plus petit bord, supérieur interne, regarderait le bord du maxillaire in-férieur.

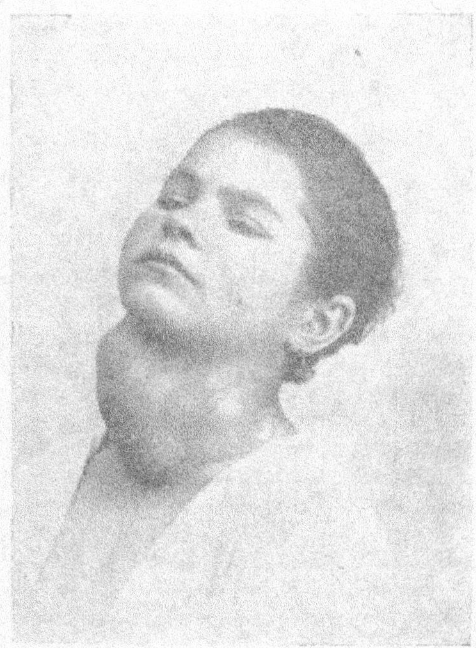

Fig. 1

En faisant exécuter à la malade des mouvements de déglutition, on constate une mobilité limitée de la région dans les sens vertical et antéro-postérieur.

La peau présente un aspect normal.

Par la palpation on reconnaît la parfaite mobilité de la peau dans toute l'étendue de la tuméfaction; dans la partie super-externe et postérieure, correspondant à l'élévation prééminente de l'ensemble qu'on note à l'inspection, on rencontre un corps lisse, dur, sphérique, bien délimité, ne cédant pas à la pression, se mouvant dans tous les sens (surtout dans le sens horizontal) sous la peau et sur un plan sous-jacent, liée par un pédicule postéro-interne à la masse qui constitue la tumeur principale.

Exactement à la partie postérieure de cette nodosité, un autre corps se rencontre dont la palpation, un peu difficile, est encore assez praticable et qui, à simple inspection, est peu apparent. Comme le premier il est mobile (un peu moins), de résistance élastique à la pression, d'une surface lisse et globuleuse.

On trouve des corps semblables mais avec des formes moins nettes et moins faciles à observer: l'un dans le bord inférieur, près de la partie gauche de la clavicule sternale; en outre de ces corps il y en a encore d'autres de moindre volume et de caractères moins accentués; l'un au bord convexe et inférieur; un autre au bord supérieur; dans la partie du milieu de la tumeur, un troisième, petit, dur, peu mobile.

Les uns et les autres se logent dans un tissu susceptible de dépression, de consistance analogue à de la chair musculaire qui constitue — *la plus grande partie du volume observé.*

Dans la région antérieure la tumeur passe un peu en bas du bord supérieur du cartilage thyroïde, de façon à permettre l'exploration facile par palpation de son échancrure médiane.

Il est possible avec les doigts d'imprimer à la tumeur des déplacements dans le sens transversal, mais non dans le vertical.

J'ai reconnu, ainsi que je l'indiquai et le fis remarquer dans ma leçon sur ce cas, que, par les caractères généraux donnés par la palpation, par la résistance élastique de quelques-unes des nodosités, dans deux desquelles la palpation bi-digitale me permit de reconnaître l'existence de liquide, que le diagnostic anatomo-pathologique de la variété de goître devait exclure les goîtres charnus, avec hypertrophie totale d'un des lobes ou de toute la glande, et que la prédominance de l'hypertrophie se réalisait sur l'élément glandulaire, et qu'on était en présence d'un goître adénomateux. Cependant, par quelques-uns des caractères indiqués, on devait voir s'affirmer la dégénérescence kystique de ce goître sans détermination exacte de la nature des kystes.

Le diagnostic devrait être enfin d'adénome kystique du lobe droit de la glande thyroïde; et dans le segment inférieur de ce lobe et de l'isthme, étant donnée la masse plus compacte et plus dure, le diagnostic devait être aussi celui de l'adéno-fibrome.

Perturbations fonctionnelles. — Aussi bien les corps globoïdes que tout le reste de la tumeur sont indolents à la pression.

On remarque à simple inspection une couleur violacée de la face, plus accentuée aux lèvres et sur les doigts des mains et des pieds.

Elle n'a pas de symptômes nets d'anémie cérébrale, cependant il y a mydriase légère et somnolence.

Les symptômes des fonctions de l'appareil respiratoire sont les dominants; la voix faible a de la raucité marquée et variable suivant l'attitude de la malade

La dyspnée, qui existe depuis deux mois, fait des progrès depuis l'entrée de la malade à l'hôpital et l'oblige parfois à s'asseoir sur le lit.

De l'ensemble de ces symptômes on doit indiquer la nécessité de la thyroïdectomie partielle, la seule qui se pratique aujourd'hui.

En traits généraux je donne la description de la technique chirurgicale suivie dans l'opération.

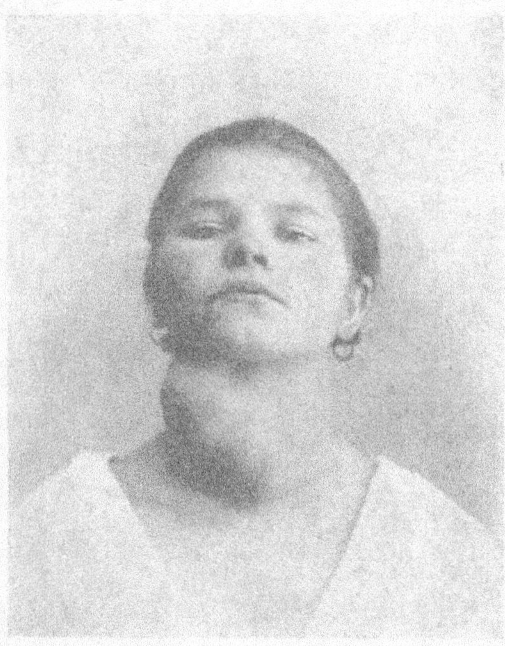

Fig. 1

La malade est chloroformisée sous la direction du professeur Elysio de Moura, après injection de morphine et de spartéine 20 minutes avant l'opération.

Mes aides sont le professeur Angelo da Fonseca et l'étudiant Almeida Ribeiro.

Je fais l'incision de la peau suivant la direction du grand axe du goitre et dans la partie du milieu, dans une direction sensiblement correspondante au bord interne du sterno-cléido-mastoïdien, et je la dissèque des deux côtés, prenant garde à la veine jugulaire antérieure droite qui acquiert un énorme volume causé par la compression intense des veines profondes; elle est saisie entre deux pinces et entre deux ligatures avant d'être sectionnée. Je dissèque l'aponévrose superficielle jusqu'au-dessous du point d'émergence de la veine vers le dehors de l'aponévrose superficielle afin d'éviter de la sectionner de nouveau et pour ouvrir d'abord un accès jusqu'à l'espace supra-sternal, à la hauteur duquel se trouve le segment inférieur du goître. Je coupe le muscle peaucier et, parce que le muscle omo-hyoïdien se présente très tendu par l'effet du grand volume du goître et que je ne puis l'écarter sans violence, je le coupe aussi. Je peux écarter le sterno-cléido-hyoïdien et le sterno-thyroïdien sans les couper.

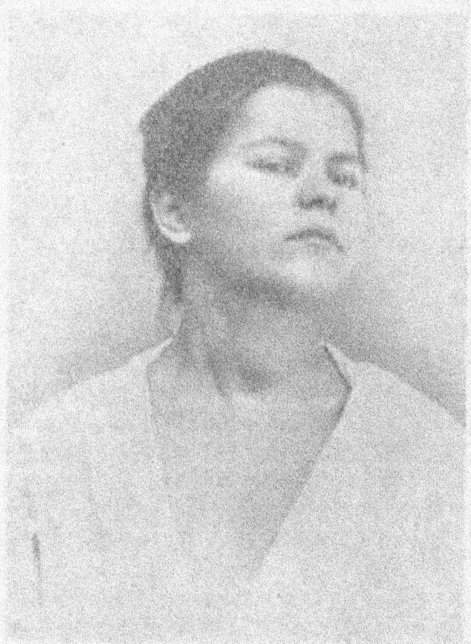

Fig. 1

J'incise alors dans la partie du milieu la gaine périthyroïdienne et la capsule propre, toutes deux dans cette région assez amincies; et prolongeant l'incision par en bas et par en dessus, je trouve en dessus une discontinuité dans la capsule. En correspondance avec les corps globuloïdes décrits il n'y a pas de capsule; à la suite de la gaine péri-thyroïdienne il y a aussi une couche très irrégulière et très discontinue, je les prends avec les doigts et je les sépare de la gangue conjonctive qui les enveloppe. Quelques-uns, plus nombreux que la palpation n'en détermina, constituent des kystes remplis d'un liquide rougeâtre qui se vident quand on les détache, d'autres restent fermés. Je fais la ligature des vaisseaux des pédicules de chacun d'eux.

La masse qui suit est plus conglomérée, mais manifestement constituée par des adénomes avec hyperplasie des cloisons capsulaires. Je me trouve dans la

hauteur où la capsule est distincte et je reconnais un plan de clivage que je vais
suivre, mais avant je fais la ligature de l'artère thyroïde supérieure qui maintenant
est visible. À l'intérieur de la capsule je détache alors une partie de la tumeur ; et
je sens, lorsque je fais le dissection à la sonde cannelée et particulièrement à l'aide
d'un doigt, qu'une partie de cette masse a encore un autre kyste de paroi moins rougeâtre et moins tendu : après l'opération je vérifie dans ce kyste un contenu colloïde.
En suivant vers la partie inférieure la tumeur adhère beaucoup à la capsule ; la

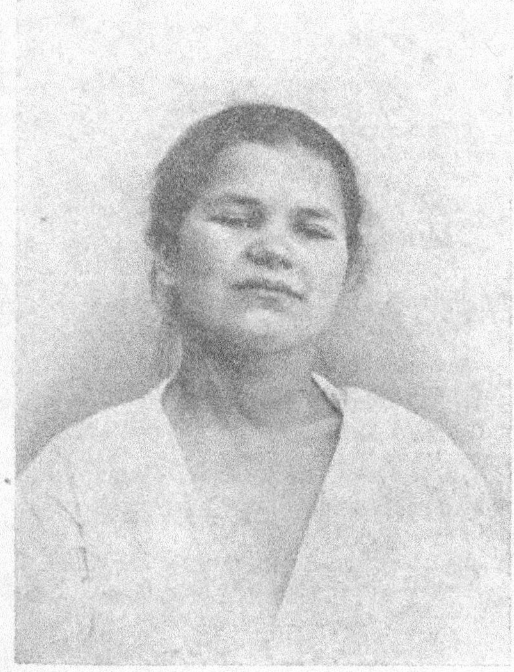

Fig. 4

pression qu'il faudrait faire pourrait infléchir la trachée. Je vais ensuite sectionner
l'isthme non seulement pour délivrer la trachée, mais dans le but de continuer à
suivre la continuité intra-capsulaire et d'avoir un plan plus favorable de sépa-
ration.

Il faut couper l'isthme au-delà de la ligne médiane près du côté gauche de
la trachée, pour la soulager définitivement de la compression, étant donnée la
dyspnée de la malade. Par l'incision de la capsule dans le lobe droit sur l'isthme
j'essais, avant d'inciser celui-ci, de l'affranchir de la capsule, ce que je reconnais
être impossible à cause de son adhérence très intime. Je le coupe donc avec la

capsule, passant à pratiquer vers l'isthme et le segment inférieur du lobe la thy-roïdectomie extra-capsulaire, plus difficile et sujette à des déboires, mais néces-saire en ce moment. Une fois l'isthme détaché, je l'écarte au dehors, ayant fait la ligature des vaisseaux rompus médiaux et découvert l'artère thyroïdienne infé-rieure, je procède à sa ligature après l'avoir mise à nu, et voyant en arrière bien nettement le nerf récurrent, qui n'est pas lésé.

Dès lors la thyroïdectomie continua à être extra-capsulaire jusqu'à la région où se terminait la dissection intra-capsulaire, et j'achevai avec facilité la sépa-ration de la tumeur.

Il restait à la méthode, comme il convenait, le lobe gauche. L'aspect du tissu dans l'incision de l'isthme était normal. Pour éviter la diffusion de substances de sécrétion du lobe vers la cavité que j'allais former, je fis la suture au catgut sur le bout de la section de l'isthme tout en façonnant la capsule de façon à ajuster la face antérieure avec la postérieure. Je suturai tous les plans de tissus divisés, et les muscles coupés en cherchant à ne pas laisser d'espaces morts. Drainage dans l'angle inférieur de la plaie.

Les résultats immédiats de cette opération furent excellents; la dysphagie disparut entièrement ainsi que toutes les perturbations fonctionnelles de la respi-ration.

La technique chirurgicale de la thyroïdectomie possède au-jourd'hui trois méthodes principales: extra-capsulaire, intra-capsu-laire et intra-glandulaire, et quoique l'on tâche de suivre de pré-férence les deux dernières méthodes, parce qu'elles sont plus simples et offrent moins de danger, on ne peut cependant s'assujet-tir d'avance, dans chaque cas, à l'emploi de l'une à l'exclusion des autres.

Leur choix d'avance et leurs modifications durant l'opéra-tion dépendent fondamentalement des variétés anatomo-pathologi-ques du goitre.

Dans cette opération, s'il est nécessaire et indispensable de posséder la connaissance précise de l'anatomie de la région, il est aussi très utile d'avoir une appréciation exacte des lésions anatomo-pathologiques qui caractérisent chaque cas où l'interven-tion chirurgicale se trouve indiquée.

DISCUSSION

M. FRANCISCO-DANTAS: Parmi nous le goitre est peu fréquent et mon ex-périence à ce sujet est très restreinte, car je n'ai opéré que 12 cas. Chez tous les malades porteurs de goitre unilatéral, la méthode employée a été celle de Kocher; dans les cas de goitre diffus, j'ai pratiqué l'énucléation. Dans le premier cas que j'ai opéré de cette façon, la masse extirpée pesait 510 grammes, et dans un autre cas plus de 600 gr.

Ce qui m'a porté à parler sur l'intéressante communication de M. le prof. Daniel de Mattos, c'est le cas d'un goitre malin, un sarcome du corps thyroïdien, que j'ai opéré il y a deux ans chez une femme de 50 ans. La plaie opératoire a cicatrisé, mais trois mois après il se montrait une reproduction suivie d'une sarcomatose des deux plèvres et du cœur; malheureusement je ne puis pas vous montrer cette pièce si rare et si curieuse.

M. FRIJÃO: Je n'ai pas pris la parole pour occuper l'attention de l'assemblée sur la thyroïdectomie, que j'ai pratiquée le premier en Portugal, mais pour appeler son attention sur un cas clinique de myxœdème. J'ai observé une dame mariée, qui n'avait jamais été réglée et chez laquelle je n'ai pu trouver aucune trace de matrice ni d'ovaires, le vagin se terminait en cul de sac. La sœur de cette dame est une jeune fille qui aussi ne fut jamais réglée. Les deux sont les seuls enfants de la mère. Chez la dame mariée il se développa un très fort myxœdème, tout son corps devint dur, énormément grossi, mais la thyroïde ne prit pas de développement remarquable. J'ai soigné cette dame avec la thyroïdine, qui au commencement apporta une amélioration, mais comme celle-ci s'arrêta, je pensai que l'absence des ovaires pourrait être pour quelque chose dans le myxœdème et j'ai donné l'ovarine avec la thyroïdine, une semaine l'une, l'autre semaine l'autre. Sous ces derniers médicaments combinés la malade est et se maintient tout à fait guérie.

M. KOHRT: J'ai dans ma clientèle une femme mariée, que j'ai vue avant le mariage, car elle n'avait pas de règles, et la mère avait des remords de marier sa fille dans ces conditions. Le fiancé savait du reste la situation et voulait être lui aussi renseigné scientifiquement, tout en admettant la stérilité obligatoire. Je n'ai pu trouver, par tous les moyens, ni utérus, ni ovaires, ni vagin. Il y a une atrésie complète vulvaire. J'ai fabriqué, avec le consentement des intéressés, un petit vagin artificiel. Le mariage s'est fait et les conséquences ont été comme on les prévoyait. La femme avait les seins bien développés et une constitution robuste. Rien dans la glande thyroïde. C'est donc un cas de plus, que l'absence des organes génitaux de la femme n'oblige pas la présence du myxœdème. Du reste l'orateur antérieur cite le même cas d'aménorrhée absolue sans pourtant pouvoir donner la preuve anatomique et clinique précise, par refus de la jeune fille, sœur du cas intéressant de myxœdème et absence des organes génitaux.

Le procédé de Mac-Burney dans l'appendicectomie

Par M. FRANCISCO GENTIL, Lisbonne.

Dans l'appendicectomie opérée à froid, on n'a parfois à craindre que le danger d'une éventration que l'on pourra empêcher au moyen de sutures bien faites, exception faite des cas où des conditions spéciales de la paroi du ventre font céder la cicatrice ou lors d'un effort violent produisant l'éventration aiguë. Il existe, cependant, un procédé qui rend impossible l'accident et évite même l'usage temporaire de la ceinture abdominale indispensable pour toute autre méthode d'ouverture du ventre; c'est le procédé de laparotomie proposé par Mac-Burney pour l'intervention regardant l'appendice. Les procédés de Wilcox, Abbe et Robson pour l'utérus et le rein, celui de Edebohls pour

l'opération des reins, voies biliaires et appendice, sont autant
de procédés semblables et qui en dérivent. L'observation des cas
que j'ai opérés par ce procédé et qui m'ont fourni des éléments
propres à garantir la solidité de la paroi abdominale éveillent
en moi le désir de faire cette communication et je serais heureux
si en quelque manière je réussissais à divulguer un très bon
procédé opératoire.

Laparotomie de Mac-Burney. Incision cutanée, longue de
deux pouces, oblique et légèrement courbe, à concavité interne,
faite un pouce en dedans de l'épine iliaque antéro-supérieure,
sensiblement perpendiculaire à la ligne qui joint cette épine
osseuse à l'ombilic. Coupe, dans le même sens, mais en ligne
droite, du grand oblique et de son aponévrose. Le petit oblique
mis à nu, on écarte ses fibres et celles du transverse, sans les
couper, selon leur direction, vers le milieu de la plaie du grand
oblique. On incise le fascia transversalis parallèlement au plan
antérieur. Une fois mise à découvert, la gaine abdominale
est écartée et le péritoine ouvert par une incision transversale.
C'est alors que l'on cherche l'appendice et on le prépare à être
sorti hors du ventre en même temps que le cœcum. Parfois on
a de la difficulté à défaire les adhérences qui se sont produites
tout autour de l'appendice, ainsi qu'il est arrivé à mes quatrième, sixième, neuvième et dixième opérés; mais, malgré tout,
l'ouverture ménagée par la laparotomie de Mac-Burney y suffit
très bien. Des écarteurs retiennent les divers plans d'ouverture
de la paroi abdominale au fur et à mesure qu'on opère. On les
ôte aussitôt que le cœcum se trouve hors du ventre. Le rapprochement des bords des différentes incisions soutient l'intestin
et permet de faire aisément la résection et le traitement du moignon appendiculaire. Après ce temps de l'opération, on tire les
écarteurs, remet en place le cœcum et reconstitue la paroi abdominale par autant de sutures isolées qu'il y a de plans d'ouverture; cette paroi reste tout à fait solide et parfaitement rétablie;
de cette façon, quinze jours après l'intervention, le patient n'a
plus besoin de porter une bande ou une ceinture abdominale.

Le premier malade que j'ai opéré par cette méthode, il y a
cinq ans, et un autre, il y a deux ans, étaient des hommes de 26
et 20 ans respectivement, qui s'adonnent à tout genre de sport,
sans avoir jamais porté de ceinture abdominale; ils n'ont jamais
rien remarqué d'anormal dans la paroi du ventre, n'importe la
force déployée lors de leurs exercices. Un autre, que j'ai opéré il

y a trois ans, fait le portefaix dans une gare de chemin de fer; c'est un métier qui oblige à de grands efforts; eh bien! il n'a jamais porté la ceinture et ne s'est jamais plaint de quoi que ce soit du côté de la paroi du ventre.

Voilà les avantages qu'offre le procédé de Mac-Burney sur tous les autres que l'on emploie couramment.

Sur les plaies par les armes modernes dans la guerre Russo-Japonaise 1904-1905 (Observations et Remarques)

Par M. A. D. Pawlowsky, Kieff.

Je me permets de communiquer à la section de chirurgie du XV Congrès International de Médecine à Lisbonne les résultats de mes observations sur les plaies occasionnées par les fusils à petit calibre modernes et par les obus dans la guerre russo-japonaise. Ayant travaillé en qualité de professeur de chirurgie dans les hôpitaux de guerre à Laoyan et dans les points de pansement au corps de l'Est dans l'armée russe, j'ai eu l'occasion d'observer, d'opérer et de panser plus de 3000 blessés.

Les principes du service d'un chirurgien et médecin dans la guerre ont été primordialement indiqués par N. Y. Pirogoff. Lui, le premier, a appliqué le pansement au gypse dans la guerre du Caucase. C'est encore lui qui pendant la guerre de Crimée (1855-56) a le premier largement appliqué l'évacuation de blessés. Il a remarqué la différence dans l'action pénétrante des balles en cuivre de petit calibre des circassiens et des grosses balles en plomb mou de l'armée russe. Il défendait le conservatisme en chirurgie, disant toujours: «Surtout ne sondez pas les plaies». Il a décrit une série de maladies infectieuses de plaies inconnues jusqu'à lui (voir *Chirurgie de Guerre*, Pirogoff).

L'aspect des plaies, avec l'introduction des fusils Lebel à poudre sans fumée Vial, a complètement changé:

L'action de la balle est définie par la force vive des balles d'après la formule $F = \frac{mx^2}{2}$ ou bien par l'énergie de la coupe transversale d'après la formule $Eg = \frac{mv^2}{2r^2 w}$, elle dépend aussi de la quantité et de la force de la poudre, du calibre et du poids de la balle et de sa matière. Tous ces éléments, y compris le calibre du fusil et la quantité de ses entailles, définissent la trajectoire de la balle et par conséquent la justesse du coup, la pénétration du but. En rencontrant un obstacle, la force vive se transforme en travail mécanique, ou, si l'obstacle est dur, en travail moléculaire avec développement de chaleur, ou enfin en action hydraulique quand elle rencontre des cavités remplies de liquide. Il est bien connu que le fusil Lebel a 8 mm. de calibre et 600 m. par seconde de vitesse initiale, ainsi que le fusil anglais Lee-Medford et le fusil russe de Mossine 7,62 mm. de calibre et 600 m. par seconde de vitesse initiale. Le fusil allemand Mauser (modèle 1896) a 7 mm. de calibre et 720 de vitesse initiale, tandis que le fusil japonais Arisaka a 6,5 mm. de calibre et 725 m. v. i. Les fusils russes et japonais ont tous les deux des mécanismes de répétition à 5 cartouches, qui ont une enveloppe de melchior et sont chargées de poudre sans fumée.

Par conséquent, les rapports entre l'armée russe et japonaise en fait d'armes étaient les mêmes qu'entre l'armée anglaise et les boërs pendant la guerre d'Afrique; mais la qualité et le caractère des plaies étaient les mêmes dans les deux armées. Il faut ajouter que chaque soldat russe était muni d'un paquet antiseptique individuel, qui rendit de grands services dans le traitement des plaies.

Quant aux caractères des plaies, il faut remarquer que dans les distances de 500 à 600 mètres, dans la première zone, on a observé des plaies perforantes avec effet explosif; dans la deuxième zone, de 600 à 1200 1500 mètres, seulement les plaies perforantes sans effet explosif comme résultat de la plus grande action de la force vive, et de 1500 à 2000 et même 3000 mètres des fractures compliquées d'éclats, des plaies déchirées ainsi que des plaies à orifice d'entrée seulement. J'ai observé que les orifices d'entrée et de sortie des plaies perforantes étaient ordinairement petits, correspondant au calibre de la balle. Pour les distances courtes l'orifice d'entrée est petit, avec bords brûlés ou écorchés; l'orifice de sortie était de forme irrégulière ou large avec les tissus mous déchirés et avec des fragments d'os écrasés et enfoncés dedans. Aux distances plus grandes l'orifice d'entrée était petit, le trajet souvent en forme *d'entonnoir*, l'orifice de sortie tantôt à forme irrégulière, tantôt grand et déchiré, avec des os brisés et fragments pénétrés. Le trajet de la balle souvent étroit et droit, presque toujours rempli de sang coagulé, quelquefois en zig-zag, ou en forme d'entonnoir, avec déchirure des tissus et fortes hémorrhagies. J'ai observé que la balle, en traversant les tissus mous, ne se déforme pas, tandis que, en pénétrant dans les os, elle se déforme tantôt en spirale ou en arc ou en angle. A la rencontre des os durs (fémur et tibia) l'enveloppe de la balle se déchire et la balle avec plomb se déforme en éventail, ou en forme de parasol, ou de champignon; la noix se déchire aussi. Quelquefois l'enveloppe se déchire en plusieurs morceaux. Dans ces cas la blessure est compliquée par les 2 ou 3 trajets et orifices de sortie. En ce qui concerne *les blessures des os*, nous avons observé que les os étaient le plus souvent brisés en morceaux, surtout les diaphyses. Les grands os (fémur, tibia et humérus) sont brisés en grands fragments avec déplacement et hémorrhagie. Les blessures des métaphyses occupent le milieu entre les blessures des diaphyses et des épiphyses. Les os plats aux distances courtes étaient brisés; aux distances moyennes, très souvent, des fractures à orifice sans altération de l'intégrité des os et avec des fissures radiaires.

Aux grandes distances, les épiphyses de l'humérus, du tibia, sont brisées le plus souvent en grands morceaux. Les blessures du crâne sont ordinairement graves ou mortelles. Aux distances courtes les os sont brisés; de larges hémorrhagies occupent les parties latérales de la tête, les orbites, les régions temporales et frontales. Le cerveau est dispersé et rejeté en dehors. Le trajet de la balle est rempli de sang. Le malade succombe de méningite et encéphalite provoquées par les staphylocoques et streptocoques. Les trépanations et débridements accomplis assez tôt ont donné de bons résultats; ils appartiennent aux opérations absolument obligatoires dans la guerre; ils doivent être accomplis le plus tôt possible, avant le commencement de l'infection.

Les trépanations et débridements accomplis pendant les périodes de développement de l'infection pyogène et de la méningite ont donné des résultats défavorables. Une série de plaies perforantes de la voûte du crâne, observées par moi, et surtout sans fissure de la base, ont fini par la guérison, en cas de cours aseptique. Tels sont les cas des blessures frontales dans les régions des tempes et frontales, de même que les blessures diagonales et tangentielles, pariéto-occipitales et vice-versa, et blessures sans orifice de sortie. J'ai observé aussi des cas de guérison de blessures sagittales perforatives. Un des cas les plus remarquables que j'ai eu l'occasion d'observer a été celui où la balle, entrée par l'os occipital, est sortie par l'os frontal, en emportant quelques fragments de l'os frontal: ce cas a fini par guérison avec des phénomènes de parésie des extrémités gauches.

Dans un cas de blessure transversale du crâne et du cerveau l'orifice d'entrée était dans la région temporale droite sans aucun orifice de sortie; le malade était en sopor; débridement sans succès, mort. En faisant l'autopsie j'ai trouvé une large hémorrhagie le long du trajet, les fragments gros dans l'os temporal gauche et la balle sous le muscle temporal gauche. Dans l'autre cas il s'agit de blessure diagonale avec prolapsus du cerveau et méningite. Après débridement et levée du cerveau, on a remarqué l'amélioration du malade, mais après un ou deux jours le collapsus et la méningite se déclaraient de nouveau et le malade succomba.

Les plaies des os de la face en général sont favorables, mais la plupart se conduisent avec brisement des os, surtout des maxillaires supérieur et inférieur. Dans les blessures frontales de la mâchoire inférieure, nous avons vu l'écrasement des dents et des branches de l'os avec de grandes hémorrhagies. Souvent les balles s'enclavent dans l'os en traversant la membrane muqueuse de la mâchoire inférieure; l'enlèvement de telles balles est très difficile. Les plaies des os du nez, traversant la basis nasi, brisent les os de la voûte nasale. Toutes ces blessures des os de la face dans des directions variables s'accompagnent très souvent d'infections pyogènes consécutives et finissent par la guérison.

Les blessures de la colonne vertébrale sont les plus graves de toutes et presque désespérées. Dans les blessures frontales les balles qui traversent le corps et la colonne vertébrale dans la région des reins provoquent la paralysie complète des extrémités inférieures, de la vessie et du rectum. Les mêmes balles qui traversent la colonne dans la région du cou provoquent la paralysie complète de toutes les 4 extrémités, de la vessie et du rectum. Les malheureux malades succombent à cause de l'intoxication et de l'infection consécutives, du marasme et décubitus, en conservant toute conscience. Dans quelques cas rares on en a observé l'amélioration et aussi la guérison. Dans les autopsies de tels cas j'ai trouvé les fractures des vertèbres, avec écrasement en grands morceaux, avec des fissures du corps des vertèbres et surtout des hémorrhagies dans les membranes de la moelle épinière. La dernière était comprimée ou brisée. Quelquefois les balles s'enclavent dans les vertèbres, en les écrasant en quelques morceaux et se déformant. Therapia nulla.

Les plaies des articulations sont le plus souvent traversées. Dans les articulations humérales, du cou, du fémur, du genou, du tibia et du tarse elles provoquent des hémorrhagies abondantes, avec fracture en grands morceaux des épiphyses des os. Elles guérissent sans fièvre après le pansement aseptique avec pression et repos complet. Sur l'articulation du genou j'ai observé les plaies traversées, sans fracture des os et avec hémorrhagie abondante dans la cavité du genou. En traitant de telles plaies par la ponction au trocart aseptique, lavage avec solution faible de sublimé et injection d'iodoforme (5 %), éther, alcool et pansement avec pression, j'ai obtenu la guérison complète avec fonctions du genou. Les plaies sagittales et surtout d'arrière en avant sont dangereuses à cause des blessures de vaisseaux et hémorrhagies primitives et consécutives, et surtout à cause d'anévrysmes traumatiques consécutifs. Les balles de ces plaies souvent s'enclavent fortement dans la rotule ou dans la tubérosité tibiale et pour les enlever il faut une grande force.

La marche des plaies des articulations, dans la majorité des cas, est très favorable; pour le pansement aseptique primitif elles se terminent par la guérison sans fièvre et avec reconstitution des fonctions, ou avec limitation jusqu'à un certain degré, ou enfin avec ankylose. Nous avons traité avec grand succès les suppurations consécutives des articulations par les ponctions, l'injection d'iodoforme-éther-alcool et surtout par le pansement avec pression et par le repos.

Les plaies du cou transversales sont très graves. Elles s'accompagnent de blessure de l'œsophage, du larynx et des grands vaisseaux. Les hémorrhagies sont larges et abondantes. Dans quelques cas l'œdème du cou, difficultant la respiration et la déglutition, exige la trachéotomie. Mais, malgré celle-ci, la fièvre, les phlegmons et la Schluckpneumonie sont des complications fréquentes de ces plaies. Beaucoup de cas de blessures du cou se guérissent aseptiquement. J'ai observé des cas de plaies du cou traversées, frontales, dans lesquelles la balle a traversé le cou entre la trachée et l'œsophage, sans toucher les vaisseaux et avec guérison rapide et aseptique. Les blessures sagittales du cou et surtout de sa partie latérale et du sommet des poumons sont très favorables.

Les plaies du thorax et des poumons sont habituellement des plaies traversées. Dans la grande majorité des cas elles sont très favorables. Les plaies sagittales, frontales et diagonales des poumons, ne rencontrant pas le cœur, les vaisseaux et le hile des poumons, finissent par la guérison sans fièvre et sans aucun inconvénient. Habituellement les malades toussent quelques jours avec du sang; on remarque quelque sonorité autour du trajet, la respiration affaiblie et des frottements de la plèvre, mais la température ne monte pas, les orifices sont bouchés par une croûte sèche et brune, sans réaction autour. Dans d'autres cas j'ai observé l'emphysème tuméfiant l'un ou l'autre côté de la poitrine et montant au cou et même au visage avec des symptômes cliniques classiques; cet emphysème trouble surtout la respiration. Mais après quelques jours il diminue peu à peu et disparaît. Les blessures des grands vaisseaux des poumons donnent l'hémothorax et l'hémopéricarde, sans coagulation de sang, avec marche lente et complications consécutives variables.

Les blessures du hile des poumons provoquent quelquefois de grandes hémorrhagies avec dépression progressive des poumons, trouble de la respiration, asphyxie progressive et mort en quelques heures. Nos essais de réséquer les côtes et de tamponner la cavité pectorale sont restés sans succès. Les complications pyogènes et surtout les empyèmes sont rares après les plaies des poumons. Dans les autopsies j'ai observé que l'orifice d'entrée est en forme de fente entre les côtes et en forme de cercle sur la plèvre viscérale; le trajet dans les poumons, irrégulier, plein de sang et entouré de sang épanché.

Je me permets de noter ici quelques cas remarquables de blessures de la poitrine et des poumons. Dans un cas, la balle a traversé la région du cœur au moment de la systole et est sortie par le dos entre le scapulum et la colonne vertébrale. L'officier blessé a guéri rapidement. Dans l'autre cas, la balle a traversé le coude gauche, la poitrine et l'articulation humérale droite. Guérison aseptique.

Les plaies de la cavité abdominale et de ses organes sont très graves. Les plaies frontales et traversées donnent ici habituellement une série d'orifices dans les intestins, et la péritonite grave très aiguë se développe comme conséquence, presque toujours avec les symptômes classiques. Les malades crient jour et nuit, avec rythme, pendant quelques jours. En ouvrant la cavité abdominale on trouve les intestins gonflés, rouges, hémorrhagiques, couverts de flocons fibrineux, exsudat pyogène avec odeur fécale. En examinant le pus, en faisant les cultures bactériologiques, j'ai trouvé dans l'exsudat toujours le bacillus coli communis. Trois laparotomies, qui ont été faites 2-3 jours après la blessure, n'ont donné aucun résultat favorable; tous les trois malades succombèrent. On trouve beaucoup d'orifices dans les intestins. Une fois j'ai suturé plus de 10 orifices dans les intestins. Notre conclusion est que la laparotomie est inutile dans ces cas, déjà 24 heures après la blessure, mais les laparotomies pendant les premières 6 heures après la blessure, dans de bonnes conditions aseptiques, sont indiquées.

Une série de blessures traversant l'abdomen dans des directions diverses se sont terminées par la guérison complète, sans péritonite et sans aucune opération; ce sont surtout les plaies sagittales et diagonales de l'abdomen. J'ai observé deux japonais blessés à l'abdomen par une balle russe: le premier une fois et l'autre deux fois. Tous les deux ont été guéris sans opération, après quelques jours d'irritation légère péritonitique locale, autour des orifices intestinaux. Ainsi, la cure d'attente est indiquée dans la majorité de ces cas et la guérison est plus assurée dans les cas où les intestins étaient vides avant la blessure.

Les plaies du bassin en général sont favorables, même si elles traversent la région de la vessie. Il y a aussi les plaies frontales avec déchirure de la vessie; la péritonite aiguë se développe ici comme conséquence. Dans un cas de plaie frontale traversant le bassin entre les épines iliaques (mort de péritonite aiguë) j'ai fait l'autopsie et j'ai trouvé que la balle avait seulement traversé la paroi antérieure de l'abdomen, sans toucher aux intestins et sans donner aucun orifice ou déchirure visibles; mais malgré cela l'hyperémie de l'intestin et l'exsudat séreux se sont développés; c'est-à-dire, les bacilles de l'intestin ont passé ici par la paroi intestinale commotionnée (après la vibration), ainsi que je l'ai démontré dans mon travail expérimental sur l'étiologie de la péritonite (v. *Virch. Arch.*, 1888 ou 1889).

Toutes les plaies des autres parties molles de l'organisme sont très favorables. Après le premier pansement, la plus grande majorité des cas guérit rapidement sans aucune réaction et, habituellement 2 ou 3 jours après la blessure, les orifices d'entrée et de sortie sont couverts de croûte brunâtre *sèche*, petite, ronde.

Les plaies des grands vaisseaux donnent: a) des fissures dans les parois; b) des orifices latéraux; c) des orifices médiaux. Elles se caractérisent par de larges et abondantes hémorrhagies sous-cutanées, par des douleurs constantes et surtout par des anévrysmes traumatiques, rapidement développés. Beaucoup de plaies des vaisseaux guérissent après des symptômes insignifiants.

Les plaies du foie et de la rate sont très dangereuses, parce que ces organes sont toujours brisés par la balle; la mort suit après de grandes hémorrhagies et la péritonite aiguë.

Les plaies des reins sont semblables à celles du foie et de la rate, mais souvent elles donnent la guérison après hématurie plus ou moins prolongée.

Dans beaucoup de cas, j'ai observé des plaies multiples — de 6 jusqu'à 8 plaies, sur un blessé, dans des régions différentes du corps; en règle générale toutes ces plaies guérissent rapidement, au-dessous de la croûte. Même des cas dans lesquels les balles traversaient le corps humain de haut en bas et vice versa: en entrant par exemple par la région supra-claviculaire et en sortant par le bassin, et au contraire, en entrant par le coude gauche, en traversant la poitrine et en sortant par l'articulation humérale droite et vice versa — tous ces cas finissaient en général par guérison aseptique ou avec symptômes légers.

Les blessures par les obus sont plus graves. L'orifice d'entrée de la balle du schrapnel est plus grand, ainsi que l'hémorrhagie autour de celui-ci, le trajet est plus court et plus irrégulier ou en zig-zag; les parois du trajet sont brisées et hémorrhagiques, non traversées. Les balles d'obus restent habituellement dans le corps; en rencontrant les os, ces balles brisent ces derniers en grands morceaux et déchirent les tissus mous. Les grands morceaux d'obus arrachent des parties de membres, en provoquant des plaies terribles, qui sont accompagnées toujours de suppurations profondes polymicrobiques et qui finissent par l'amputation.... Les plaies occasionnées par les petits éclats d'obus et par des parcelles de poudre donnent de petites déchirures dans la peau, une sorte de dessin semblable aux lignes de tatouage ou de la foudre.

Les recherches bactériologiques que j'ai faites dans mon laboratoire à Laoyan et ensuite à Kieff m'ont montré que les microbes habituels, provoquant les maladies infectieuses chez les blessés dans la guerre, sont toujours les microbes pyogènes: staphylocoques, streptocoques et, après, le bacille pyocyanique. Dans les péritonites perforatives j'ai trouvé toujours le bacillus coli communis, comme cause de la péritonite générale et surtout de la colibacillose générale. Dans un cas d'un phlegmon à gaz j'ai trouvé aussi le colibacillus en culture pure avec des bulles de gaz, dans la gélose. La grande majorité des cas guérissaient aseptiquement sans suppuration et sans aucun signe d'irritation, grâce à la qualité et au calibre des balles, au paquet individuel placé le plus tôt possible sur la plaie et grâce au traitement conservateur. En examinant les croûtes des orifices d'entrée et de sortie par les mé-

thodes bactériologiques, j'ai trouvé dans la majorité des cas les
staphylocoques blancs (les dorés étaient plus rares), mais malgré
leur présence la guérison s'opérait sans aucun symptôme d'irritation locale et sans fièvre. J'ai toujours trouvé les staphylocoques
blancs et dans les croûtes molles et dans les orifices; mais cela
aussi ne dérangeait pas la guérison rapide, surtout après avoir
touché avec la teinture d'iode.

Dans les infections graves des blessés, j'ai observé quelques
cas de tétanos général. Tous les cas finissaient par la mort. Le
sérum antitétanique de Behring ne donna aucun succès; de même
les larges incisions de ces plaies avec curettage, injection et dés-
infection énergique par la teinture d'iode ne donnaient aucun résultat favorable. Les bacilles du tétanos évidemment existent dans
le sol de Mandchourie, et des cas de cette terrible maladie ont été
observés assez souvent après les plaies d'obus.

Il y a eu aussi des cas de charbon, surtout en forme d'œdème
charbonneux, chez les soldats destinés à la garde des chevaux.

En résumé, les signes caractéristiques et fondamentaux des
plaies modernes, provoquées par les fusils à répétition et par les
balles à petit calibre, sont les suivants:

1) ces plaies sont pénétrantes, traversantes et de petit calibre;

2) dans la majorité des cas, elles sont légères et guérissent
aseptiquement et rapidement au-dessous de la croûte;

3) la guérison aseptique est le résultat du petit calibre de la
balle; celle-ci traverse les vêtements en les perçant seulement, sans
en emporter des lambeaux dans le trajet;

4) la quantité de microbes pyogènes apportés dans le trajet
est petite, sans grande virulence;

5) le paquet individuel antiseptique de l'armée russe, placé
tout de suite après la blessure, protège parfaitement la plaie contre les infections consécutives; les plaies guérissent habituellement
aseptiquement par le collage du trajet et par l'action du bouche-
ment des orifices par une croûte sèche et brunâtre;

6) les plaies du crâne, de la colonne vertébrale et surtout de
l'abdomen, sont très graves et, dans la grande majorité des cas,
mortelles.

Sur l'humanité des balles modernes, en comparaison avec les
balles anciennes à grand calibre, je dois dire que la balle moderne
donne plus de tués à la place même de la bataille et aux points
de pansement et aussi plus de blessés. La relation entre les tués
et les blessés, dans les guerres passées, était 1:4 à 1:5; dans la

guerre russo-japonaise: elle était 1:3. Mais à présent plus de blessés guérissent qu'autrefois; les maladies infectieuses chirurgicales sont très diminuées, et ont presque disparu les septicémies, les pyohémies et les gangrènes nosocomiales, dont Pirogoff a décrit les espèces et quelques familles dans sa *Chirurgie de guerre*. La période de traitement est devenue à présent plus courte et les souffrances des blessés sont aussi abrégées et amoindries grâce à l'asepsie dans la guerre, grâce au grand conservatisme dans le traitement, aux recherches bactériologiques, aux paquets individuels, aux rayons de Röntgen et en général, par conséquent, grâce à la position plus haute et plus précise de la science médicale et grâce à nos connaissances des causes des maladies et de leur traitement, plus larges, plus précises et plus claires.

La chirurgie moderne de la guerre doit être profondément conservatrice. Le travail du chirurgien sur le champ de bataille, à présent, est, dans la majorité des cas, le pansement aseptique précoce bien réglé. Le nombre des grandes opérations est diminué à présent. Sur un chiffre de 3000 blessés, j'ai observé seulement trois amputations faites. Le pansement au plâtre reçoit de nouveau tous ses droits. À son côté j'ai pratiqué aussi le pansement d'amidon, qui est très pratique, surtout dans la guerre; j'ai pratiqué la plupart des opérations avec anesthésie locale, provoquée par la cocaïne.

DISCUSSION

M. NAPALKOFF: Les armes à feu contemporaines sont employées à de grandes distances, et même dans ces conditions les blessures sont affreuses. En dehors de la guerre japonaise, nous avons rappelé une autre guerre à petites distances à Moscou. Les blessures de cette guerre sont incroyables par leur gravité. Les balles traversaient les hommes à travers les parties osseuses les plus fortes. Tous les malades qui furent apportés dans notre clinique avec des blessures de l'abdomen et du crâne sont morts. Nous protestons contre l'emploi des armes à feu contemporaines à la guerre et partout. (Vifs applaudissements.)

Excision of Os Calcis

Par M. Edward Wolfenden Collins, Londres.

The subject which I wish to bring briefly before you is «Excision of the Os Calcis illustrated by two cases in which I have completely removed the bone, in order that I may demonstrate the utility of this simple operation in preserving a perfectly useful foot, notwithstanding the removal of what appears to be so material a support of the body as the bone of the heel. I do so also because I have reason to know that this conservative operation has not received at the hands of some operating surgeons in high places the attention which it deserves.

I. My first case is that of a boy, aged 7 years, who was admitted into the Children's Infirmary, Sydenham, during September 1895, suffering from well marked caries of the left Os Calcis with a discharging sinus. The disease had been slowly progressing for 15 months.

Suffice it to say that, after sending him for some months to the Seaside Convalescent Home attached to the Infirmary, I gouged the cavity without advantage four times, at intervals of several months, before I came to the conclusion that such procedures were futile to arrest the progress of the tubercular mischief which had attacked the bone. Further evidence of tubercular disease was afforded by a caseating gland below the chin, which was removed at the time of the first gouging operation; and subsequently by suppuration, as the result of glandular implication, in the popliteal space. The popliteal infection gradually extended to the adjacent knee joint, which became the seat of steadily progressive pulpy thickening of its synovial membrane. I excised the disorganized knee joint, a year and a half after the boy's admission, immediately on his return from another prolonged sojourn of six months at the seaside. Three months later I excised the diseased Os Calcis — thus bringing to an end quite a series of operations. When he was convalescent, a further stay of six months at the seaside consolidated his recovery; and he left the Infirmary after a sojourn in it extending over three years.

Five years have elapsed since then, during which period he has enjoyed excellent health, and he possesses a perfectly useful, tho' shortened, limb and foot.

The history of this case led me to the conclusion that the progress and spread of the tubercular mischief might have been arrested much earlier had the Os Calcis in the first instance been completely removed; and I resolved in the next case of advanced disease of this bone to deal with it at once by excision.

II. When, in March last, another diseased Os Calcis came under my care, I had no hesitation in advising the parents of the little girl, aged 4 years, to permit me without delay to excise the bone.

So progressive had been the disease during six months' sojourn in a leading Metropolitan Hospital that finally permission had been asked to amputate the foot; and it was the refusal of this permission, with consequent discharge from the Hospital, which led to the child being transferred to the Sydenham Children's Infirmary.

From the photograph of this child's foot it will be seen that, owing to the considerable swelling in front of the astragalus, it was by no means improbable that the disease implicated that bone as well as the Os Calcis. Hoping that the X-Rays might clear up this important point, I had a skiagram taken by our Radiologist, Dr. Batten, without however a solution of the difficulty. The parents readily gave their consent to removal of the diseased Os Calcis — as well as of the astragalus, if necessary — as a desirable alternative to amputation of the foot. So, a week after the child's admission, I excised the Os Calcis — and it alone, as I found the under surface of the astragalus quite healthy. Uneventful hea-

ling gradually took place without any further manifestation of disease. After a
stay at the seaside, she returned to her home within six months from the date of
her admission into the Infirmary, to the delight of her parents, from whom I have
received a letter expressing their gratitude that, owing to this operation, the child
is now able to be on her feet all day long and walk perfectly well.

The removal of the bone is easily and safely effected from its
outer side by two continuous incisions carried directly down to
the bone - the first horizontal, along its upper border, extending
from the inner edge of the tendo Achillis to, and slightly beyond,
the calcaneo cuboid joint, which is found about midway between the
outer malleolus and the projection of the fifth metatarsal bone —
the second incision vertical, extending downwards from the anterior end of the first to about one third across the sole of the
foot. After the flaps have been dissected back in their thickness,
the articulation with the cuboid is opened in front, and then that
with the astragalus above. The lion forceps is now of essential
service, its firm grip being utilized for twisting the bone outwards,
so that its further separation from the astragalus above, as well
as from the important structures on its inner side, can be accom-
plished with safety by keeping the knife close to the bone. No ill
effect follows the unavoidable division on the outer surface of the
Os Calcis of the two peroneal tendons.

CLÔTURE DES TRAVAUX DE LA SECTION

M. FEIJÃO: Mesdames et Messieurs. Nos travaux sont finis,
mais avant de clore la dernière séance de la IX Section du
Congrès de Lisbonne, je prends à cœur de vous remercier de votre présence à nos séances, et de la présentation des études et
des travaux très intéressants auxquels est dû tout l'éclat dont
nos séances ont été revêtues. A vous, chers collègues, qui êtes venus de très loin illuminer cette salle avec le vif éclat de vos ta-
lents, à vous revient tout l'honneur du grandiose que nos séances
ont atteint. Je vous remercie de cette coopération brillante; vous
emporterez du Portugal le jugement juste de ce qu'il est; nous res-
tons avec le regret de vous voir partir, mais aussi avec le bonheur
d'avoir reserré avec vous des relations amicales, qui seront toujours, comme j'ai dit, en ouvrant les séances de cette section, un
des plus agréables souvenirs de votre présence et du Congrès de
Lisbonne. Au revoir. La séance est close.

TABLE DES MATIERES

Première partie — Rapports officiels

Deuxième partie — Comptes rendus des séances

Erratum

Page 90, le morceau qui commence par *J'ai colligé* (ligne 12) et finit à *pendant le temps nécessaire* (lignes 20-21) doit être placé en entier entre les lignes 3 et 4.

guérison par l'intervention chirurgicale, même sans sympathectomie; en outre, il y avait du liquide dans le péritoine, liquide qu'on a retiré, en faisant après la toilette de la membrane.

Il n'y a contre cela que l'impression personnelle de l'opérateur, mais en science ce n'est pas assez.

Tuttavia credo di poter asserire cosa nota a quanti hanno pratica di chirurgia addominale, che non incontro ogni giorno un'ammalata laparotomizzata, che nella sera medesima dell'operazione dichiari di sentirsi completamente sollevata dei suoi dolori, ciò che si deve quindi attribuire non già all'estirpazione dell'ovario, in se stessa, ma sibbene alla resezione del plesso.

Dans la seconde observation de Cavazzani nous retrouvons les mêmes conditions que celles des deux premières de Ruggi; et l'on doit attribuer le résultat à l'intervention sur le sympathique et non à l'extirpation de l'autre ovaire:

Va notato che le sofferenze di questa paziente erano costantemente a destra e que l'ovario rimasto era a sinistra, ma ovario e tuba erano in completa fase di involuzione e non esisteva traccia di processo morboso in corso o progresso.

La troisième observation est plus démonstrative par l'inefficacité des opérations antérieures.

Dans la quatrième la démonstration de la valeur de la sympathectomie est plus claire; la guérison de cette malade a été obtenue en respectant les annexes et l'utérus qui étaient sains, et on remarque une modification frappante dans l'état psychique du malade.

Dans la dernière opération, l'extirpation des deux ovaires, en atrophie, ôte quelque valeur au cas comme pièce à conviction. Nous pouvons supposer seulement que la sympathectomie a eu des avantages, par la fréquence de l'inutilité de l'ovariotomie bilatérale, sur des malades avec des manifestations névralgiques aussi intenses que celles de la malade dont je parle.

Voyons les trois observations de Ruggi.

Dans la première, le résultat a été meilleur du côté où l'on n'a fait que l'opération de Ruggi que du côté où l'on a retiré l'ovaire. Dans la seconde, les douleurs continuèrent, après la castration utéro-ovarienne, vaginale, et il y eut des attaques hystériques; mais on a obtenu la guérison radicale, observée pendant deux années, en appliquant le système de Ruggi.

Dans la troisième on n'a fait que l'opération de Ruggi, laissant les annexes, et la malade a été guérie des douleurs et des attaques.

En résumé: Nous avons 14 opérations (j'en exclus la première et la dernière de Cavazzani) dans lesquelles l'intervention sur le sympathique a été favorable. De celles-ci les plus démonstratives sont une de Ruggi, une de Cavazzani et une autre de Foschini, dans lesquelles on a conservé les organes génitaux internes.

Mais, si l'observation de Ruggi et la troisième de Foschini perdent une partie de leur valeur, parce qu'on peut faire intervenir en elles la suggestion — car la malade de Ruggi tombait en syncope avec facilité, ce qui pourrait être en rapport avec l'hystérie, et celle de Foschini a eu des attaques hystériques —, la 21ᵉ de Cavazzani est, au contraire, très démonstrative, et l'idée de suggestion doit être entièrement mise de côté, la malade ayant déjà souffert des traitements antérieurs, et même avec un intervalle de trois mois. On peut dire la même chose de la 2ᵉᵐᵉ opération de Foschini. Dans les autres, l'insuccès d'interventions considérées comme radicales montre également que, dans cet ordre de faits (même s'il y a des lésions supposées des annexes), la sympathectomie du plexus utéro-ovarien est un puissant élément de guérison.

Quant à la douleur, m'appuyant seulement sur un si petit nombre de cas, je crois pouvoir conclure que: 1.º — Au cas où l'on intervient sur des lésions utéro-ovariennes ou annexiales douloureuses, avec des irradiations, l'extirpation du plexus utéro-ovarien est un complément de l'opération qui donnera à celle-ci plus de garanties de guérison; 2.º — Attendu le peu de gravité de l'intervention chez les malades avec des névralgies annexiales et qui irradient jusqu'à l'abdomen et aux cuisses, etc., cas où l'intervention sur les annexes est contre-indiquée, parce qu'ils sont sains, la sympathectomie doit être tentée en désespoir de cause, avec quelques probabilités de succès.

Si, sans aucun doute, les 16 opérations que j'ai citées nous mènent à poursuivre dans cette voie, pleine d'espoir, nous manquons de la sanction du temps et d'un plus grand nombre d'observations pour avoir une opinion solide sur la stabilité de la guérison. Les cas de Foschini, suivis pendant une ou deux années, et ceux de Ruggi, suivis plus longtemps, nous permettent de la prophétiser; et je terminerai en transcrivant quelques lignes de Ruggi, où il parle de ses observations:

> I fatti tutti annotati sono oltremodo eloquenti, essendo destinati a far conoscere che l'operazione di simpatectomia da me consigliata in questi speciali

aventi, riesce sempre efficace perchè quando non guarì perfetamente le ammalate ne migliorò in modo sensibilissimo le loro condizioni.

In tute le predette inferme finalmente la mia operazione riuscì del tutto innocua, essendo tutte le malate guarite senza complicazioni e fatti successivi fastidiosi.

Table

XV Congrès International de Médecine

Lisbonne — 19-26 Avril 1906

Section IX

CHIRURGIE

2.ᵐᵉ FASCICULE

LISBONNE
IMPRIMERIE ADOLPHO DE MENDONÇA
1907

www.ingramcontent.com/pod-product-compliance
Lightning Source LLC
La Vergne TN
LVHW010607180726
843502LV00001B/175